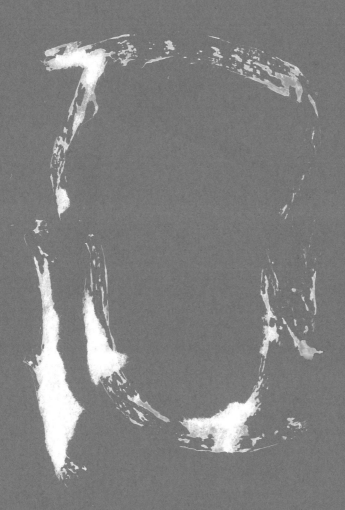

# HYPERTENSION IN PREGNANCY

# HYPERTENSION IN PREGNANCY

Edited by

## J. J. Walker

*Professor of Obstetrics and Gynaecology*
*Department of Obstetrics and Gynaecology*
*St James's University Hospital,*
*Leeds,*
*UK*

## N. F. Gant

*Professor of Obstetrics and Gynecology*
*Department of Obstetrics and Gynecology*
*The University of Texas*
*Southern Medical Center*
*Dallas*
*USA*

**CHAPMAN & HALL MEDICAL**
London · Weinheim · New York · Tokyo · Melbourne · Madras

**Published by Chapman & Hall, 2–6 Boundary Row, London SE1 8HN, UK**

Chapman & Hall, 2–6 Boundary Row, London SE1 8HN, UK

Chapman & Hall GmbH, Pappelallee 3, 69469 Weinheim, Germany

Chapman & Hall USA, 115 Fifth Avenue, New York, NY 10003, USA

Chapman & Hall Japan, ITP-Japan, Kyowa Building, 3F, 2-2-1 Hirakawacho, Chiyoda-ku, Tokyo 102, Japan

Chapman & Hall Australia, 102 Dodds Street, South Melbourne, Victoria 3205, Australia

Chapman & Hall India, R. Seshadri, 32 Second Main Road, CIT East, Madras 600 035, India

© 1997 Chapman & Hall

Typeset in Palatino 10/12pt by Saxon Graphics Ltd, Derby

Printed in Great Britain by Alden Press, Oxford

ISBN 0 412 30910 6

A catalogue record for this book is available from the British Library

Library of Congress Catalog Card Number: 96-70877

∞ Printed on acid-free text paper, manufactured in accordance with ANSI/NISO Z39.48-1992 (Permanence of Paper).

# CONTENTS

# CONTRIBUTORS

JOHN R. BARTON, MD
Director, Maternal – Fetal Medicine,
Central Baptist Hospital,
Perinatal Diagnostic Center,
1740 Nicholasville Road,
Lexington, Kentucky, USA

CHRISTINE BAYLIS, PhD
Professor of Physiology,
West Virginia University,
Morgantown, West Virginia, USA

DAVID B. COTTON, MD, FACOG
Professor, Department of Obstetrics and
Gynecology,
Wayne State University,
Detroit, Michigan, USA

JOHN DAVISON, MD, FRCOG
Professor of Obstetric Medicine, University of
Newcastle-upon-Tyne and Consultant
Obstetrician and Gynaecologist,
Royal Victoria Infirmary,
Newcastle-upon-Tyne, UK

GUSTAAF A. DEKKER MD, PhD
Senior Lecturer, Division of Maternal–Fetal
Medicine,
Department of Obstetrics and Gynecology,
Free University Hospital,
Amsterdam,
Netherlands

FIONA M. FAIRLIE MD, MRCOG
Consultant in Obstetrics and Gynaecology,
Jessop Hospital,
Sheffield, UK

J. STEWART FORSYTH MD, FRCP, DCH,
DObstRCOG
Consultant Pediatrician,
Ninewells Hospital and Medical School,
Dundee, UK

EILEEN GALLERY MD, FRACP
North Shore Hospital,
Sydney, Australia

NORMAN F. GANT MD, FACOG
Professor of Obstetrics and Gynecology,
University of Texas
Southwestern Medical Center,
Dallas, Texas, USA

LARRY C. GILSTRAP, MD
Professor of Obstetrics and Gynecology and
Director, Maternal–Fetal Medicine Fellowship
and Clinical Genetics,
Southwestern Medical School,
University of Texas,
Dallas, Texas, USA

WESLEY LEE, MD FACOG
Department of Obstetrics and Gynecology,
William Beaumont Hospital,
Royal Oak, Michigan, USA
Associate Professor of Obstetrics/Gynecology,
Wayne State University,
Detroit, Michigan, USA

RONALD R. MAGNESS, PhD
Professor of Obstetrics/Gynecology and
Meat/Animal Sciences,
University of Wisconsin–Madison,
Madison, Wisconsin, USA

JACK MOODLEY MD
Director, Natal University/Medical Research
Council Pregnancy Hypertension Research
Unit,
Durban, Natal, South Africa

LAWRENCE NATHAN MD
Fellow in Maternal–Fetal Medicine,
Department of Obstetrics and Gynecology,
University of Texas Southwestern Medical
Center, Dallas, Texas, USA

BAHA M. SIBAI MD
Chief, Maternal–Fetal Medicine,
Department of Obstetrics and Gynecology,
University of Tennessee,
Memphis, Tennessee, USA

JAMES J. WALKER MD, FRCPGlasg, FRCOG
Professor of Obstetrics and Gynaecology,
St James's Univesity Hospital,
Leeds, UK

# PREFACE

In summing up this section, it is evident that the cause of eclampsia has not been discovered, and that the peace of mind of all concerned would have been increased, had many of the so-called contributors never written, or at least had withheld their contributions sufficiently long to subject them to ordinary self-criticism.

*Whitridge Williams*

Much time has passed since the conception of this book. The idea for it was developed after attending meetings of experts in the field and finding so many areas of difference and disagreement. People had fixed views about the risks of the condition, the medications that should be used and the management regimes that should be followed. This book has attempted to bring together workers from different parts of the world to present the problems as they see them, to describe the methods of care that they have developed and to try and show the areas of agreement rather than the areas of controversy. Hypertension in pregnancy is a multifaceted disease, presenting in many ways with various levels of seriousness. It remains a major cause of maternal and fetal mortality and morbidity. The aims of the different management systems are the same, that is to reduce the effects of the condition on the pregnant population. It is hoped that after reading this book, it will be easier to understand why people do what they do and help can be gained in developing the management protocols that are so important to the successful outcome for the women dependent on our care. It is impossible to cover every possibility available but an attempt has been made to get contributions from those who are actively involved in the areas they have written about. It is an evolving subject and recently there has been major advances in the techniques of assessment and investigation and management. However, the principals of care remain the same.

James J. Walker and Norman F. Gant
Leeds and Dallas, July 1996

# INTRODUCTION

*James J. Walker and Norman F. Gant*

Although the association of convulsions and maternal death has been known since ancient times, there remains confusion and controversy concerning the hypertension and convulsions in pregnancy. The word 'eclampsia' comes from the Greek verb eklampein meaning 'to flash out'. This relates to its sudden onset or to the flashing hallucinations experienced in the prodromal phase. Hippocrates described the condition in *On The Sacred Disease*. Unfortunately he did not distinguish eclampsia from epilepsy, but stated that 'it proves fatal to women in the state of pregnancy' (Chesley, 1980). Over the centuries, it was noted that the presence of convulsions and coma were ominous signs in the presence of difficult labor and often resulted in the death of both mother and fetus (Chesley, 1980). In the 16th century, Gabelchoverus noted that pregnancy was a cause of epilepsy and described the epigastric pain associated with this. He felt that the pain was a sign that the cause of the convulsion came from the uterus (Chesley, 1980). Mauriceau (1668) refers to eclampsia, as does Denman (1768) in a book dedicated to the problem along with puerperal fever. He recognized eclampsia as a major cause of morbidity and mortality.

Once it was realized that the condition was specific to pregnancy, it was thought by many to be a form of renal disease. In 1843, Lever found that patients with eclampsia had proteinuria (Lever, 1843). Although he realized that eclampsia was different from renal dis-ease since the proteinuria disappeared after delivery, others thought that the condition was very similar to that seen in glomerulonephritis. Simpson, who found proteinuria at about the same time, saw contracted kidneys in one of his patients and felt that this was the cause of the problem (Simpson, 1843). This became the popular opinion for some time. It was not until the development of methods of assessment of renal function and finally the renal histology studies of Sheehan (1950) and McCartney (1964), that the timing of the stages of the disease was realized. Both Sheehan and McCartney stated that renal lesions were present only when the patient had proteinuria and, since this was a late manifestation of the condition called preeclampsia, it could not be a primary cause of the condition.

It was not until the late 19th century that hypertension was first noted to be associated with eclampsia (Ballantyne, 1885; Cook and Briggs, 1903). In 1896, essential hypertension was first differentiated from renal hypertension. However, as it was originally called 'senile plethora', many obstetricians felt that none of their (mostly young) patients could have this condition (Chesley, 1980). It was not until the 1940s that the possibility of essential hypertension as a cause of hypertension in pregnancy was accepted. From this time it was realized that renal disease was a relatively rare cause of hypertension in pregnancy. Although pregnancy could occur in a patient

*Hypertension in Pregnancy*
Edited by J.J. Walker and N.F. Gant. Published by Chapman & Hall, 1997 ISBN 0 412 30910 6

with preexisting essential hypertension, renal disease or other hypertensive disorder, there was a specific hypertensive syndrome arising in pregnancy that disappeared when the pregnancy was over and apparently carried no long-term sequelae (Chesley, Annitto and Cosgrove, 1976).

The realization that this pregnancy-'associated' hypertension often precedes convulsions led to the term 'preeclampsia'. This term was initially used for the immediate prodromal stage of eclampsia but is now applied to patients with milder forms of the disease. Although eclampsia is associated with hypertension it is not an obligatory endpoint of the condition. Convulsions are independent of the severity of the disease. 'Mild' preeclampsia may be associated with convulsions and 'severe' may not. Between 15 and 20% of the patients suffering from 'eclampsia' had no record of hypertension prior to the seizure (Cruickshank, 1923; Cruickshank, Hewitt and Couper, 1927) Although these early findings could partly be due to inadequate records, the results have been confirmed by more recent workers (Sibai et al., 1981).

Over 100 names have been used in the past to define the different forms of hypertension in pregnancy and efforts have been made to simplify this (Rippman, 1968; Hughes, 1972; Nelson, 1955). However, hypertension in pregnancy is not a single disorder but has multivariate causes, dependent on different etiologies and on the mother's varying response to the stimuli. It is often not possible to be sure to which group a patient belongs at the time of presentation. Postnatal follow-up may demonstrate, for example, renal pathology causative of the hypertension. The term preeclampsia implies an inevitable progression to convulsion. This has influenced the management of the condition for a generation of obstetricians. The more recent term of 'pregnancy-induced hypertension' is no great improvement, as it implies etiology.

Until the underlying etiology is understood the disease will continue to be described in the clinical way it presents or develops. The 'Organization Gestosis', or EPH-Gestosis, the first international organization formed for the study of this clinical condition, used the clinical signs of edema, proteinuria and hypertension as the basis of the diagnosis. The presence of any two of these signs is all that is required for the diagnosis of 'gestosis' but the dominance of the edema as the presenting sign is overstressed and the hypertension is given little prominence (Rippman, 1968). The 'International Society for the Study of Hypertension in Pregnancy' (ISSHP) is devoted to the study of all aspects of the pregnancy conditions associated with hypertension, with the emphasis on hypertension arising for the first time during pregnancy and its various manifestations (Davey and MacGillivray, 1988). These methods of classification lead to confusion, as some patients with 'gestosis' do not have 'preeclampsia'. It is important to realize that these societies are describing different groups of patients, although there is a considerable degree of overlap.

The problems with the definitions of the condition make comparison of the apparent incidence and risks difficult. It would appear that hypertension in human pregnancy occurs in around 25% of primigravid and in 10% of multigravid mothers but the incidence varies with the experience of different authors (Chamberlain et al., 1978; Nelson, 1955; MacGillivray, 1958; Common Services Agency, 1986). In Western society, despite improved environmental conditions, improved maternal health, greatly improved antenatal care and reduction in perinatal loss in association with hypertensive syndromes, the rate of maternal death attributed to pregnancy hypertension in the UK has changed little for 30 years (DHSS, 1969, 1974, 1979, 1991, 1994; Turnbull, 1987; Turnbull et al., 1989; Scottish Home and Health Department, 1978, 1987, 1989).

The confidential inquiries into these deaths found that in 75–81% of cases, avoidable factors can be found. Most of these were associated with failure to recognize early warning signs. There was also failure to initiate proper therapy rather than the use of inadequate or wrong therapy. The reduction in the incidence of the severe forms of hypertensive disease in pregnancy in the western world has led to reduction in the exposure of obstetricians to the problem and a lowering of their ability to manage severe cases as they arise. Eclampsia is now rare in the UK, which has led to a rethink on the role of anticonvulsants in the management of pregnancy hypertension. In other parts of the world, eclampsia is still a common presentation and is associated with a high mortality.

The modern clinician is caught in a clinical dilemma. Because the incidence of severe forms of the condition appears to be reducing in the developed world and the overall incidence of all forms of hypertension appears to be unchanged, the risk of the condition to the mother and baby of hypertension in pregnancy would appear to be diminishing. Therefore, it is difficult to justify continued admission to hospital for all cases of hypertension in pregnancy, especially when the risks appear to be small and the patient feels so well. However, hypertension in pregnancy is still one of the main causes of maternal death throughout the world and it remains a significant contributor to the perinatal mortality rate (Common Services Agency, 1986; Scottish Home and Health Department, 1989). This has allowed continuation of the more cautious approach of admission to hospital for observation. Since pregnancy has a finite length and the admission will be only for a short stay, the price to pay for hospitalization is small and the rewards of success appear to be great. Every satisfactory outcome following admission to hospital for the management of this condition leads to a further positive reinforcement that it is the best approach (De Swiet, 1985). A logical approach to the management of pregnancy hypertension is difficult because of the emotional and deep-seated feelings it can produce (De Swiet, 1985; Hodgson, 1985). Anything that is thought to put the mother or baby at risk is rejected in return for the tried and tested 'status quo'. However, there has been no randomized study carried out proving that admission to hospital is beneficial to mother or baby (Crowther and Chalmers, 1989). Since the situation is confused, and experience limited, there has been a call for the setting up of specialized teams of clinicians to manage and study all patients who present with hypertension in pregnancy (Turnbull et al., 1989).

This book aims to study the factors associated with pregnancy hypertension and the different approaches to its care. The chapters discuss the incidence of hypertensive problems in the hospital practice, the maternal and fetal morbidity associated with the hypertension, specific aspects of etiology, the role of screening tests for hypertensive risk, the role of early intervention therapy using hospital admission or hypotensive regimes in both mild to moderate and severe pregnancy hypertension and the development of standardized protocols to simplify patient management. Although the regimes used are varied, it is clear that there are many common threads to the managements used. There are, however, still areas of controversy, especially around the use of anticonvulsants and antihypertensive drugs. It is hoped that the reader will gain some understanding into the management regimes described by the authors and the reason for their use.

## REFERENCES

Ballantyne, J. W. (1885) Sphygmographic tracings in puerperal eclampsia. *Edin. Med. J.*, **30**, 1007–1011.

Chamberlain, G. V. P., Phillip, E., Howlett, B. and Masters, K. (1978) *British Births 1970, 2: Obstetric Care*, Heinemann, London, p. 80–84.

Chesley, L. C. (1980) Evolution of concepts of eclampsia, in *Pregnancy Hypertension*, (eds J. Bonnar, I. MacGillivray and E. M. Symonds), MTP Press, Lancaster, p. 1–4.

Chesley, L. C., Annitto, J. E. and Cosgrove, R. A. (1976) The remote prognosis of eclamptic women. Sixth periodic report. *Am. J. Obstet. Gynecol.*, **124**, 446–450.

Common Services Agency (1986) *Scottish Stillbirth and Neonatal Death Report*, Scottish Home and Health Department, Edinburgh.

Cook, H. W. and Briggs, J. C. (1903) Clinical observations on blood pressure. *Johns Hopkins Hosp. Rep.*, **11**, 451–455.

Crowther, C. A. and Chalmers, I. (1989) Bed rest and hospitalisation during pregnancy, in *The Effective Care in Pregnancy and Childbirth*, vol. 1, (eds I. Chalmers, M. Enkin and M. J. N. C. Kerse), Oxford University Press, Oxford, p. 624–632.

Cruickshank, J. M. (1923) Studies of the toxaemias of pregnancy as they occur in Glasgow. *J. Obstet. Gynaecol. Br. Emp.*, **30**, 541–545.

Cruickshank, J. M., Hewitt, R. and Couper, J. (1927) *The Toxaemias of Pregnancy: A Clinical and Biochemical Study*, Medical Research Council Special Report Series 117, Medical Research Council, London, p. 47–51.

Davey, D. A. and MacGillivray, I. (1988) The classification and definition of the hypertensive disorders of pregnancy. *Am. J. Obstet. Gynecol.*, **158**, 892–898.

Denman, T. (1768) *Essays on the Puerperal Fever and on Puerperal Convulsions*. Walter, London.

De Swiet, M. (1985) Antihypertensive drugs in pregnancy. *Br. Med. J.*, **291**, 365–369.

DHSS (1969) *Report on Confidential Enquiries into Maternal Deaths in England and Wales 1964–66*, HMSO, London.

DHSS (1974) *Report on Confidential Enquiries into Maternal Deaths in England and Wales1970–72*, HMSO, London.

DHSS (1979) *Report on Confidential Enquiries into Maternal Deaths in England and Wales 1973–75*, HMSO, London.

DHSS, Welsh Office, Scottish Home and Health Department (1991) *Report on Confidential Enquiries into Maternal Deaths in the United Kingdom 1985–87* HMSO, London.

DHSS, Welsh Office, Scottish Home and Health Department (1994) *Report on Confidential Enquiries into Maternal Deaths in the United Kingdom 1988–90* HMSO, London.

Hodgson, P. (1985) Antihypertensive treament in pregnancy. *Br. Med. J.*, **295**, 936–940.

Hughes, E. C. (1972) Obstetrics–Gynecological Terminology, F. A. Davis, Philadelphia, PA, p. 422–423.

Lever, J. C. W. (1843) Cases of puerperal convulsions with remarks, in *Guy's Hospital Reports*, vol. 1, 2nd edn, (ed. G. H. Barlow), Samuel Highley, London, p. 495–506.

MacGillivray, I. (1958) Some observations on the incidence of pre-eclampsia. *J. Obstet. Gynaecol. Br. Emp.*, **65**, 536–540.

McCartney, C. P. (1964) Pathological anatomy of acute hypertension of pregnancy. Circulation 30 37–41.

Mauriceau, F. (1668) *Des Maladies des Femmes Grosses et Accouches avec la Bonne et Veritable*, Cercle du Livre Precieux, Paris.

Nelson, T. R. (1955) A clinical study of pre-eclampsia, part 1. *J. Obstet. Gynaecol. Br. Emp.*, **62**, 48–52.

Rippman, E. T. (1968) Gestosis of late pregnancy. *Gynaecologia*, **165**, 12–16.

Scottish Home and Health Department (1978) *A Report on an Enquiry into Maternal Deaths in Scotland, 1972–1975*, HMSO, Edinburgh.

Scottish Home and Health Department (1987) *A Report on an Enquiry into Maternal Deaths in Scotland, 1976–1980*, HMSO, Edinburgh.

Scottish Home and Health Department (1989) *A Report on an Enquiry into Maternal Deaths in Scotland, 1981–1986*, HMSO, Edinburgh.

Sheehan, H. L. (1950) Pathological lesions in the hypertensive toxaemias of pregnancy, in *Toxaemias of Pregnancy*, (eds J. Hammond, F. J. Browne and G. E. W. Wolstenholme), J & A Churchill, London.

Sibai, B. M., McCubbin, J. H., Anderson, H. D. *et al.* (1981) Eclampsia. 1 Observations from 67 recent cases. *Obstet. Gynecol.*, **58**, 609–613.

Simpson, J. Y. (1843) Contributions to the pathology and treatment of diseases of the uterus. *Edin. Monthly J. Med. Sci.*, **3**, 1009–1013.

Turnbull, A. C. (1987) Maternal mortality and present trends, in *Hypertension in Pregnancy. Proceedings of the Sixteenth Study Group of the Royal College of Obstetricians and Gynaecologists*, (eds F. Sharp and E. M. Symonds), Perinatology Press, Ithaca, NY, p. 135–144.

Turnbull, A., Tindall, V. R., Beard, R. W. *et al.* (1989) *Report on Confidential Enquiries Into Maternal Deaths in England and Wales 1982–1984*, DHSS, London, vol. 34, p. 1–166.

# NORMAL VASCULAR ADAPTATIONS IN PREGNANCY: POTENTIALS CLUES FOR UNDERSTANDING PREGNANCY-INDUCED HYPERTENSION

*Ronald R. Magness and Norman F. Gant*

## 2.1 INTRODUCTION

Multiple hypotheses have been presented in an attempt to explain the etiology and progression of pregnancy-induced hypertension (PIH)/preeclampsia. Despite a wide diversity of opinions regarding this disease, we and others generally have accepted the central thesis that this pathophysiological process is characterized by vasospasm, hypertension and different degrees of impaired regional perfusion to multiple organs. Our purpose in this chapter is to review normal cardiovascular adaptations to pregnancy and when possible to emphasize normal pregnancy adaptations which might offer insights into the etiology and/or development of the clinical symptoms and signs of PIH/preeclampsia. The work largely concentrates on our work in the renin/angiotensin system. Chapter 7 covers other aspects of vasoactivity and the pathogenesis of preeclampsia.

## 2.2 NORMAL CARDIOVASCULAR CHANGES IN PREGNANCY

Normal pregnancy is characterized by dramatic alterations in the maternal cardiovascular system (Wilson *et al.*, 1980; Cunningham, MacDonald and Gant, 1989; Magness and Rosenfeld, 1993a). These changes include profound vasodilation accompanied by increases in blood volume; decreases in blood pressure; and increases in cardiac output. If these massive increases in blood volume and cardiac output were to occur in non-pregnant subjects, without the normal peripheral vasodilation of pregnancy, severe hypertension surely would ensue.

Each of the above pregnancy-related cardiovascular changes are 'time-dependent' events varying from week to week throughout gestation. For example, increases in plasma volume begin at about 6 weeks and plateau between 30 and 34 weeks of gestation (Lund and Donovan, 1967). In addition, the 'hypotensive' effects of pregnancy commence at approximately six to eight weeks gestation and become significant by twelve weeks (Gant *et al.*, 1973; Wilson *et al.*, 1980; Cunningham, MacDonald and Gant, 1989). The nadir in blood pressure is reached at around 20 weeks of gestation and blood pressure remains low until about 30–32 weeks gestation. After this time, blood pressure slowly returns to near non-pregnant values

*Hypertension in Pregnancy*
Edited by J.J. Walker and N.F. Gant. Published by Chapman & Hall, 1997 ISBN 0 412 30910 6

by term. Moreover, greater decreases in diastolic than systolic pressures have been reported (Wilson *et al.*, 1980), an observation consistent with the view that significant decreases in vascular tone are involved in these cardiovascular alterations. These observations also are consistent with the hypothesis that pregnancy is a state manifested by elevations in local and/or systemic vasodilators, rather than the removal of vasoconstrictors. Accompanying these peripheral vascular alterations, heart rate increases in a nearly linear fashion from eight weeks of gestation until a plateau is reached at about twenty-eight to thirty-two weeks (Wilson *et al.*, 1980; Cunningham, MacDonald and Gant, 1989). These increases in heart rate are paralleled by elevations in cardiac output (Lees *et al.*, 1967; Ueland *et al.*, 1969; Cunningham, MacDonald and Gant, 1989), which also are frequently accompanied by increases in stroke volume (Magness and Zheng, 1996). Because resistance is calculated as pressure divided by flow, decreases in blood pressure and the progressive increases in cardiac output are accompanied by quite dramatic falls in peripheral vascular resistance (Wilson *et al.*, 1980; Cunningham, MacDonald and Gant, 1989; Magness and Zheng, 1996). Furthermore, changes in peripheral vascular resistance can be estimated by dividing the mean arterial blood pressure by the cardiac output and should be considered as the 'best index' of systemic vasoconstriction (or vasodilation) because it accounts for alterations in both pressure as well as systemic flow (Naden and Rosenfeld, 1981; Magness and Rosenfeld, 1988; Magness and Zheng, 1996). Curiously, in women with PIH/preeclampsia, cardiac output often remains elevated; however peripheral vascular resistance is abnormally increased suggesting the development of severe vasoconstriction or a substantial loss of peripheral vasodilatory mechanisms (Werko, 1950; Assali, Holm and Parker, 1964; Lees *et al.*, 1967; Ueland *et al.*, 1969).

Since elevations in peripheral vascular resistance can occur either through increases in blood pressure or decreases in cardiac output, or both (Magness and Zheng, 1996) and cardiac output is not decreased consistently in women with PIH/preeclampsia, it is important to better understand those factors believed to alter increases in vascular reactivity which can lead to vasoconstriction and elevated peripheral vascular resistance. As early as 1937, Dieckman and Michel reported that vascular reactivity to the pressor effects of an infused 'vasoactive agent', which consisted of a crude posterior pituitary extract (likely to be arginine vasopressin), was greater in women with preeclampsia than in normotensive pregnant subjects. Nearly 20 years later, Raab *et al.* (1956), reported analogous results for another a class of vasoconstrictor, the catecholamines (noradrenalin/norepinephrine and adrenalin/epinephrine). Neither of these investigative groups observed dramatic differences in pressor responses between non-pregnant and normal pregnant control subjects. However, Raab *et al.* (1956) did report data suggesting that when the same pregnant patients were infused during the postpartum period with these alpha-adrenergic sympathomimetic agents, blood pressure responses were increased compared with their own pregnancy responses. This observation was virtually ignored in their report as well as in subsequent reviews of their work. Moreover, similar conflicting conclusions of decreased or no changes in vascular reactivity to alpha-adrenergic agents in normal pregnancy were later reported by others in pregnant women (Chesley *et al.*, 1965; Lumbars, 1970) and sheep (Magness and Rosenfeld, 1986, 1988). In contrast to alpha-adrenergic agents, more consistent responses have been observed for another pressor agent, angiotensin II (ANG II). Studies involving ANG II have therefore dominated the focus of our studies of PIH/preeclampsia for the last 20 years.

## 2.3 VASCULAR REACTIVITY IN NORMAL AND HYPERTENSIVE PREGNANT WOMEN

Abdul-Karim and Assali reported in 1961 that pregnant women were refractory to the pressor effects of infused ANG II when compared with results observed after delivery. Subsequently, Talledo, Chesley and Zuspan (1968), reported that subjects with preeclampsia did not exhibit this pregnancy-associated blunted vascular response to ANG II. They suggested that the attenuated pressor effects to infused ANG II that characterize normal pregnancy might result from elevated endogenous plasma concentrations of ANG II. From the above studies, it is likely that the vascular refractoriness to vasoconstrictors observed in normal pregnancy and the loss of these attenuated vascular responses which occurs in preeclampsia may be a somewhat generalized phenomenon seen with many, if not all, vasoconstrictor agonists. It must be emphasized, however, that during pregnancy the mechanisms responsible for these alterations in vascular responsiveness to each of the above classes of agonists have not yet been established conclusively to be the same for either normotensive or hypertensive pregnant women. For example, there appears to be a major cardiac component, via a baroreceptor-mediated mechanism, controlling the reduced vascular reactivity to infused alpha-adrenergic agent (Magness and Rosenfeld, 1988); however, the refractoriness described for ANG II may involve a greater peripheral vascular involvement (Gant *et al.*, 1974; Cunningham, Cox and Gant, 1975; Everett *et al.*, 1978a; Naden and Rosenfeld, 1981; Naden *et al.*, 1984; Magness and Rosenfeld, 1990).

Because of the interesting studies of Abdul-Karim and Assali (1961) and those of Talledo, Chesley and Zuspan (1968), a prospective study of vascular responsiveness to ANG II throughout pregnancy was conduced (Gant *et al.*, 1973). These studies were designed in order to establish during which week of pregnancy vascular refractoriness to the pressor effects of ANG II developed and also to define when this normal and progressive phenomenon was interrupted in gestations destined to develop PIH/preeclampsia. The results of this study are illustrated in Figure 2.1.

The 192 primigravid women in this prospective study were 16 years of age or younger and were studied sequentially from as early in gestation as possible and throughout the remainder of their pregnancy (Gant *et al.*, 1973). At each clinic visit, patients received an ANG II infusion which was sufficient to increase baseline diastolic blood pressure by 20 mmHg. This dose of ANG II (ng/kg/min) required to elevate diastolic blood pressure by 20 mmHg was defined as 'the effective pressor dose' of ANG II. As observed for the normal pregnant women, those subjects destined to develop PIH/preeclampsia initially became refractory to the pressor effects of infused ANG II; however, the future hypertensive women subsequently lost this refractoriness and became progressively more sensitive to the pressor effects of infused ANG II. The increased sensitivity commenced after the 18th week of gestation; i.e. the effective pressor dose to infused ANG II decreased substantially. In addition, 90% of those women whose effective pressor dose to infused ANG II was less than 8 ng/kg/min between the 28th and 32nd weeks of gestation ultimately developed PIH/preeclampsia by term. Conversely, over 90% of women whose effective pressor dose to infused ANG II was greater than 8 ng/kg/min during the same time period remained normotensive for the duration of pregnancy.

## 2.4 RENIN–ANG II–ALDOSTERONE SYSTEM IN NORMAL AND HYPERTENSIVE PREGNANCY

From these and other studies, the renin–ANG II–aldosterone system appears to be altered dramatically in normal pregnancy and PIH/preeclampsia when compared with normotensive non-pregnant women. Specifically,

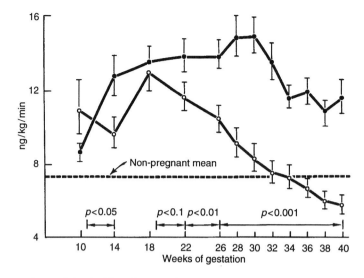

**Figure 2.1** Comparison of the ANG II dose (ng/kg/min) required to elicit a pressor response (increase in diastolic blood pressure of 20 mmHg) in 120 primigravid women (769 infusions; black circles) who remained normotensive and 72 primigravid women who subsequently developed pregnancy-induced hypertension (421 infusions; open circles). The non-pregnant mean is shown as a broken line. Values are the means ± one standard error. The difference between the two groups was significant after 22 weeks gestation ($p < 0.01$), and the two groups continued to diverge widely after 26 weeks gestation ($p < 0.001$). (Source: reprinted with permission from Gant *et al.*, 1973.)

during normotensive pregnancies, there are dramatic two- to fivefold increases in plasma renin concentrations, plasma renin activity, renin substrate, ANG II and aldosterone levels (Broughton Pipkin and Symonds, 1977; Chesley, 1978; Broughton Pipkin *et al.*, 1982; Hanssens *et al.*, 1991a, b). In contrast to normotensive pregnancies, those complicated by PIH/preeclampsia are associated with lower levels of plasma renin concentration, plasma renin activity, ANG II levels and aldosterone concentrations (Weir *et al.*, 1973; Chesley, 1978; Hanssens *et al.*, 1991a, b). As described above, women who either presently have or are destined to develop PIH/preeclampsia require substantially less exogenously administered ANG II to elicit a similar pressor response than do normotensive pregnant women (Gant *et al.*, 1973). Thus, it appears that this early divergence of the effective pressor dose to infused ANG II between normal

and subsequently hypertensive patients probably results from significant modifications in the physiological processes controlling this normal cardiovascular adaptive response to pregnancy. Therefore, a series of studies were conducted in normal pregnant women in order to test the hypothesis that reductions in circulating plasma renin activity (an indicator of the circulating levels of plasma ANG II) by volume loading would decrease the effective pressor dose to infused ANG II.

## 2.5 CONTROL OF VASCULAR REACTIVITY IN NORMOTENSIVE AND HYPERTENSIVE PREGNANT WOMEN

In these studies, control samples for baseline hematocrit and plasma renin activity levels were obtained; then the effective pressor response was measured. These measurements were then repeated. The volume loads included one liter of normal saline, 500 ml of Dextran, 950 ml of packed red blood cells or 200 ml of 5% sodium chloride (hypertonic saline). Results from these studies are summarized in Figure 2.2 (Gant *et al.*, 1974; Cunningham, Cox and Gant, 1975).

Following volume expansion, and in spite of the significant reductions in volume deficits (increases in blood volume) associated with decreases in circulating plasma renin activity (indicative of decreases in plasma ANG II levels), no significant changes in the effective pressor dose to infused ANG II could be detected in pregnant women. This was in contrast to the results in non-pregnant women, in whom blood volume expansion significantly decreased the effective pressor dose to infused ANG II. Similar responses to plasma volume expansion and ANG II were obtained in non-pregnant and pregnant sheep (Matsuura *et al.*, 1981). From these results, it was concluded that a primary factor controlling vascular refractoriness/sensitivity

to infused ANG II during pregnancy was a component other than circulating levels of ANG II, e.g. individual vessel wall refractoriness to infused ANG II. This supposition was supported by the observation that, following the infusion of hypertonic saline, there was a consistent and significant increase in the pressor response to infused ANG II. Brunner *et al.* (1972) proposed the possibility that increases in vascular reactivity after hypertonic saline treatments might result from alterations of ANG II binding to specific ANG II receptors on the vascular endothelium; this has not yet been tested critically.

The attenuated pressor responses to infused ANG II in normal pregnant women are likely to be the consequence of the collective refractoriness of many individual vascular beds to this vasoconstrictor agent (Figure 2.3).

From the results reported above it appears that, in women destined to develop PIH/preeclampsia, or in women who are

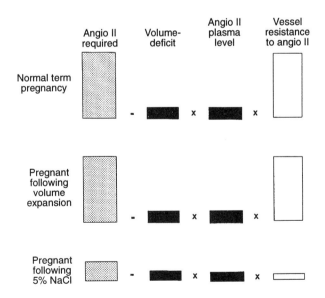

**Figure 2.2** Hypothetical model of physiological determinants of ANG II dose requirements necessary to evoke a pressor response, diagrammatically represented according to their apparent physiological importance in normal pregnancy and in normal pregnancy following volume expansion and hypertonic saline administration. (Source: reprinted with permission from Gant *et al.*, 1974.)

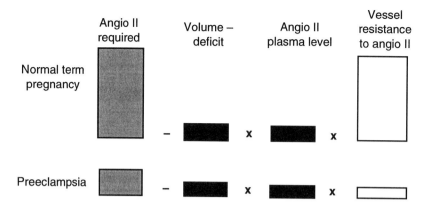

**Figure 2.3**   Hypothetical model of physiological and pathological determinants of ANG II dose requirements necessary to evoke a pressor response diagrammatically represented according to their physiological importance in normal pregnancy and in preeclampsia. (Reprinted with permission from Gant *et al.,* 1974).

already acutely ill with this disease, the increased sensitivity to ANG II results from alterations in the local responsiveness of the vessel wall of individual vascular beds rather than from changes in blood volume or circulating renin–ANG II levels, both of which may be secondary phenomena. This hypothesis is supported by the studies of Aalkjaar and co-workers (1984), who reported that the *in vitro* vasoconstrictor responses to ANG II were increased in omental arteries obtained from women with PIH/preeclampsia as compared with those obtained from normotensive pregnant women.

Even after evaluating these studies of blood volume expansion, it still was not known what mediated the vascular refractoriness to ANG II observed during normal human pregnancy. McGiff and Itskovitz (1973) proposed prostaglandins as possible candidates as potent modulators of vascular reactivity in several different organs under a variety of conditions. Terragno *et al.* (1974) supported this thesis when they reported that, late in canine pregnancy, elevated uterine blood flow was associated with a high concentration of prostaglandin E in the uterine venous blood. These investigators also observed that the intravenous infusion of ANG II into pregnant dogs led to an increase in uterine blood flow and to a rise in the concentration of prostaglandin E in the uterine venous effluent. Magness *et al.* (1992) reported that, in the chronically-instrumented pregnant sheep, ANG II also will increase the *de novo* synthesis of prostacyclin ($PGI_2$), the primary eicosanoid produced by blood vessels, and in particular, the vascular endothelium (Terragno *et al.*, 1978; Magness *et al.*, 1985, 1996; Magness, 1991; Magness and Rosenfeld, 1993) of the uterine vascular bed. In these studies, Magness *et al.* (1992) also reported that the local inhibition of ovine uterine horn prostaglandin production *in vivo*, using indomethacin infusions directly into the uterine circulation, locally increased the uterine vascular responsiveness to infused ANG II. Data from these studies will be presented in greater detail later, in order now to focus more closely on the control of systemic pressor responses rather than on regional responses to infused ANG II in pregnancy.

Prostaglandin-related substances such as prostaglandin E and $PGI_2$ also appear to be involved in the regulation of systemic vascular reactivity during normal human pregnancy. This hypothesis was tested in studies evaluating the effects of the prostaglandin synthetase inhibitors indomethacin and aspirin on the effective pressor dose of infused ANG II in normal pregnant women after the 28th week of pregnancy (Everett *et al.*, 1978a). Each woman had been normotensive throughout pregnancy, had no history of hypertension and was on a diet of her own choice from the hospital menu. Patients were not permitted to take any non-steroidal anti-inflammatory medication prior to study.

After establishing the control effective pressor dose to infused ANG II before treatment, each subject was administered either 25 mg of indomethacin or 10 grains of aspirin (650 mg; two adult aspirins) at 6-hour intervals. Two hours after the second dose of indomethacin or aspirin, the effective pressor dose to infused ANG II was again measured. Patients were allowed to engage in usual hospital activities between the ANG II infusion tests. It is clear from the data illustrated in Figure 2.4 that the administration of high doses of these prostaglandin synthetase inhibitors to normal pregnant women resulted in significant reductions in the amount of infused ANG II required to evoke a 20 mmHg rise in diastolic blood pressure.

In the same year that we (Everett *et al.*, 1978a) published this study, McLaughlin, Brennan and Chez (1978) also reported that indomethacin increased the systemic pressor response to infused ANG II in late-pregnant sheep. Therefore, it is likely that the attenuated pressor responses to infused ANG II normally observed in human pregnancy are mediated, at least in part, by the production of prostaglandin-related substances. We hypothesized that these prostaglandins were produced *in situ* in the blood vessels (Everett *et al.*, 1978a; Magness *et al.*, 1985) or more specifically the endothelium (Magness, 1991; Magness and Rosenfeld, 1990). It is not known if ANG II refractoriness, which is characteristic of nor-

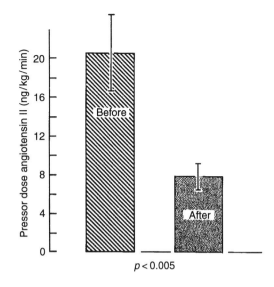

**Figure 2.4** The mean effective pressor dose of ANG II before and during indomethacin treatment of 11 normotensive women studied during late gestation. (Source: reprinted with permission from Everett *et al.*, 1978a.)

mal pregnancy, results from the increased basal production of vasodilatory prostanoids reported during normal gestation (Magness, Mitchell and Rosenfeld, 1990; Magness and Rosenfeld, 1990) or from an ANG II-stimulated increase in these prostaglandins during the steady-state infusion of this potent pressor agent (Magness and Rosenfeld, 1990; Magness *et al.*, 1992, 1996).

Contrasting the above observations in normal pregnancy with those observed in women destined to develop hypertension has uncovered several cardiovascular characteristics that have potential significant clinical importance. Specifically, these are the observations that, in pregnant women who are destined to develop or have already developed PIH/preeclampsia, there are not only decreases in the rate of prostaglandin synthesis (or increases in the rate of prostaglandin catabolism) in the mother (Goodman *et al.*, 1982; Fitzgerald *et al.*, 1987a) and placenta (Walsh,

1985), but also dramatic increases in systemic vascular pressor responsiveness to infused ANG II (Gant *et al.*, 1973; Figure 2.3). The data of Everett *et al.* (1978a) would suggest that a 'cause and effect' relationship is present during pregnancy.

## 2.6 PHARMACOLOGICAL MANIPULATION OF VASCULAR REACTIVITY AND THE PREVENTION OF PIH

The relationships discussed above are consistent with the studies reported by Walsh (1985), who observed that in normotensive pregnancies the placenta produces approximately equivalent amounts of prostacyclin ($PGI_2$; a potent vasodilator and platelet anti-aggregating prostanoid) and thromboxane ($TxA_2$; a vasoconstrictor and platelet proaggregating eicosanoid). Walsh (1985) reported that in hypertensive gravidas an imbalance was evident between $PGI_2$ and $TxA_2$, i.e. in women with preeclampsia the placenta produced seven times less $PGI_2$ than $TxA_2$. For example, in normal pregnancy, arachidonic acid, the obligate precursor of both $PGI_2$ and $TxA_2$, is predominantly directed towards $PGI_2$ (Figure 2.5), i.e. there is a relatively high or equal $PGI_2$ to $TxA_2$ ratio.

In the patient with PIH/preeclampsia, however, arachidonic acid is probably directed more towards $TxA_2$, thus resulting in substan-

tial reductions in the ratio of $PGI_2$ to $TxA_2$. An extension of this interpretation is that $PGI_2$ and $TxA_2$ are derived from different cellular sources which produce these eicosanoids, e.g. endothelium, platelets and/or trophoblast, which are differently inhibited or stimulated during the progression of the disease that ultimately results in PIH/preeclampsia. This is difficult to address because the interactions of locally produced vasoactive substances, such as these eicosanoids, act in autocrine or paracrine fashions within or between the cells that produce them, and the disruption of their close proximity will alter the interactions between these cell types.

In the studies of Everett *et al.* (1978a), it was reported that, in the normotensive pregnant woman who was refractory to infused ANG II, indomethacin and high-doses of aspirin therapy (at levels that will inhibit the production of both $PGI_2$ and $TxA_2$) would concomitantly render them 'sensitive' to the pressor effects of infused ANG II. The level of ANG II sensitivity (< 8 ng/kg/min) after cyclooxygenase enzyme inhibition (Everett *et al.*, 1978a) was similar to what was observed in either the non-pregnant woman or those subjects who were 'sensitive' to ANG II and destined to develop PIH/preeclampsia (Gant *et al.*, 1973). This may occur, in part, by reversing the normal $PGI_2$-dominated or 'protective' condition. In fact, this proposal has been the basis for the 'alleged' beneficial therapeutic effects of low-dose aspirin; i.e. by virtue of low-dose aspirin's 'selective' blockade of $TxA_2$ it will increase the ratio of plasma $PGI_2$ to $TxA_2$ (Masotti *et al.*, 1979). Specifically, low-dose aspirin therapy as proposed by Beaufils *et al.* (1985) and Wallenburg *et al.* (1986) was based on the assumption that low-dose aspirin's beneficial effects in decreasing the incidence of proteinuric hypertension would be due to a decrease in the overproduction of $TxA_2$ while sparing $PGI_2$ production; however this hypothesis was not proved in their reports.

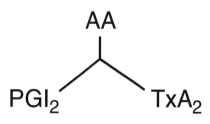

**Figure 2.5** Arachidonic acid (AA) is the obligate precursor converted to either prostacyclin ($PGI_2$) or thromboxane $A_2$ ($TxA_2$) by the actions of the enzyme cyclooxygenase.

Subsequently, we (Spitz *et al.*, 1988), and others (Caruso *et al.*, 1988) reported that low-dose aspirin restored vascular refractoriness in ANG-II-sensitive women; i.e. the effective pressor dose to infused ANG II increased from $5.9 \pm 2.4$ to $10.2 \pm 5.5$ ng/kg/min after 1 week of low-dose aspirin therapy (81 mg or one baby aspirin daily for 1 week; Spitz *et al.*, 1988; Figure 2.6).

In these patients, this treatment inhibited $TxA_2$ production (serum/platelet-derived $TxB_2$ $1804 \pm 1771$–$132 \pm 206$ pg/ml; plasma $TxB_2$ $130 \pm 107$ to $19 \pm 12$ pg/ml, mean $\pm$ s.d.). In contrast to the proposed hypothesis, $PGI_2$ production was only partially spared; i.e. it was reduced 25–30% from $243 \pm 90$ to $163 \pm 90$ pg/ml, mean $\pm$ s.d. (Figure 2.7).

This inhibition of $PGI_2$, however, was not as great as the inhibition of $TxA_2$ (70–90%).

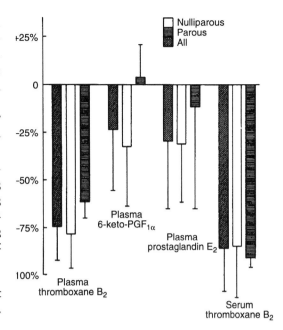

**Figure 2.7** Relative inhibition of serum and plasma thromboxane $B_2$ and plasma 6-keto-prostaglandin $F1_\alpha$ and prostaglandin $E_2$ after 1 week of 81 mg aspirin treatment. Values are illustrated as means $\pm$ one standard deviation. (Redrawn with permission from Spitz *et al.*, 1988, in *Am. J. Obstet. Gynecol.*, **159**, 1035–43.)

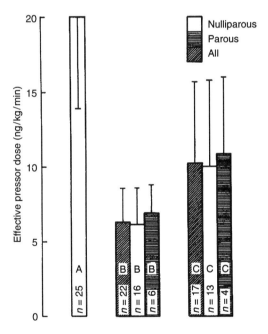

**Figure 2.6** Effective pressor dose of ANG II in non-sensitive (*A*) and sensitive women before (*B*) and after (*C*) low-dose aspirin treatment. (A > B, p < 0.001; B < C, $p = 0.037$; C < A, $p < 0.001$). Values are illustrated as means $\pm$ one standard deviation. (Redrawn with permission from Spitz *et al.*, 1988, in *Am. J. Obstet. Gynecol.*, **159**, 1035–43.)

Therefore, the ratio of $PGI_2$ to $TxA_2$ increased dramatically: nearly fourfold (Figure 2.8).

Subsequently, these observations were confirmed by Schiff *et al.* (1989) and Sabai *et al.* (1989). It is possible that using a lower dose of aspirin (for example 40 or 60 mg per day) we would have demonstrated selective inhibition of $TxA_2$ with complete sparing of the $PGI_2$ production (Hanley *et al.*, 1981; Sabai *et al.*, 1989).

In these studies, a 'favorable' response to low-dose aspirin was considered to be an increase in the effective pressor dose to infused ANG II, a selective inhibition of $TxA_2$ with sparing of the $PGI_2$, and the prevention of PIH/preeclampsia while on this treatment. Upon further analysis of our data (Spitz et al., 1988), we were concerned that certain subsets

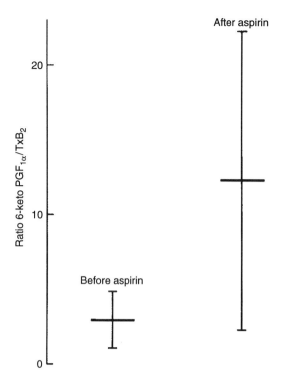

**Figure 2.8** Effect of low-dose aspirin on the ratio of plasma 6-keto-prostaglandin $F_{1\alpha}$/$TxB_2$ in ANG-II-sensitive pregnant women. Values are illustrated as means $\pm$ one standard deviation. (Redrawn with permission from Spitz *et al.*, 1988, in *Am. J. Obstet. Gynecol.*, **159**, 1035–43.)

of patients did not appear to respond in a totally 'favorable' fashion while on this low-dose aspirin therapy. We expanded this analysis and reported these and additional data in a subsequent report (Brown et al., 1990) of 40 nulliparous pregnant women (28–32 weeks gestation) who were given low-dose aspirin therapy (81 mg per day) from the time of enrollment and throughout gestation until delivery. The ANG II pressor responses (effective pressor dose to infused ANG II) and circulating eicosanoid levels were measured before and after one week of low-dose aspirin therapy. The subsequent clinical outcome after the patients remained on low-dose aspirin therapy throughout the remainder of gestation was correlated with these pressor

and eicosanoid results. All women receiving this aspirin treatment had significant reductions in serum and plasma $TxB_2$ levels demonstrating therapy compliance ($p < 0.01$). In Figure 2.9 are illustrated the changes in effective pressor dose to infused ANG II after 1 week of low-dose aspirin therapy in these 40 patients.

Data were stratified according to the patient's effective pressor dose to infused ANG II before and after one week of low-dose aspirin. Eleven women remained 'sensitive' to the pressor effects of ANG II (effective pressor dose $< 10$ ng/kg/min) after 1 week of low-dose aspirin treatment. These women also exhibited significant decreases ($p < 0.05$) in plasma $PGI_2$ levels (6-keto-prostaglandin $F_{1\alpha}$; $264 \pm 119$ versus $161 \pm 31$ pg/ml, mean $\pm$ s.d.) and prostaglandin $E_2$ ($476 \pm 174$ versus $351 \pm 112$ pg/ml) levels. In contrast, patients who were either 'non-sensitive' (refractory) to ANG II ($n = 18$; $X^2 \geqslant 10$ ng/kg/min) before and after low-dose aspirin or became 'non-sensitive' after aspirin administration ($n = 11$) had no significant changes in either plasma 6-keto-prostaglandin $F_{1\alpha}$ or prostaglandin $E_2$ concentrations. The clinical relevance of this study is evident also by examining Figure 2.9. We observed that the occurrence of PIH/preeclampsia was 100% in women who remained sensitive to the pressor effects of infused ANG II during low-dose aspirin therapy as compared with an occurrence of 36% and 39% in the other two groups ($\chi^2 = 16.14$; $p < 0.001$).

The severity of this disease also was exacerbated in the group of women who were sensitive to the pressor effects of ANG II before and after treatment with low-dose aspirin. Thus, based on these limited numbers of patients during low-dose aspirin therapy, a failure to develop refractoriness to infused ANG II is associated with a non-selective inhibition of eicosanoids and a virtual certainty of developing PIH/preeclampsia. Another way in which we evaluated these data, in a *post hoc* fashion, is seen in Table 2.1.

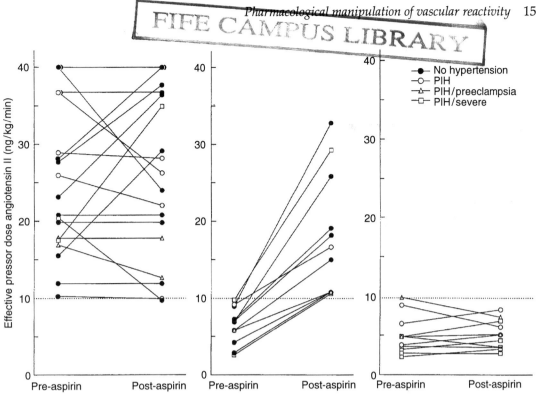

**Figure 2.9** Effective pressor dose and clinical outcome in ANG-II-non-sensitive and -sensitive women before and after low-dose aspirin therapy. The occurrence of hypertension was (**a**) non-sensitive 7/18, (**b**) sensitive/non-sensitive 4/11, (**c**) sensitive/sensitive 11/11; $X^2 = 16.14$, $p < 0.001$. (Redrawn with permission from Brown *et al.*, 1990, in *Am. J. Obstet. Gynecol.*, **163**, 1853–61.)

**Table 2.1** Eicosanoid concentrations (pg/ml) after one week of low-dose aspirin therapy in serum and plasma obtained from pregnant women who remained normotensive or became hypertensive; values are means ± s.d. (Source: Brown *et al.*, 1990, in *Am. Obstet. Gynecol.*, **163**, 1853–61.)

|  | Normotensive | | Hypertensive | |
|---|---|---|---|---|
|  | *Control* | *Aspirin* | *Control* | *Aspirin* |
| **Plasma** |  |  |  |  |
| 6-keto-prostaglandin $F_{1\alpha}$ | 175 ± 113 | 153 ± 80 | 202 ± 111 * | 154 ± 32 |
| Thromboxane $B_2$ | 338 ± 165 *** | 132 ± 59 | 288 ± 187 *** | 102 ± 55 |
| 6-keto-$PGF_{1\alpha}$/$TxB_2$ | 0.52 ± 0.22 ** | 1.46 ± 1.42 | 0.88 ± 0.53 ** | 2.62 ± 0.85 |
| Prostaglandin $E_2$ | 360 ± 173 | 367 ± 186 | 390 ± 203 * | 294 ± 130 |
| **Serum** |  |  |  |  |
| Thromboxane $B_2$ | 1430 ± 1161 *** | 1031 ± 72 | 1307 ± 0.53 *** | 135 ± 165 |

$*p < 0.05$; $**p < 0.01$; $***p < 0.001$

Specifically, regardless of the initial ANG II sensitivity at the time of entry into this study, women who subsequently developed PIH/preeclampsia exhibited decreases in plasma $TxB_2$, 6-keto-prostaglandin $F_{1\alpha}$ and prostaglandin $E_2$ concentrations. In contrast, those women who did not become hypertensive only had an isolated decrease in $TxB_2$ with low-dose aspirin therapy while both 6-keto-prostaglandin $F_{1\alpha}$ and prostaglandin $E_2$ were completely 'spared'.

It was proposed (Brown *et al.*, 1990) that these observations might reflect a basic defect in vascular adaptation to pregnancy manifested by a greater low-dose-aspirin-induced cyclooxygenase inhibition in numerous tissues because these eicosanoids are derived primarily from several tissue sites, e.g. endothelium ($PGI_2$; Magness, 1991; Magness and Rosenfeld, 1993b), platelets ($TxA_2$; Fitzgerald *et al.*, 1987b; Spitz *et al.*, 1988), and placenta (prostaglandin $E_2$; Yoshimura, Rosenfeld and Magness, 1991). Although other tissue and cellular sources of prostanoids also have been reported, for illustrative purposes only these three will be discussed in this review. Since it is believed that aspirin functions to inhibit prostanoid synthesis by irreversible acetylation of the enzyme cyclooxygenase, the continuation and subsequent resumption of prostanoid production must occur by transcription and translation of new enzyme. It is therefore not surprising that $TxA_2$ levels were decreased in all patients studied because the platelets from which $TxA_2$ is primarily derived (Fitzgerald *et al.*, 1987b; Spitz *et al.*, 1988) are no more than fragments of megakaryoblast plasma membrane, containing cytoplasm but no nucleus from which new cyclooxygenase mRNA can be synthesized. In contrast, endothelium-derived $PGI_2$ (Magness, 1991; Magness and Rosenfeld, 1993b) or placenta-derived prostaglandin $E_2$ (Yoshimura, Rosenfeld and Magness, 1991) will transcribe new mRNA within the nucleus of individual cells in order to maintain and restore production of these eicosanoids.

Moreover, because the half-life of the mRNA for cyclooxygenase is rather short (< 10 min), the importance of transcriptional regulation of this enzyme becomes exceedingly evident, especially when one considers the complexity of the clinical results presented in these studies. For example, in a situation such as PIH/preeclampsia many tissues and/or vascular beds all containing cyclooxygenase and producing various types of eicosanoids are affected during the progression of this disease, and each may have a slightly different regulation or response to this inhibitor.

Thus, it is possible, but not proved, that the relationships observed in our studies between differences in vascular reactivity, different patterns of prostaglandin responses to low-dose aspirin, and clinical outcome are related to the same overall underlying systemic pathophysiology. The most attractive single unifying hypothesis is that a metabolic and/or enzymatic defect renders some women incapable of maintaining an appropriate balance of factors, such as eicosanoids, that act to modulate vascular reactivity.

Although prostaglandins may play a role in the pathogenesis of PIH/preeclampsia (Everett *et al.*,1978a; McLaughlin, Brennan and Chez, 1978; Friedman, 1988) other factors, e.g. endothelium-derived relaxing factor/nitric oxide (Magness, 1991; Magness *et al.*, 1996) or progesterone (Everett *et al.*, 1978b) may work in concert with them to contribute to the maintenance of normal vascular reactivity and vasodilation; these will be discussed below in greater detail. Metabolic or enzymatic defects are often genetically determined in an autosomal recessive manner, and a number of investigators have suggested that the pre- disposition for PIH/preeclampsia may reflect this type of defect (Cooper and Liston, 1979; Chesley, 1980; Sutherland *et al.*, 1981). Whether or not the associations observed in the study of Brown *et al.* (1990) between the two or three subpopulations based on the pregnant patients' responses to low-dose aspirin treatment (Figure 2.9) are due to a single enzyme defect, such as cyclooxygenase, or a more complex situation of several enzymes remains to be ascertained. After the time we published the work of Brown *et al.* (1990) another isoform of cyclooxygenase, an 'inducible form' named PGH synthase 2, has been discovered and cloned. Therefore, the physiological, pharmacological and clinical changes noted in our studies could potentially relate to the differential effects of low-dose aspirin on the inhibition or the subsequent transcriptional regulation of either the 'constitutive' (PGH synthase 1) or inducible (PGH synthase 2) isoforms of cyclooxygenase. This hypothesis as yet has not been tested. Regardless of the mechanism of action of this therapy, our studies regarding low-dose aspirin therapy support the thesis that this agent is not 'the answer' for the prevention of preeclampsia in all women, at least in the setting and dosage used in these studies.

## 2.7 FACTORS OTHER THAN PROSTAGLANDINS WHICH ALTER ANG II RESPONSES

Another endothelium-derived vasodilator that has recently received a considerable amount of attention because of its local paracrine regulation of vascular tone is endothelium-derived relaxing factor/nitric oxide (Magness, 1991; Magness *et al.*, 1996). This highly labile substance is produced by the endothelial nitric oxide synthase enzyme, which synthesizes nitric oxide from the guanidine group of l-arginine. Indeed structural analogues of l-arginine such as Nω-nitro-l-arginine have been shown to increase basal blood pressure in normotensive and spontaneously hypertensive pregnant rats (Ahokas, Mercer and Sibai, 1991; Molnar and Hertelendy, 1992). Baylis and Engels (1992) recently reported that the chronic blockade of nitric oxide synthase in the pregnant rat causes hypertension, inhibits the systemic and renal vasodilatory effects of normal pregnancy and is associated with significant protein-

uria and fetal morbidity late in gestation. Moreover, Molnar and Hertelendy (1992) demonstrated that the *in vivo* inhibition of this enzyme also increased pressor responses to infused ANG II, noradrenalin and arginine vasopressin, such that they were 'virtually identical' to those of non-pregnant postpartum control rats. The specificity of this response was demonstrated, since this inhibitor-induced increase in pressor response sensitivity was reversed by treatment of these animals with l-arginine, the endogenous substrate for the enzyme nitric oxide synthase. Taken together these data provide evidence that endothelium-derived relaxing factor/nitric oxide may be involved in the normal cardiovascular adaptation to pregnancy and that it may also be involved in some of the adverse cardiovascular alterations that we and others have noted in PIH/preeclampsia.

Factors other than the $PGI_2$ to $TxA_2$ ratio and endothelium-derived relaxing factor/nitric oxide also appear to participate in modulating vascular reactivity in response to infused ANG II during normal gestation. We have noted that normal pregnant women lose their pregnancy-associated vascular refractoriness to infused ANG II within 15–30 minutes after the placenta is delivered. These data are suggestive that a rapidly cleared substance of placental origin could potentially be responsible for promoting refractoriness to the pressor effects of infused ANG II, either directly or by stimulating the production of vasodilatory factors such as $PGI_2$ or nitric oxide by the vessel wall. Among the rapidly cleared hormones of placental origin which could be a likely candidate for this role is progesterone, or one of its metabolites. Progesterone, which is a mediator of uterine smooth muscle quiescence, may also have profound actions on the modulation of vascular relaxation. Indeed, intramuscular administration of large amounts of progesterone to the gravid woman during the later stages of labor delays the loss of refractoriness to ANG II that follows delivery (Gant, Worley, Chand, unpublished observations). In contrast, intravenous administration of progesterone did not restore ANG II refractoriness to women with PIH/preeclampsia (Figure 2.10).

From these observations, we suggest that a progesterone metabolite, formed in significant amounts after intramuscular injection but less prominently after intravenous administration of the hormone, might be responsible for delaying the loss of vascular refractoriness to ANG II after delivery. This supposition was supported by results obtained in earlier studies, in which we observed that plasma concentrations of 5α-pregnane-3,20-dione (5α-DHP) were strikingly elevated during human pregnancy and that the concentration of this progesterone

metabolite appeared to parallel the effective pressor dose to infused ANG II (Everett *et al.*, 1978b). In fact, the infusion of 5α-DHP into ANG-II-sensitive women with mild PIH/preeclampsia restored vascular refractoriness to ANG II to a response similar to those we had observed in normal pregnancy (Figure 2.10).

Although the mechanism by which 5α-DHP restored ANG II vascular refractoriness to women with PIH/preeclampsia is not known, infusion of this steroid hormone metabolite into five normal pregnant women who had been rendered ANG-II-sensitive by administration of indomethacin (Everett *et al.*, 1978a) also restored vascular refractoriness to ANG II (Figure 2.11; Everett *et al.*, 1978b).

It is possible, therefore, that a progestin-induced mechanism may modulate the expression of prostaglandin-mediated vascular responsiveness to the pressor effects of infused ANG II in normal pregnancy. Alternatively under these circumstances, this steroid may act independently of prostaglandins as a smooth muscle relaxant.

We reported another observation that may have added additional information regarding the physiological mechanisms controlling vascular responsiveness to ANG II in pregnancy (Everett *et al.*, 1978c). Administration of the cyclic nucleotide (e.g., cyclic AMP) phosphodiesterase inhibitor, theophylline, to women with mild PIH who were sensitive to ANG II late in gestation, more than doubled the mean effective pressor dose to infused ANG II, restoring the vascular refractoriness characteristic of normal pregnancy (Figure 2.12; Everett *et al.*, 1978c).

Whether this treatment was of therapeutic benefit in lowering blood pressure could not be ascertained from this study, because the mildly hypertensive women had become normotensive while at bed rest before the study was performed. It should be emphasized, however, that, despite a return of normotensive blood pressure readings associated with decreased physical activity, these women

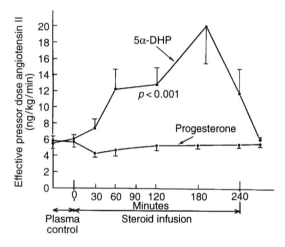

**Figure 2.10** The effect of intravenously infused progesterone (150 μg/min) and 5α-dihydroprogesterone (5α-DHP, 12–15 μg/min) on the amount of administered ANG II required to elicit a standard pressor response in women with mild pregnancy-induced hypertension. The effective pressor dose of ANG II required at all time periods during 5α-DHP infusion was significantly greater ($p < 0.001$) than that required before infusion of this steroid. The infusion of progesterone was not associated with a change in the effective pressor dose of ANG II. (Source: reproduced with permission from Everett *et al.*, 1978b.)

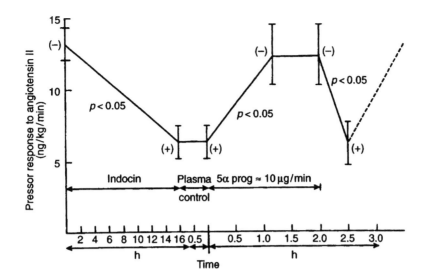

**Figure 2.11** The effect of 5α-dihydroprogesterone (5α-DHP) infusions on the amount of ANG II required to elicit a standard pressor response in indomethacin-treated normal pregnant women. The amounts of ANG II required to raise diastolic pressure by 20 mmHg before indomethacin treatment, after indomethacin treatment and during 5α-DHP treatment are illustrated. (Source: reproduced with permission from Everett *et al.*, 1978b.)

remained 'sensitive' to infused ANG II until treated with theophylline.

It is likely that this vascular effect of theophylline resulted from its inhibition of the enzyme cyclic nucleotide phosphodiesterase, a known action of theophylline. We cannot exclude, however, another known action of theophylline. Specifically, theophylline can inhibit adenosine receptor function. If the former is the mechanism of action, then inhibition of phosphodiesterase, a principal regulator in intracellular cyclic nucleotide accumulation, would promote cyclic AMP accumulation within vascular smooth muscle. Increases in cyclic AMP within the myocyte would lead to sequestration of calcium in the cytoplasmic reticulum. The resulting reductions in intracellular free calcium ion concentration would be expected to promote vascular smooth muscle relaxation (Figure 2.13).

This proposed mechanism in pregnancy is supported by the reports of elevated urinary cyclic AMP levels in normal human pregnancy (Kopp, Paradiz and Tucci, 1977). More recently, we reported that during ovine pregnancy vascular smooth muscle production of cyclic AMP is increased in uterine arteries obtained

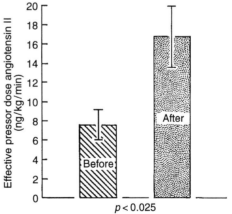

**Figure 2.12** The mean effective pressor dose to infused ANG II before and during theophylline treatment of seven women with pregnancy-induced hypertension. (Source: reproduced with permission from Everett *et al.*, 1978c.)

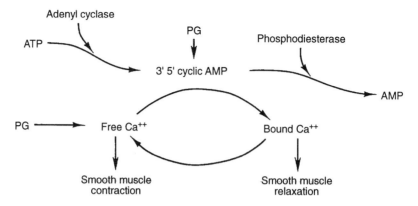

**Figure 2.13** Schematic model of the proposed role of prostaglandin and cyclic 3′,5′-adenosine monophosphate in pregnancy-associated vascular refractoriness to the pressor effects of ANG II. (Source: reproduced with permission from Everett *et al.*, 1978c.)

from pregnant compared with non-pregnant sheep (Magness *et al.*, 1996). We also reported that this pregnancy-associated increase in cyclic AMP was controlled by the local production of endothelium-derived $PGI_2$, and that both $PGI_2$ and cAMP are also specifically stimulated *in vitro* by ANG II.

To summarize, these studies describing the modulation of vascular reactivity in human pregnancy are consistent with the following suggestions:

1. The relative vascular refractoriness to ANG II that characterizes normal pregnancy probably results from the action of a prostaglandin(s) or prostaglandin-related substance(s) on vascular smooth muscle.
2. This prostaglandin effect may be modified or modulated by the actions of a steroid (presumably placental in origin), most probably a progesterone metabolite; however, the effects of estrogens or androgens or their metabolites have not been critically studied.
3. The mechanism whereby prostaglandins, presumably of endothelial origin, alter vascular sensitivity to ANG II may involve the

mediation of the cyclic nucleotide (e.g. cyclic AMP) system of the vascular smooth muscle.

It was apparent from a consideration of the foregoing studies on vascular reactivity in normal pregnancy and PIH/preeclampsia that the pressor effects of ANG II could be readily manipulated. This led Gant and Worley (1980) to propose that 'if loss of vascular refractoriness to ANG II plays a central role in the pathogenesis of PIH/preeclampsia, it is now possible that a simple, fruitful means for restoring ANG II refractoriness, or preventing its loss altogether, will some day be found'.

The concept of restoring ANG II vascular refractoriness to the 'future hypertensive' ANG-II-sensitive woman or, even better, by preventing its loss altogether would be of critical importance to a pregnant woman and her fetus. Although blood pressure can most often be controlled with a variety of antihypertensive pharmaceutical agents, the effects of these agents upon fetal growth, and even survival, have not usually been well studied. Furthermore, it now appears likely, from studies in animals, that the action of some of these hypotensive agents, while beneficial to the mother, may be acutely or chronically detrimental to the fetus (see below).

## 2.8 VASCULAR REACTIVITY IN PREGNANCY AND PIH/PREECLAMPSIA IN RELATION TO UTEROPLACENTAL BLOOD FLOW

The gravid sheep has been shown to be an excellent animal model in which to study vascular reactivity to ANG II and other vasopressors in normal pregnancy (Rosenfeld and Gant, 1981; Rosenfeld, 1984). That is, as in the gravid women, the pregnant sheep is refractory to the pressor effects of infused ANG II. Using an animal model of this size also allows for studies of regional blood flow and/or vascular reactivity that obviously could not be performed in humans. This, therefore, led to studies of direct comparisons of systemic with uteroplacental blood flows, and the contrasting of systemic and uterine vascular resistances/reactivities in this animal model (Figure 2.14).

There is a marked refractoriness of systemic blood pressure and vascular resistance responses to infused ANG II (Rosenfeld and Gant, 1981; Naden and Rosenfeld, 1981, 1984; Rosenfeld, 1984). In addition to these systemic alterations, uterine vascular resistance responses are even more blunted in response to infused ANG II than is systemic vascular resistance (Naden and Rosenfeld, 1981). The differences in the reactivity between these two vascular beds results in the maintenance or even increases in uteroplacental blood flow noted during the infusion of lower, less 'pharmacological', doses of ANG II, i.e. when the uterine perfusion pressures (mean arterial blood pressure) exceed the relative rise in uterine vascular resistance. Moreover, similar relationships between blood pressure, resistance and uterine blood flow estimates have been confirmed in the human using Doppler ultrasound measurements (Erkkola and Pirhonen, 1990).

As Everett *et al.* (1978a) and McLaughlin, Brennan and Chez (1978) observed for the

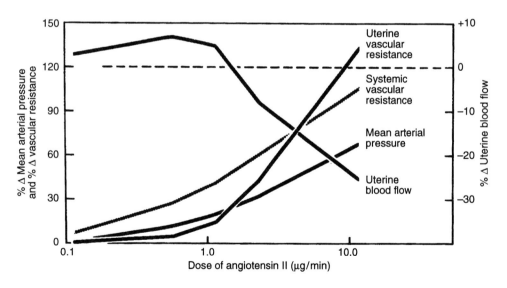

**Figure 2.14**   The relative steady-state changes in uterine blood flow, mean arterial pressure (perfusion pressure), systemic vascular resistance, and uterine vascular resistance during the systemic infusion of ANG II in term pregnant ewes. Responses were recorded after 4–5 min of stabilization at each dose of ANG II. (Source: reproduced with permission from Rosenfeld, 1984.)

systemic ANG II pressor responses, we recently reported that the reduced uteroplacental vasoconstrictive effects to ANG II compared with the systemic vasculature also result, at least in part, from a prostaglandin-mediated mechanism (Magness *et al.*, 1992; Figure 2.15).

In these studies, we observed that the unilateral uterine arterial infusion (ipsilateral) of indomethacin locally increased uterine vascular sensitivity to the vasoconstrictor effects of systemically infused ANG II in association with the local ipsilateral, but not contralateral,

inhibition of uterine $PGI_2$ production. Systemic pressor and cardiac responses to infused ANG II were unaltered by uterine arterial infusion of indomethacin. When comparing the local effects of indomethacin on ANG II responses in ipsilateral uterine blood flow with data presented both in Figure 2.14 and with the pre-indomethacin data illustrated in Figure 2.15, it is quite evident that the local uterine vascular effects of prostaglandins manifest a parallel shift in the relationship between uterine vascular resistance and uterine perfusion pressure (mean arterial blood

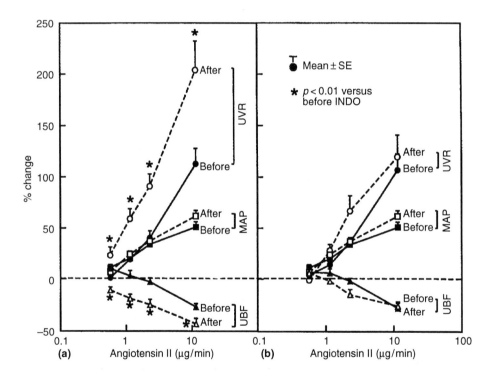

**Figure 2.15** Effects of systemic ANG II infusions on the relative steady-state changes (%) in uterine perfusion pressure (MAP), uterine vascular resistance (UVR) and uterine blood flow (UBF) before and after the local infusion of indomethacin ipsilateral (a) and contralateral (b) to the indomethacin infusion. (Source: reproduced with permission from Magness *et al.*, 1992.)

pressure). Specifically, during the systemic infusion of ANG II prior to indomethacin treatment, whenever the relative rise in uterine vascular resistance was less than the rise in perfusion pressure, uterine blood flow was either increased or unchanged. In contrast, after local uterine treatment with indomethacin, at all doses of systemically infused ANG II, the relative rise in ipsilateral uterine vascular resistance always exceeded that of perfusion pressure and uterine blood flow was observed to decrease. The control of this local uterine refractory response to infused ANG II probably results in an initial potential advantage to the fetus when there is a loss in refractoriness to ANG II pressor responses (increased systemic sensitivity), as occurs in women destined to develop PIH/preeclampsia (Gant *et al.*, 1973). In fact, this transient advantage of an increase or maintenance in uteroplacental blood flow developing in cases of future hypertension has been shown actually to occur in human pregnancies (Gant *et al.*, 1972, 1976). It is also likely that as the disease worsens and an increase in uterine vascular reactivity occurs, a further rise in uterine vascular resistance will exceed the relative rise in perfusion pressure and result in reductions in uteroplacental blood flow.

It was concluded that the gravid sheep is a valid animal model, with respect to responses in uterine blood flow and vascular reactivity to pressor agents, and that this animal model is useful in studying normal cardiovascular adaptations to pregnancy. From these studies in the sheep, it also is apparent that any hypotensive pharmacological agent that significantly decreases mean arterial blood pressure will also result in a 'serious' decrease in uterine blood flow. From the above discussion of the control of vascular reactivity in pregnancy, it seems likely that early-gestational attempts to prevent the development of PIH/preeclampsia will prove more advantageous to the fetus than will 'rescue' attempts to treat the hypertension once it has devel-

oped. This should not, however, prevent the development of mechanism-based prospective placebo-controlled clinical trials of antihypertensive agents that can be used to treat both chronic hypertension and PIH/preeclampsia in pregnant women. Such studies to establish effective and safe agents for both mother and fetus are of utmost importance and long overdue.

## REFERENCES

Aalkjaer, C., Johannesen, P., Pederson, E. B. *et al.* (1984) Morphology and angiotensin II responsiveness of isolated resistance vessels from patients with pre-eclampsia. *Scan. J. Clin. Lab. Invest. Suppl.*, **169**, 57–62.

Abdul-Karim, R. and Assali, N. S. (1961) Pressor response to angiotensin in pregnant and non-pregnant women. *Am. J. Obstet. Gynecol.*, **82**, 246–248.

Ahokas, R. A., Mercer, B. M. and Sabai, B. M. (1991) Enhanced endothelium-derived relaxing factor activity in pregnant, spontaneously hypertensive rats. *Am. J. Obstet. Gynecol.*, **165**, 801–804.

Assali, N. S., Holm, L. W. and Parker, H. R. (1964) Systemic and regional hemodynamic alterations in toxemia. *Circulation*, **30(Suppl 2)**, 53–58.

Baylis, C. and Engels, K. (1992) Adverse interactions between pregnancy and a new model of systemic hypertension produced by chronic blockade of endothelium derived relaxing factor (EDRF) in the rat. *Clin. Exper. Hypertens. Pregn.*, **B11**(2&3), 117–121.

Beaufils, M., Uzan, S., Donsimoni, R. and Colau, J. C. (1985) Prevention of pre-eclampsia by early antiplatelet therapy. *Lancet*, **i**, 840–845.

Brown, C. E. L. Gant, N. F., Cox, K. *et al.* (1990) Low-dose aspirin. II. Relationship of angiotensin II pressor responses, circulating eicosanoids, and pregnancy outcome. *Am. J. Obstet. Gynecol.*, **163**, 1853–1861.

Broughton Pipkin, F. and Symonds, E. M. (1977) The renin–angiotensin system in the maternal and fetal circulation in pregnancy hypertension. *Clin. Obstet. Gynecol.*, **4**, 65–77.

Broughton Pipkin, F., Hunter, J. C., Turner, S. R. and O'Brien, P. M. S. (1982) Prostaglandin E$_2$ attenuates the pressor response to angiotensin II in pregnant subjects but not in non-pregnant subjects. *Am. J. Obstet. Gynecol.*, **142**, 168–171.

Brunner, H. R., Chang, P., Wallach, R *et al.* (1972) Angiotensin II vascular receptors. Their avidity in relationship to sodium balance, the autonomic nervous system and hypertension. *J. Clin. Invest.*, **51**, 58–61.

Caruso, A., Ferrazzani, S., DeCarolis, S. *et al.* (1988) Effects of low-dose aspirin on vascular sensitivity to angiotensin II and on 24 hours arterial blood pressure in pregnancy. *Clin. Exp. Hypertens. – Hypertens. Pregn.*, **B7**, 171–174.

Chesley, L. C. (1978) Renin, angiotensin and aldosterone in pregnancy, in *Hypertensive Disorders in Pregnancy*, (ed. L. C. Chesley), Appleton-Century-Crofts, New York, p. 236.

Chesley, L. C. (1980) Hypertension in pregnancy: definitions, familial factor, and remote prognosis. *Kidney Int., Suppl.*, **18**, 234–246.

Chesley, L. C., Talledo, E., Bohler, C. S. and Zuspan, F. P. (1965) Vascular reactivity to angiotensin II and norepinephrine in pregnant and non-pregnant women. *Am. J. Obstet. Gynecol.*, **91**, 837–841.

Cooper, D. W. and Liston, W. A. (1979) Genetic control of severe pre-eclampsia. *J. Med. Genet.*, **16**, 409–412.

Cunningham, F. G., Cox, K. and Gant, N. F. (1975) Further observations on the nature of pressor responsivity to angiotensin II in human pregnancy. *Obstet. Gynecol.*, **46**, 581–584.

Cunningham, F. G., MacDonald, P. C. and Gant, N. F. (1989) Chapter 7, in *Williams Obstetrics*, 18th edn, (eds L. M. Hellman and J. A. Pritchard), Appleton & Lange, Norwalk, CT.

Dieckmann, W. J. and Michel, H. L. (1937) Vascular-renal effects of posterior pituitary extracts in pregnant women. *Am. J. Obstet. Gynecol.*, **33**, 131–134.

Erkkola, R. U. and Pirhonen, J. P. (1990) Flow velocity waveforms in uterine and umbilical arteries during the angiotensin II sensitivity test. *Am. J. Obstet. Gynecol.*, **162**, 1193–1197.

Everett, R. B., Worley, R. J., MacDonald, P. C. and Gant, N. F. (1978a) Effect of prostaglandin synthetase inhibitors on pressor response to angiotensin II in human pregnancy. *J. Clin. Endocrinol. Metab.*, **46**, 1007–1011.

Everett, R. B., Worley, R. J., MacDonald, P. C. and Gant, N. F. (1978b) Modification of vascular responsiveness to angiotensin II in pregnant women by intravenously infused 5α-dihydroprogesterone. *Am. J. Obstet. Gynecol.*, **131**, 352–356.

Everett, R. B., Worley, R. J., MacDonald, P. C. and Gant, N. F. (1978c) Oral administration of theophylline to modify pressor responsiveness to angiotensin II in women with pregnancy-induced hypertension. *Am. J. Obstet. Gynecol.*, 132, 359–363.

Fitzgerald, D. J., Entmann, S. S., Mulloy, K. and Fitzgerald, G. A. (1987a) Decreased prostacyclin biosynthesis preceding the clinical manifestation of pregnancy-induced hypertension. *Circulation*, 75, 956–959.

Fitzgerald, D. J. Mayo, G., Catella, F. *et al.* (1987b) Increased thromboxane biosynthesis in normal pregnancy is mainly derived from platelets. *Am. J. Obstet. Gynecol.*, **157**, 325–329.

Friedman, S. A. (1988) Preeclampsia: a review of the role of prostaglandins. *Obstet. Gynecol.*, **71**, 122–127.

Gant, N. F. and Worley, R. J. (1980) Maternal vascular reactivity to pressor agents, in *Hypertension in Pregnancy: Concepts and Management*, (eds N. F. Gant and R. J. Worley), Appleton-Century-Crofts, New York, ch. 2.

Gant, N. F., Madden, J. D., Siiteri, P. K. and MacDonald, P. C. (1972) A sequential study of the metabolism of dehydroisoandrosterone sulfate in primigravid pregnancy. *Excerpta Medica International Congress Series 273*, Excerpta Medica, Amsterdam, p. 1026–1031.

Gant, N. F., Daley, G. L., Chand, S. *et al.* (1973) A study of angiotensin II pressor response throughout primigravid pregnancy. *J. Clin. Invest.*, **52**, 2682–2686.

Gant, N. F., Chand, S., Whalley, P. J. and MacDonald, P. C. (1974) The nature of pressor responsiveness to angiotensin II in human pregnancy. *Obstet. Gynecol.*, **43**, 854–858.

Gant, N. F., Madden, J. D., Chand, S. *et al.* C. (1976) Metabolic clearance rate of dehydroisoandrosterone sulfate. V. Studies of essential hypertension complicating pregnancy. *Obstet. Gynecol.*, **47**, 319–343.

Goodman, R. P., Killam, A. P., Brash, A. R. and Branch, R. A. (1982) Prostacyclin production during pregnancy: comparison of production during normal pregnancy and pregnancy complicated by hypertension. *Am. J. Obstet. Gynecol.*, **142**, 817–821.

Hanley, S. P., Cockbill, S. R., Bevan, J. and Heptinstall, S. (1981) Differential inhibition by low-dose aspirin in human venous prostacyclin synthesis and platelet thromboxane synthesis. *Lancet*, **i**, 969–972.

Hanssens, M., Keirse, M. J. N. C., Spitz, B. and Van Assche, F. A. (1991a) Measurement of individual plasma angiotensins in normal pregnancy and pregnancy-induced hypertension. *J. Clin. Endocrinol. Metab.*, **73**, 489–493.

Hanssens, M., Keirse, M. J. N. C., Spitz, B. and Van Assche, F. A. (1991b) Angiotensin II levels in hypertensive and normotensive pregnancies. *Br. J. Obstet. Gynaecol.*, **98**, 155–159.

Kopp, L., Paradiz, G. and Tucci, J. R. (1977) Urinary excretion of cyclic 3′,5[[PRIME-adenosine monophosphate and cyclic 3′,5[[PRIME-guanosine monophosphate during and after pregnancy. *J. Clin. Endocrinol. Metab.*, **44**, 590–593.

Lees, M. M., Taylor, S. H., Scott, D. B. and Kerr, M. G. (1967) A study of cardiac output at rest throughout pregnancy. *J. Obstet. Gynaecol. Br. Commonw.*, **74**, 319–324.

Lumbars, E. R. (1970) Peripheral vascular reactivity to angiotensin II and noradrenaline in pregnant and non-pregnant women. *Aust. J. Exp. Biol. Med. Sci.*, **48**, 493–498.

Lund, C. J. and Donovan, J. C. (1967) Blood volume changes during pregnancy. Significance of plasma and red cell volume. *Am. J. Obstet. Gynecol.*, **98**, 393–398.

McGiff, J. C. and Itskovitz, H. D. (1973) Prostaglandins and the kidney. *Circ. Res.*, **33**, 479.

McLaughlin, M. K., Brennan, S. C. and Chez, R. A. (1978) Effects of indomethacin on sheep uteroplacental circulations and sensitivity to angiotensin II. *Am. J. Obstet. Gynecol.*, **132**, 430–435.

Magness, R. R. (1991) Endothelium-derived vasoactive substances and uterine blood vessels. *Semin. Perinatol.*, **5**, 68–78.

Magness, R. R., Mitchell, M. D. and Rosenfeld, C. R. (1990) Uteroplacental production of eicosanoids in ovine pregnancy. *Prostaglandins*, **39**, 75–78.

Magness, R. R. and Rosenfeld, C. R. (1986) Systemic and uterine responses to α-adrenergic stimulation in pregnant and non-pregnant sheep. *Am. J. Obstet. Gynecol.*, **155**, 897–901.

Magness, R. R. and Rosenfeld, C. R. (1988) Mechanisms for attenuated pressor responses to α-agonists in ovine pregnancy. *Am. J. Obstet. Gynecol.*, **159**, 252–257.

Magness, R. R. and Rosenfeld, C. R. (1990) Eicosanoids and the regulation of uteroplacental hemodynamics, in *Eicosanoids in Reproduction*, (ed. M. D. Mitchell), CRC Uniscience Series, CRC Press, Boca Raton, FL, p. 139–167.

Magness, R. R. and Zheng, J. (1996) Maternal cardio-vascular alterations during pregnancy, in *Paediatric and Perinatal Perspective. The Scientific Basis* (eds P. Gluckman and M. Heyman), Edward Arnold, London, 762–772.

Magness, R. R. and Rosenfeld, C. R. (1993b) Calcium modulation of endothelium-derived prostacyclin production in ovine pregnancy. *Endocrinology*, **132**, 2446–2452.

Magness, R. R., Osei-Boaten, K., Mitchell, M. D. and Rosenfeld, C. R. (1985) *In vitro* prostacyclin production by ovine uterine and systemic arteries: Effects of angiotensin II. *J. Clin. Invest.*, **76**, 2206–2211.

Magness, R. R., Rosenfeld, C. R., Hassan, A. and Shaul, P. W. (1996) Endothelial vasodilator production by uterine and systemic arteries. I. Effects of Ang II on $PGI_2$ and No in pregnancy. *Am. J. Physiol.*, **270**, H1914–H1923.

Magness, R. R., Rosenfeld, C. R., Faucher, D. J. and Mitchell, M. D. (1992b) Uterine prostaglandin production in ovine pregnancy: Effects of angiotensin II and indomethacin. *Am. J. Physiol.*, **263**, H188–H197.

Masotti, G., Poggesi, L., Galanti, G. *et al.* (1979) Differential inhibition of prostacyclin production and platelet aggregation by aspirin. *Lancet*, **ii**, 1213–1217.

Matsuura, S., Naden, R. P., Gant, N. F. Jr *et al.* (1981) Effect of volume expansion on pressor response to angiotensin II in pregnant ewes. *Am. J. Physiol.*, **240**, H908–H913.

Molnar, M. and Hertelendy, F. (1992) N[[omega]]-nitro-l-arginine, an inhibitor of nitric oxide synthesis, increases blood pressure in rats and reverses the pregnancy-induced refractoriness to vasopressor agents. *Am. J. Obstet. Gynecol.*, **166**, 1560–1567.

Naden, R. P. and Rosenfeld, C. R. (1981) Effect of angiotensin II on uterine and systemic vasculature in pregnant sheep. *J. Clin. Invest.*, **68**, 469.

Naden, R. P., Gant, N.F. and Rosenfeld, C. R. (1984) The pressor response to angiotensin II: The roles of peripheral and cardiac responses in pregnant and non-pregnant sheep. *Am. J. Obstet. Gynecol.*, **148**, 450–457.

Raab, W., Schroeder, G., Wagner, R. and Gigee, W. (1956) Vascular reactivity and electrolytes in normal and toxemic pregnancy. *J. Clin. Endocrinol.*, **16**, 1196–1214.

Rosenfeld, C. R. (1984) Consideration of the uteroplacental circulation in intrauterine growth. *Semin. Perinatol.*, **8**, 42–51.

Rosenfeld, C. R. and Gant, N. F. Jr (1981) The chronically instrumented ewe. A model for studying vascular reactivity to angiotensin II in pregnancy. *J. Clin. Invest.*, **67**, 486–492.

Schiff, E., Peleg, E., Goldenberg, M. *et al.* (1989) The use of aspirin to prevent pregnancy-induced hypertension and lower the ratio of thromboxane $A_2$ to prostacyclin in relatively high risk pregnancies. *N. Engl. J. Med.*, **321**, 351–356.

Sibai, B. M., Mirro, R., Chesney, C. M. and Leffler, C. (1989) Low-dose aspirin in pregnancy. *Obstet. Gynecol.*, **74**, 551–557.

Spitz, B., Magness, R. R., Cox, S. M. *et al.* (1988) Low-dose aspirin. I. Effect on angiotensin II pressor responses and blood prostaglandin concentrations in pregnant women sensitive to angiotensin II. *Am. J. Obstet. Gynecol.*, **159**, 1035–1043.

Sutherland, A., Cooper, D. W., Howie, P. W. *et al.* (1981) The incidence of severe pre-eclampsia amongst mothers and mothers-in-law of pre-eclamptics and controls. *Br. J. Obstet. Gynaecol.*, **88**, 785–791.

Talledo, D. E., Chesley, L. C. and Zuspan, F. P. (1968) Renin-angiotensin system in normal and toxemic pregnancies. III. Differential sensitivity to angiotensin II and norepinephrine in toxemia of pregnancy. *Am. J. Obstet. Gynecol.*, **100**, 218–221.

Terragno, N. A., Terragno, D. A., Pacholczyk, D. and McGiff, J. C. (1974) Prostaglandins and the regulation of uterine blood flow in pregnancy. Nature, **249**, 57–58.

Terragno, N. A., McGiff, J. C., Smigel, M. and Terragno, A. (1978) Patterns of prostaglandin production in the bovine fetal and maternal vasculature. *Prostaglandins*, **16**, 847–865.

Ueland, K., Novy, M. J., Peterson, E. N. and Metcalfe, J. (1969) Maternal cardiovascular dynamics. IV. The influence of gestational age on the maternal cardiovascular response to posture and exercise. *Am. J. Obstet. Gynecol.*, **104**, 856–864.

Wallenburg, H. C. S., Dekker, G. A., Makovitz, J. W. and Rotmans, P. (1986) Low-dose aspirin prevents pregnancy-induced hypertension and pre-eclampsia in angiotensin-sensitive primigravidae. *Lancet*, **i**, 1–3.

Walsh, S. W. (1985) Preeclampsia: an imbalance in placental prostacyclin and thromboxane production. *Am. J. Obstet. Gynecol.*, **152**, 335.

Weir, R. J., Brown, J. J., Fraser, R. *et al.* (1973) Plasma renin, renin substrate, angiotensin II and aldosterone in hypertensive disease in pregnancy. *Lancet*, **i**, 291–294.

Werko, L. (1950) Studies in the problems of circulation in pregnancy, in *Toxemias of Pregnancy Human and Veterinary*, (eds J. Hammond, F. J. Brown and G. E. W. Wolstenholm), Blakiston, Philadelphia, PA, p. 155.

Wilson, M., Morganti, A. A., Zervoudakis, I. *et al.* (1980) Blood pressure, the renin–aldosterone system and sex steroids throughout normal pregnancy. *Am. J. Med.*, **68**, 97–104.

Yoshimura, T., Rosenfeld, C. R. and Magness, R. R. (1991) Angiotensin II and $\alpha$-agonist. III. *In vitro* fetal–maternal placental prostaglandins. *Am. J. Physiol.*, **260**, E8–E13.

# A SIMPLIFIED DEFINITION OF PREGNANCY HYPERTENSION FOR CLINICAL PRACTICE

*James J. Walker*

## 3.1 INTRODUCTION

Accurate disease definition is important to allow assessment of the risk that the disease entails and for comparison between investigating centers. It is important to set the limits of the disease groups under scientific study. For the definition to be useful, it must be easy to implement and reproducible in any environment without need for specialist knowledge or equipment. To be accurate, it should be partly related to the etiology of the condition and partly to the clinical presentation.

Over 100 different names have been used to define hypertension in pregnancy (Rippman, 1968). This is because the etiology is still largely unknown and the clinical picture is so variable. If the classification is based on clinical presentation alone it becomes less specific and more like a syndrome than a disease state. Hypertension in pregnancy is largely defined using the main presenting signs of hypertension, edema, proteinuria and convulsions. More recently 'subdefinitions' have been produced based on laboratory findings. HELLP syndrome (Weinstein, 1982, 1985) consisting of **h**emolysis, **e**levated **l**iver enzymes and **l**ow **p**latelets, is one such example. This may describe a higher-risk group but it does little to 'help' the understanding of the problem (Greer, Cameron and Walker, 1985) and such taxonomy has been criticized (Redman, 1989).

There has been some improvement over the centuries. When Hippocrates first described eclampsia, he did not differentiate it from epilepsy. Similarly, Gabelchoverus, in the 16th century, felt that pregnancy was a cause of epilepsy. This is because the clinical presentation of epilepsy and eclampsia can be very similar if other factors such as blood pressure and proteinuria are not taken into account (Chesley, 1980). By the end of the 18th century, there was a realization that the condition was specific to pregnancy and the term 'toxemia' of pregnancy was introduced (Beker, 1948). This further confused the situation, as it implied the presence of a toxin causing the condition. Years of fruitless research followed but no toxin has been found despite the description of the 'worm' (Lueck *et al.*, 1983a, b; Aladjem, Lueck and Brewer *et al.*, 1983; Sibai and Spinnato, 1983; Perkins and Cauchi, 1983). Another problem was that several conditions came under the term 'toxemia', including hypertension and eclampsia, albuminuria alone, acute yellow atrophy and hyperemesis gravidarum (Munro Kerr, 1933). This makes the interpretation of studies reported from that time difficult. When Lever

*Hypertension in Pregnancy*
Edited by J.J. Walker and N.F. Gant. Published by Chapman & Hall, 1997 ISBN 0 412 30910 6

(1843) and Simpson (1843) found proteinuria in the urine in the 19th century, they wrongly assigned the blame for the condition to the kidney. It was not until the histological findings of Baird and Shaw Dunn (1933), Sheehan (1950), Sheehan and Lynch (1973) and McCartney (1964) that the separation of renal disease from the preeclamptic lesion became accepted.

It therefore became obvious that there were two main groups with hypertension in pregnancy (Chesley, Annitto and Cosgrove, 1976):

1. hypertension occurring for the first time during the pregnancy, labor or puerperium and returning to normal after the end of the pregnancy;
2. pregnancy occurring in patients with preexisting essential hypertension, renal disease or other hypertensive disease, diagnosed by previous history prior to pregnancy, high blood pressure at the booking clinic or persistent hypertension after the pregnancy is over.

The problems do not stop here. What is hypertension? What is the relevance of the other two main clinical signs of proteinuria and edema? Where does eclampsia fit into the criteria? If a patient has preexisting disease, is it renal in origin or has the patient essential hypertension? Can such a patient develop 'superimposed' preeclampsia and, if so, is this important? Is there any reason to attempt to diagnose the problem before the pregnancy is over as the clinical condition may worsen, so altering the classification (Redman, 1989)?

## 3.2 WHAT IS HYPERTENSION?

Blood pressure is not an absolute value but a variable physiological measurement. In a large population it forms a normal Gaussian distribution. Pickering (1968) stated that arterial pressure is a quantity and should be treated as such. The diagnosis of hypertension is fairly arbitrary and there should not be a rigid cut-off point taken to diagnose abnormality. Hypertension is not a disease in itself but a reflection of an individual's response to an underlying stimulus. It can therefore be used as a marker of risk. Obviously, in any disease situation, the risk that a given value produces is an important parameter in determining whether that value is abnormal or not. It should be remembered that discovery of an association of high blood pressure and a detrimental outcome does not imply cause, only a relationship.

Studies by Friedman and Neff (1975) and Page and Christianson (1976) suggested that the risk to the baby increased significantly once the diastolic blood pressure was above 95 or 90 mmHg respectively (Table 3.1).

**Table 3.1** Fetal loss rates per 1000 births associated with diastolic blood pressure and gestational age, taken from a study of 35 486 pregnancies by Friedman and Neff (1977). The increase in fetal loss rate seen in association with diastolic blood pressures above 95 mmHg was significant ($p < 0.01$) in all gestations, although the difference was less in gestations above 36 weeks. This is true despite the fact that the numbers in the earlier gestation group are inevitably small.

| Diastolic BP (mmHg) | Weeks gestation | | | | | |
|---|---|---|---|---|---|---|
| | 24–27 | 28–32 | 33–34 | 35–36 | 37–38 | 39–41 |
| 65–74 | 8 | 7 | 6 | 4 | 5 | 5 |
| 75–84 | 10 | 8 | 6 | 6 | 4 | 3 |
| 85–94 | 9 | 9 | 8 | 6 | 5 | 5 |
| > 95 | 26 | 21 | 19 | 16 | 9 | 9 |

Friedman and Neff (1975, 1976, 1978) found that this was true at all gestations. This finding is surprising. In many women, the diastolic blood pressure rises to above 90 mmHg as they approach term when blood pressure reaches prepregnancy levels. These patients are at low risk of fetal loss (MacGillivray, 1961; Friedman and Neff, 1978). These studies confirmed the findings of the British Birth Survey of 1958 (Butler and Bonham, 1963), that a single diastolic blood pressure above 90 mmHg was associated with an increased perinatal mortality rate. However, the more recent British Births Survey 1970 (Chamberlain *et al.*, 1978) did not demonstrate this, as a rise in perinatal mortality rate was not associated with diastolic blood pressure until it was either above 110 mmHg, or above 90 mmHg with significant proteinuria (Table 3.2).

Similar findings were seen if the end point was neonatal neurological complications. The report concluded that raised arterial pressure in pregnancy, whether due to preexisting hypertension or to preeclampsia, increases the risks that the fetus will grow poorly, die *in utero* or be delivered prematurely (Chamberlain *et al.*, 1978). This would appear to be an overstatement from their data, as it would seem that, in the absence of severe disease, the outcome is no worse than in the normal population. Differences in the outcome of pregnancies between these studies may well be due to management variations rather than disease disparity.

The risks to the mother are more difficult to assess. Pregnancy hypertension is one of the largest causes of maternal death in England and Wales in the last 20 years. Cerebral vascular accident (CVA) was the commonest mode of death in this group (DHSS, 1969, 1974, 1979, 1991, 1994; Turnbull, 1987; Turnbull *et al.*, 1989; Scottish Home and Health Department, 1978, 1987, 1989). It was often difficult to discover the maternal blood pressure before this event occurred as many patients presented only after the occurrence of the CVA. It can, however, be assumed that the risk is associated with a rise of blood pressure to abnormally high levels for that given patient. Blood pressures of 170–180/110–120 mmHg or greater are equivalent levels to those that produce vascular damage in experimental animals (Goldby and Beilin, 1972). The association with other complications is not so clear.

In many studies there has not been an absolute correlation between blood pressure rise and eclampsia. Cruickshank, Hewitt and Couper (1927) in a review of patients in the Glasgow Royal Maternity Hospital, showed that 18.5% of the women who had eclampsia had a systolic blood pressure below 140 mmHg. In the Johns Hopkins Hospital between 1924 and 1943, in 2418 cases of preeclampsia only 92 (3.2%) of the patients

**Table 3.2** Data from the British Birth Survey showing that the perinatal mortality is increased only in association with severe proteinuric preeclampsia (Chamberlain *et al.*, 1978). It is important to note that even in these patients the perinatal mortality is only 175% of normal and in 96.6% of the pregnancies the fetus survived.

|  | *No. women* | *No. perinatal deaths* | *Perinatal mortality rate/1000* |
|---|---|---|---|
| Normotensive | 10 787 | 207 | 19.2 |
| Preeclampsia |  |  |  |
|     Mild | 2459 | 48 | 19.5 |
|     Moderate | 610 | 11 | 18.1 |
|     Severe | 830 | 28 | 33.7 |
| Total | 14 686 | 294 | 20.0 |

developed eclampsia (Chesley, 1971). Therefore, the risk of eclampsia would appear to relatively low for the preeclamptic.

In the 1930s, over 75% of all cases of abruptio placentae were associated with preeclampsia (Munro Kerr, 1933). More recent studies suggest that that is no longer true since now more than two thirds of the cases occur in patients with normal blood pressure (Chamberlain, 1981). Although the British Birth Survey 1970 shows a slight increase of abruption in hypertensive patients (1.38%) compared with normotensive patients (1.05%) (Chamberlain *et al.*, 1978), there was no increase in the perinatal mortality rate in these cases unless the abruption accompanied severe hypertension. Again, hypertension should not be classified as a risk factor for abruption.

The absolute level of blood pressure measured may be less important than the absolute rise and the temporal aspect of that rise. Some workers believe that a rise of blood pressure of 30/20 mmHg to whatever level is sufficient for a diagnosis of preeclampsia (Chesley, 1978; Zuspan, 1966). Redman states that the sudden increases of blood pressure that occurs in severe preeclampsia and eclampsia are the most likely cause of the associated neurological signs and cerebral pathology (Redman, 1980).

Therefore, a rise in diastolic blood pressure to levels above 90 mmHg would appear to put a patient into an 'at risk' group, particularly for the fetus, implying the need for increased monitoring and surveillance. A diastolic BP of above 110 mmHg would signify a more severe risk, particularly for the mother, meriting some form of management decision and potential intervention. It would be reasonable to use these measurements as differential markers of disease severity. If the rise in the blood pressure has been acute, the risk is consequently higher. However, it is important to remember that maternal risk does not necessarily represent a fetal risk and the risk is not absolute as most of the patients,

even in these higher risk groups, will have a successful outcome.

## 3.3 BLOOD PRESSURE MEASUREMENT

All these studies presume that the measurement of the blood pressure is accurate. Some workers take one reading only to classify the patients. There is a wide degree of inherent variation in the blood pressure itself (Munro Kerr, 1933; Pickering, 1968; Redman, Beilin and Bonnar, 1977b). There is also a variation found in the methodology and it is probably important to standardize the method of blood pressure assessment to allow comparison between centers (O'Brien; and O'Malley, 1979). In the non-pregnant patient the fifth Korotkoff sound corresponds to the intra-arterial measurement (Kirkendall, 1967). However, in pregnancy, the fifth sound may continue down to zero because of the hyper-dynamic circulation, and the fourth Korotkoff sound is more reproducible (MacGillivray, Rose and Rowe, 1969) This is taken by most centers in Europe to measure the diastolic blood pressure in the pregnant woman. Many of the older studies used the fifth sound and this is still the recommended method in the United States. This often leads to false comparisons, as obviously more patients will have a diastolic blood pressure over 90 mmHg if measurement is by the fourth sound rather than by the fifth sound.

MacGillivray (1961), in his study of blood pressure throughout pregnancy, showed that there was no difference in the diastolic blood pressure with the patient in the lying position or sitting at an angle of 30–45° from the horizontal (MacGillivray, 1961). The blood pressure should be taken in the right arm with the sphygmomanometer at the level of the heart. The patient should be rested prior to the measurement. The practice of lying the patient on their left side to rest and then taking the blood pressure in the right (upper) arm can produce a BP that is falsely low by as much as 15 mmHg because of the hydrostatic pressure differences between the sphygmomanometer cuff and the heart.

Most workers use a single diastolic blood pressure reading above 110 mmHg as being adequate for a diagnosis of severe preeclampsia (Hughes, 1972; Nelson, 1955b; Gant *et al.*, 1980) although a repeated measurement is probably sensible. For the diagnosis of mild or moderate hypertension, two readings above 90 mmHg diastolic at least 6 h apart are accepted. It is important that these readings are close enough together to imply a definite relationship (Nelson, 1955b).

## 3.4 PROTEINURIA

The definition of 'proteinuria' depends on the methods used. Protein excretion goes up in pregnancy from a level of around 18 mg in 24 hours in the non-pregnant to over 300 mg total protein. Albumin represents about 55% of this. The Committee on Terminology of the American College of Obstetricians and Gynecologists recommends that a total daily protein excretion over 300 mg should be taken as abnormal (Hughes, 1972). When 'dip' sticks are used, the false-positive rate is around 25%

with 'a trace' and 6% with 'one +'. This is probably due to the fluctuation in the concentration of protein in the urine and the presence of vaginal contamination or urinary infection. Therefore, if proteinuria is suspected, 24-hour urine collections should be made.

The importance of proteinuria has been known since the 19th century, although it was considered to be due to renal disease. Nelson used the presence of proteinuria as his main differentiate of mild and severe disease (Nelson, 1955b). Friedman and Neff (1977), in a study of over 32 000 pregnancies, showed that proteinuria is associated with increased perinatal mortality even in the absence of hypertension (Table 3.3).

Unfortunately they defined hypertension as blood pressure above 95 mmHg diastolic. It is possible that some of these proteinuric non-hypertensive patients had a diastolic blood pressure of above 90 mmHg and would be defined by many as preeclamptic. In the same patient group, they showed that, in combination with hypertension, proteinuria increases the risk of perinatal loss, neonatal cerebral signs and intrauterine growth retardation (Table 3.4) (Friedman and Neff, 1975).

**Table 3.3** Fetal loss rates per 1000 births associated with proteinuria without hypertension by gestational age, taken from a study of 35 486 pregnancies by Friedman and Neff (1977). The increase in fetal loss rate seen in association with proteinuria alone was seen in all gestations. The figures in bold are significantly different ($p < 0.001$). The relevance of these findings is difficult to assess. Unfortunately, the authors took a diastolic of 95 mmHg as the cut-off point of hypertension. Some of these patients may have had a diastolic blood pressure of between 90 and 95 mmHg and would have been classified as severely hypertensive in many centers in the presence of proteinuria. The numbers associated with proteinuria +++ were so small that the results were not statistically significant.

| | | *Weeks gestation* | | | | | |
| Proteinuria | *n* | *24–27* | *28–32* | *33–34* | *35–36* | *37–38* | *39–41* |
|---|---|---|---|---|---|---|---|
| None | 15 365 | 10 | 10 | 8 | 6 | 5 | 4 |
| Trace | 6631 | 14 | 11 | 11 | 10 | 8 | 10 |
| + | 2712 | 14 | 6 | 10 | 16 | 11 | 6 |
| ++ | 597 | 26 | 40 | 44 | 17 | 25 | 41 |
| +++ | 183 | 71 | 58 | 56 | 24 | 19 | 22 |

Table 3.4   Fetal loss rate per 1000 births by diastolic blood pressure and proteinuria. This data was taken from a study of 58 906 pregnancies by Friedman and Neff (1976). The figures marked † are significantly increased ($p < 0.01$). It can be seen that, although, each parameter appears to exert an independent influence, the diastolic blood pressure is the major factor associated with increased fetal loss.

| Diastolic BP (mmHg) | Proteinuria | | | | | | |
| --- | --- | --- | --- | --- | --- | --- | --- |
| | None | Trace | + | ++ | +++ | ++++ | Total |
| <65 | 15.5 | 13.64 | 6.20 | — | — | — | 13.60 |
| 65–74 | 9.30 | 8.06 | 5.58 | 32.86 | 41.54 | — | 8.84 |
| 75–84 | 6.20 | 7.44 | 6.20 | 19.22 | — | — | 6.80 |
| 85–94 | 8.68 | 9.30 | 23.56† | — | 22.32 | — | 10.20 |
| 95–104 | 19.22† | 17.36† | 26.66† | 55.80† | 115.32† | 143.22† | 25.16 |
| 105+ | 20.46† | 27.90† | 62.62† | 68.82† | 125.24† | 110.98† | 41.48 |
| Total | 8.60 | 9.46 | 12.94 | 23.22 | 41.96 | 56.76 | |

It is difficult to explain why proteinuria is associated with this increased risk to the fetus. It is almost always associated with the 'pathognomonic' preeclamptic glomerular lesions (Sheehan and Lynch, 1973). Rather than being associated with a worsening disease risk, it may be that the presence of proteinuria increases the probability of the patient having 'true' preeclampsia. The risk to the fetus is therefore higher because the pregnancy is complicated by preeclampsia rather than 'simple' hypertension.

Although proteinuria is associated with increased risk to the baby, there is less evidence that it is associated with an increased risk to the mother. Gibberd is quoted as presenting a series 300 patients with albuminuria out of 8000 pregnancies (Gibberd, 1928). Only 3.7% of these patients developed eclampsia. These results are similar to those found with raised blood pressure alone. However, the few maternal deaths seen in the United Kingdom are almost always associated with proteinuric hypertension. This again may be due to the presence of proteinuria confirming the diagnosis of preeclampsia.

These studies suggest that the presence of proteinuria implies the presence of the specific renal lesion confirming the diagnosis of preeclampsia. It is associated with an increased risk to the fetus of both IUGR and death. The effect on the risk to the mother is less clear, but it is an obvious sign that increased vigilance is required.

## 3.5 EDEMA

Edema is a common finding in normal pregnancy. Some 64% of normal women have edema of the face and hands (Dexter and Weiss, 1941) and this is associated with no adverse affects (Chamberlain *et al.*, 1978; Dexter and Weiss, 1941) Although Hamlin (1952) reported edema in the fingers of almost every primigravida who developed preeclampsia 6 weeks later, the additional presence of edema does not increase the risk of hypertension (MacGillivray and Campbell, 1980).

## 3.6 ROLE OF PARITY

'Pure' preeclampsia is defined by Nelson as a diastolic blood pressure over 90 mmHg with proteinuria of over 300 mg in 24 hours occurring in a primigravid patient where there is no evidence of preexisting hypertensive disease (Nelson, 1955b) This definition is widely accepted and was validated by the biopsy studies of McCartney (1964). This study showed that the majority of primigravid patients with proteinuric preeclampsia had the pathognomonic renal lesion. However, the results also showed that, although most of the multigravid patients with proteinuric disease had underlying renal disease, some patients did have the classic renal lesions. Therefore, the diagnosis of pure preeclampsia is more likely in primigravidae but it cannot be excluded in a later pregnancy (McCartney, 1964). If it does occur it tends to be less severe but the women can still suffer from serious complications such as convulsions and HELLP syndrome. Therefore, multigravid women are unlikely to develop the disease for the first time but the diagnosis of preeclampsia is still possible. If a patient has preeclampsia in her first pregnancy, she is more likely to have problems in her next pregnancy. However, if apparent 'mild preeclampsia' is found in a multigravid patient, the patient may be demonstrating a tendency towards 'latent' hypertension which recurs in subsequent pregnancies and she will have an increased chance of developing hypertension in later life. Such women often have a strong family history of essential hypertension (Chesley, 1978, 1980; Nelson, 1955b; Gibberd, 1928). Nelson, in a study of 5251 booked married primigravidae between 1948 and 1953, showed that this 'latent hypertension' increased in incidence with increasing age (Nelson, 1955b). This was not true of 'pure' preeclampsia. Proteinuric hypertension occurring for the first time in pregnancy in a primigravid patient is almost certainly preeclampsia. To be surer of this diagnosis, post-pregnancy follow-up is also required to make sure that normality returns.

## 3.7 ECLAMPSIA

Eclampsia can be defined as a convulsive state occurring for the first time during pregnancy, associated with hypertension prior to or after the fit has taken place. Although eclampsia is often associated with severe preeclampsia, as the name suggests (Hamlin, 1952; Dawson, 1953), this is not always so. Convulsions may occur in the presence of mild preeclampsia and most severe cases of preeclampsia are not complicated by eclampsia (Cruickshank, 1923; Nelson, 1955a). The seizure threshold of the patient probably has as much to do with the occurrence of the seizure as the hypertension (Nelson, 1955a; MacIntosh, 1952). In Nelson's studies (1955a, b), all the baby deaths associated with eclampsia occurred in patients with severe preexisting preeclampsia, and none in the patients where the preexisting preeclampsia was mild. In fact, he states that a case of eclampsia occurring with mild preeclampsia was probably less dangerous to mother and baby than a case of severe preeclampsia with no convulsions. The grading of the patient should be related to preexisting preeclampsia rather than an automatic inclusion of all patients in the severe group or a separate group (Nelson, 1955a).

## 3.8 PREEXISTING HYPERTENSIVE DISEASE

Once it was accepted that young women could have essential hypertension, it was realized that renal disease was not as common as was once thought. If the blood pressure was known to be elevated prior to pregnancy, the diagnosis of a form of preexisting hypertension is obvious. However, as most patients presenting in their first pregnancy will probably never have had their blood pressure checked before, this may not be known. If the blood pressure is found to be elevated in the first half of pregnancy, a diagnosis of preexisting hypertension can be assumed. But since the diastolic blood pressure may fall by as much as 15 mmHg in the second trimester (MacGillivray, 1961), a diastolic of 85 mmHg at 16 weeks may hide a non-pregnant equivalent of 100 mmHg. This patient might have been diagnosed correctly if she had presented earlier in the pregnancy. Therefore, only a normal first trimester blood pressure can be used to exclude essential hypertension accurately. With the rise of blood pressure towards term, a false diagnosis of preeclampsia may be made if the diastolic rises over 90 mmHg on its way back to prepregnancy levels (MacGillivray, 1961). Many of the 'latent' hypertensive group probably fall into this category. If the blood pressures remain in the mild-to-moderate range, this will have little clinical relevance but would interfere with any 'pure' group studies.

Most patients with renal disease are known prior to pregnancy but the differentiation between renal disease and essential hypertension has been made easier with the development of methods of assessment of renal function. The presence of proteinuria in early pregnancy should alert the obstetrician to possible renal problems, which can be confirmed by plasma creatinine estimation, urinalysis for infection and casts, and ultrasound of the kidneys looking for evidence of renal scarring.

### 3.9 'SUPERIMPOSED' PREECLAMPSIA

This is described as an exacerbation of hypertension or the development of proteinuria in previously observed hypertension or a rise in uric acid to high levels in a patient with known essential hypertension (Redman, Beilin and Bonnar, 1977a). These criteria are useful in cases of essential hypertension but it is more difficult to differentiate 'superimposed' preeclampsia from a deterioration in renal disease. Whatever the reason for the worsening of the underlying cause of the hypertension, the risk to both the mother and the fetus is significantly increased (Chamberlain *et al.*, 1978).

### 3.10 NOMENCLATURE

Over the years many names have been used to describe hypertension in pregnancy (Rippman, 1968). Although much effort has been made to simplify the problem, the situation is still confused. In order to be able to discuss and compare cases with hypertension in pregnancy, it is important that terms are used that all can accept and understand.

The Organization Gestosis was set up to attempt to clarify the diagnosis. Since they decided to use a symptomatic method of nomenclature based on edema as the cardinal sign (Table 3.5), their recommendations have not been universally accepted.

The full name of their condition is EPH-gestosis, using the signs edema, proteinuria and hypertension as the method of diagnosis. Each sign is classified numerically according to the severity and the diagnosis is made. e.g. E1P2H2-gestosis for a patient with mild edema, moderate proteinuria and moderate hypertension. The method is simplistic and relatively reproducible and transferable. Its

**Table 3.5** The definitions used by Organization Gestosis. The patient is then classified by score such as E1P2H2 for someone with pretibial edema, between 2 and 5 g/dl of proteinuria and a blood pressure of 160–180/100–110 mmHg

|  | 0 | 1 | 2 | 3 |
|---|---|---|---|---|
| Edema | none | pretibial | generalized | |
| Proteinuria | | | | |
|   g/dl | < 0.5 | 0.5–2 | 2–5 | > 5 |
|   Stix' | nil | + | + + | + + + |
| Systolic BP | < 140 | 140–160 | 160–180 | > 180 |
| Diastolic BP | < 90 | 90–100 | 100–110 | > 110 |

main drawback is the importance placed on the edema. The presence of edema and proteinuria constitutes 'gestosis' even in the absence of hypertension. There is also a further category of 'imminent' eclampsia.

The other main international group studying hypertension in pregnancy (the International Society for the Study of Hypertension in Pregnancy, or ISSHP) concentrates on hypertension as the main diagnostic factor, along with proteinuria, but ignores the presence of edema (Table 3.6) (Davey and MacGillivray, 1988).

This is similar to Nelson's criteria (Nelson, 1955b). This is now the most widely accepted nomenclature. It is clear that 'true preeclampsia' should only be used for the primigravid patient with no preexisting disease who

---

**Table 3.6**   The definitions as used by the ISSHP (Davey and MacGillivray, 1988)

**A. Gestational hypertension and/or proteinuria**
Hypertension and/or proteinuria developing during pregnancy, labor or the puerperium in a previously normotensive non-proteinuric women and subdivided into:
*(1) Gestational hypertension (without proteinuria)*
   developing during pregnancy (antenatal), developing for the first time in labor or developing for the first time in the puerperium
*(2) Gestational proteinuria (without hypertension)*
   developing during pregnancy (antenatal), developing for the first time in labor or developing for the first time in the puerperium
*(3) Gestational proteinuric hypertension (preeclampsia)*
   developing during pregnancy (antenatal), developing for the first time in labor or developing for the first time in the puerperium

**B. Chronic hypertension and chronic renal disease**
Hypertension and/or proteinuria in pregnancy in a woman with chronic hypertension or chronic renal disease diagnosed either before, during or persisting after pregnancy and subdivided into
*(1) Chronic hypertension (without proteinuria)*
*(2) Chronic renal disease (proteinuria and hypertension)*
*(3) Chronic hypertension with superimposed preeclampsia (proteinuria developing for the first time during pregnancy in a woman with known chronic hypertension)*

**C. Unclassified hypertension and/or proteinuria**
Hypertension and/or proteinuria found:
(a) at first 'booking' examination after the 20th week of pregnancy (140 days) in a woman without known chronic hypertension or chronic renal disease, or
(b) during pregnancy, labor or the puerperium with insufficient information
   is provisionally regarded as unclassified and subdivided into unclassified hypertension, unclassified proteinuria or unclassified proteinuric hypertension

**D. Eclampsia**
is regarded as one of the complications of the hypertensive disorders of pregnancy and should be included in a separate classification of complications.

**Hypertension is defined as either:**
- One measurement of DBP of 110 mmHg or above
- Two consecutive measurements of DBP of 90 mmHg or above

**Proteinuria is defined as:**
- Total protein excretion of 300 mg or more in 24 h

develops proteinuric hypertension in the second half of pregnancy. This implies that hypertension occurring in pregnancy without proteinuria is not preeclampsia but some other kind of 'pregnancy-induced hypertension'. This is not true but, although preeclampsia can exist in the multigravid patient, its diagnosis is less sure and the term pregnancy-induced hypertension (PIH) is generally used. The main criticism of this term is the implication of etiology, which is unproven. Pregnancy-associated hypertension (PAH) is a similar term without the etiological suggestion. 'Gestational hypertension' is the same as 'latent' hypertension and implies late-onset mild to moderate PIH in a multigravid patient. The assumption is that the patient is demonstrating a hypertensive tendency which will become apparent in later life (Nelson, 1955b; Chesley, Annitto and Cosgrove, 1976; Dieckmann, 1952).

Despite the simplification of the classification it is often difficult to define the condition at first presentation. All forms of definition include an unclassified group of patients who present too late or are 'unbooked' at the time of admission, making accurate diagnosis impossible. Also, many patients classified under one group may need to be reclassified as pregnancy continues, since the condition may worsen or preexisting disease may become apparent after delivery.

## 3.11 CONCLUSIONS

It is clear that there are major problems in the clinical diagnosis of hypertension in pregnancy. Proteinuric hypertension occurring for the first time in a primigravid pregnancy can be accurately diagnosed as preeclampsia but all other forms of hypertension could be preeclampsia or due to other etiologies. Therefore, if a 'pure group' is to be studied for the etiology of preeclampsia, a primigravid proteinuric group should be chosen. Although preeclampsia can occur in the multigravid patient, the diagnosis is less accu-

rate. Mild or moderate preeclampsia will often be confused with latent or essential hypertension in any pregnancy. However, in clinical practice, none of this really matters. What is important is the risk in any given pregnancy.

It would appear that, although problems of hypertension in pregnancy are indeed polysymptomatic, high blood pressure is the primary sign of danger to the mother. The presence of proteinuria significantly increases the risks for the fetus and edema appears to have little significance at all. It would seem reasonable to classify the problem for the mother on the basis of hypertension and the fetal risk on the presence of proteinuria or some more specific method of fetal monitoring.

## REFERENCES

Aladjem, S., Lueck, J. and Brewer, J. I. (1983) Experimental induction of a toxemia-like syndrome in the pregnant beagle. *Am. J. Obstet. Gynecol.*, **145**, 27–38.

Baird, D. and Shaw Dunn, J. (1933) Renal lesions in eclampsia and nephritis of pregnancy. *J. Path. Bact.*, **37**, 291–295.

Beker, J. C. (1948) Aetology of eclampsia. *J. Obstet. Gynaecol. Br. Emp.*, **55**, 756–760.

Butler, N. R. and Bonham, D. G. (1963) *First Report of the British Perinatal Mortality Survey 1958*, E. & S. Livingstone, Edinburgh.

Chamberlain, G. V. P. (1981) Raised blood pressure in pregnancy. The fetus in hypertension. *Br. J. Hosp. Med.*, **26**, 127–131.

Chamberlain, G. V. P., Phillip, E., Howlett, B. and Masters, K. (1978) *British Births 1970, 2: Obstetric Care*, Heinemann, London, p. 80–84.

Chesley, L. C. (1971) Johns Hopkins Hospital figures, quoted in Hypertensive disorders of pregnancy, in *Williams Obstetrics*, 14th edn, (eds L. M. Hellman and J. A. Pritchard), Appleton-Century-Crofts, New York, p. 747–747.

Chesley, L. C. (ed.) (1978) *Hypertensive Disorders in Pregnancy*, Appleton-Century-Crofts, New York.

Chesley, L. C. (1980) Evolution of concepts of eclampsia, in *Pregnancy Hypertension*, (eds J. Bonnar, I. MacGillivray and E. M. Symonds), MTP Press, Lancaster, p. 1–4.

Chesley, L. C., Annitto, J. E. and Cosgrove, R. A. (1976) The remote prognosis of eclamptic women. Sixth periodic report. *Am. J. Obstet. Gynecol.*, **124**, 446–450.

Cruickshank, J. M. (1923) Studies of the toxaemias of pregnancy as they occur in Glasgow. *J. Obstet. Gynaecol. Br. Emp.*, **30**, 541–545.

Cruickshank, J. M., Hewitt, R. and Couper, J. (1927) *The Toxaemias of Pregnancy: A Clinical and Biochemical Study*, Medical Research Council Special Report Series 117, Medical Research Council, London, p. 47–51.

Davey, D. A. and MacGillivray, I. (1988) The classification and definition of the hypertensive disorders of pregnancy. *Am. J. Obstet. Gynecol.*, **158**, 892–898.

Dawson, B. (1953) The prevention of eclampsia, an Australian experiment. *J. Obstet. Gynaecol. Br. Emp.*, **60**, 80–84.

Dexter, L. and Weiss, S. (1941) *Preeclamptic and Eclamptic Toxaemia of Pregnancy*, Little, Brown & Co., Boston, MA.

DHSS (1969) *Report on Confidential Enquiries into Maternal Deaths in England and Wales 1964–66*, HMSO, London.

DHSS (1974) *Report on Confidential Enquiries into Maternal Deaths in England and Wales 1970–72*, HMSO, London.

DHSS (1979) *Report on Confidential Enquiries into Maternal Deaths in England and Wales 1973–75*, HMSO, London.

DHSS, Welsh Office, Scottish Home and Health Department (1991) *Report on Confidential Enquiries into Maternal Deaths in the United Kingdom 1985–87*, HMSO, London.

DHSS, Welsh Office, Scottish Home and Health Department (1994) *Report on Confidential Enquiries into Maternal Deaths in the United Kingdom 1988–90*, HMSO, London.

Dieckmann, W. J. (1952) *The Toxemias of Pregnancy*, 2nd edn, C. V. Mosby, St Louis, MO, p. 305–311.

Friedman, E. A. and Neff, R. K. (1975) Pregnancy outcome as related to hypertension, edema and proteinuria, in *Hypertension in Pregnancy*, (eds M. D. Lindheimer, A. I. Katz and F. P. Zuspan), John Wiley, New York, p. 13–17.

Friedman, E. A. and Neff, R. K. (1976) Pregnancy outcome as related to hypertension, edema, and proteinuria. *Perspect. Nephrol. Hypertens.*, **5**, 13–22.

Friedman, E. A. and Neff, R. K. (1977) Pregnancy outcome as related to hypertension, edema and proteinuria, in *Hypertension in Pregnancy*, (eds M. D. Lindheimer, A. I. Katz and F. P. Zuspan), John Wiley, New York.

Friedman, E. A. and Neff, R. K. (1978) Hypertension–hypotension in pregnancy. Correlation with fetal outcome. *J. A. M. A.*, **239**, 2249–2251.

Gant, N. F., Worley, R. J., Everett, R. B. and MacDonald, P. C. (1980) Control of vascular responsiveness during human pregnancy. *Kidney Int.*, **18**, 253–257.

Gibberd, G. F. (1928) Consideration of results of albuminuria occuring during pregnancy with special reference to the relationship between pregnant kidney and chronic nephritis. *Proc. Roy. Soc. Med.*, **21**, 39–43.

Goldby, F. S. and Beilin, L. J. (1972) Relationship between arterial pressure and the permiability of arterioles to carbon particles in acute hypertension. *Cardiovasc. Res.*, **6**, 384–388.

Greer, I. A., Cameron, A. D. and Walker, J. J. (1985) HELLP syndrome: pathological entity or technical inadequacy? *Am. J. Obstet. Gynecol.*, **152**, 113–117.

Hamlin, R. H. J. (1952) The prevention of eclampsia and pre-eclampsia. *Lancet*, **i**, 64–68.

Hughes, E. C. (1972) *Obstetrics–Gynecological Terminology*, F. A. Davis, Philadelphia, PA, p. 422–423.

Kirkendall, W. M. (1967) Recommendations for human blood pressure determination by sphygmomanometers. *Circulation*, **36**, 980–983.

Lever, J. C. W. (1843) Cases of puerperal convulsions with remarks, in *Guy's Hospital Reports, vol. 1*, 2nd edn, (ed. G. H. Barlow), Samuel Highley, London, p. 495–506.

Lueck, J., Brewer, J. I., Aladjem, S. and Novotny, M. (1983a) Hydatoxi lualba: organism or artifact? *Am. J. Obstet. Gynecol.*, **146**, 742–744.

Lueck, J., Brewer, J. I., Aladjem, S. and Novotny, M. (1983b) Observation of an organism found in patients with gestational trophoblastic disease and in patients with toxemia of pregnancy. *Am. J. Obstet. Gynecol.*, **145**, 15–26.

McCartney, C. P. (1964) Pathological anatomy of acute hypertension of pregnancy. *Circulation*, **30**, 37–41.

MacGillivray, I. (1961) Hypertension in pregnancy and its consequences. *J. Obstet. Gynaecol. Br. Emp.*, **68**, 557–561.

MacGillivray, I. and Campbell, D. M. (1980) The effect of hypertension and oedema on birth weight, in *Pregnancy Hypertension*, (eds J. Bonnar, I. MacGillivray and E. M. Symonds), University Park Press, Baltimore, MD, p. 307–311.

MacGillivray, I., Rose, G. and Rowe, B. (1969) Blood pressure survey in pregnancy. *Clin. Sci.*, **37**, 395–399.

MacIntosh, R. R. (1952) The significance of fits in eclampsia. *J. Obstet. Gynaecol. Br. Emp.*, **59**, 197–201.

Munro Kerr, J. M. (1933) *Maternal Morbidity and Mortality: A Study of Their Problems*, E. & S. Livingstone, Edinburgh.

Nelson, T. R. (1955a) A clinical study of pre-eclampsia, part 2. *J. Obstet. Gynaecol. Br. Emp.*, **62**, 58–62.

Nelson, T. R. (1955b) A clinical study of pre-eclampsia. Part 1. *J. Obstet. Gynaecol. Br. Emp.*, **62**, 48–52.

O'Brien, E. and O'Malley, K. (1979) ABC of blood pressure measurement. *Br. Med. J.*, **ii**, 982–986.

Page, E. W. and Christianson, R. (1976) Influence of blood pressure changes with and without proteinuria upon outcome of pregnancy. *Am. J. Obstet. Gynecol.*, **126**, 821–825.

Perkins, D. and Cauchi, M. N. (1983) Hydatoxi lualba – an artifact. *Am. J. Obstet. Gynecol.*, **147**, 469.

Pickering, G. (1968) *High Blood Pressure*, 2nd edn, Grune & Stratton, New York.

Redman, C. W. (1980) Treatment of hypertension in pregnancy. *Kidney Int.*, **18**, 267–271.

Redman, C. W. (1989) Classification of hypertensive disorders of pregnancy. *Lancet*, **i**, 935–936.

Redman, C. W., Beilin, L. J. and Bonnar, J. (1977a) Treatment of hypertension in pregnancy with methyldopa: blood pressure and control and side effects. *Br. J. Obstet. Gynaecol.*, **84**, 419–423.

Redman, C. W., Beilin, L. J. and Bonnar, J. (1977b) Variability of blood pressure in normal and abnormal pregnancy, in *Hypertension in Pregnancy*, (eds M. D. Lindheimer, A. I. Katz and F. P. Zuspan), John Wiley, New York, p. 53–57.

Rippman, E. T. (1968) Gestosis of late pregnancy. *Gynaecologia*, **165**, 12–16.

Scottish Home and Health Department (1978) *A Report on an Enquiry into Maternal Deaths in Scotland, 1972–1975*, HMSO, Edinburgh.

Scottish Home and Health Department (1987) *A Report on an Enquiry into Maternal Deaths in Scotland, 1976–1980*, HMSO, Edinburgh.

Scottish Home and Health Department (1989) *A Report on an Enquiry into Maternal Deaths in Scotland, 1981–1986*, HMSO, Edinburgh.

Sheehan, H. L. (1950) Pathological lesions in the hypertensive toxaemias of pregnancy, in *Toxaemias of Pregnancy*, (eds J. Hammond, F. J. Browne and G. E. W. Wolstenholme), J & A Churchill, London.

Sheehan, H. L. and Lynch, J. B. (1973) *Pathology of Toxaemia of Pregnancy*, Churchill Livingstone, Edinburgh.

Sibai, B. M. and Spinnato, J. A. (1983) Hydatoxi lualba: artifact produced by sulfation. *Am. J. Obstet. Gynecol.*, **147**, 854.

Simpson, J. Y. (1843) Contributions to the pathology and treatment of diseases of the uterus. *Edin. Monthly J. Med. Sci.*, **3**, 1009–1013.

Turnbull, A. C. (1987) Maternal mortality and present trends, in *Hypertension in Pregnancy. Proceedings of the Sixteenth Study Group of the Royal College of Obstetricians and Gynaecologists*, (eds F. Sharp and E. M. Symonds), Perinatology Press, Ithaca, NY, p. 135–144.

Turnbull, A., Tindall, V. R., Beard, R. W. *et al.* (1989) *Report on Confidential Enquiries Into Maternal Deaths in England and Wales 1982–1984*, DHSS, London, vol. 34, p. 1–166.

Weinstein, L. (1982) Syndrome of Hemolysis, elevated liver enzymes and low platelet count; A severe consequence of hypertension in pregnancy. *Am. J. Obstet. Gynecol.*, **142**, 159–163.

Weinstein, L. (1985) Pre-eclampsia/eclampsia with hemolysis, elevated liver enzymes, and thrombocytopenia. *Obstet. Gynecol.*, **66**, 657–661.

Zuspan, F. P. (1966) Treatment of severe preeclampsia and eclampsia. *Clin. Obstet. Gynecol.*, **9**, 954–958.

# THE ETIOLOGY AND PATHOPHYSIOLOGY OF HYPERTENSION IN PREGNANCY

*James J. Walker and Gustaaf A. Dekker*

## 4.1 INTRODUCTION

In order to understand the disease process and the relevance of the clinical signs at presentation, it is important to understand the etiology and pathophysiology of the condition. If the etiology were elucidated, early diagnosis and potential prevention might be possible. Unfortunately, the etiology of hypertension in pregnancy is still largely unknown. There has been much confusion over the role of the many pathological findings in this condition. It is important to distinguish the signs caused by disease progression from those that are markers of the underlying process. If this can be done, and if there are recognizable stages in the disease process, it may be possible to use these changes as predictors of patient risk.

Since the 18th century, when the term 'toxemia of pregnancy' was first used, it has been known that there was a specific disease of pregnancy that could be characterized by edema, hypertension, albuminuria and convulsions (Chesley, 1980a). Since then, much has been written about the etiology of preeclampsia. The main problem is that many of the theories that have been put forward for the cause of eclampsia describe the pathological features found in end-stage disease (Chesley, 1976). These may be the result of the disease process rather than the cause. Hypertension in pregnancy may not lead to eclampsia. Therefore signs found after maternal death from eclampsia may have little relevance to the earlier stages of the preeclampsia.

In 1916, Zweifel first termed it 'the disease of theories' (Zweifel, 1916). Zweifel states that any cause of preeclampsia must explain the following points:

1. the predisposing influence of nulliparity, multiple pregnancy, hydatidiform mole and hydramnios;
2. higher incidence in certain geographical areas;
3. increasing incidence as term approaches;
4. rarity of repeated problems in subsequent pregnancies;
5. improvement after death of the fetus;
6. hypertension, edema, proteinuria, convulsions and coma;
7. the hepatic and renal lesions.

These factors will be considered in turn.

*Hypertension in Pregnancy*
Edited by J.J. Walker and N.F. Gant. Published by Chapman & Hall, 1997 ISBN 0 412 30910 6

## 4.2 THE PREDISPOSING INFLUENCE OF NULLIPARITY, MULTIPLE PREGNANCY, HYDATIDIFORM MOLE AND HYDRAMNIOS

### 4.2.1 NULLIPARITY

Until the histological studies in the 1950s and 1960s (Sheehan, 1950; McCartney, 1964; Sheehan and Lynch, 1973) there was no clear method of accurate diagnosis. It was already known that hypertension was more common in the primigravida (Nelson, 1955b; Munro Kerr, 1933; MacGillivray, 1961) but the renal histological studies showed that the majority of primigravidae with proteinuria had a specific renal lesion while many of the multigravidae were found to have renal disease (Sheehan, 1950; McCartney, 1964; Sheehan and Lynch, 1973). This suggested that preeclampsia is mostly a disease of the primigravida and a normal first pregnancy can be seen to protect the patient from any future preeclampsia (Chesley, 1978). Even an earlier abortion may protect the patient (MacGillivray, 1958). However, if the patient changes partner, the incidence increases to that of a primigravida. If she has had a prior blood transfusion, she is also at reduced risk of developing preeclampsia (Feeney *et al.*, 1977). There is no evidence that blood group incompatibilities make any difference although some recent studies suggest that a male baby predisposes some women to preeclampsia (Arngrimsson *et al.*, 1993).

All these findings suggest that the condition is associated with the patient's first exposure to certain antigens carried by the fetus. Prior exposure to these antibodies would appear to protect the patient from disease development. This implies an immunological factor in the etiology of the condition.

### 4.2.2 HYPERPLACENTOSIS

Another factor influencing the development of preeclampsia is hyperplacentosis (Jeffcoatte and Scott, 1959). This may occur with hydatidiform mole, diabetes, multiple pregnancies, erythroblastosis fetalis and triploidy. Polyhydramnios has also been suggested as a risk factor but the association of polyhydramnios in the absence of other accepted risk factors is probably unlikely (Jeffcoatte and Scott, 1959). Polyhydramnios due to fetal abnormality alone is not associated with a higher incidence and is only associated with preeclampsia if there is another influencing factor involved (Desmedt, Henry and Beischer, 1990). Diabetic pregnancies have a higher incidence of the disease, especially if there is poor control (Siddiqi *et al.*, 1991). Hydatidiform mole is associated with classic preeclampsia and eclampsia, but this rarely develops before 16 weeks (Page, 1939; Chesley, Cosgrove and Preece, 1946). Twins are reported to carry a fourfold increase in incidence compared to singleton pregnancies. However, there is no difference in the incidence between monozygotic and dizygotic twins (Campbell, MacGillivray and Thompson, 1977). Therefore, it would appear that it is the presence of the placental tissue rather than polyhydramnios that is associated with preeclampsia. This again suggests an immunological basis to the disease, as both molar and multiple pregnancy will produce a higher immunological load than a normal pregnancy.

### 4.2.3 IMMUNOLOGICAL FACTORS (TABLE 4.1)

Both these findings suggest that immunological factors may be involved, with some form of maternal and fetal incompatibility producing an abnormal immunological response. This may be due to an imperfect maternal response to pregnancy which improves in the next pregnancy or an inability to recognize paternal antigens displayed by the fetus. The first pregnancy would then help to 'immunize' the patient against any future pregnancy to the same partner (Sutherland *et al.*, 1981). If this is true, there may be differences found in immunological investigations. No increase in ABO-, HLA- or Y-linked compatibility was

> **Table 4.1** Evidence for and against an immunological basis to preeclampsia
>
> **For**
> - More common in primigravidae
> - More common in twin pregnancies
> - A higher incidence of HLA homozygosity
> - There are abnormalities of lymphocyte function
> - There is activation of circulating neutrophils
> - VCAM-1 is elevated in the serum
> - There is an abnormality of adhesion molecule expression
>
> **Against**
> - No increase in ABO-, HLA- or Y-linked compatibility
> - The incidence is similar in monozygotic and dizygotic twin pregnancies
> - Similar placental findings are found in intrauterine growth retardation

found in couples with a preeclamptic pregnancy by Scott and Beer (1976). Redman *et al.* (1978) showed that there was a higher incidence of HLA homozygosity in couples where the women suffered from preeclampsia. This would increase the chances of antigen-sharing by preeclamptic women and their husbands. This may lead to the mother failing to mount the normal immunological response to the implanting placenta and developing fetus. Abnormality of the action of the maternal recessive immune-response genes may contribute to the development of preeclampsia (Redman, Bonnar and Beilin, 1978).

Chen *et al.* (1994a, b) found abnormalities of lymphocyte function in women with pregnancy-induced hypertension. Other studies have demonstrated activation of neutrophils within the maternal circulation in preeclampsia (Greer *et al.*, 1991a, b). Immunocytochemical studies have localized neutrophil elastase in term placenta decidua and myometrium in women with pregnancy-induced hypertension (Butterworth *et al.*, 1991). The cell-adhesion molecule VCAM-1 is elevated in serum in preeclamptic women, Neutrophil activity is partly mediated through this adhesion molecule, which encourages adhesion to the vascular endothelium (Lyall *et al.*, 1994). This could be part of the mechanism of endothelial cell

dysfunction discussed later. These changes may be by direct cellular effects or through release of cytokines, which affect cellular function. Cytokines have been shown to affect the production of prostacyclin and thromboxane in human mononuclear cells (Chen *et al.*, 1993a, 1994c)

Therefore, there is evidence of an immunological abnormality in preeclampsia interfering with the normal maternal response to her fetus, but the exact mechanism is still obscure (Petrucco, 1981). The abnormality may be either an increased response to fetal antigens or a reduction in the suppressive effect normally seen in pregnancy. The greatly increased incidence of preeclampsia in twin pregnancies without any difference between monozygotic and dizygotic pregnancies (Campbell, MacGillivray and Thompson, 1977) suggest increased immune-response suppression rather than increased maternal–fetal incompatibility.

Implantation of the developing embryo is influenced by immunologically active cells in the decidua. During the luteal phase of the menstrual cycle, large granular lymphocytes migrate into the endometrium. These disappear after 20 weeks and would appear to play a critical role in the implantation process. Although it was thought that the trophoblast was immunologically neutral, it is now known that the trophoblast expresses MHC class I antigens at specific times related to the stages of implantation. These cells are in close contact with maternal immunologically active cells and trophoblastic cells can be found deep within the stroma of the decidua and the maternal vessels as far as the myometrium. It has been postulated that blocking antibodies are formed by the mother under the influence of these trophoblastic cells. These antibodies then suppress T-lymphocyte activation (Currie and Bagshawe, 1967). Although most of this action takes place in the uterine cavity, Schmorl and Veit showed the presence of placental villi in the circulation as early as 1933. Therefore, antibody production would be expected. Insufficient production of blocking antibody could lead an increased maternal immunological activity, placental damage and preeclampsia. However, although circulating antibodies to the placenta have been found in preeclamptic patients, this has not been confirmed by all workers (Currie and Bagshawe, 1967). Various studies have shown complement activation in the placenta (Faulk, Carbonara and Jeannot, 1973; Kitzmiller and Benirschke, 1973) but no definitive findings of immunological damage have been described.

There may also be a role for some of the placental proteins, such as PAPP-A or hCG, in immunosuppression, as they are known to have an immunodepressant effect (Bischof, 1981). These hormones are produced in high amounts by the implanting trophoblast and it is likely that they have local effects around the areas of implantation. The fact that embryos can successfully implant outwith the uterine cavity also suggests that the implanting embryo must influence its close environment.

Therefore, although there is strong circumstantial evidence of an immunological basis to preeclampsia, its exact mechanism and site of action is still unclear. The immunological role of the decidual tissue is to allow the trophoblast to invade but also to control the depth of invasion. Any immunological abnormality is probably associated with alterations

of the implantation process. Zhou *et al.* (1993) have demonstrated that there is abnormality in the expression of the adhesion molecules in the extravillus trophoblast in preeclamptic pregnancies. There is a failure in the expression of those associated with successful invasion into the myometrium. This could explain the failure of the secondary invasion that is associated with the classic placental lesion of preeclampsia.

A further complication to this work is that the placental lesion is not specific to preeclampsia. Similar findings are found in intrauterine growth retardation (IUGR) (Sheppard and Bonnar, 1981). This may imply that both the placental lesion and the immunological lesion may not be unique to preeclampsia and other specific etiological factors are required before preeclampsia occurs. It is now thought that in preeclampsia the placenta produces a substance or substances that causes the systemic disease. This factor, termed factor X, is the link between the placental pathology and the systemic manifestations of preeclampsia (Table 4.2).

## 4.3 HIGHER INCIDENCE IN CERTAIN GEOGRAPHICAL AREAS

Differences have been seen between racial groups. In Israel, Jews have a higher incidence than Africans or Asians. However, different geographical incidence of the condition and its severity may be due to environmental differences, particularly diet, genetics and other factors including the standard of health care and the timing of presentation (Davies, 1971). There are also problems with the accuracy of case recording and diagnosis of hypertension in the Third World. Many studies are based on hospital reports which suggest a higher incidence in the urban areas. This could be explained by the differences in the reporting of the condition, in the standard of antenatal care available and the access patients have to medical help. There is no doubt, however, that the disease is a major

Increasing incidence as term approaches 43

---

**Table 4.2** Possible sequence of events that leads to preeclampsia

**Implantation**
- Immunological abnormality at implantation
- Deficient Implantation
- Placental ischemia

**Systemic spread**
- Production of factor X'
- Systemic neutrophil/cytokine activity
- Increased lipid peroxide production
- Increased free radical activity/decreased protection

**Systemic effects**
- Generalized membrane instability
- Diminished vascular endothelial function
- Platelet–vessel-wall interaction

**Physiological changes**
- Increased vascular resistance
- Vasoconstriction
- Systemic tissue hypoxia
- Eclampsia
- HELLP syndrome
- Renal impairment

---

case of maternal mortality in these countries and that eclampsia is a more common presentation than it is in the developed world.

These variances make the assessment of the difference in incidence between the racial groups difficult. Despite this, differences obviously exist, and the explanation of this could be related to the environmental and familial factors discussed later (Chesley, Annitto and Cosgrove, 1961, 1968; Cooper *et al.*, 1988; Cooper and Liston, 1979; Arngrimsson *et al.*, 1990).

**4.4 INCREASING INCIDENCE AS TERM APPROACHES**

The blood pressure rises towards term in most pregnancies (MacGillivray, 1961) and Nelson found that mild or 'latent' hypertension is more common in the later gestations (Nelson, 1955b). The epidemiology of hypertension without proteinuria has several characteristic features which suggest that it should

not always be regarded as mild preeclampsia (MacGillivray, 1961). The incidence rises sharply over the age of 30 at a time when essential hypertension is also becoming more common (Nelson, 1955b). The risks to mother and baby of late-onset mild to moderate hypertension are much lower when compared with hypertension in pregnancy as a whole (Nelson, 1955a). Mild hypertension occurring during late pregnancy is not associated with poor fetal growth (Baird, Thomson and Billewicz, 1955). Women who had hypertension without proteinuria were found to have a higher risk of hypertension in later life compared with those with true preeclampsia (Chesley, 1978; Browne and Dodds, 1939). These findings suggest that the finding of an increasing incidence of preeclampsia towards term may be a reflection of the demonstration of the 'latent' hypertension described by Dieckmann (1952), Nelson (1955b) and Browne and Shaimich (1956). This is supported by the lack of pathology, the association with increasing age and the higher incidence of essential hypertension in later life.

In areas where antenatal care is well established, the incidence of severe late-onset preeclampsia is rare. Most of the management problems are in those presenting before 30 weeks gestation. This implies that presentation later in pregnancy is more easily controlled. It has been suggested that preeclampsia occurring before 34 weeks has a different etiology and inherent pathological process than that presenting later (Moore and Redman, 1983)

## 4.5 RARITY OF REPEATED PROBLEMS IN SUBSEQUENT PREGNANCIES

MacGillivray showed that if the first pregnancy was normal the incidence in a subsequent pregnancy was low. If the first pregnancy was complicated by severe preeclampsia, the incidence was found to be similar to that of a primigravida (MacGillivray, 1981). The protection in the multipara may be related to the immunological factors previously mentioned. The first pregnancy immunizes the woman against her husband's antigens and allows a normal immunological response in subsequent pregnancies. This argument is supported by Feeney, who found that, after a blood transfusion, a woman had a lower incidence of preeclampsia (Feeney, Tovey and Scott, 1977). However, Lopez Llera followed up 110 patients with a history of eclampsia. In the next pregnancy 35.4% of the patients had repeated preeclampsia, although he was less specific in his diagnosis (Lopez Llera and Hernandez Horta, 1974). Therefore, the protection of a first pregnancy is not absolute and appears to be most effective if preeclampsia does not develop. This suggests a degree of susceptibility in those patients in whom the disease is manifest. Therefore, rather than protect against the disease, a normal first pregnancy may 'screen out' those who are not susceptible. This susceptibility may be related to the familial tendencies already alluded to.

## 4.6 IMPROVEMENT AFTER DEATH OF THE FETUS

Beker stated that 'if the foetus dies *in utero* the general condition of the mother generally improves' (Beker, 1948) However, fetal death is not always followed by immediate clinical improvement. Dexter and Weiss found this in less than one third of cases (Dexter and Weiss, 1941). Therefore, although there may be an improvement, it is not absolute and the susceptibility remains.

## 4.7 HYPERTENSION, EDEMA, PROTEINURIA, CONVULSIONS AND COMA

The clinical hallmarks of preeclampsia in the mother are hypertension, proteinuria, edema and the tendency to convulsions and coma. The physiological characteristics are an increase in peripheral resistance (Larkin *et al.*, 1980; Lim and Walters, 1979) exaggerated responses to pressor agents (Talledo, Chesley and Zuspan, 1968; Gant *et al.*, 1973, 1980; Zuspan, 1979), activation of the coagulation system (Howie, Prentice and McNicol, 1971), largely manifest by a reduced platelet count (Redman, Bonnar and Beilin, 1978), and decreased utero-placental blood flow (Lunell *et al.*, 1982). There is also an impairment of the normal increase of plasma volume and cardiac output (Lim and Walters, 1979; Gallery, Hunyor and Gyory, 1979). A full review of the normal and abnormal cardiovascular changes in pregnancy is found in Chapters 2 and 5.

### 4.7.1 CHANGES IN THE CARDIOVASCULAR SYSTEM IN NORMAL PREGNANCY

Normal pregnancy is associated with a number of alterations in the cardiovascular system which start to occur early in pregnancy. Cardiac output increases by around 40% during the first trimester and this increase is maintained throughout the rest of the pregnancy. Blood pressure starts to fall in the first trimester, reaches a nadir in mid-pregnancy, then slowly rises during the third trimester to levels comparable with those in the non-pregnant state at term (MacGillivray, Rose and Rowe, 1969). As arterial pressure is determined by cardiac output and total peripheral resistance, the decrease in blood pressure must be due to a fall in the latter. Since these changes occur early in pregnancy, they must reflect a change in systemic vascular resistance, as the utero-placental circulation is not sufficiently large to account for such a reduction in peripheral resistance at this stage of pregnancy.

The fall in peripheral resistance in normal pregnancy is associated with a relative insensitivity to the pressor effects of exogenous angiotensin II (AII) (Gant et al., 1973), which is detectable as early as 8 weeks gestation and reaches a peak in mid-pregnancy. The mechanism underlying this insensitivity may be prostaglandin-dependent. The pressor effects of angiotensin II may be balanced in normal pregnancy by prostaglandin $E_2$ and prostacyclin, which have vasodilator effects. It is obvious that changes in vascular reactivity may be at the center of the etiology of the hypertension changes in preeclampsia. The clinical signs of hypertension may be due to the loss of the normal vasodilator responses rather than to an increase in the vasoconstriction.

### 4.7.2 VASCULAR SENSITIVITY AS A CAUSE OF HYPERTENSION

Beker postulated that 'toxemia' of pregnancy was not due to a toxin but was related to an upset in the circulatory system (Beker, 1948). Hertig suggested that the disease was one of widespread vasospasm (Hertig, 1945). However, this vascular constriction would only contribute towards the vascular hypertension as the blood flow to the major organs, apart from the uterus, liver and kidney, would continue to be normal unless there is severe cardiac compromise. There is not a general reduction in peripheral blood flow. Burt showed increased blood flow to the hand and

the forearm in preeclampsia, but this may be related to muscle blood flow rather than the true periphery (Burt, 1950). Since that time, there has been much work on the causes of the hypertension. Studies have shown that the vascular system in preeclampsia is hypersensitive to several pressor agents. The first studies used various pituitary extracts (De Valera and Kellar, 1948; Browne, 1946). Browne showed that this sensitivity disappeared after delivery. Raab et al. (1956) found it with noradrenalin (norepinephrine) and Talledo, Chesley and Zuspan (1968), Chesley et al. (1965) and Zuspan (1979) found it with noradrenaline and angiotensin. Gant et al. (1973), Wallenburg et al. (1986) and Dekker, Makovitz and Wallenburg (1990) have shown that the angiotensin infusion test can select out patients who are destined to develop preeclampsia by demonstrating sensitivity at 16–18 weeks although a more recent studies have failed to confirm this (Baker, Broughton Pipkin and Symonds, 1992). This suggests that the sensitivity is present prior to the disease presentation, implying susceptibility to the condition. It is now widely accepted that vasoconstriction is the basic cause of the hypertension in preeclampsia (Gant et al., 1980; Hardy and Williams, 1988; Gilstrap and Gant, 1990) and this is partly due to changes in vascular endothelial function (see later). However, since the hypertension develops later in the pregnancy and it is known that the sensitivity is an early sign, a further stimulus would seem to be required and the vasoconstriction would then be a secondary effect following this stimulus.

### 4.7.3 SALT AND WATER RETENTION

Sodium and water retention could be an explanation for the arterial hypertension. Sodium is retained in preeclampsia (Chesley, 1966; Plentl and Gray, 1959). Harding and Van Wyck (1930) gave sodium solutions to preeclamptic women with disastrous results: one patient developed fulminating preeclampsia within 24 hours with a BP rise from 128/100 to 200/140. Dieckmann (1952) showed that a high salt intake in preeclamptic women produced a deterioration of the symptoms and there was a reduced ability to concentrate salt in the urine. However, spironolactone, a drug useful in other salt-retaining conditions, has no effect on the blood pressure in preeclamptic women (MacGillivray, 1981). Salt restriction has been a commonly used therapy, particularly in Holland, but prophylactic salt restriction has little benefit on the development of the disease although it may have an effect on the sensitivity of the peripheral vasculature by altering AII receptor activity. These factors have led on to the interest in the renin–angiotensin system.

### 4.7.4 THE RENIN–ANGIOTENSIN SYSTEM

Salt excretion is controlled by the renin–angiotensin system. As already stated, the response to a angiotensin infusion is abnormal in preeclampsia (Chesley *et al.*, 1965; Gant *et al.*, 1973, 1980). Gant feels that if levels of angiotensin are low, receptor site occupancy will be low and sensitivity to angiotensin will be raised. The results of studies of blood levels are confusing. Massiani *et al.* (1967) found angiotensin levels to be normal, Weir *et al.* (1973) found them to be severely depressed and Symonds, Broughton Pipkin and Craven (1975) found them to be raised. All the studies were on patients of apparently similar severity.

Both adrenalin/epinephrine and noradrenalin/norepineprine can cause vasoconstriction and increased sensitivity to infusions of these substances have been demonstrated (Talledo, Chesley and Zuspan, 1968; Chesley *et al.*, 1965; Zuspan, 1979) but levels of noradrenaline have been found to be low (Tunbridge and Donnia, 1981).

Broughton Pipkin (1976) has demonstrated that the fetal placental unit can produce angiotensin II and the levels in the cord venous blood of babies from mothers with

preeclampsia are found to be significantly elevated above levels seen in normal pregnancy. Symonds, Broughton Pipkin and Craven (1975) found that the levels of AII in plasma in late pregnancy in over 50 primigravidae were in direct relationship to diastolic blood pressure. He feels that the fetal placental unit produces angiotensin in response to hypoxia. This, in turn, can produce hypertension in susceptible patients. This production of angiotensin II may act as the trigger to the blood pressure rise. The susceptibility of the patient to respond to this stimulation may be related to the level of prostaglandin activity by the peripheral vasculature. Therefore, abnormalities of vascular endothelial function are associated with preeclampsia.

### 4.7.5 THE RELEVANCE OF EDEMA

As already discussed, edema is found in 85% of women with preeclampsia (Thomson, Hytten and Billewicz, 1967) and it may be severe. The edema fluid is an ultrafiltrate of plasma and is associated with reduced plasma albumin and oncotic pressure, and with retention of sodium and potassium. Although Hamlin (1952) found that all patients who developed PIH had been noted to show edema during the preceding 6 weeks, others have found that patients with edema had an incidence of PIH which was similar to patients without edema (MacGillivray and Campbell, 1980). In fact, retention of fluid is associated with heavier babies (Duffus *et al.*, 1969).

Therefore, edema is of little value as a specific diagnostic sign as it occurs in 64% of normal pregnancies (Thomson, Hytten and Billewicz, 1967; Dexter and Weiss, 1941) and is associated with no increase in the incidence of preeclampsia or perinatal mortality (Thomson, Hytten and Billewicz, 1967; Chamberlain *et al.*, 1978). Physiological edema develops gradually, is associated with a smooth rate of weight gain and usually affects the lower parts of the body. In some normotensive pregnancies up to 5 liters of water can be retained, giving a more generalized edema. Physiological edema is caused by an increase of capillary hydrostatic pressure that results from a lowering of the precapillary resistance.

Pathological edema is not caused by an increased intracapillary hydrostatic pressure. Because of the increase in the precapillary resistance in preeclampsia, the intracapillary hydrostatic pressure is significantly decreased. Pathological edema is caused by an increased microvascular permeability to plasma proteins, a reduction in plasma colloid osmotic pressure and an increase in interstitial protein mass (Oian and Maltau, 1987). Because of this loss of plasma fluid, there is loss of intravascular volume. Hemoconcentration also occurs (Zangemeister, 1903). Dieckmann, in his monograph *The Toxemias of Pregnancy* (1952) states that serum protein concentration rises at least 2 days prior to the development of eclampsia, as does the hematocrit and hemoglobin. This demonstrates the association of the hypertension with a reduced plasma volume (Gallery, Hunyor and Gyory, 1979).

### 4.7.6 PROTEINURIA

The proteinuria in pregnancy-induced hypertension is related to disease severity (MacGillivray, 1961; Nelson, 1955b). It is moderately selective in terms of size of the filtered proteins, but can be heavy, with more than 5 g of protein per day being lost. It is due to a glomerular protein leak, signifying glomerular involvement in the disease process. As this is always associated with the pathognomonic renal lesion, this will be discussed under renal pathology.

### 4.7.7 CONVULSIONS AND COMA

Severe hypertension causes arterial damage and this has been demonstrated in animals (Goldby and Beilin, 1972). This arterial damage may explain the convulsions and cerebral hemorrhage seen in untreated severe preeclampsia. Cerebral hemorrhage is the commonest cause

of death in pregnancy-induced hypertension (DHSS, 1969, 1974, 1979, 1991, 1994; Turnbull, 1987; Turnbull *et al.*, 1989). Postmortem studies of the brain show edema, hyperemia, focal lesions, thrombosis and hemorrhage (Sheehan and Lynch, 1973; Smorl and Veit, 1933). As these lesions were found at post mortem, they may be end-stage changes rather than causal lesions. The length of time after death that the studies were carried out may also contribute. Sheehan (1950) studied 48 cases within 1 hour of death. Hemorrhages were the most common findings. There was little edema at this time. Govan (1961) showed that the cause of death in 39 of 110 women who died of PIH was cerebral hemorrhage. In a further 47 it was cardiorespiratory failure, with small hemorrhages found in 85% of them. Fibrinoid changes were regular findings in the walls of the cerebral vessels. Because of the lymphocyte reactions around the lesions with infiltration by pigmented macrophages, they appeared to have been present for some time. This could suggest that these lesions antedate the fit and are not caused by the seizure itself. Whether these lesions are the cause of the neurological symptoms and the convulsions is more difficult to discover. The relevant factor concerning whether a patient does or does not convulse appears to be her own fitting threshold (Nelson, 1955b). The degree of pathological damage found may well be related to the amount of prodromal preeclampsia. It may be that only some of the pathology results from the damage due to the seizure itself.

### 4.8 HEPATIC LESIONS

The most characteristic feature of the hepatic lesion in eclampsia is its variability in extent and severity. Many cases are described with no hepatic necrosis at all (Acosta Sison, 1931; Bell, Dieckmann and Eastmann, 1940; Theobald, 1933). The classic hepatic lesion associated with severe preeclampsia is periportal or focal parenchymal necrosis and periportal lake hemorrhages. Fibrin–fibrinogen deposition in the hepatic sinusoids has been noted to occur as an early feature of preeclampsia. In severe preeclampsia large deposits of fibrin-like material may obstruct blood flow in sinusoids and cause hepatic capsular distention. Hepatic capsular distention may cause upper epigastric pain, 'stomach upset', a feeling of upper abdominal pressure or banding. The changes seen within the liver are not related to severity, although the pathological damage can be quite extensive (Sheehan and Lynch, 1973; Dieckmann, 1929). Therefore, it is thought that the lesions are caused by the condition and do not contribute to the etiology of the disease. In biopsies of five patients who survived eclampsia, a normal liver was found in two. In a further two patients, the lesions were found to be worse than those found in the patients who died (Ingerslev and Teilum, 1946). The hepatic findings are mostly related to end-stage disease and are found at postmortem. Because most of the early studies were carried out on patients who had died, this led to the opinion held in the 1930s that hemorrhagic necrosis in the periphery of the lobules is the characteristic lesion of eclampsia (Acosta Sison, 1931).

The lesions are most commonly found in the right lobe of the liver. The areas of hemorrhage begin around a periportal space and are usually associated with extensive thrombosis in the smallest vessels in the periportal connective tissue. Sheehan and Lynch (1973) thought that the primary lesion was the escape of blood or plasma into the peripheral base of the hepatic cell cords. Focal fibrosis is usually seen. Lesions of the center of the hepatic lobule are also seen (Acosta Sison, 1931). Hemorrhage beneath the liver capsule may be so extensive as to cause rupture of the capsule, with massive hemorrhage into the peritoneal cavity (Golan and White, 1979). This remains one of the rare but severe causes of maternal mortality. It would appear that hepatic lesions are patient-specific rather than related directly to disease severity.

## 4.9 RENAL LESIONS

There is ongoing debate whether the kidney is the culprit, the victim or just an innocent bystander in preeclampsia. The involvement of the kidneys is one of the most consistent features of preeclampsia, and the changes in kidney function are essential in the pathogenesis of at least three of the major signs: hypertension, proteinuria and hyperuricemia. In pregnancy-induced hypertensive disorders a deficient intrarenal release of local vasodilator autocoids may result in unopposed intrarenal effects of angiotensin II and other vasoconstrictor autocoids (De Jong, Dekker and Sibai, 1991), in this way causing an impaired ability to excrete sodium. The impaired ability to excrete sodium causes a shift to the right in the renal-pressure–natriurese curve and in this way an increase in vascular tone and blood pressure (Guyton *et al.*, 1990). This also leads to increasing fluid retention and edema.

The normal pregnancy-induced changes in renal function are remarkable. The renal plasma flow (ERPF) increases by 50–75% and glomerular filtration rate (GFR) increases by 50% over non-pregnant values (Dunlop, 1981). Significant elevation of the creatinine clearance, used clinically to estimate GFR, is apparent as soon as 4 weeks after conception. This leads to a reduction in the plasma urea and creatinine concentrations. In preeclampsia, GFR and ERPF average respectively 30% and 20% lower as compared to matched normotensive control pregnancies; the preeclamptic values for GFR and ERPF usually fall in the ranges that would be considered to be normal for non-pregnant women, but the decrease may be as much as 50% or more (Chesley and Lindheimer, 1988). The decreased GFR is caused by the decrease in ERPF and in the filtration fraction (Chesley, 1978).

In severe preeclampsia there is a characteristic increase in the amount of protein excreted by the kidney into the measurable range (above 300 mg/l). In the presence of proteinuria, renal lesions are usually found (Sheehan,

1980; McCartney, 1964) Altchek, Albright and Sommers (1968) showed that the typical biopsy lesions are:

1. Glomerular lesions
2. Juxtaglomerular cellular hyperplasia
3. Lesions of the loop of Henle
4. Afferent arteriolar spasm.

Glomeruli were enlarged by 20%, with cellular swelling and glomerular capillary endotheliosis. All glomeruli appeared affected but the distribution within the glomeruli was patchy. There was an increase of the number of cells and thickening of the capillary endothelium between the capillaries, explaining the appearance of the splitting of the basement membrane seen by light microscopy. This is really an increase in the mesangial matrix. Capillary endothelial cells were swollen and many lumina appeared empty or absent. Deposition of fibrin protein strands were seen within Bowman's capsule. Vassalli, Morris and McClusky (1963) have found fibrinogen within these lesions. Immunofluorescent studies suggested that the deposits seen on the basement membrane are fibrinogen derivatives. This supports the view that an upset in the coagulation system is involved in preeclampsia. The epithelium of Henle's loop was severely desquamated, with fragments of nuclei and cells evident. In other areas regeneration was apparent. The afferent arterioles showed marked vasospasm.

Tubular lesions are also common and casts are seen in the urine. Chesley and Duffus (1971) showed that the kidney has a decreased ability to secrete uric acid in preeclampsia, hence the increase in the concentration of uric acid and a fall in bicarbonate concentration. Uric acid is filtered completely by glomeruli, reabsorbed completely by proximal tubules and then secreted by distal convoluted tubules. Therefore, in preeclampsia, the initial filtering may be reduced by glomerular impairment or the secretion may be deficient as a result of tubular damage. In support of the latter possibility,

Altchek, Albright and Sommers (1968) have reported a lesion in the loop of Henle, the severity of which is related to the level of uric acid. They and Pollak and Nettles (1960) have shown hyperplasia of the juxtaglomerular apparatus (JGA) and apparent cellular hyperactivity. The JGA was swollen, with an increase in the number of cells and vacuolation. There is an increase in renin, angiotensin and aldosterone activity. This could lead to retention of sodium and water. However these lesions appear to be progressive with the disease and may be secondary to the volume depletion rather than being an etiological factor. Dieckmann (1952) has reported the rare lesion of cortical necrosis, which was fatal although it can now be managed by renal dialysis. The lesion is caused by spasm of the renal arteries and anemic infarcts. This lesion is not specific to pregnancy.

After delivery, the changes disappear quickly (Sheehan, 1950) with occasional traces of increased mesangial matrix. Petrucco *et al.* (1974) did not see the changes of the JGA or the loop of Henle but their samples were taken from the recovery phase post delivery while the findings of Altchek (1961, 1964; Altchek, Albright and Sommers, 1968) and others came from renal biopsies taken during the active phase.

### 4.9.1 URIC ACID

Uric acid is formed from xanthine by the action of xanthine oxidase, and is the chief end product of purine metabolism. In nonpregnant subjects, daily excretion varies between 500 and 800 mg of urate, and plasma uric acid levels vary between 0.24 and 0.36 mmol/l. Urate clearance varies between 6 and 12 ml/min. Renal handling of urate and subsequent urinary excretion is estimated to cover two-thirds of the daily elimination of uric acid. The bulk of plasma urate is freely filterable. Most (98%) is initially reabsorbed and the largest part of excreted urate (80–85%) derives from secondary tubular secretion.

Tubular secretion of urate is dependent on renal tubular blood flow. In addition, a variety of factors influence the renal excretion of uric acid: these include volume status, the renin–angiotensin system, catecholamines, urinary solute excretion, plasma ketoacids, plasma glucose and plasma cortisol.

Production of uric acid during pregnancy has been described as unaltered, but pregnant women excrete considerably more uric acid than when they are not pregnant. During pregnancy, urate clearance increases to between 12 and 20 ml/min and plasma levels decrease to 0.18–0.26 mmol/l. This increase in uric acid excretion is probably mainly caused by the physiological hypervolemia of pregnancy and increased renal blood flow. Sodium restriction and use of diuretics are known to cause an increase in serum uric acid levels. In the third trimester, plasma uric acid levels may increase to concentrations equivalent to non-pregnant values (Chesley, 1978; Lindheimer and Katz, 1991). The hyperuricemia of pregnancy-induced hypertensive disorders was first described by Slemons and Bogert (1917), and was later confirmed by many other investigators (Dekker and Sibai, 1991). The placenta is not the source of the hyperuricemia because placental tissue lacks the enzyme xanthine dehydrogenase/xanthine oxidase (Hayashi *et al.*, 1964). Also, the fetus is not involved in the causation of hyperuricemia in pregnancy-induced hypertensive disorders (Wallenburg and van Kreel, 1978). Cadden and Stander (1939) found similar urinary uric acid excretion (130–750 mg/24 h) in their normotensive and hypertensive patients. Because these authors did not appreciate the fact that urinary excretion is not an adequate method to assess kidney function, they concluded that kidney function was apparently normal in preeclampsia, and thought that the hyperuricemia was caused by liver cell injury.

Chesley (1950) calculated uric acid clearance from the data presented in the data from Cadden and Stander, and clearly demonstrated that preeclamptic hyperuricemia is caused largely by a decreased urate clearance by the kidneys. In addition, Chesley clearly demonstrated that uric acid clearance drops disproportionally in preeclampsia as compared to urea clearance. In contrast, pure renal disease is characterized by equal depression of urate and urea clearance. Initially, Chesley proposed the clearance ratio of urate to urea as a differential diagnostic test, but Chesley and Valenti (1958) reported that this test had a diagnostic error of about 20%. The pathophysiological explanation for this specific decrease in urate clearance is based on the biphasic pattern of renal involvement in preeclampsia. The tubular function is the first to be involved and it is late in the disease process that the glomerular function is impaired. The impairment of tubular physiology results in a reduced renal clearance of uric acid and thus an increase of plasma uric acid levels. Later, about the time proteinuria appears, glomerular function and thus urea and creatinine clearance become impaired. Therefore, the decrease in urate clearance occurs earlier and is more profound than the decrease in GFR; therefore the urate/creatinine clearance ratio falls (Chesley and Williams, 1945; Lindheimer and Katz, 1991).

In the non-pregnant and pregnant kidney, an increase in plasma volume inhibits proximal tubular reabsorption and increases distal tubular urate secretion. Hypovolemia induces opposite changes in tubular function. Preeclamptic hyperuricemia has been shown to correlate more or less with the decrease in plasma volume and plasma renin activity (Beaufils *et al.*, 1981; Gallery, Hunyor and Gyory, 1979). Preeclamptic hyperuricemia is probably caused by a combination of intrarenal (peritubular) vasoconstriction and hypovolemia, both an expression of the increased systemic vasoconstriction, resulting from deficient endothelial release of vasodilator substances (Fadel, Northrop and Nisenhimer, 1976; Dekker and Sibai, 1992; Zeeman *et al.*, 1992). In preeclampsia, a rise in uric acid can be seen to be a marker of the underlying disease process rather than simply a sign of renal involvement.

## 4.10 PLACENTAL LESIONS

The fetus depends on the placenta for its survival. The ability of the placenta to exchange nutrients and gases between the fetus and the mother is largely dependent on blood flow, both from the mother and the fetus. It has been known for some years that the blood flow to the placenta is reduced in maternal hypertension (Browne and Veall, 1953; Dixon and Robertson, 1958; Assali *et al.*, 1954). Campbell *et al.* (1986) has show abnormalities in the uterine artery Doppler velocity wave form as early as 18 weeks in patients who are destined to develop preeclampsia and IUGR. Some workers have suggested that this could be used as a screening test to select those women that might benefit from intervention therapy (McParland, Pearce and Chamberlain, 1990)

These observations might be explained by the pathology in the terminal segments of the uterine spiral arteries. Within the placenta, these become obstructed by fibrin and platelet aggregates. Placental infarcts are also seen. However, these 'so-called' infarcts are found in about 60% of normal pregnancies. Tenney and Parker (1940) believe that the characteristic placental change is one of premature aging. Fox (1978) disregards this term and calls the lesions ischemic villus necrosis. Tenney and Parker (1940) found that in preeclampsia most of the villi show syncytial degeneration, a finding in only 10–50% of normal pregnancy . Extensive infarcts of more than 5% of the placental area are not found in normal pregnancy (Fox, 1978) but are found in increasing frequency in patients with worsening hypertension. This lesion is not specific to preeclampsia and occurs in essential hypertension without evidence of superimposed preeclampsia. It is likely that these changes are those of hypertensive damage of what-

ever cause (Fox, 1978). The work of Dixon and Robertson (1958), Brosens, Robertson and Dixon (1970); Brosens, Dixon and Robertson (1977), Robertson, Brosen and Dixon (1967) and Robertson (1976) showed the obvious differences between normal and preeclamptic pregnancies.

The fundamental lesions of preeclampsia are in the spiral arterioles of the placental bed. There is a failure of the normal invasion of these vessels by the invading trophoblastic cells. This invasion is necessary to destroy the musculo-elastic tissue in the media to allow vasodilatation of the spiral arterioles. There is then failure of the normal vasodilatation of these vessels, leading to a reduced placental blood flow in later pregnancy. The trigger for failure of the normal physiological changes in the maternal blood vessels is unknown but could be due to the previously discussed immunological abnormality, which interferes with the normal trophoblastic invasion (Zhou, 1993). In order for invasion to occur, both the maternal tissue and the trophoblast need to express specific molecules on the cell surface. These allow the cells to recognize each other, invade and adhere. There is an abnormality of these adhesion molecules on the surface of the cells taken from trophoblastic tissue taken from preeclamptic pregnancies.

Studies by Sheppard and Bonnar (1981) suggest that the placental pathological changes are not specific to preeclampsia but are found in the vessels from pregnancies with intrauterine growth retardation with or without hypertension. Therefore, some other factor is required to produce the systemic changes found ('factor X').

The placental changes give rise to interference with fetal growth and oxygenation. Bastiaanse and Mastboom (1950) claimed that utero-placental ischemia was responsible for preeclampsia. Therefore, the maternal changes seen in pregnancy-induced hypertension may be secondary to placental ischemia. Animal models of the disease depend on procedures that cause placental ischemia (Cavanagh *et al.*,

1977). This theory would support Symonds's belief that uteroplacental stimulation of the renin/angiotensin system secondary to placental ischemia plays a central role in the development of hypertension (Symonds, 1981). Others have suggested alternative candidates for this 'factor X' (Table 4.3).

## 4.11 ABNORMALITIES OF THE COAGULATION SYSTEM

During pregnancy, major changes occur in the coagulation system and to a lesser extent in platelets (Table 4.4).

Evidence of this includes the increased concentrations of all clotting factors, except factors XI and XIII. Particularly marked increases occur in the levels of fibrinogen and factors VII, VIIIc, VIIIrag and X. In contrast, plasma levels of the coagulation inhibitors antithrombin III (ATIII) and protein C remain normal, while protein S may decrease to levels as low as those observed in patients with congenital protein S deficiency (Comp *et al.*, 1986; Hathaway and Bonnar, 1987; Fernandez *et al.*, 1989).

Pregnancy-induced hypertensive disorders are associated with alterations in this normal physiological response of the homeostatic system during pregnancy. Whether these changes are primary or secondary to a basic trigger mechanism or mechanisms is a matter of active investigation and debate. Until recently many investigators have proposed

---

**Table 4.3** Possible candidates for factor X'; these substances may be increased in production secondarily to placental ischemia and contribute to the systemic disease

- Angiotensin II
- Lipid peroxides
- Cytokines
- Free radicals
- Neutrophil activity
- Immunocomplexes

---

that disseminated intravascular coagulation (DIC) is either a prominent event in the pathogenesis of preeclampsia or an important consequence of the advanced syndrome (McKay *et al.*, 1953; Page, 1972). Probably neither is the case (Wallenburg, 1987). Chesley (1978) stated: 'Many women with the diagnosis of eclampsia and of preeclampsia, even of severe degree, show no detectable signs of increased coagulation and fibrinolysis. DIC, if it does occur, does not appear to be a fundamental feature of the disease.' The confusion may be related to cases studied with coexisting abruptions.

The 'real' disease of preeclampsia is probably a microangiopathy, with extensive endothelial cell damage and subsequent platelet activation (Zeeman *et al.*, 1992). Only in certain organs, such as the uteroplacental vascular bed, the liver and the kidneys, is there local increase of thrombin formation and fibrin deposition. In Table 4.5 the major differences between DIC and microangiopathy are presented in a schematic way (Speroff, Glass and Kase, 1983).

Manifestations of endothelial cell damage in preeclampsia are increased levels of factor VIII-related antigen (Fournie *et al.*, 1981), increased levels of fibronectin and ED1+ fibronectin (Ballegeer *et al.*, 1989; Lockwood and Peters, 1990), a disturbance of tissue-plasminogen activator and plasminogen-activator inhibitor (de Boer *et al.*, 1988), a disturbance of the prostacyclin/thromboxane balance (Friedman, 1988; Dekker and Sibai, 1992; Greer *et al.*, 1985a), and an increase in plasma endothelin levels (Dekker and Sibai, 1991). Vascular damage and platelet aggregation precede the increase in thrombin and fibrin formation (Ballegeer *et al.*, 1992). The concept of surface-mediated platelet activation and consumption in the uteroplacental vessels fully explains the platelet and coagulation changes observed in preeclampsia (Wallenburg, 1987; Dekker, 1989).

**Table 4.4** Changes in the coagulation system in normal pregnancy and preeclampsia

**Normal pregnancy**
- An increase in the concentrations of all clotting factors, except factors XI and XIII
- Particular increase in the levels of fibrinogen, factors VII, VIIIc, VIIIrag and X
- Increase in factor VIII-related antigen/factor VIIIc ratio
- Marginal decrease in ATIII, with an increase in levels TAT
- Protein C stays the same although protein C inhibitor increases
- Protein S demonstrates a significant reduction
- Levels of fibrinogen gradually increases
- Levels of fibronectin are similar or only slightly increased

**Preeclampsia**
- Increased platelet activation with increased volume and reduced lifespan
- Increased levels of factor VIII-related antigen
- Further increase in factor VIII-related antigen/factor VIIIc ratio
- Increased levels of fibronectin
- A reduction in the prostacyclin–thromboxane balance
- Increase in plasma endothelin levels
- Increase in thrombin and fibrin formation
- Decreased ATIII with an increase in levels of thrombin–ATIII complexes
- Levels of protein C are reduced in severe disease

### 4.11.1 FACTOR VIII-RELATED ANTIGEN/FACTOR VIIIC (FVIIIRAG/FVIIIC)

The ratio of factor VIII-related antigen to factor VIII coagulant activity (fVIIIrag/fVIIIc) in healthy subjects is 1. Stress, physical exercise and catecholamine infusion elevate both fVIIIrag and fVIIIc; under these circumstances the ratio will remain about 1. A decrease in the denominator, fVIIIc, is an expression of circulating thrombin. Malignancy, thromboembolic processes and DIC increase the fVIIIrag/fVIIIC ratio by lowering fVIIIc. Thrombin inactivates fVIIIc but not fVIIIrag.

An increase in the numerator of this ratio, the fVIIIrag, is associated with endothelial release of this antigen (Hoyer, 1987).

During normal pregnancy the levels of fVIIIc and fVIIIrag show an approximately proportional rise in the first half of pregnancy, but then, according to some authors, diverge because of a greater increase in fVIIIrag. Therefore, according to some authors, the ratio remains around 1 (Bennett and Ratnoff, 1972; Fournie *et al.*, 1981; Scholtes, Gerretsen and Haak, 1983), but most investigators describe an increase in this ratio from 1.0

**Table 4.5** Basic differences between DIC and microangiopathy

|  | *DIC* | *Microangiopathy* |
| --- | --- | --- |
| Etiology | Thromboplastins, thrombin, fibrin | Endothelial cell damage, platelet activation, deficient production of vasodilator autocoids |
| Pathology | Intravascular fibrin | Intravascular platelet aggregation and deposition |
| Fibrinogen levels | Low | Normal or high |
| Platelet count | Mildly to moderately decreased | Moderately to markedly decreased |
| Red cells | Slight to moderate fragmentation | Moderate to marked fragmentation |

(non-pregnant value) in the first half of pregnancy to around 2.0 near term (Hellgren and Blomback, 1981; Inglis *et al.*, 1982; Stirling *et al.*, 1984; van Royen and ten Cate, 1973).

Several authors have demonstrated an early rise of the fVIIIrag/fVIIIc ratio in pregnancy-induced hypertensive disease; a positive correlation between the magnitude of increase of the ratio and the severity of the disease, the degree of hyperuricemia, placental infarcts, adverse perinatal outcome; and a strong negative correlation between this ratio and platelet lifespan (Thornton and Bonnar, 1977; Redman *et al.*, 1977; Fournie *et al.*, 1981; Whigham *et al.*, 1980; Scholtes, Gerretsen and Haak, 1983). Thornton and Bonnar (1977) longitudinally followed the fVIIIrag/fVIIIc ratio in ten normotensive pregnant women and in ten patients who ultimately developed preeclampsia. In the normotensive women the ratio was 1.02–1.32 at 16–20 weeks and 1–1.45 at 36 weeks gestation. At 16–20 weeks the women who developed preeclampsia had a ratio similar to the normotensive patients; at 29–30 weeks the ratio had increased to 1.5–2.6 and at 36 weeks gestation to 1.69–3.1. In all patients who reached a ratio of < 2.5, pregnancy had to be terminated within 10 days because of severe preeclampsia and/or fetal distress. At first, the increase in fVIIIrag/ fVIIIc ratio in pregnancy-induced hypertensive disorders was interpreted as a sign of increased intravascular coagulation (Fournie *et al.*, 1981). However, fVIIIc levels are not decreased in preeclampsia (Dunlop *et al.*, 1978; Lazarchick, Stubbs and Romein, 1986). In addition, Scholtes, Gerretsen and Haak (1983) demonstrated that the increase in the fVIIIrag/fVIIIc ratio is not caused by an increased consumption of fVIIIc, by reporting ATIII levels that were completely in the normal range at a time the fVIIIrag/fVIIIc ratio was significantly elevated. Factor VIIIrag is a glycoprotein produced by endothelial cells. It is this factor, the von Willebrand factor, that is essential for platelet adhesion (Tschopp, Weiss and Baumgarter, 1974). The increase in the

fVIIIrag/fVIIIc ratio in hypertensive disorders of pregnancy is caused by increased endothelial release of fVIIIrag. This thought to be an expression of endothelial cell damage. A minor portion of the circulating fVIIIrag may be derived from aggregating platelets (Boneu *et al.*, 1975; Nachman and Jaffe, 1980; Ruggeri, 1980; Scholtes, Gerretsen and Haak, 1983). The increase of fVIIIrag and thereby the ratio is most pronounced in preeclampsia associated with fetal growth retardation (Scholtes, Gerretsen and Haak, 1983). Endothelial release of fVIIIrag is not increased in chronic hypertension. In conclusion, measuring fVIIIrag or the fVIIIrag/fVIIIc ratio is a sensitive indicator of both the severity and the degree of endothelial cell damage, and the extend of placental insufficiency in pregnancy-induced hypertensive disorders. The ratio correlates with fetal growth retardation and perinatal morbidity and mortality. The increase in fVIIIrag runs parallel with the increase in serum uric acid levels and the increase in blood pressure (Boneu *et al.*, 1980; Whigham *et al.*, 1980). These changes are likely to be the result of the endothelial dysfunction in preeclampsia and are not the underlying cause of the disease. They may be associated with many of the other pathological findings seen.

### 4.11.2 ANTITHROMBIN III (ATIII)

Antithrombin III (ATIII), a serine protease inhibitor, is produced by the liver, and is active against all activated coagulation factors except factor VIIIa. The activity of ATIII is dramatically increased by heparin. *In vivo* endothelial heparin-like molecules accelerate the inhibitory activity of ATIII. Because activation of the soluble clotting cascade cannot occur without ATIII consumption, ATIII is a sensitive indicator of excess clotting activity (Harpel, 1987; Weiner, 1991). When assayed immunologically, no relation exists between the level of ATIII and thromboembolic disease. However, decreased ATIII activity does occur in diseases characterized by an increase in intravascular thrombin production, such as thromboembolic diseases and DIC, and after major surgery. ATIII activity is also low in chronic liver disease and protein-losing renal disease (Hirsch, 1987).

In uncomplicated pregnancy, ATIII activity levels show no changes or only a marginal decrease. However, the 'reserve' or the ability of the pregnant woman to maintain a normal level of activity when challenged is reduced. Decreased ATIII activity levels have been demonstrated to exist in a majority of patients with preeclampsia (Weiner and Brandt, 1980, 1982; Hellgren and Blomback, 1981; Weenink *et al.*, 1983, 1984; Stirling *et al.*, 1984; Weiner, 1991; Perry and Martin, 1992). ATIII activity levels are normal in chronic hypertension in pregnancy, and thus this measurement can be used for differential diagnosis. The decline in ATIII activity in preeclampsia is not a consequence of liver function disturbances, or increased extrinsic loss (proteinuria), but is caused by increased consumption (Weiner, 1991). A decrease in ATIII activity levels is not useful for early diagnosis (Dekker, 1989; Scholtes, Gerretsen and Haak, 1983; Dekker and Sibai, 1991), although occasionally a patient may show a decrease in ATIII activity more than 10 weeks prior to the development of clinical manifestations (Weiner and Brandt, 1982). Exacerbations and remissions of the disease process are closely reflected in fluctuations of ATIII activity levels. Low ATIII activity levels are strongly associated with placental infarction and adverse perinatal outcome (Weenink *et al.*, 1984; Weiner and Brandt, 1982; Maki, 1983; Graninger *et al.*, 1985).

Preeclampsia may be confused with thrombotic thrombocytopenic purpura (TTP) and hemolytic uremic syndrome (HUS). The differences in maternal serum ATIII activity may aid in the differential diagnosis. ATIII activity is decreased in case of severe preeclampsia–HELLP syndrome, but remains stable in almost all cases of TTP and HUS (Sipes and Weiner, 1992).

Considerable progress has been made in developing enzyme-linked immunoassays that measure complexes of ATIII and thrombin. Thrombin, the key enzyme that converts fibrinogen to fibrin, is gradually inactivated by ATIII. This inactivation proceeds by 1:1 molecular complex formation and concurrent inactivation of the thrombin serine-esterase activity. Therefore, *in vivo* generation of thrombin–ATIII complexes (TAT complexes) is a molecular marker of thrombin formation and thus of activation of the coagulation system and consumption of a major coagulation inhibitor. De Boer *et al.* (1989) and Reinthaller, Mursch-Edlmayr and Tatra (1990) observed an increase in levels of thrombin–ATIII complexes (TAT) in the second and third trimester of normotensive pregnancies. In established preeclampsia TAT levels were more than twice as high as those in gestational age-matched normotensive control women. Further studies are necessary to evaluate if measuring TAT levels is a better way of monitoring preeclampsia than measuring just ATIII activity levels. According to Terao *et al.* (1991), there is no additional gain in measuring TAT complexes as compared to the diagnostic efficacy of ATIII activity as parameter of disease severity.

### 4.11.3 ACTIVATED PROTEIN C (APC) AND PROTEIN S

Activated protein C (aPC), a vitamin-K-dependent serine protease, plays an important regulatory role in blood coagulation through its ability to degrade coagulation factors V and VIII. In addition, aPC activates the fibrinolytic system, probably by destroying fast-acting inhibitors of plasminogen activator. Protein C is activated by thrombin. The activation process is many thousandfold enhanced by interaction of thrombin with an endothelial cell surface factor known as thrombomodulin. Plasma also contains an inhibitor of aPC, which in turn limits the duration of its action. Protein C is highly sensitive to consumption, as may be caused by systemic thrombosis or surgery. Protein C levels are reduced in patients with disseminated intravascular coagulation and liver disease, and patients that use vitamin K antagonists.

Protein S, another vitamin K-dependent protein, has a role as a cofactor for aPC by promoting its binding to lipid and platelet surface, thus localizing the reaction. Protein S normally exists in plasma in two forms: the functionally active free protein S and protein S complexed with C4b-binding protein, which is functionally inactive. Thrombin degrades the protein S–C4b-binding protein complex and releases active free protein S.

In normal pregnancy immunological and functional levels of protein C are similar to non-pregnant women, although protein C inhibitor increases significantly (Stirling *et al.*, 1984; Aznar *et al.*, 1986). Functional and immunological levels of protein S demonstrate a significant reduction during normal pregnancy (third trimester mean = 38%, Comp *et al.*, 1986; Fernandez *et al.*, 1989; de Boer *et al.*, 1989). The reduction in activity appears to be due to a reduction in total protein S as measured antigenically rather than a change in C4b-binding protein.

Only in severe preeclampsia are the immunological and functional levels of protein C reduced (Aznar *et al.*, 1986; Gilabert *et al.*, 1988; de Boer *et al.*, 1989). However, because protein C inhibitor is increased in mild, moderate, and severe preeclampsia, it is likely that functional protein C is also already decreased in mild preeclampsia (Gilabert *et al.*, 1988; de Boer *et al.*, 1989). Because protein C is involved in the tPA-mediated fibrinolysis, the decrease in protein C may be important in causing the hypofibrinolysis found in preeclampsia. Protein S levels in preeclampsia are similar to levels found in uncomplicated pregnancy (Gilabert *et al.*, 1988; de Boer *et al.*, 1989). In the near future, sophisticated methods, such as the measurement of aPC/a1-antitrypsin complex, may turn out to be of help in the early identification of coagulation abnor-malities in the development of preeclampsia (Espana *et al.*, 1991).

### 4.11.4 FIBRINOGEN

In non-pregnant women, the concentration of fibrinogen in plasma is, on the average, about 3 g/l, ranging from about 1.7–4.1 g/l. During uncomplicated pregnancy, the concentration of fibrinogen gradually increases to values of about 4.5 g/l at term. Although the turnover of fibrinogen has been reported to be increased in preeclampsia, fibrinogen levels are normal or even slightly increased in nearly all cases of preeclampsia (Howie, Prentice and McNicol, 1971; Davies and Prentice, 1992). This supports the concept of a compensated localized increased intravascular coagulation in preeclampsia. In very severe cases of HELLP syndrome, and in some cases of eclampsia, especially the post-ictal stage, lowered fibrinogen levels suggest that consumption is exceeding production, and thus implicate the presence of significant DIC and thereby a critical maternal condition. However, most cases of frank hypofibrinogemia in cases of severe preeclampsia–eclampsia are seen in association with placental abruption (Pritchard, Cunningham and Mason, 1976).

### 4.11.5 FIBRINOPEPTIDE A

The action of thrombin on fibrinogen is the crucial step in the coagulation cascade. Thrombin splits two molecules of fibrinopeptide A and two molecules of fibrinopeptide B from fibrinogen. The remaining molecule is called a fibrin monomer and polymerizes rapidly to fibrin. Fibrinopeptide A has a half-life in blood of approximately 3 minutes. Free fibrinopeptides in the blood are a specific measure of thrombin activity and high levels of fibrinopeptide A have been shown to be associated with DIC in pregnancy. Levels of fibrinopeptide A have been reported to be elevated or unchanged in normotensive pregnancy (Douglas *et al.*, 1982a; Maki, 1983;

Wallmo, Karlsson and Teger-Nilsson, 1984; Stirling *et al.*, 1984). Patients with mild to moderate pregnancy-induced hypertensive disorders appear to have normal or slightly increased levels of fibrinopeptide A. In most patients with severe preeclampsia, marked increases in concentrations of fibrinopeptide A are apparent (Douglas *et al.*, 1982a; Wallmo, Karlsson and Teger-Nilsson, 1984; Borok *et al.*, 1984). This suggests that there is an increased activity of the coagulation cascade only in severe disease.

### 4.11.6 FIBRIN MONOMER

After the release of fibrinopeptide A and B from fibrinogen a part of the fibrinogen molecule remains; this part is termed fibrin monomer. Fibrin monomer binds to other monomers or to native fibrinogen and remains in solution until the polymers increase in size and precipitate as fibrin. Until recently, soluble fibrin monomers could only be detected by protamine sulfate or ethanol precipitation assays or by precipitation in the cold (cryofibrinogen). The finding of cryofibrinogen is a rather non-specific finding. Cryofibrinogen may be elevated in severe preeclampsia and the protamine sulfate and ethanol gelation test have been reported to give variable results in pregnancy-induced hypertensive disorders (Howie, Prentice and McNicol, 1971; Gibson *et al.*, 1982; Wallmo, Karlsson and Teger-Nilsson, 1984; Wallenburg, 1987). Specific commercial assays for measuring fibrin monomers are now available. Soluble fibrin complexes made up of fibrin–fibrinogen dimers are increased in conditions of low-grade DIC (Aznar *et al.*, 1982). Soluble fibrin monomer complexes are slightly increased during normal pregnancy (Maki, 1983). Chromatographic study of levels of soluble fibrin complexes demonstrated a further increase of soluble fibrin monomer complexes in pregnancy-induced hypertensive disorders (McKillop *et al.*, 1976; Gibson *et al.*, 1982).

### 4.11.7 FIBRINOLYSIS

Fibrinolysis is caused by the proteolytic enzyme plasmin, which splits polymerized fibrin strands. Plasmin arises from plasminogen by the action of plasminogen activators. There are two types of plasminogen activator: the tissue type (tPA), a serine protease released by endothelial cells, and the urokinase type, which can be found in the plasma as a single-chain proenzyme (scu-PA) and which is converted into a two-chain molecule (tcu-PA) upon activation. tPA is a poor plasminogen activator, except in the presence of fibrin, which increases its activity by a factor of approximately 100. Therefore, all plasminogen activation by tPA is localized inside the fibrin clot. tPA is released into the circulation following a variety of stimuli such as exercise, mental stress, venous occlusion, hypoxia, and the presence of thrombin, vasopressin, adrenaline and bradykinin. Patients with arterial thrombosis, advanced atherosclerotic disease and diabetic vasculopathy have an impaired endothelial tPA release. In plasma, tPA activity is almost negligible. This is due to an excess of free plasminogen activator inhibitor-1 (PAI-1). Up to now at least four immunologically distinct molecules with PAI activity have been identified. These include: PAI-1, the endothelial cell-derived PAI, which is present in plasma and platelets; PAI-2, the placental-type PAI, identified in plasma from pregnant women; PAI-3, which is identical to protein C inhibitor; and finally protease nexin (de Boer *et al.*, 1988). PAI reacts with tPA, scu-PA and aPC.

### 4.11.8 FIBRONECTIN

Fibronectin is a major cell-surface glycoprotein distributed widely in the extracellular matrix of mesenchymal tissues. The soluble form in plasma (mol. wt 450 000) is mainly synthesized by endothelial cells and hepatocytes. Plasma half-life has been estimated to be 24 hours. Fibronectin plays an important role in cell–cell interaction and a wide range of processes vital to homeostasis and tissue repair. Levels of fibronectin decrease in diseases characterized by an increase in intravascular thrombin action and fibrin deposition (Graninger *et al.*, 1985; Eriksen *et al.*, 1987). In contrast to many other laboratory parameters used in obstetrics, fibronectin levels as reported in the literature are remarkably similar. The nephelometric method for measuring plasma fibronectin is a laboratory procedure that is suitable for the average hospital laboratory (van Helden *et al.*, 1985).

In normal pregnancy plasma levels of fibronectin are similar or just slightly increased as compared to non-pregnant individuals. The upper range of normal is 300 mg/l (Stubbs, Lazarchick and Horger, 1984; Graninger *et al.*, 1985; Eriksen *et al.*, 1987; Dekker and Kraayenbrink, 1991).

In pregnancy-induced hypertensive disorders plasma fibronectin levels are elevated. In established preeclampsia most studies show an approximately two- to threefold increase in plasma fibronectin levels. There is almost no overlap in plasma fibronectin levels between normotensive and hypertensive pregnancy. The high fibronectin levels are probably mainly caused by the endothelial cell damage and subsequent repair processes that occur in the uteroplacental vascular bed, kidneys, liver, etc. Platelets contain only 0.5% of the total circulating fibronectin, so the marked increase in plasma fibronectin levels cannot be explained on the basis of accelerated platelet utilization. Pregnancies in women with chronic hypertension have normal fibronectin levels, so the increase in plasma fibronectin is not simply a consequence of hypertension (Taylor *et al.*, 1991). Thus, measuring fibronectin is of great help in the differential diagnosis of high blood pressure in pregnancy (Stubbs, Lazarchick and Horger, 1984; Lazarchick, Stubbs and Romein, 1986; Dekker and Kraayenbrink, 1991; Zeeman *et al.*, 1992). In established preeclampsia, fibronectin levels correlate with low ATIII lev-

els and the degree of proteinuria (Graninger *et al.*, 1985; Stubbs, Lazarchick and Horger, 1984; Lazarchick, Stubbs and Romein, 1986; Saleh *et al.*, 1987). Because fibronectin levels decrease in case of DIC, the increased levels of fibronectin in preeclampsia once again demonstrate that DIC is not involved in the pathogenesis of preeclampsia. Saleh *et al.* (1988) compared the diagnostic accuracy of fibronectin and ATIII in pure preeclampsia and concluded that plasma fibronectin levels are superior to ATIII activity levels in the diagnosis and differential diagnosis of preeclampsia and superimposed preeclampsia. In addition, it is worthwhile to use plasma fibronectin levels for trend detection in established preeclampsia. Patients with severe preeclampsia may demonstrate a sudden further increase in fibronectin level several days before the development of the first laboratory features of HELLP syndrome. A sudden decrease in previously elevated fibronectin levels may indicate DIC.

### 4.11.9 PLATELET ACTIVITY

The platelet count does not change significantly during pregnancy, although there may be a slight fall during the last 8 weeks of pregnancy. This decrease is probably caused by hemodilution and/or a slight, but not significant, decrease in the platelet life-span (Wallenburg and van Kessel, 1978; Rakoczi *et al.*, 1979; Douglas *et al.*, 1982; Fay, Hughes and Farron, 1983; Sill, Lind and Walker, 1985). During uncomplicated pregnancy the platelet count remains within the accepted non-pregnant range (Sejeny, Eastham and Baker, 1975; Fenton, Saunders and Cavill, 1977; Beal and de Masi, 1985; Sill, Lind and Walker, 1985). The peripheral blood platelet count for both non-pregnant and pregnant adults normally ranges from 150 000–400 000/mm$^3$. In term patients, Burrows and Kelton (1988) reported a mean platelet count of 225 × 10$^9$/l with 95% confidence intervals being 109–341 × 10$^9$/l. These levels are below accepted non-pregnant normals. A recent analysis of 6715 deliveries indicated that about 5% of all healthy women will have mild to moderate thrombocytopenia. The platelet count can be as low as $50 \times 10^9/l$ but tends to be above $80 \times 10^9/l$, without consequences for mother and/or baby (Burrows and Kelton, 1990). Burrows and Kelton (1992) stated that it remains uncertain whether any of these patients have mild ITP, but the issue is moot, i.e. all are well and have well infants without any special precautions being taken.

Platelet lifespan is significantly shorter in pregnancy-induced hypertensive disorders, in particular when complicated by fetal growth retardation, as compared to uncomplicated pregnancy (Rakoczi *et al.*, 1979; Wallenburg and van Kessel, 1979; Wallenburg and Rotmans, 1982). There is a good correlation between platelet lifespan, hyperuricemia and the fVIIIrag/fVIIIc ratio (Boneu *et al.*, 1980).

Studies of platelet volume in normal pregnancy have yielded conflicting results, Giles (1981) reported no alteration in platelet numbers or mean platelet volume (MPV) in 1087 normal pregnant women compared to non-pregnant controls. In contrast, Hsieh and Cauchi (1983) reported a fall in MPV in normal pregnancy, most profound in the first trimester but sustained throughout normal pregnancy. Fay, Hughes and Farron (1983) have reported a significant drop in platelet numbers in the last 8 weeks associated with a rise in the MPV in the last 4 weeks of normal gestation, and Sill, Lind and Walker (1985) reported increased MPV and platelet distribution width (PDW) between 34 and 37 weeks. Many studies in women with pregnancy-induced hypertension and preeclampsia have reported changes in platelet numbers, platelet survival and MPV, which have been interpreted as evidence of increased platelet consumption (Singer *et al.*, 1986; Redman, Bonnar and Beilin, 1978, Wallenburg and Rotmans, 1980; Giles, 1981; Hsieh and Cauchi, 1983).

Thrombocytopenia is a common finding (Birmingham Eclampsia Study Group, 1971), is associated with progressive disease (Redman, Bonnar and Beilin, 1978, Trudinger, 1976), and has been shown to be related to disease severity (Howie, Prentice and McNicol, 1971). Changes in platelet size may antedate the clinical findings (Walker *et al.*, 1989). Platelet life span is known to be reduced in PIH (Rakoczi *et al.*, 1979) and this is thought to be secondary to intravascular platelet aggregation and increased adhesion to damaged vascular endothelium. If platelets are activated, betathromboglobulin and serotonin are often increased in the plasma. Increased betathromboglobulin has been found (Douglas *et al.*, 1982b; Socol *et al.*, 1985) but Lang *et al.* (1984) found no increase. Serotonin levels have been found to be raised (Jelen, Fananapazir and Crawford, 1979) in pregnancy-induced hypertension and intraplatelet serotonin levels are decreased (Whigham *et al.*, 1978). Page (1972) suggested that there is varying activation of the coagulation system and platelet aggregation but the trigger to this activity is unknown. It is also not known whether this is a primary or secondary effect. The differences seen may be related to differing disease severities in the study groups. These changes seen in the platelet function are associated with changes seen in the prostaglandin system.

## 4.12 THE ROLE OF THE PROSTAGLANDINS AND VASOACTIVE SUBSTANCES

It is thought that the local effects of the prostanoids, prostacyclin and thromboxane, have a major role to play in the pathophysiology of this disease.

### 4.12.1 PROSTACYCLIN

Prostacyclin ($PGI_2$) is the major product of the arachidonic acid cascade in vascular tissue, and is a potent vasodilator and inhibitor of platelet aggregation (Moncada *et al.*, 1977;

Ritter *et al.*, 1983). It has a short half-life and is usually measured as one of its stable metabolites, such as 6-keto-$PGF_{1\alpha}$. In normal pregnancy, levels of $PGI_2$ rise with gestation (Greer *et al.*, 1985b). In preeclampsia, production of $PGI_2$ from both maternal and fetal vascular tissue has been shown to be reduced (Downing, Shepherd and Lewis, 1980; Remuzzi *et al.*, 1980; Jogee, Myatt and Elder, 1983) and lower levels of amniotic fluid prostacyclin compared to normal pregnancy have also been found (Bodzenta, Thomson and Pollier, 1980; Ylikorkala and Makali, 1985). This reduction in $PGI_2$ may be seen prior to the disease presentation (Greer *et al.*, 1985a; Fitzgerald *et al.*, 1987). High levels of prostacyclin stimulating factor have also been found in patients with pregnancy-induced hypertension suggesting a reduced end-organ response (Remuzzi *et al.*, 1981).

### 4.12.2 THROMBOXANE

Thromboxane $A_2$ is a powerful vasoconstrictor and platelet-aggregating agent (Ylikorkala and Makali, 1985). It is the major product of the arachidonic acid cascade in platelets, and is synthesized and released when platelets aggregate. Increased $TxA_2$ production from placentas and platelets has been shown to occur in pregnancy-induced hypertension (Makila, Viinikka and Ylikorkala, 1984; Fitzgerald *et al.*, 1990; Walsh, 1989).

### 4.12.3 PROSTACYCLIN/THROMBOXANE INTERACTION

Thromboxane $A_2$ and prostacyclin oppose each other through regulation of adenylate cyclase (Tateson, Moncada and Vane, 1977). The proaggregatory substances thromboxane $A_2$ and the endoperoxides $PGG_2$ and $PGG_2$ inhibit adenylate cyclase allowing free intraplatelet $Ca^{++}$ to rise. They also have a direct effect, promoting $Ca^{++}$ release from intracellular storage sites (Gerrard *et al.*, 1977). Platelet inhibitory prostaglandins stimulate

adenylate cyclase, increasing cyclic AMP and reducing $Ca^{++}$ (Tateson, Moncada and Vane, 1977; Gorman, Bunting and Miller, 1977). An increase in intracellular calcium would increase the sensitivity of smooth muscle cells to contract and platelets to aggregate. An increase in intracellular calcium has been found in pregnancy-induced hypertension (Kilby *et al.*, 1990).

It has been suggested that normally a balance exists between $PGI_2$ and $TxA_2$, and that this balance may be upset in pregnancy-induced hypertension (Walsh, 1985). A reduced prostacyclin/thromboxane ratio would account for the increased platelet consumption and the increasing sensitivity to vasoconstrictors and peripheral constriction found in patients with pregnancy-induced hypertension. Experimentally, this increased sensitivity to angiotensin II can be produced in normal pregnancy by the administration of indomethacin, a prostaglandin synthetase inhibitor (Everett *et al.*, 1978).

An imbalance between PGI and TxA could lead to platelet aggregation and the formation of platelet thrombi, and fibrin deposition in the kidney and placenta, causing impairment of these organs. The renal effects of sodium retention and reduced glomerular filtration rates seen in pregnancy-induced hypertension could also be due to the lack of vasodilator and natriuretic $PGE_2$ and $PGI_2$ in the kidney.

Therefore, pregnancy-induced hypertension could be largely a consequence of a prostaglandin deficiency. This could be from either a deficiency of precursors, reduced production or defective action. O'Brien and Broughton Pipkin (1979) showed that, in pregnant rabbits, a restriction of the dietary essential fatty acid precursors of prostaglandins leads to an increased sensitivity towards angiotensin II. However, studies have shown that no more 50% of the patients sensitive to AII infusions will develop preeclampsia (Gant *et al.*, 1973; Wallenburg *et al.*, 1986). This suggests that PGI$_2$ deficiency may not be the primary cause of the disease but may play an important role in the pathophysiology of the condition by altering the patient's response to vasopressor agents.

Prostacyclin infusions have been used successfully in severe pregnancy-induced hypertension (Fidler *et al.*, 1981) where both its vasodilator and antiplatelet effects have been of value. However, PGI$_2$ requires a continuous intravenous infusion and has not been shown to be an efficient antihypertensive agent.

### 4.12.4 OTHER PROSTAGLANDINS

Other prostaglandins have been implicated but the picture is less clear. Demers and Gabbe (1976) showed that PGF$_{2\alpha}$ was elevated and PGE$_2$ low in preeclampsia. Hiller and Smith (1981) found no change and Robinson *et al.* (1979) found both PGE and PGF to be reduced.

### 4.12.5 NITRIC OXIDE

There is no doubt that there is an upset in the prostaglandin biochemistry, most probably related to changes in production of prostacyclin, but similar changes have been implicated in nitric oxide and endothelin production, particularly in the control of placental bed vasculature (Myatt, 1992). Nitric oxide production appears to be increased in normal pregnancy (Weiner *et al.*, 1994; Morris *et al.*, 1994), similar to the changes seen in the levels of prostacyclin (Greer *et al.*, 1985a). There are probably nitric-oxide-dependent and nitric-oxide-independent mechanisms of vasodilatation in pregnancy (Beilin and Chu, 1993).

Animal studies have shown that prolonged blockade of nitric oxide synthesis in gravid rats produces sustained hypertension, proteinuria, thrombocytopenia, and intrauterine growth retardation (Molnar *et al.*, 1994; Yallampalli and Garfield, 1993). Inhibition of nitric oxide augments the vascular angiotensin II reactivity in the pregnant rat hindlimb (Ahokas *et al.*, 1992).

### 4.12.6 SUMMARY OF THE PROSTAGLANDIN AND VASOACTIVE SYSTEMS

Therefore, it may be that there is a general reduction, or lack of increase, in the vasodilator substances in preeclampsia compared with normal pregnancy. The exact timing of these changes may vary. It would appear that deficiency of vasodilator substances is more fundamental to the disease process and the changes in vasoconstrictor substances are pathogenic as the disease progresses. These changes have convinced many that preeclampsia is a vascular endothelial disease (Roberts *et al.*, 1989; Zeeman *et al.*, 1992)

### 4.13 GENERAL CELLULAR ABNORMALITY

Although the above evidence is suggestive of a vascular cell disorder, other changes are suggestive of disorders in function of other cells in the body. These include hepatic cells, platelets, vascular smooth muscle cells, neutrophils, neurons and red cells. This suggests that there may be more fundamental dysfunction of all cellular membranes related to this circulating 'factor X' (Rodgers, Taylor and Roberts, 1988). This may be related to changes in free radical activity and the ability of the different cells to protect themselves against free radical attack (Zeeman *et al.*, 1992; Wisdom *et al.*, 1991). Studies have shown that the red cell in women with preeclampsia is deficient in intracellular free radical scavengers opening them to increased damage and membrane instability (Wisdom *et al.*, 1991; Chen *et al.*, 1994d). Levels of antioxidant activity correlate with plasma levels of prostacyclin and thromboxane in women with pregnancy-induced hypertension (Chen *et al.*, 1993b). These changes, particularly those found with superoxide dismutase (SOD), have also been found in neutrophils. However, normal superoxide-dismutase gene activity has been found in pregnancy-induced hypertension. Therefore, the decreased SOD activity would appear to be a secondary phenomenon (Chen *et al.*, 1994e). Changes in the membrane stability can lead to an influx of calcium into the cell, producing increased activity of the cell and changes in membrane rigidity. These changes in the membrane of the red cell can alter blood rheology.

## 4.14 CHANGES IN RHEOLOGY

Preeclampsia and intrauterine growth retardation are both associated with abnormal hemostasis which may be related to histological evidence of placental intravascular changes (Bonnar, McNicol and Douglas, 1971; Sheppard and Bonnar, 1976; Brosens, Dixon and Robertson, 1977, Howie *et al.*, 1976). Blood flow, and changes in blood rheology that may reduce blood flow, are important factors in determining the amount of oxygen and nutrients transferred across the placenta. Abnormal blood rheology has been found in both preeclampsia and IUGR (Inglis *et al.*, 1982; Buchan, 1982; Hobbs *et al.*, 1982; Thorburn *et al.*, 1982). Lang *et al.* (1984) showed that blood viscosity was increased at high shear rate, due in part to high hematocrit. Blood viscosity was also increased at low shear rate. Some studies (Thorburn *et al.*, 1982) have found reduced red cell deformability when filtration of cells was performed in native plasma but not in donor plasma. This would imply that a plasma factor may be responsible (Inglis *et al.*, 1982). Whole blood viscosity (i.e. red cells in native plasma) at high shear was still elevated after correction to standard hematocrit (Lang *et al.*, 1984). This suggests that red cells are less deformable in preeclampsia, since high shear viscosity is influenced by red cell deformation under high shear conditions. Therefore, the consensus of opinion is that blood viscosity is increased and red cell deformability in native plasma is decreased in preeclampsia (Thorburn *et al.*, 1982; Lang *et al.*, 1984). These

changes will influence blood flow and tissue perfusion. They may also be responsible for some of the changes seen in Doppler ultrasound studies.

## 4.15 HEREDITARY FACTORS

There is increasing evidence that severe preeclampsia is a familial disease (Adams and Finlayson, 1961; Chesley, Annitto and Cosgrove, 1968; Cooper and Liston, 1979). Chesley, Annitto and Cosgrove (1968) traced 96% of the grown daughters of the women who had had eclampsia at the Margaret Hague Maternity Hospital. The incidence of preeclampsia in daughters was 26%. It was 32% in sisters and 16% in granddaughters. Adams and Finlayson (1961), in a study of sisters, found a strong family association. Humphries (1960) looked at the mothers of women who had eclampsia in the Johns Hopkins Hospital in Baltimore. There was an incidence of 28% in the mothers compared with 13% in other random patients. Sutherland *et al.* (1981) studied the mothers and mothers-in-law of patients with severe preeclampsia. The study showed that mothers-in-law did not have an incidence higher than expected (4%) but mothers did (14%). So the condition appears to be passed from mother to daughter and is not transmitted by the husband. Therefore, a single recessive gene in the mother and not the fetus could be responsible for the development of pregnancy-induced hypertension (Cooper and Liston, 1979). This is unlikely to be true, as other factors are undoubtedly involved. It is more likely that the hereditary factors are dominant in nature, with only 50% penetrance. This would allow for the other factors to influence the disease penetration and reduce the incidence of the carrier gene required in the population to support the single recessive gene theory. Incomplete penetrance is very difficult to distinguish from multifactorial inheritance.

Recent studies in Iceland has confirmed this family linkage and the results are consistent with a single-gene dominant inheritance with 48% inheritance (Arngrimsson *et al.*, 1990). This work has led on to investigations of gene linkage within the family groups.

### 4.15.1 ANGIOTENSINOGEN: A CANDIDATE GENE INVOLVED IN PREECLAMPSIA?

Ward *et al.* (1993) reported an association between preeclampsia and a molecular variant (M235T) in the angiotensinogen gene (AGT) on chromosome 1q42-43 in 54 patients from USA and Japan. These was a cohort study. In a study of several generations of women Arngrimsson *et al.* (1993) found further evidence for the role of AGT or a neighboring gene in the predisposition to this heterogeneous condition. The affected pedigree member method was used to study the segregation of a highly informative dinucleotide repeat, from the 3' flanking region of AGT in 22 families with preeclampsia and eclampsia from Iceland and Scotland. This method was developed to detect distortion of independent segregation of the marker and the disease within families. It is robust, depends only on the marker phenotypes of the affected individuals, requires no prior assumption about the mode of inheritance and can accommodate reduced penetrance and heterogeneity in the sample.

The results showed that when women with preeclampsia both with and without proteinuria were classified as affected, a significant allele sharing amongst affected sibs was observed in the total sample. The results from the extended families showed a significant distortion of allele-sharing in families where the proband had preeclampsia. The results from separate analysis of the Scottish and Icelandic data were in good agreement; however, in the five families where the proband had eclampsia no significant distortion was observed. This suggests that the genetic factor may be related to preeclampsia and that eclampsia is related to another, perhaps genetic, cause.

When the more homogenous group of women with only proteinuric preeclampsia was classified as affected, an increased significance level was observed in the families of the preeclamptic probands. The results from the whole sample, i.e. the combined families of pre-eclamptic and eclamptic probands, were also statistically significant. The results for the few affected members in the eclampsia families alone were not statistically significant. The results in the Icelandic and the Scottish preeclamptic families were both significant.

In these families, analysis of allele sharing among affected family members supports the conclusion that molecular variation in AGT or a closely linked gene on chromosome 1q may predispose to preeclampsia. The replication of this finding in samples from two populations in different countries is of relevance in evaluating this evidence. The significance of the results using the affected pedigree member method was most marked when the diagnosis was restricted to proteinuric preeclampsia. This is consistent with the view that women with proteinuric preeclampsia constitute a more homogeneous group compared with the wider definition of preeclampsia where women with high blood pressure alone are included. Moreover the diagnosis of preeclampsia is less ambiguous when it is accompanied by proteinuria (Chesley, 1980b). Inclusion of less severely affected subjects may have led to greater etiological heterogeneity in the sample but it does suggest that at least some of those with non-proteinuric hypertension in pregnancy have a similar etiology and that it may be the same disease in a less severe form.

These observations complement those of Ward *et al.* (1993), who described an association between preeclampsia and angiotensinogen in two other populations. Not only did they use a different approach, namely association analysis in cases and controls, but also a different marker genotype within the angiotensinogen gene. They have shown that a molecular variant in AGT, which has previously been shown to be associated with elevated concentrations of angiotensinogen, higher blood pressure and the risk of essential hypertension (Jeunemaitre *et al.*, 1992), is more frequent in preeclamptic women than in controls and have suggested that the same mechanism may be involved in preeclampsia. This hypothesis is supported by a prospective study which shows that women who develop preeclampsia have higher blood pressure in the first trimester than those who are normotensive and this difference in blood pressure remains throughout the pregnancy (Moutquin *et al.*, 1985). Although not universally agreed, it has also been shown in several studies that women who develop severe preeclampsia or eclampsia are at higher risk of developing essential hypertension than normotensive women, particularly if preeclampsia occurred early in the pregnancy (Sibai *et al.*, 1986; Lindeberg *et al.*, 1988). Furthermore, subjects with preeclampsia are more likely to have a family history of essential hypertension than normotensive women (Lindeberg *et al.*, 1988) and their offspring have higher blood pressure (Seidman *et al.*, 1991). Angiotensinogen may, however, represent a linked marker for a neighboring gene. Study of further families with preeclampsia and eclampsia with a battery of polymorphic markers for this region on chromosome 1 will help to exclude genetic heterogeneity and allow confirmation of this finding and precise identification of the gene, which may be one of several factors involved in the development of preeclampsia.

## 4.16 MISCELLANEOUS FACTORS

The condition is thought to be more frequent in the obese (Oats *et al.*, 1983) and it appears to be related to the weight at the start of pregnancy (Peckham and Christianson, 1971). However, fat women have higher blood pressure and it is difficult to measure as the arm is too big for a normal sphygmomanometer cuff.

There are no differences in the incidence of preeclampsia in the different social classes (Duffus and McGillivray, 1968) except for a slight increase found in social class III. Women who smoke have a lower incidence of disease (Duffus and McGillivray, 1968) but if preeclampsia develops, it tends be of a more severe form than average. Although it has been advocated that eclampsia was partly due to dietary deficiencies (MacGillivray and Johnstone, 1978), there is little evidence of this. Brewer (1969) agreed but based his argument on the fact that the incidence of preeclampsia was higher in underprivileged black groups. This difference found in social groups is not universal (Duffus and McGillivray, 1968) and some of the changes may be racial rather than social. Others found that diet has no effect on the incidence but may affect outcome (MacGillivray, 1981).

## 4.17 DISCUSSION

Much of what has been described are epiphenomena that relate to each other. They are not in themselves causes of preeclampsia. There are however two basic abnormalities that are persistently found.

1. **Abnormalities of placentation**, evidence of which can be found early in pregnancy before the clinical manifestations of the disease are apparent. Preeclampsia is also associated with excessive placentation, as in twin and molar pregnancies. It is obvious that patients may carry the susceptibility to vascular reactivity, as described by Wallenburg *et al.* (1986), without developing preeclampsia. What is required is a further trigger which would come from the placenta. The stimulus would be produced either from the ischemic, small, poorly implanted placenta of classic preeclampsia or from a large placenta found in a multiple pregnancy. This suggests that the placenta is the source of a 'factor X' that can cause the systemic manifestations of the

condition. The vascular reactivity is also associated with other vessel wall functional abnormalities such as changes in the coagulation system and platelet activation.

2. **Abnormalities of platelet–vessel-wall interaction**, leading to increased vascular sensitivity and platelet consumption. The vascular activity also appears to antedate the clinical signs of preeclampsia. These changes may be mediated through a dysfunction of the vascular endothelial cell which is part of a generalized cellular dysfunction.

There appears to be no difference between the placental changes found in preeclampsia and IUGR. The reason that some patients present with high blood pressure probably involves their hereditary tendencies. The risk of convulsion appears to be related to the patient's seizure threshold as it is not directly related to the blood pressure alone.

Therefore, most of the clinical signs found in this condition can be explained from these two main 'primary' problems: placentation and vascular endothelial dysfunction.

This does not explain why these events occur.

There is strong evidence that there is an immunological role in preeclampsia. The immunological influence is most likely to be involved in the initial implantation abnormalities leading to the spiral artery pathology related to placental insufficiency.

There is also strong evidence of an hereditary role. This could be involved in the vascular sensitivity seen by Gant *et al.* (1973) and Wallenburg *et al.* (1986) . If this was true, it could not be an autosomal recessive disorder but is more likely to be an autosomal dominant with incomplete, around 50%, penetrance. This would fit the results described by Wallenburg *et al.* (1986) and Arngrimsson *et al.* (1990).

Many of these pathological findings relate to the risks of the condition to the mother and baby described in Chapter 3 and can be used

in the monitoring of the mother (Chapter 7) and fetus (Chapter 8).

## REFERENCES

Acosta Sison, H. (1931) Clinicopathologic study of eclampsia based upon 38 autopsied cases. *J. Obstet. Gynaecol.*, **22**, 35–39.

Adams, E. M. and Finlayson, A. (1961) Familial aspects of pre-eclampsia and hypertension in pregnancy. *Lancet*, **ii**, 1375–1379.

Ahokas, R. A. and Sibai, B. M. (1992) Endothelium-derived relaxing factor in hibition augments vascular angiotensin-II reactivity in the pregnant rat hind limb. *Am. J. Obstet. Gynecol.*, **167**, 1053–1058.

Altchek, A. (1961) Electron microscopy of renal biopsies in toxemia of pregnancy. *J. A. M. A.*, **175**, 791–795.

Altchek, A. (1964) Renal biopsy and its clinical correlation in toxemia of pregnancy. *Circulation*, **30**, 43–47.

Altchek, A., Albright, N. L. and Sommers, S. C. (1968) The renal pathology of toxaemia of pregnancy. *Obstet. Gynecol.*, **31**, 594–598.

Arngrimsson, R., Bjornsson, S., Geirsson, R. T. *et al.* (1990) Genetic and familial predisposition to eclampsia and pre-eclampsia in a defined population. *Br. J. Obstet. Gynaecol.*, **97**, 762–769.

Arngrimsson, R., Purandare, S., Connor, M. *et al.* (1993) Angiotensinogen – a candidate gene involved in preeclampsia. *Nat. Genet.*, 4, 114–115.

Assali, N. S., Douglass, R. A., Baird, W. W. and Nicholson, D. B. (1954) Measurement of uterine blood flow and uterine metabolism with the $N_2O$ method in normotensive and toxemic pregnancies. *Clin. Res. Proc.*, **2**, 102–106.

Aznar, J., Gilabert, J., Estelles, A. *et al.* (1982) Evaluation of the soluble fibrin monomer complexes and other coagulation parameters in obstetric patients. *Thromb. Res.*, **27**, 691–701.

Aznar, J., Gilabert, J., Estelles, A. *et al.* (1986) Fibrinolytic activity and protein C in preeclampsia. *Thromb. Haemostasis*, **55**, 314–317.

Baird, D., Thomson, A. M. and Billewicz, W. Z. (1955) Birth weight and placental weight in preeclampsia. *J. Obstet. Gynaecol. Br. Emp.*, **64**, 370–374.

Baker, P. N., Broughton Pipkin, F. and Symonds, E. M. (1992) Comparative-study of platelet angiotensin-II binding and the angiotensin-II sensitivity test as predictors of pregnancy-induced hypertension. *Clin. Sci.*, **83**, 89–95.

Ballegeer, V., Spitz, B., Kieckens, L., *et al.* (1989) Predictive value of increased plasma levels of fibronectin in gestational hypertension. *Am. J. Obstet. Gynecol.*, **161**, 432–436.

Ballegeer, V. C., Spitz, B., De Baene, L. A. *et al.*, (1992) Platelet activation and vascular damage in gestational hypertension. *Am. J. Obstet. Gynecol.*, **166**, 629–633.

Bastiaanse, N. A. and Mastboom, J. L. (1950) Ischaemia of the gravid uterus as a possible factor in the causation of toxaemia of pregnancy, in *Toxaemia of Pregnancy, Human and Veterinary*, (eds J. Hammond, F. J. Browne and G. E. W. Wolstenholme), J. & A. Churchill, London, p. 182–191.

Beal, D. W. and de Masi, A. D. (1985) Role of the platelet count in the management of the high-risk obstetric patient. *J. A. O. A.*, **85**, 252–255.

Beaufils, M., Uzan, S., Don Simoni, R. *et al.* (1981) Metabolism of uric acid in normal and pathologic pregnancy. *Contr Nephrol.*, **25**, 132–136.

Beilin, L. J. and Chu, Z. M. (1993) Nitric-oxide-dependent and nitric-oxide-independent mechanisms of vasodilation in pregnancy. *J. Hypertens.*, **11**, S148–S149.

Beker, J. C. (1948) Aetology of eclampsia. *J. Obstet. Gynaecol. Br. Emp.*, **55**, 756–760.

Bell, E. T., Dieckmann, W. J. and Eastmann, J. (1940) Classification of the toxaemias of pregnancy. *Mother*, **1**, 13–17.

Bennett, B. and Ratnoff, O. D. (1972) Changes in AHF procoagulant activity and AHF-like antigen in normal pregnancy and following exercise and pneumoencephalography. *J. Lab. Clin. Med.*, **80**, 256–263.

Birmingham Eclampsia Study Group (1971) Intravascular coagulation and abnormal lung scans in pre-eclampsia and eclampsia. *Lancet*, **ii**, 889–893.

Bischof, P. (1981) Pregnancy associated plasma protein A – an inhibitor of the complement system. *Placenta*, **2**, 29–33.

Bodzenta, A., Thomson, G. M.,and Pollier, L. (1980) Prostacyclin activity in amniotic fluid in pre-eclampsia. *Lancet*, **ii**, 650–654.

Boneu, B., Durand, D., Counilla, F. *et al.* (1975) Factor VIII complex and endothelial damage. *Lancet*, **i**, 1430.

Boneu, B., Fournie, A., Sie, P. *et al.* (1980) Platelet production time, uricemia, and some hemostasis tests in pre-eclampsia. *Eur. J. Obstet. Gynecol. Reprod. Biol.*, **11**, 85–94.

Bonnar, J., McNicol, G. P. and Douglas, A. S. (1971) Coagulation and fibrinolytic systems in pre-eclampsia and eclampsia. *Br. Med. J.*, **ii**, 12–16.

Borok, Z., Weitz, J., Owen, J. *et al.* (1984) Fibrinogen proteolysis and platelet α-granule release in preeclampsia/eclampsia. *Blood*, **63**, 525–531.

Brewer, T. (1969) Nutrition and preeclampsia. *Obstet. Gynecol.*, **33**, 448–449.

Brosens, I., Dixon, H. G. and Robertson, W. B. (1977) Fetal growth retardation and the arteries of the placental bed. *Br. J. Obstet. Gynaecol.*, **84**, 656–663.

Brosens, I., Robertson, W. B. and Dixon, H. G. (1970) The role of the spiral arteries in the pathogenesis of pre-eclampsia. *J. Pathol.*, **101**, 6–10.

Broughton Pipkin, F. (1976) The renin–angiotensin system in normal and abnormal pregnancy. *Anaesthesia*, **31**, 848–852.

Browne, F. J. (1946) Sensitization of the vascular system in pre-eclampsic toxaemia and eclampsia. *J. Obstet. Gynaecol. Br. Emp.*, **53**, 510–514.

Browne, F. J. and Dodds, G. H. (1939) Remote prognosis of toxaemias of pregnancy based on follow-up study of 40 patients in 589 pregnancies for periods varying from 6 months to 12 years. *J. Obstet. Gynaecol. Br. Emp.*, **46**, 443–447.

Browne, F. J. and Shaimich, D. R. (1956) Chronic hypertension following preeclampsic toxaemia. The influence of familial hypertension on its causation. *J. Obstet. Gynaecol. Br. Emp.*, **63**, 573–576.

Browne, J. C. M. and Veall, N. (1953) The maternal placental blood flow in normotensive and hypertensive women. *J. Obstet. Gynaecol. Br. Emp.*, **60**, 141–145.

Buchan, P. C. (1982) Preeclampsia – a hyperviscosity syndrome. *Am. J. Obstet. Gynecol.*, **142**, 111–112.

Burrows, R. F. and Kelton, J. G. (1988) Incidentally detected thrombocytopenia in healthy mothers and their infants. *N. Engl. J. Med.*, **319**, 142–145.

Burrows, R. F. and Kelton, J. G. (1990) Thrombocytopenia at delivery. A prospective survey of 6,715 deliveries. *Am. J. Obstet. Gynecol.*, **162**, 731–734.

Burrows, R. F. and Kelton, J. G. (1992) Thrombocytopenia during pregnancy, in *Haemostasis and Thrombosis in Obstetrics and Gynaecology*, 1st edn, (eds I. A. Greer, A. G. G. Turpie and C. D. Forbes), Chapman & Hall, London, p. 408–429.

Burt, C. C. (1950) The peripheral circulation in pregnancy. *Edin. Med. J.*, **57**, 18–22.

Butterworth, B. H., Greer, I. A., Liston, W. A. *et al.* (1991) Immunocytochemical localization of neutrophil elastase in term placenta decidua and myometrium in pregnancy-induced hypertension. *Br. J. Obstet. Gynaecol.*, **98**, 929–933

Cadden, J. F. and Stander, H. J. (1939) Uric acid metabolism in eclampsia. *Am. J. Obstet. Gynecol.*, **37**, 37–47.

Campbell, D. M., MacGillivray, I. and Thompson, B. (1977) Twin zygosity and pre-eclampsia. *Lancet*, **ii**, 97–101.

Campbell, S. Pearce, J. M., Hackett, G. *et al.* (1986) Qualitative assessment of uteroplacental blood flow: early screening test for high-risk pregnancies. *Obstet. Gynecol.*, **68**, 649–653.

Cavanagh, D., Rao, P. S., Tsai, C. C. and O'Connor, T. C. (1977) Experimental toxemia in the pregnant primate. *Am. J. Obstet. Gynecol.*, **128**, 75–85.

Chamberlain, G. V. P., Phillip, E., Howlett, B. and Masters, K. (1978) *British Births 1970, 2: Obstetric Care*, Heinemann, London, p. 80–84.

Chen, C., Wilson, R., Cumming, G. *et al.* (1993a) Production of prostacyclin and thromboxane A$_2$ in mononuclear cells from preeclamptic women. *Am. J. Obstet. Gynecol.*, **169**, 1106–1111.

Chen, G., Wilson, R., Cumming, G. *et al.* (1993b) Prostacyclin, thromboxane and antioxidant levels in pregnancy-induced hypertension. *Eur. J. Obstet. Gynecol. Reprod. Biol.*, **50**, 243–250.

Chen, G., Wilson, R., Cumming, G. *et al.* (1994a) Immunological changes in pregnancy-induced hypertension. *Eur. J. Obstet. Gynecol. Reprod. Biol.*, **53**, 21–25.

Chen, G., Wilson, R., Cumming, G. *et al.* (1994b) Antioxidants and immunological markers in pregnancy-induced hypertension and essential hypertension in pregnancy. *J. Maternal–Fetal Med.*, **3**, 132–138.

Chen, G., Wilson, R., McKillop, J. H. and Walker, J. J. (1994c) The role of cytokines in the production of prostacyclin and thromboxane in human mononuclear cells. *Immunol. Invest.*, **23**, 269–279.

Chen, G., Wilson, R., Cumming, G. *et al.* (1994d) Intracellular and extracellular antioxidant buffering levels in erythrocytes from pregnancy-induced hypertension. *J. Hum. Hypertens.*, **8**, 37–42.

Chen, G., Wilson, R., Boyd, P. *et al.* (1994e) Normal superoxide-dismutase (*sod*) gene in pregnancy-induced hypertension – is the decreased *sod* activity a secondary phenomenon? *Free Radical Res.*, **21**, 59–66.

Chesley L. C. and Williams, L. O. (1945) Renal glomerular and tubular functions in relation to the hyperuricemia of pre-eclampsia and eclampsia. *Am. J. Obstet. Gynecol.*, **50**, 367–375.

Chesley, L. C. (1950) Simultaneous renal clearances of urea and uric acid in the differential diagnosis of the late toxemias. *Am. J. Obstet. Gynecol.*, **59**, 960–969.

Chesley, L. C. (1966) Sodium retention and pre-eclampsia. *Am. J. Obstet. Gynecol.*, **95**, 127–131.

Chesley, L. C. (1976) False steps in the study of preeclampsia. *Perspect. Nephrol. Hypertension*, **5**, 1–10.

Chesley, L. C. (ed. ) (1978) *Hypertensive Disorders in Pregnancy*, Appleton-Century-Crofts, New York.

Chesley, L. C. (1980a) Evolution of concepts of eclampsia, in *Pregnancy Hypertension*, (eds J. Bonnar, I. MacGillivray and E. M. Symonds), MTP Press, Lancaster, p. 1–4.

Chesley, L. C. (1980b) The remote prognostic significance of the level of blood pressure in pregnancy. *Clin. Exp. Hypertension*, **2**, 777–801.

Chesley, L. C., Annitto, J. E. and Cosgrove, R. A. (1961) Pregnancy in the sisters and daughters of eclamptic women. *Pathol. Microbiol.*, **24**, 662–666.

Chesley, L. C., Annitto, J. E. and Cosgrove, R. A. (1968) The familial factor in toxemia of pregnancy. *Obstet. Gynecol.*, **32**, 303–307.

Chesley, L. C., Cosgrove, S. A. and Preece, J. (1946) Hydatidiform mole with special reference to recurrence and associated eclampsia. *Am. J. Obstet. Gynecol.*, **52**, 311–315.

Chesley, L. C. and Duffus, G. M. (1971) Preeclampsia, posture and renal function. *Obstet. Gynecol.*, **38**, 1–5.

Chesley, L. C., Lindheimer, M. D. (1988) Renal hemodynamics and intravascular volume in normal and hypertensive pregnancy, in *Handbook of Hypertension, vol. 10: Hypertension in Pregnancy*, 1st edn, (ed. P. C. Rubin), Elsevier, Amsterdam, p. 38–65.

Chesley, L. C., Talledo, E., Bohler, C. S. and Zuspan, F. P. (1965) Vascular reactivity to angiotensin II and norepinephrine in pregnant and non-pregnant women. *Am. J. Obstet. Gynecol.*, **91**, 837–841.

Chesley, L. C. and Valenti, C. (1958) The evaluation of tests to differentiate pre-eclampsia from hypertensive disease. *Am. J. Obstet. Gynecol.*, **75**, 1165–1173.

Comp, P. C., Thurnau, G. R., Welsh, J. *et al.* (1986) Functional and immunologic protein S levels are decreased during pregnancy. *Blood*, **68**, 881–885.

Cooper, D. W. and Liston, W. A. (1979) Genetic control of severe pre-eclampsia. *J. Med. Genet.*, **16**, 409–413.

Cooper, D. W., Hill, J. A., Chesley, L. C. and Bryans, C. I. (1988) Genetic control of susceptibility to eclampsia and miscarriage. *Br. J. Obstet. Gynaecol.*, **95**, 644–653.

Currie, G. A. and Bagshawe, K. D. (1967) The masking of antigens on ttrophoblastic and cancer cells. *Lancet*, **ii**, 708–712.

Davies, A. M. (1971) *Geographical Epidemiology of the Toxemias of Pregnancy*, Charles C. Thomas, Springfield, IL.

Davies, J. A. and Prentice, C. R. M. (1992) Coagulation changes in pregnancy-induced hypertension and growth retardation, in *Haemostasis and Thrombosis in Obstetrics and Gynaecology*, 1st edn, (eds I. A. Greer, A. G. G. Turpie and C. D. Forbes), Chapman & Hall, London, p. 143–162.

de Boer, K., ten Cate, J. W., Struk, A. *et al.* (1989) Enhanced thrombin generation in normal and hypertensive pregnancy. *Am. J. Obstet. Gynecol.*, **160**, 95–100.

de Boer, K., Lecander, I., ten Cate, J. W. *et al.* (1988) Placental-type plasminogen activator inhibitor in preeclampsia. *Am. J. Obstet. Gynecol.*, **158**, 518–522.

Dekker, G. A. (1989) Prediction and prevention of pregnancy-induced hypertensive disorders: a clinical and pathophysiologic study. Academic Thesis, Erasmus University Rotterdam.

Dekker, G. A. and Kraayenbrink, A. A. (1991) Oxygen free radicals in preeclampsia. *Am. J. Obstet. Gynecol.*, **S164**, 273.

Dekker, G. A., Makovitz, J. W. and Wallenburg, H. C. (1990) Prediction of pregnancy-induced hypertensive disorders by angiotensin II sensitivity and supine pressor test. *Br. J. Obstet. Gynaecol.*, **97**, 817–821.

Dekker, G. A. and Sibai, B. M. (1991) Early detection of preeclampsia. *Am. J. Obstet. Gynecol.*, **165**, 160–172.

Dekker, G. A. and Sibai, B. M. (1992) Pathophysiology of hypertensive disorders, in *Principles and Practice of Medical Therapy in Pregnancy*, 2nd edn, (ed. N. Gleicher), Appleton & Lange, Norwalk, CT, p. 845–852.

Demers, L. M. and Gabbe, S. G. (1976) Placental prostaglandin levels in pre-eclampsia. *Am. J. Obstet. Gynecol.*, **126**, 137–141.

Desmedt, E. J., Henry, O. A. and Beischer, N. A. (1990) Polyhydramnios and associated maternal and fetal complications in singleton pregnancies. *Br. J. Obstet. Gynaecol.*, **97**, 1115–1122.

De Valera, E. and Kellar, R. J. (1948) On the effects of vasopressin on toxaemias of pregnancy. *J. Obstet. Gynaecol. Br. Emp.*, **55**, 815–819.

Dexter, L. and Weiss, S. (1941) *Preeclamptic and Eclamptic Toxaemia of Pregnancy*, Little, Brown & Co., Boston, MA.

DHSS (1969) *Report on Confidential Enquiries into Maternal Deaths in England and Wales 1964–66*, HMSO, London.

DHSS (1974) *Report on Confidential Enquiries into Maternal Deaths in England and Wales 1970–72*, HMSO, London.

DHSS (1979) *Report on Confidential Enquiries into Maternal Deaths in England and Wales 1973–75*, HMSO, London.

DHSS, Welsh Office, Scottish Home and Health Department (1991) *Report on Confidential Enquiries into Maternal Deaths in the United Kingdom 1985–87*, HMSO, London.

DHSS, Welsh Office, Scottish Home and Health Department (1994) *Report on Confidential Enquiries into Maternal Deaths in the United Kingdom 1988–90*, HMSO, London.

Dieckmann, W. J. (1929) The hepatic lesions in eclampsia. *Am. J. Obstet. Gynecol.*, **17**, 454–458.

Dieckmann, W. J. (1952) *The Toxemias of Pregnancy*, 2nd edn, C. V. Mosby, St Louis, MO, p. 305–311.

Dixon, H. G. and Robertson, W. B. (1958) A study of the vessels of the placental bed in normotensive and hypertensive women. *J. Obstet. Gynaecol. Br. Emp.*, **65**, 803–807.

Douglas, J. T., Shah, M., Lowe, G. D. O. *et al.* (1982a) Plasma fibrinopeptide A and beta-thromboglobulin in pre-eclampsia and pregnancy hypertension. *Thromb. Haemostasis*, **47**, 54–55.

Douglas, J. T., Lowe, G. D., Forbes, C. D. and Prentice, C. R. (1982b) Beta-thromboglobulin and platelet counts – effect of malignancy, infection, age and obesity. *Thromb. Res.*, **25**, 459–464.

Downing, I., Shepherd, G. L. and Lewis, P. J. (1980) Reduced prostacyclin production in pre-eclampsia. *Lancet*, **ii**, 1374–1378.

Duffus, G. M. and McGillivary, I. (1968) The incidence of pre-eclampsia in smokers and non-smokers. *Lancet*, **i**, 994–998.

Duffus, G. M., Tunstall, N. E., Condie, R. G. and MacGillivray, I. (1969) Chlormethiazole in the prevention of eclampsia and the reduction of perinatal mortality. *J. Obstet. Gynaecol. Br. Commonw.*, **76**, 645–649.

Dunlop, W. (1981) Serial changes in renal hemodynamics during normal human pregnancy. *Br. J. Obstet. Gynaecol.*, **88**, 1–9.

Dunlop, W., Hill, L. M., Landon, M. J. *et al.* (1978) Clinical relevance of coagulation and renal changes in pre-eclampsia. *Lancet*, **ii**, 346–348.

Eriksen, H. O., Hansen, P. K., Brocks, V. *et al.* (1987) Plasma fibronectin concentration in normal pregnancy and pre-eclampsia. *Acta Obstet. Gynecol. Scand.*, **66**, 25–28.

Espana, F., Gilabert, J., Aznar, J. *et al.* (1991) Complexes of activated protein C with α1-antitrypsin in normal pregnancy and in severe preeclampsia. *Am. J. Obstet. Gynecol.*, **164**, 1310–1316.

Everett, R. B., Worley, R. J., MacDonald, P. C. and Gant, N. F. (1978) Effect of prostaglandin synthetase inhibitors on pressor response to angiotensin II in human pregnancy. *J. Clin. Endocrinol. Metab.*, **46**, 1007–1010.

Fadel, H. E., Northrop, G. and Misenhimer, H. R. (1976) Hyperuricemia in pre-eclampsia: a reappraisal. *Am. J. Obstet. Gynecol.*, **125**, 640–647.

Faulk, W. P., Carbonara, A. and Jeannet, M. (1973) Immunological studies of the human placenta, in *Immunology of Reproduction*, (eds K. Bartanova, R. G. Edwards, V. H. Vulchanova *et al.*), Bulgarian Academy of Sciences, Sofia, p. 405–409.

Fay, R. A., Hughes, A. O.and Farron, N. T. (1983) Platelets in pregnancy: hyperdestruction in pregnancy. *Obstet. Gynecol.*, **61**, 238–240.

Feeney, J. G., Tovey, L. A. D. and Scott, J. S. (1977) Influence of previous blood tranfusions on incidence of pre-eclampsia. *Lancet*, **i**, 874–878.

Fenton, V., Saunders, K. and Cavill, I. (1977) The platelet count in pregnancy. *J. Clin. Pathol.*, **30**, 68–69.

Fernandez, J. A., Estelles, A., Gilabert, J. *et al.* (1989) Functional and immunologic protein S in normal pregnant women and in full term neonates. *Thromb. Haemostasis*, **61**, 474–478.

Fidler, J., Bennet, M. J., DeSweit, M. *et al.* (1981) Treatment of pregnancy hypertension with prostacyclin. *Lancet*, **ii**, 31–35.

Fitzgerald, D. J., Entman, S. S., Mulloy, K. and FitzGerald, G. A. (1987) Decreased prostacyclin biosynthesis preceding the clinical manifestation of pregnancy-induced hypertension. *Circulation*, **75**, 956–963.

Fitzgerald, D. J., Rocki, W., Murray, R. *et al.*. (1990) Thromboxane A$_2$ synthesis in pregnancy-induced hypertension. *Lancet*, **335**, 751–754.

Fournie, A., Monrozies, M., Pontonnier, G. *et al.* (1981) Factor VIII complex in normal pregnancy, pre-eclampsia and fetal growth retardation. *Br. J. Obstet. Gynaecol.*, **88**, 250–254.

Fox, H. (1978) *Pathology of the Placenta*, W. B. Saunders, London.

Friedman, S. A. (1988) Preeclamsia: a review of the role of prostaglandins. *Obstet. Gynecol.*, **71**, 122–137.

Gallery, E. D. M., Hunyor, S. N. and Gyory, A. Z. (1979) Plasma volume contraction: a significant factor in both pregnancy-associated hypertension (pre-eclampsia) and chronic hypertension in pregnancy. *Q. J. Med.*, **48**, 593–602.

Gant, N., Daley, G., Chand, S. *et al.* (1973) A study of angiotensin II, pressor response throughout primigravida pregnancy. *J. Clin. Invest.*, **52**, 2682–2686.

Gant, N. F., Worley, R. J., Everett, R. B. and MacDonald, P. C. (1980) Control of vascular responsiveness during human pregnancy. *Kidney Int.*, **18**, 253–257.

Gerrard, J. M., Peller, J. D., Krick, T. P. and White, J. G. (1977) Cyclic AMP and platelet prostaglandin synthesis. *Prostaglandins*, **14**, 39–50.

Gibson, B., Hunter, D., Neame, P. B. *et al.* (1982) Thrombocytopenia in preeclampsia and eclampsia. *Semin. Thromb. Haemostasis*, **8**, 234–247.

Gilabert, J., Fernandez, F., Espana, F. *et al.* (1988) Physiological coagulation inhibitors (protein S, protein C and antithrombin III) in preeclamptic states and in users of oral contraceptives. *Thromb. Res.*, **49**, 319–329.

Giles, C. (1981) The platelet count and mean platelet volume. *Br. J. Haematol.*, **48**, 31–37.

Gilstrap, L. C. and Gant, N. F. (1990) Pathophysiology of preeclampsia. *Semin. Perinatol.* **14**, 147–151.

Golan, A. and White, R. G. (1979) Spontaneous rupture of the liver associated with pregnancy. A report of 5 cases. *S. Afr. Med. J.*, **56**, 133–136.

Goldby, F. S. and Beilin, L. J. (1972) Relationship between arterial pressure and the permiability of arterioles to carbon particles in acute hypertension. *Cardiovasc. Res.*, **6**, 384–388.

Gorman, R. R., Bunting, S. and Miller, O. V. (1977) Modulation of human platelet adenylate cyclase by prostacyclin (PGX). *Prostaglandins*, **13**, 377–388.

Govan, A. D. T. (1961) The pathogenesis of eclamptic lesions. *Pathol. Microbiol.*, **24**, 561–565.

Graninger, W., Tatra, G., Pirich, K. *et al.* (1985) Low antithrombin III and high plasma fibronectin in pre-eclampsia. *Eur. J. Obstet. Gynecol. Reprod. Biol.*, **19**, 223–229.

Greer, I. A., Walker, J. J., Cameron, A. D. *et al.* (1985a) A prospective longitudinal study of immunoreactive prostacyclin and thromboxane metabolites in normal and hypertensive pregnancy. *Clin. Exp. Hypertension (B)*, B4, nos 2&3–2&4.

Greer, I. A., Walker, J. J., McLaren, M. *et al.* (1985b) Immunoreactive prostacyclin and thromboxane metabolites in normal pregnancy and the puerperium. *Br. J. Obstet. Gynaecol.*, **92**, 581–585.

Greer, I. A., Dawes, J., Johnston, T. A. and Calder, A. A. (1991a) Neutrophil activation is confined to the maternal circulation in pregnancy-induced hypertension. *Obstet. Gynecol.*, **78**, 28–32.

Greer, I. A., Leask, R., Hodson, B. A. *et al.* (1991b) Endothelin, elastase, and endothelial dysfunction in preeclampsia. *Lancet*, **337**, 558.

Guyton, A. C., Hall, J. E., Coleman, T. G. *et al.* (1990) The dominant role of the kidneys in the long-term regulation of arterial pressure in normal and hypertensive states, in *Hypertension: Pathophysiology, Diagnosis, and Management*, 1st edn, (eds J. H. Laragh and B. M. Brenner), Raven Press, New York, p. 1029–1052.

Hamlin, R. H. J. (1952) The prevention of eclampsia and pre-eclampsia. *Lancet*, **i**, 64–68.

Harding, V. J. and Van Wyck, H. B. (1930) Effects of hypertonic saline in the toxaemias of pregnancy. *Br. Med. J.*, **ii**, 589–593.

Hardy, T. J. and Williams, P. B. (1988) Pre-eclampsia: a hypothesis for its etiology. *Med. Hypotheses*, **27**, 157–162.

Harpel, P. C. (1987) Blood proteolytic enzyme inhibitors: their role in modulating blood coagulation and fibrinolytic enzyme pathways, in *Hemostasis and Thrombosis. Basic Principles and Clinical Practice*, 2nd edn, (eds R. W. Colman, J. Hirsch, V. J. Marder and E. W. Salzman), J. B. Lippincott, Philadelphia, PA, p. 219–234.

Hathaway, W. E. and Bonnar, J. (1987) Physiology of coagulation in pregnancy, in *Hemostatic Disorders of the Pregnant Woman and Newborn Infant*, 1st edn, John Wiley, Chichester, p. 39–56.

Hayashi, T., Baldrigde, R. C., Olmsted, P. S. *et al.* (1964) Purine nucleotide catabolism in placenta. *Am. J. Obstet. Gynecol.*, **88**, 470–478.

Hellgren, M. and Blomback, M. (1981) Studies on blood coagulation and fibrinolysis in pregnancy, during delivery and in the puerperium. I. Normal condition. *Gynecol. Obstet. Invest.*, **12**, 141–154.

Hertig, A. T. (1945) Vascular pathology in the hypertensive albuminuric toxaemias of pregnancy. *Clinics*, **4**, 602–606.

Hiller, K. and Smith, M. D. (1981) Prostaglandin E and F concentrations in placentae of normal hypertensive and pre-eclamptic patients. *Br. J. Obstet. Gynaecol.*, **88**, 274–278.

Hirsch, J. (1987) Laboratory diagnosis of thrombosis, in *Hemostasis and Thrombosis. Basic Principles and Clinical Practice*, 2nd edn, (eds R. W. Colman, J. Hirsch, V. J. Marder and E. W. Salzman), J. B. Lippincott, Philadelphia, PA, p. 1165–1183.

Hobbs, J. B., Oats, J. N., Palmer, A. A. *et al.* (1982) Whole blood viscosity in preeclampsia. *Am. J. Obstet. Gynecol.*, 142, 288–292.

Howie, P. W., Prentice, C. R. M. and McNicol, G. P. (1971) Coagulation fibrinolysis and platelet function in pre-eclampsia, essential hypertension and placental insufficiency. *J. Obstet. Gynecol. Br. Commonw.*, **78**, 992–1003.

Howie, P. W., Begg, C. B., Purdie, D. W. and Prentice, C. R. (1976) Use of coagulation tests to predict the clinical progress of pre-eclampsia. *Lancet*, **ii**, 323–325.

Hoyer, L. W. (1987) Factor VIII, in *Hemostasis and Thrombosis. Basic Principles and Clinical Practice*, 2nd edn, (eds R. W. Colman, J. Hirsch, V. J. Marder and E. W. Salzman), J. B. Lippincott, Philadelphia, PA, p. 48–59.

Hsieh, C. and Cauchi, M. N. (1983) Platelet and complement changes in preeclampsia. *J. Obstet. Gynaecol.*, **3**, 165–196.

Humphries, J. O. (1960) A recurance of hypertensive toxaemia of pregnancy in mother–daughter pairs. *Bull. John Hopkins Hosp.*, **107**, 271–275.

Ingerslev, M. and Teilum, G. (1946) Biopsy studies of the liver in pregnancy. *Acta Obstet. Gynecol. Scand.*, **25**, 339–343.

Inglis, T. C. M., Stuart, J., George, A. J. *et al.* (1982) Haemostatic and rheological changes in normal pregnancy and pre-eclampsia. *Br. J. Obstet. Haematol.*, **56**, 461–465.

Jeffcoatte, T. N. A. and Scott, J. S. (1959) Some observations on the placental factor in pregnancy toxemia. *Am. J. Obstet. Gynecol.*, **77**, 475–479.

Jelen, I., Fananapazir, L. and Crawford, T. B. B. (1979) The possible relationship between late pregnancy hypertension and 5-hydroxytryptamine in maternal blood. *Br. J. Obstet. Gynaecol.*, **86**, 468–472.

Jeunemaitre, X., Soubrier, F., Kotelevtsev, Y. V. *et al.* (1992) Molecular-basis of human hypertension – role of angiotensinogen. *Cell*, **71**, 169–180.

Jogee, M., Myatt, L. and Elder, M. G. (1983) Decreased prostacyclin production by placental cells in culture form pregnancies complicated by fetal growth retardation. *Br. J. Obstet. Gynaecol.*, **90**, 247–251.

Jong de, C. L. D., Dekker, G. A. and Sibai, B. M. (1991) The renin–angiotensin system in preeclampsia; a review. *Clin. Perinatol.*, **18**, 683–711.

Kilby, M. D., Pipkin, F. B., Cockbill, S. *et al.* (1990) A cross-sectional study of basal platelet intracellular free calcium concentration in normotensive and hypertensive primigravid pregnancies. *Clin. Sci.*, **78**, 75–80.

Kitzmiller, K. L. and Benirschke, K. (1973) Immunofluorescent study of the placental bed vessels in pre-eclampsia of pregnancy. *Am. J. Obstet. Gynecol.*, **115**, 248–252.

Lang, G. D., Lowe, G. D., Walker, J. J. *et al.* (1984) Blood rheology in pre-eclampsia and intrauterine growth retardation: effects of blood pressure reduction with labetalol. *Br. J. Obstet. Gynaecol.*, **91**, 438–443.

Larkin, H., Gallery, E. D., Hunyor, S. N. *et al.* (1980) Haemodynamics of hypertension in pregnancy assessed by M-mode echocardiography. *Clin. Exp. Pharmacol. Physiol.*, **7**, 463–468.

Lazarchick, J., Stubbs, T. M. and Romein L. A. (1986) Factor VIII procoagulant antigen levels in normal pregnancy and preeclampsia. *Ann. Clin. Lab. Sci.*, **16**, 395–398.

Lim, Y. L. and Walters, W. A. W. (1979) Haemodynamics of mild hypertension in pregnancy. *Br. J. Obstet. Gynaecol.*, **86**, 198–202.

Lindeberg, S., Axelsson, O., Jorner, U. *et al.* (1988) *Acta Obstet. Gynecol. Scand.*, **67**, 605–609.

Lindheimer, M. D. and Katz, A. I. (1991) The kidney and hypertension in pregnancy, in *The Kidney*, 3rd edn, (eds B. M. Brenner and F. C. Rector), W. B. Saunders, Philadelphia, PA, p. 1551–1595.

Lockwood, C. J. and Peters, J. H. (1990) Increased plasma levels of ED1+ cellular fibronectin precede the clinical signs of preeclampsia. *Am. J. Obstet. Gynecol.*, **162**, 358–362.

Lopez Llera, M. and Hernandez Horta, J. L. (1974) Pregnancy after eclampsia. *Am. J. Obstet. Gynecol.*, **119**, 193–198.

Lunell, N. O., Njemdahl, P., Fredholm, B. B. *et al.* (1982) Acute effects of labetalol on maternal metabolism and uteroplacental circulation in hypertension in pregnancy, in *The Investigation of Labetalol in the Management of Hypertension in Pregnancy*, (eds A. Riley and E. M. Symonds), Excerpta Medica, Amsterdam, p. 34–8.

Lyall, F., Greer, I. A., Boswell, F. *et al.* (1994) The cell adhesion molecule, VCAM-1, is selectively elevated in serum in pre-eclampsia: does this indicate the mechanism of leucocyte activation? *Br. J. Obstet. Gynaecol.* 101, 485–487.

McCartney, C. P. (1964) Pathological anatomy of acute hypertension of pregnancy. *Circulation*, **30**, 37–41.

MacGillivray, I. (1958) Some observations on the incidence of pre-eclampsia. *J. Obstet. Gynaecol. Br. Emp.*, **65**, 536–540.

MacGillivray, I. (1961) Hypertension in pregnancy and its consequences. *J. Obstet. Gynaecol. Br. Emp.*, **68**, 557–561.

MacGillivray, I. (1981) Raise blood pressure in pregnancy. Aetiology of preeclampsia. *Br. J. Hosp. Med.*, August, 110–114.

MacGillivray, I. and Campbell, D. M. (1980) The relevance of hypertension and oedema in pregnancy. *Clin. Exp. Hypertension*, **2**, 897–914.

MacGillivray, I. and Johnstone, F. D. (1978) Dietary protein and pre-eclampsia, in *Hypertensive Disorders of Pregnancy*, (eds F. K. Beller and I. MacGillivray), Georg Theime, Stuttgart, p. 81–85.

MacGillivray, I., Rose, G. and Rowe, B. (1969) Blood pressure survey in pregnancy. *Clin. Sci.*, **37**, 395–399.

McKay, D. G., Merrill, S. J., Weiner. A. E. *et al.* (1953) The pathologic anatomy of eclampsia, bilateral renal cortical necrosis, pituitary necrosis, and other acute fatal complications of pregnancy, and its possible relationship to the generalized Schwartzman phenomenon. *Am. J. Obstet. Gynecol.*, **66**, 507–539.

McKillop, C., Howie, P. W., Forbes, C. D. *et al.* (1976) Soluble fibrinogen/fibrin complexes in pre-eclampsia. *Lancet*, i, 56–58.

McParland, P., Pearce, J. M. and Chamberlain, G. V. (1990) Doppler ultrasound and aspirin in recognition and prevention of pregnancy-induced hypertension. *Lancet*, **335**, 1552–1555.

Maki, M. (1983) Coagulation, fibrinolysis, platelet and kinin forming systems during toxemia of pregnancy. *Biol. Res. Pregn. Perinat.*, **4**, 152–154.

Makila, U. M., Viinikka, L. and Ylikorkala, O. (1984) Increased thromboxane A$_2$ production but normal prostacyclin by the placeta in hypertensive pregnancies. *Prostaglandins*. **27**, 87–91.

Massiani, Z. M., Sanguinetti, R., Gallegos, R. and Raimondi, D. (1967) Angiotensin blood levels in normal and toxaemic pregancy. *Am. J. Obstet. Gynecol.*, **313**, 99–103.

Molnar, M., Suto, T., Toth, T. and Hertelendy, F. (1994) Prolonged blockade of nitric-oxide synthesis in gravid rats produces sustained hypertension, proteinuria, thrombocytopenia, and intrauterine growth-retardation. *Am. J. Obstet. Gynecol.*, **170**, 1458–1466.

Moncada, S., Herman, A. G., Higgs, E. A. and Vane, J. R. (1977) Differential formation of prostacyclin (PGX or PGI$_2$) by layers of the arterial wall: an explanation for the anti-thrombotic properties of vascular endothelium. *Thromb. Res.*, **11**, 323–327.

Moore, M. P. and Redman, C. W. (1983) Case control study of severe pre-eclampsia of early onset. *Br. Med. J.*, **2**, 580–584.

Morris, N. H., Carroll, S. Nicolaides, K. H. *et al.* (1994) Nitric-oxide production during human pregnancy assessed in amniotic fluid and exhaled breath. *J. Physiol. (Lond.)*, **477P**, P34.

Moutquin, J. M., Rainville, C., Giroux, L. *et al.* (1985) A prospective study of blood pressure in pregnancy: prediction of preeclampsia. *Am. J. Obstet. Gynecol.*, **151**, 191–196.

Munro Kerr, J. M. (1933) Maternal morbidity and mortality: a study of their problems, E. & S. Livingstone, Edinburgh.

Myatt, L. (1992) Current topic – control of vascular resistance in the human placenta. *Placenta*, **13**, 329–341.

Nachman, R. L., Jaffe, E. A. (1980) Platelet–endothelial cell–VIII axis, in *Hemostasis, Prostaglandins and Renal Disease*, (eds G. Remuzzi, G. Mecca and G. de Gaetano), Raven Press, New York, p. 5–10.

Nelson, T. R. (1955a) A clinical study of pre-eclampsia. Part 2. *J. Obstet. Gynaecol. Br. Emp.*, **62**, 58–62.

Nelson, T. R. (1955b) A clinical study of pre-eclampsia. Part 1. *J. Obstet. Gynaecol. Br. Emp.*, **62**, 48–52.

Oats, J. N., Abell, D. A., Andersen, H. M. and Beischer, N. A. (1983) Obesity in pregnancy. *Compr. Ther.*, **9**, 51–55.

O'Brien, P. M. and Broughton Pipkin, F. (1979) The effects of deprivation of prostaglandin precursors on vascular sensitivity to angiotensin II and on the kidney in the pregnant rabbit. *Br. J. Pharmacol.*, **65**, 29–34.

Oian, P. and Maltau, J. M. (1987) Calculated capillary hydrostatic pressure in normal pregnancy and preeclampsia. *Am. J. Obstet. Gynecol.*, **157**, 102–106.

Page, E. W. (1939) The relation between hydatid moles, relative ischaemia of the gravid uterus, and the placental origin of eclamsia. *Am. J. Obstet. Gynecol.*, **37**, 291–295.

Page, E. W. (1972) On the pathogenesis of pre-eclampsia and eclampsia. *J. Obstet. Gynaecol. Br. Commonw.*, **79**, 883–894.

Peckham, C. H. and Christianson, R. E. (1971) The relationship between prepregnancy weight and certain obstetric factors. *Am. J. Obstet. Gynecol.*, **111**, 1–7.

Perry, K. G. and Martin, J. N. (1992) Abnormal hemostasis and coagulopathy in preeclampsia and eclampsia. *Clin. Obstet. Gynecol.*, **35**, 338–350.

Petrucco, O. M. (1981) Aetiology of pre-eclampsia, in *Progress in Obstetrics and Gynaecology 1*, (ed. J. W. W. Studd), Churchill Livingstone, Edinburgh, p. 51–58.

Petrucco, O. M., Thomson, N. M., Lawrence, J. R. and Weldon, M. W. (1974) Immunofluorescent studies in renal biopsies in pre-eclampsia. *Br. Med. J.*, **i**, 473–476.

Plentl, A. A. and Gray, M. J. (1959) Total body water, sodium space and total exchangeable sodium in normal and toxaemic pregnant women. *Am. J. Obstet. Gynecol.*, **78**, 472–476.

Pollak, V. E. and Nettles, J. B. (1960) The kidney in toxaemia of pregnancy. A clinical and pathologic study based on renal biopsies. *Medicine*, **39**, 469–473.

Pritchard, J. A., Cunningham, F. G. and Mason, R. A. (1976) Coagulation changes in eclampsia: their frequencies and pathogenesis. *Am. J. Obstet. Gynecol.*, **124**, 855–864.

Raab, W., Schroeder, G., Wagner, R. and Giegee, W. (1956) Vascular reactivity and electrolytes in normal and toxaemic pregnancy. *J. Clin. Endocrinol.*, **16**, 1196–1200.

Rakoczi, I., Tallian, F., Bagdany, S. and Gati, I. (1979) Platelet life-span in normal pregnancy and pre-eclampsia as determined by a non-radioisotope technique. *Thromb. Res.*, **15**, 553–556.

Redman, C. W., Bonnar, J. and Beilin, L. J. (1978) Early platelet consumption in pre-eclampsia. *Br. Med. J.*, **i**, 146–150.

Redman, C. W. G., Denson, K. W. E., Beilin, L. J. *et al.* (1977) Factor VIII consumption in pre-eclampsia. *Lancet*, **ii**, 1249–1252.

Redman, C. W., Bodmer, J., Bodmer, W. F. *et al.* (1978) HLA antigens in severe pre-eclampsia. *Lancet*, **ii**, 397–401.

Reinthaller, A., Mursch-Edlmayr, G. and Tatra, G. (1990) Thrombin-antithrombin III complex in normal pregnancy with hypertensive disorders and after delivery. *Br. J. Obstet. Gynaecol.*, **97**, 506–510.

Remuzzi, G., Marchesi, B., Zoja, S. B. *et al.* (1980) Reduced umbilical and placental vascular prostacyclin in severe pre-eclampsia. *Prostaglandins*, **20**, 105–109.

Remuzzi, G., Zoja, C., Marchesi, D. *et al.* (1981) Plasmatic regulation of the vascular prostacyclin in pregnancy. *Br. Med. J.*, **282**, 512–516.

Ritter, J. M., Blair, I. A., Barrow, S. E. and Dollery, C. T. (1983) Release of prostacyclin *in vivo* and its role in man. *Lancet*, **i**, 317–321.

Roberts, J. M., Taylor, R. N., Musci, T. J. *et al.* (1989) Preeclampsia: an endothelial cell disorder. *Am. J. Obstet. Gynecol.*, **161**, 1200–1204.

Robertson, W. B. (1976) Utero-placental vasculature. *J. Clin. Pathol. Suppl.*, **29**, 1009–1014.

Robertson, W. B., Brosens, I. and Dixon, H. G. (1967) The pathological response of the vessels of the placental bed to hypertensive pregnancy. *J. Pathol. Bacteriol.*, **93**, 581–585.

Robinson, J. S., Redman, C. W., Clover, L. and Mitchell, M. D. (1979) The concentrations of the prostaglandins E and F, 13 14-dihydro-15-oxo-prostaglandin F and thromboxane $B_2$ in tissues obtained from women with and without pre-eclampsia. *Prostaglandins Med.*, **3**, 223–234.

Rodgers, G. M., Taylor, R. N. and Roberts, J. M. (1988) Preeclampsia is associated with a serum factor cytotoxic to human endothelial cells. *Am. J. Obstet. Gynecol.*, **159**, 908–914.

Ruggeri, Z. M. (1980) Endothelium, fVIII/ von Willbrand factor, in *Hemostasis, Prostaglandins and Renal Disease*, (eds G. Remuzzi, G. Mecca and G. de Gaetano), Raven Press, New York, p. 11–20.

Saleh, A. A., Bottoms, S. F., Welch, R. A. *et al.* (1987) Preeclampsia, delivery and the hemostatic system. *Am. J. Obstet. Gynecol.*, **157**, 331–336.

Saleh, A. A., Bottoms, S. F., Norman, G. *et al.* (1988) Hemostasis in hypertensive disorders of pregnancy. *Obstet. Gynecol.*, **71**, 719–722.

Schmorl, R. and Veit, P. (1933) Quoted in *Maternal Mortality and Morbidity*, (ed. J. M. Munro Kerr), E. & S. Livingstone, Edinburgh, p. 361–365.

Scholtes, M. C. W., Gerretsen, G. and Haak, H. L. (1983) The factor VIII ratio in normal and pathological pregnancies. *Eur. J. Obstet. Gynecol. Reprod. Biol.*, **16**, 89–95.

Scott, J. R. and Beer, A. A. (1976) Immunologic aspects of pre-eclampsia. *Am. J. Obstet. Gynecol.*, **125**, 418–422.

Seidman, D. S., Laor, A., Gale, R. *et al.* (1991) Pre-eclampsia and offspring's blood pressure, cognitive ability and physical development at 17 years of age. *Br. J. Obstet. Gynaecol.*, **98**, 1009–1014.

Sejeny, S. A., Eastham, R. D., Baker, S. R. (1975) Platelet counts during normal pregnancy. *J. Clin. Pathol.*, **28**, 812–813.

Sheehan, H. L. (1950) Pathological lesions in the hypertensive toxaemias of pregnancy, in *Toxaemias of Pregnancy*, (eds J. Hammond, F. J. Browne and G. E. W. Wolstenholme), J & A Churchill, London.

Sheehan, H. L. (1980) Renal morphology in preeclampsia. *Kidney Int.*, **18**, 241–252.

Sheehan, H. L. and Lynch, J. B. (1973) *Pathology of Toxaemia of Pregnancy*, Churchill Livingstone, Edinburgh.

Sheppard, B. L. and Bonnar, J. (1976) The ultrastructure of the arterial supply of the human placenta in pregnancy complicated by fetal growth retardation. *Br. J. Obstet. Gynaecol.*, **83**, 948–959.

Sheppard, B. L. and Bonnar, J. (1981) An ultrastructural sudy of uteroplacental spiral arteries in hypertensive and normotensive pregnancy and fetal growth retardation. *Br. J. Obstet. Gynaecol.*, **88**, 695–699.

Sibai, B. M., El-Nazer, A. and Gonsalez-Ruiz, A. (1986) *Am. J. Obstet. Gynecol.*, 155, 1011–1016.

Siddiqi, T., Rosenn, B., Mimouni, F. *et al.* (1991) Hypertension during pregnancy in insulin-dependent diabetic women. *Obstet. Gynecol.*, **77**, 514–519.

Sill, P. R., Lind, T. and Walker, W. (1985) Platelet values during normal pregnancy. *Br. J. Obstet. Gynaecol.*, **92**, 480–483.

Singer, C. R. J., Walker, J. J., Cameron, A. D. and Fraser, C. (1986) Platelet studies in normal pregnancy and pregnancy-induced hypertension. Clin Lab Haem **8**, 27–31.

Sipes, S. L. and Weiner, C. P. (1992) Coagulation disorders in pregnancy, in *Medicine of the Fetus and Mother*, 1st edn, (eds E. A. Reece, J. C. Hobbins, M. J. Mahoney and R. H. Petrie), J. B. Lippincott, Philadelphia, PA, p. 1111–1138.

Slemons, J. M. and Bogert, L. J (1917) The uric acid content of maternal and fetal blood. *J. Biol. Chem.*, **32**, 63–69.

Socol, M. L., Weiner, C. P., Louis, G. *et al.* (1985) Platelet activation in preeclampsia. *Am. J. Obstet. Gynecol.*, **151**, 494–497.

Speroff, L., Glass, R. H. and Kase, N. G. (1983) Prostaglandins, in *Clinical Gynecologic Endocrinology and Infertility*, 2nd edn, Williams & Wilkins, Baltimore, MD, p. 307–333.

Stirling, Y., Woolf, L., North, W. R. S. *et al.* (1984) Haemostasis in normal pregnancy. *Thromb. Haemostasis*, **52**, 176–182.

Stubbs, T. M., Lazarchick, J. and Horger, E. O. III (1984) Plasma fibronectin levels in pre-eclampsia: a possible marker for vascular endothelial damage. *Am. J. Obstet. Gynecol.*, **150**, 885–889.

Sutherland, A., Cooper, D. W., Howie, P. W. *et al.* (1981) Incidence of severe pre-eclampsia amongst mothers and mothers-in-law of pre-eclampsics and controls. *Br. J. Obstet. Gynaecol.*, **88**, 75–79.

Symonds, E. M. (1981) The renin–angiotensin system in pregnancy. *Obstet. Gynecol. Annu.*, **10**, 45–67.

Symonds, E. M., Broughton Pipkin, F. and Craven, D. J. (1975) Changes in the renin angiotnesin system in primigravidae with hypertensive disease of pregnancy. *Br. J. Obstet. Gynaecol.*, **82**, 643–647.

Talledo, O. E., Chesley, L. C. and Zuspan, F. P. (1968) Renin–angiotensin system in normal and toxaemic pregnancies. *Am. J. Obstet. Gynecol.*, **100**, 218–222.

Tateson, J. E., Moncada, S. and Vane, J. R. (1977) Effects of prostacyclin (PGX) on cyclic AMP concentrations in human platelets. *Prostaglandins*, **13**, 389–397.

Taylor, R. N., Crombleholme, W. R., Friedman, S. A. *et al.* (1991) High plasma cellular fibronectin levels correlate with biochemical and clinical features of preeclampsia but cannot be attributed to hypertension alone. *Am. J. Obstet. Gynecol.*, **165**, 895–901.

Tenney, B. and Parker, F. (1940) The placenta in toxaemia of pregnancy. *Am. J. Obstet. Gynecol.*, **39**, 1000–1004.

Terao, T., Maki, M., Ikenoue, T *et al.* (1991) The relationship between clinical signs and hypercoagulable state in toxemia of pregnancy. *Gynecol. Obstet. Invest.*, **31**, 74–85.

Theobald, G. W. (1933) The relationship of the albuminuria of pregnancy to chronic nephritis. *Lancet*, **i**, 626–630.

Thomson, A. M., Hytten, F. E. and Billewicz, W. Z. (1967) The epidemiology of oedema during pregnancy. *J. Obstet. Gynaecol. Br. Commonw.*, **74**, 1–10.

Thorburn, J., Drummond, M. M., Wigham, K. A. *et al.* (1982) Blood viscosity and haemostatic factors in late pregnancy, pre-eclampsia and fetal growth retardation. *Br. J. Obstet. Gynaecol.*, **89**, 117–121.

Thornton, C. A. and Bonnar, J. (1977) Factor VIII-related antigen and factor VIII coagulant activity in normal and pre-eclamptic pregnancy. *Br. J. Obstet. Gynaecol.*, **84**, 919–923.

Trudinger, B. J. (1976) Platelets and intrauterine growth retardation in pre-eclampsia. *Br. J. Obstet. Gynaecol.*, **83**, 284–286.

Tschopp, T. B., Weiss, H. J. and Baumgarter, H. R. (1974) Decreased adhesion of platelets to subendothelium in Von Willebrand's disease. *J. Lab. Clin. Med.*, **83**, 296–300.

Tunbridge, R. D. G. and Donnia, P. (1981) Plasma noradrenaline in normal pregnancy and in hypertension of late pregnancy. *Br. J. Obstet. Gynaecol.*, **88**, 105–109.

Turnbull, A. C. (1987) Maternal mortality and present trends, in *Hypertension in Pregnancy. Proceedings of the Sixteenth Study Group of the Royal College of Obstetricians and Gynaecologists*, (eds F. Sharp and E. M. Symonds), Perinatology Press, Ithaca, NY, p. 135–144.

Turnbull, A., Tindall, V. R., Beard, R. W. *et al.* (1989) *Report on Confidential Enquiries Into Maternal Deaths in England and Wales 1982–1984*, DHSS, London, vol. 34, p. 1–166.

van Helden, W. C. H., Kok-Verspuy, A., Harff, G. A. *et al.* (1985) Rate-nephelometric determination of fibronectin in plasma. *Clin. Chem.*, **31**, 1182–1184.

van Royen E. A. and ten Cate, J. W. (1973) Antigen-biological activity ratio for factor VIII in late pregnancy. *Lancet*, **ii**, 449–450.

Vassalli, P., Morris, R. H. and McClusky, R. T. (1963) The pathologenic role of fibrin deposition in the glomerular lesions of toxaemia of pregnancy. *J. Exper. Med.*, **118**, 467–471.

Walker, J. J., Cameron, A. D., Bjornsson, S. *et al.* (1989) Can platelet volume predict progressive hypertensive disease in pregnancy? *Am. J. Obstet. Gynecol.*, **161**, 676–679.

Wallenburg, H. C. S. (1987) Changes in the coagulation system and platelets in pregnancy-induced hypertension and preeclampsia, in *Hypertension in Pregnancy. Proceedings of the Sixteenth Study Group of the Royal College of Obstetricians and Gynaecologists*, (eds F. Sharp and E. M. Symonds), Perinatology Press, Ithaca, NY, p. 227–248.

Wallenburg, H. C. S. and Rotmans, N. (1980) Circulating large platelets and platelet turnover in normotensive and hypertensive pregnancies with insufficient fetal growth, in *Pregnancy Hypertension*, (eds M. B. Sammour, E. M. Symonds, F. P. Zuspan and N. El Tomi), Aim Shams University Press, Cairo.

Wallenburg, H. C. S. and Rotmans, N. (1982) Enhanced reactivity of the platelet thromboxane pathway in normotensive and hypertensive pregnancies with insufficient fetal growth. *Am. J. Obstet. Gynecol.*, **144**, 523–528.

Wallenburg, H. C. S. and van Kessel, P. H. (1978) Platelet lifespan in normal pregnancy as determined by a nonradioisotopic technique. *Br. J. Obstet. Gynaecol.*, **85**, 33–36.

Wallenburg, H. C. S. and van Kessel, P. H. (1979) Platelet life span in pregnancies resulting in small-for-gestational age infants. *Am. J. Obstet. Gynecol.*, **134**, 739–742.

Wallenburg, H. C. S. and van Kreel, B. K. (1978) Transfer and dynamics of uric acid in the pregnant rhesus monkey. I. Transplacental and renal uric acid clearances. *Eur. J. Obstet. Gynecol. Reprod. Biol.*, **8**, 211–217.

Wallenburg, H. C. S., Dekker, G. A., Makovitz, J. W. and Rotmans, P. (1986) Low dose aspirin prevents pregnancy induced hypertension and pre-eclampsia in angiotensin sensitive primigravidae. *Lancet*, **i**, 1–5.

Wallmo, L., Karlsson, K. and Teger-Nilsson, A. C. (1984) Fibrinopeptide and intravascular coagulation in normotensive and hypertensive pregnancy and parturition. *Acta Obstet. Gynecol. Scand.*, **63**, 637–640.

Walsh, S. W. (1985) Preeclampsia: an imbalance in placental prostacyclin and thromboxane production. *Am. J. Obstet. Gynecol.*, **152**, 335–340.

Walsh, S. W. (1989) Thromboxane production in placentas of women with preeclampsia. *Am. J. Obstet. Gynecol.*, **160**, 1535–1536.

Ward, K., Hata, A., Jeunemaitre, X. *et al.* (1993) A molecular variant of angiotensinogen associated with preeclampsia. *Nat. Genet.*, **4**, 59–61.

Weenink, G. H., Borm, J. J. J., Cateten, J. W. *et al.* (1983) Antithrombin III levels in normotensive and hypertensive pregnancy. *Gynecol. Obstet. Invest.*, **16**, 230–242.

Weenink, G. H., Treffers, P. E., Vijn, P. *et al.* (1984) Antithrombin III levels in preeclampsia correlate with maternal and fetal mobidity. *Am. J. Obstet. Gynecol.*, **148**, 1092–1097.

Weiner, C. P. (1991) Preeclampsia–Eclampsia Syndrome and Coagulation. *Clin. Perinatol.*, **18**, 713–726.

Weiner, C. P. and Brandt, J. (1980) Plasma antithrombin III activity in normal pregnancy. *Obstet. Gynecol.*, **56**, 601–603.

Weiner, C. P. and Brandt, J. (1982) Plasma antithrombin III activity: an aid in the diagnosis of preeclampsia–eclampsia. *Am. J. Obstet. Gynecol.*, **142**, 275–281.

Weiner, C. P., Knowles, R. G. and Moncada, S. (1994) Induction of nitric-oxide synthases early in pregnancy. *Am. J. Obstet. Gynecol.*, **171**, 838–843.

Weinstein, L. (1982) Syndrome of hemolysis, elevated liver enzymes, and low platelet count: a severe consequence of hypertension in pregnancy. *Am. J. Obstet. Gynecol.*, **142**, 159–167.

Weir, R. J., Brown, J. J., Fraser, R. *et al.* (1973) Plasma renin substrate angiotensin II and aldosterone in hypertensive disease of pregnancy. *Lancet*, **i**, 291–295.

Whigham, K. A., Howie, P. W., Drummond, A. H. and Prentice, C. R. (1978) Abnormal platelet function in pre-eclampsia. *Br. J. Obstet. Gynaecol.*, **85**, 28–32.

Whigham, K. A. E., Howie, P. W., Shah, M. M. *et al.* (1980) Factor VIII related antigen/coagulant activity ratio as a predictor of fetal growth retardation: a comparison with hormone and uric acid measurements. *Br. J. Obstet. Gynaecol.*, **87**, 797–803.

Wisdom, S. J., Wilson, R., McKillop, J. H. and Walker, J. J. (1991) Antioxidant systems in normal pregnancy and in pregnancy-induced hypertension. *Am. J. Obstet. Gynecol.*, **165**, 1701–1704.

Yallampalli, C. and Garfield, R. E. (1993) Inhibition of nitric-oxide sythesis in rats during pregnancy produces signs similar to those of preeclampsia. *Am. J. Obstet. Gynecol.*, **169**, 1316–1320.

Ylikorkala, O. and Makali, U. M. (1985) Prostacyclin and thromboxane in gynecology and obstetrics. *Am. J. Obstet. Gynecol.*, **152**, 318–322.

Zangemeister, W. (1903) Untersuchungen über die Blutbeschaffenheit und die Harnsekretion bei Eclampsie. *Zentralbl. Gynäkol.*, **50**, 385–389.

Zeeman, G. G., Dekker, G. A., van Geijn, H. P. and Kraayenbrink, A. A. (1992) Endothelial function in normal and pre-eclamptic pregnancy: a hypothesis. *Eur. J. Obstet. Gynecol. Reprod. Biol.*, **43**, 113–122.

Zhou, Y., Damsky, C. H., Chiu, K., Roberts, J. M. and Fisher, S. J. (1993) Preeclampsia is associated with abnormal expression of adhesion molecules by invasive cytotrophoblasts. *J. Clin. Invest.*, **91**, 950–960.

Zuspan, F. P. (1979) Catecholamines. Their role in pregnancy and the development of pregnancy-induced hypertension. *J. Reprod. Med.*, **23**, 143–147.

Zweifel, P. (1916) Eklampsie, in *Handbuch der Gerburtshilfe, II*, (ed. A. Doderlein), Bergman, Wiesbaden, p. 672–676.

# HEMODYNAMIC CHARACTERIZATION OF SEVERE PREGNANCY-INDUCED HYPERTENSION

*Wesley Lee and David B. Cotton*

## 5.1 INTRODUCTION

Over recent years, investigators have studied maternal circulatory alterations to improve our understanding about severe pregnancy-induced hypertension (PIH). We will summarize current concepts about these changes and outline clinical indications for hemodynamic monitoring in patients with severe PIH. Much of the information obtained by pulmonary artery catheterization and non-invasive Doppler ultrasound have suggested a broad spectrum of hemodynamic findings in these patients. However, a detailed review of these observations must consider gestational age, severity of disease, and the potential effect of medical therapy before one can better understand the natural history of this disorder

## 5.2 INVASIVE STUDIES

Central hemodynamic measurements from severely preeclamptic women appear to represent a broad spectrum of hemodynamic findings The most comprehensive series include hypertensive gravidas from Baylor College of Medicine (Houston, TX), University of Tennessee (Memphis, TN), and Erasmus University School of Medicine (Rotterdam, Netherlands) These studies provide important information about cardiac output, systemic vascular resistance and left ventricular performance associated with severe PIH. The major findings, similarities and differences between these investigations are outlined below to provide a framework for interpreting the results.

Cotton *et al.* (1988) prospectively studied 45 gravidas by right heart catheterization at Baylor College of Medicine to characterize the hemodynamic profile of severe PIH. All patients had been started on intravenous magnesium sulfate for at least 1 hour prior to baseline measurements. No antihypertensive medications were administered before pulmonary artery catheterization. Intravenous fluids were minimized at 75 ml/h. The mean gestational age of this group was $35.4 \pm 6$ weeks (range 27–41.5 weeks); 14 women (31%) had eclamptic seizures prior to baseline measurements; six women had chronic hypertension with superimposed PIH; 13 women were in early labor; only two women experienced pulmonary edema. Hemodynamic measurements are summarized in Table 5.1.

*Hypertension in Pregnancy*
Edited by J.J. Walker and N.F. Gant. Published by Chapman & Hall, 1997 ISBN 0 412 30910 6

**Table 5.1**   Hemodynamic profile of severe PIH – Baylor College of Medicine (Source: Cotton *et al.*, 1988, Hemodynamic profile of severe pregnancy-induced hypertension. *Am. J. Obstet. Gynecol.*, *158*, 523–9)

| Parameter | Measurement | Range |
|---|---|---|
| Systolic BP (mmHg) | 193 ± 3 | (150–236) |
| Diastolic BP (mmHg) | 110 ± 2 | (65–140) |
| CVP (mmHg) | 4 ± 1 | (0–12) |
| PCWP (mmHg) | 10 ± 1 | (4–30) |
| Heart rate (beats/min) | 95 ± 2 | (69–129) |
| SV index (ml/beat/min) | 44 ± 1 | (24–65) |
| Cardiac index (l/min/m$^2$) | 4.14 ± 0.13 | (2.43–5.91) |
| PVRI (dyne.sec. cm$^{-5}$) | 127 ± 9 | (43–304) |
| SVRI (dyne.sec. cm$^{-5}$) | 2726 ± 120 | (1146–4996) |

These measurements were further stratified into low, normal and high categories based upon estimated normal ranges for pregnant women (Figure 5.1).

Normal ranges included:

1. cardiac index (CI): 3–5 l/min/m$^2$;
2. systemic vascular resistance index (SVRI): 1500–2200 dyn.s/cm$^5$;
3. pulmonary capillary wedge pressure (PCWP): 6–12 mmHg;

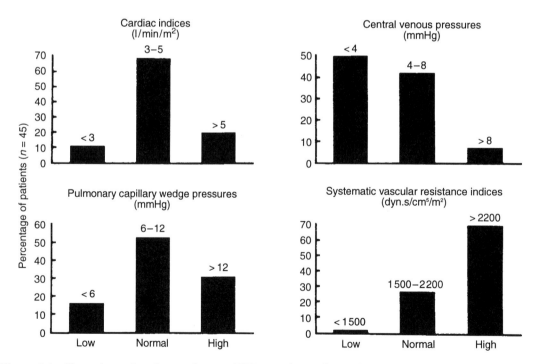

**Figure 5.1**   Hemodynamic subsets of severe PIH – Baylor College of Medicine. (Redrawn with permission from Cotton et al., 1988, Hemodynamic profile of severe pregnancy-induced hypertension. *Am. J. Obstet. Gynecol.*, **158**, 523-9.)

When summarized in this manner, 69% of these women had a normal CI. Nine women (20%) had an elevated CI as compared to only five women (11%) with low values. A total of 32 women (71%) had increased SVRI with the majority of the remaining patients having high normal values. The majority of women were also observed to have normal to high PCWP measurements and low to normal CVP values. Some 80% (35 women) demonstrated hyperdynamic left ventricular function and a Starling curve shifted upward and to the left (Figure 5.2).

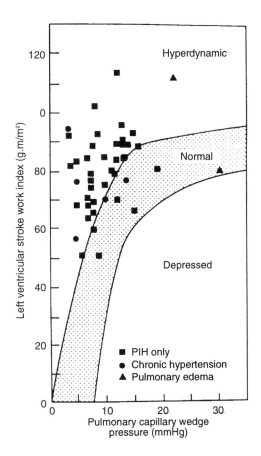

**Figure 5.2** Left ventricular function with severe PIH – Baylor College of Medicine. (Redrawn with permission from Cotton et al., 1988, Hemodynamic profile of severe pregnancy-induced hypertension. *Am. J. Obstet. Gynecol.*, **158**, 523-9.)

Only a modest correlation between CVP and PCWP was observed ($r = 0.59$). The Baylor study found that the majority of women with severe PIH had normal to slight elevated cardiac indices and pulmonary capillary wedge pressures accompanied by normal or hyperdynamic left ventricular function.

Another study involving 49 women was also reported by Mabie, Ratts and Sibai (1989) from the University of Tennessee at Memphis (Table 5.2).

The mean gestational age was $32.4 \pm 0.5$ weeks (range 27–40 weeks). However, 22 women (45%) were in early labor with cervical dilatation less than 4 cm and 16 (33%) had received hydralazine within the 7-hour period preceding pulmonary arterial catheterization. Further stratification using estimated normal criteria for hemodynamic values during pregnancy led to results that were quite similar to the Baylor study. Table 5.3 demonstrates that the majority (88%) of their patients had normal left ventricular filling pressures.

Most patients (80%) had normal CI, with the majority of the remaining values being elevated. Approximately half of the women had SVR values in the normal range, with others being primarily elevated. Patients with chronic hypertension and superimposed PIH were hemodynamically indistinguishable from cases presenting with PIH alone. A total

**Table 5.2** Hemodynamic profile of severe PIH – University of Tennessee (Source: Mabie, Ratts and Sibai, 1989 *Am. J. Obstet. Gynecol.*, **161**, 1443-8.)

| Parameter | Measurement | Range |
|---|---|---|
| Systolic BP (mmHg) | $175 \pm 3$ | (132–219) |
| Diastolic BP (mmHg) | $106 \pm 2$ | (74–130) |
| CVP (mmHg) | $4.8 \pm 0.4$ | (0–10) |
| PCWP (mmHg) | $8.3 \pm 0.3$ | (3–13) |
| Heart rate (beats/min) | $94 \pm 2$ | (65–122) |
| SV index (ml/beat/min) | $48 \pm 1$ | (33–65) |
| Cardiac index (l/min/m²) | $4.4 \pm 0.1$ | (3.1–6.2) |
| PVRI (dyn.s/cm⁵) | $121 \pm 7$ | (33–207) |
| SVRI (dyn.s/cm⁵) | $2293 \pm 65$ | (1637–3336) |

**Table 5.3**  Hemodynamic subsets of severe PIH – University of Tennessee (Source: adapted with permission from Mabie, Ratts and Sibai, 1989)

|  | *Low* | *Normal* | *High* |
|---|---|---|---|
| Pulmonary capillary wedge pressure (mmHg) | < 6 | 6–12 | > 12 |
| n (%) | 3 (7) | 36 (88) | 2 (5) |
| Cardiax index (l/min/m²) | < 3 | 3–5 | > 5 |
| n (%) | 0 (0) | 33 (80) | 8 (20) |
| Systemic vascular resistance (dyn.s/cm⁵) | < 800 | 800–1200 | > 1200 |
| n (%) | 0 (0) | 18 (44) | 23 (56) |

of 73% of patients exhibited hyperdynamic left ventricular function by Starling curve analysis. The Memphis study suggests that severe PIH is generally characterized by normal to high cardiac output state with inappropriately high peripheral vascular resistance. Again, most of the cardiac output values observed in their preeclamptic women were not significantly different from similar measurements taken from normal pregnancies.

The Baylor and University of Tennessee studies underscored the spectrum of hemodynamic measurements from severely preeclamptic patients presenting to tertiary care centers. However, the heterogeneity of these circulatory findings could have been related to various fluid and drug therapies. In order to better understand this possibility, Visser and Wallenburg (1991) prospectively studied 134 consecutive patients with preeclampsia (Table 5.4).

All subjects having gestational ages less than 34 weeks were stratified according to treatment and parity. These values were also compared to ten normotensive women who consented to right heart catheterization between 28 and 31 weeks gestation. None of the women was in labor. Severe preeclampsia was defined by diastolic blood pressure being 100 mmHg or more on two occasions at least 4 hours apart, with proteinuria of 0.5 g/l or more.

Some 47 women met their criteria for treated severe preeclampsia. These patients had received a variety of therapies, including dihydralazine, magnesium sulfate and diazepam.

Treated nulliparous women had slightly higher cardiac indices on the basis of higher HR and slightly elevated SVI when compared to untreated women. Treated parous women had slightly increased CI when compared to untreated parous women, primarily on the basis of higher SVI alone. The treated and untreated severe PIH cases were compared to ten normotensive parous women between 28 and 31 weeks gestation (Table 5.5).

Untreated preeclamptic women had lower HR and CI when compared to the normal group. However, CI in treated preeclamptics was similar to normotensive controls. Analysis of their left ventricular function curves again revealed values that were shifted upward and to the left for the majority of preeclamptic patients. The treated women demonstrated much more heterogeneity in their left ventricular function (Figure 5.3).

### 5.3 COMPARISON OF INVASIVE STUDIES

The Baylor College of Medicine and University of Tennessee studies examined the presenting hemodynamic profile of pregnant women with acute signs and symptoms of severe PIH. Most patients presenting with severe PIH had normal to elevated pulmonary capillary wedge pressures, cardiac indices and systemic vascular indices. Furthermore, hyperdynamic left ventricular function curves were usually shifted upward and to the left.

However, some potentially significant differences exist between these two studies. For

Table 5.4 Treated and untreated severe PIH – the Netherlands; values given are median (range) (Reproduced by permission of the American Heart Association, Inc. from Visser and Wallenburg, 1991)

| | Untreated | | | Treated | | |
|---|---|---|---|---|---|---|
| | Nulliparous (n = 74) | p | Parous (n = 13) | Nulliparous (n = 32) | p | Parous (n = 15) |
| **Systemic circulation** | | | | | | |
| Heart rate (beats/min) | 74 (57–110) | NS | 78 (51–95) | 84 (64–131)* | NS | 87 (62–135) |
| Mean intra-arterial pressure (mmHg) | 125 (92–156) | NS | 123 (96–143) | 120 (80–138)* | NS | 120 (105–154) |
| Cardiac index (l/min/m²) | 3.4 (2.1–5.3) | NS | 3.1 (2.0–4.2) | 4.3 (3.0–7.6)* | NS | 3.8 (2.4–7.0)† |
| Stroke volume index (ml/beat/m²) | 48 (25–75) | <0.05 | 35 (29–56) | 52 (32–82)* | NS | 52 (33–65)* |
| Systemic vascular resistance index (dyn.s/cm⁵/m²) | 2951 (1771–5225) | NS | 3331 (1827–4753) | 2162 (1057–3325)* | NS | 2581 (1177–3688)† |
| Left ventricular stroke work index (J/beat/m²) | 0.71 (0.40–1.16) | NS | 0.63 (0.45–0.85) | 0.81 (0.48–1.27) | NS | 0.72 (0.52–1.06) |
| **Pulmonary circulation** | | | | | | |
| Mean pulmonary arterial pressure (mmHg) | 12 (3–26) | NS | 12 (3–18) | 13 (5–29) | NS | 12 (1–30) |
| Pulmonary capillary wedge pressure (mmHg) | 7 (–1–20) | NS | 5 (0–13) | 7 (1–20) | NS | 6 (0–25) |
| Right atrial pressure (mmHg) | 2 (–4–10) | NS | 1 (–3–6) | 1 (–3–12) | NS | 2 (–3–12) |
| Pulmonary vasular resistance index (dyn.s/cm⁵/m²) | 130 (47–278) | NS | 153 (48–379) | 99 (29–181)* | NS | 114 (8–317) |
| Right ventricular stroke work index (J/beat/m²) | 0.06 (0.01–0.20) | NS | 0.05 (0.01–0.10) | 0.08 (0.03–0.22)* | NS | 0.07 (0.08–0.15) |

* $p < 0.05$ versus untreated nulliparous patients; † $p < 0.05$ versus untreated parous patients

**Table 5.5** Severe PIH: comparison with normals – the Netherlands; values given are median (range) (Reproduced by permission of the American Heart Association, Inc. from Visser and Wallenburg, 1991)

| | Preeclamptics, untreated (n = 87) | p* | Normotensive controls (n = 10) | p† | Preeclamptics, treated (n = 47) |
|---|---|---|---|---|---|
| **Systemic circulation** | | | | | |
| Heart rate (beats/min) | 74 (51–110) | < 0.05 | 82 (68–93) | NS | 85 (62–135)‡ |
| Mean intra-arterial pressure (mmHg) | 125 (92–156) | < 0.001 | 83 (81–29) | < 0.001 | 120 (80–154)‡ |
| Cardiac index (l/min/m²) | 3.3 (2.0–5.3) | < 0.001 | 4.2 (3.5–4.6) | NS | 4.3 (2.4–7.6)‡ |
| Stroke volume index (ml/beat/m²) | 46 (25–75) | NS | 51 (38–61) | NS | 52 (32–82)‡ |
| Systemic vascular resistance index (dyn.s/cm⁵/m²) | 3003 (1771–5225) | < 0.001 | 1560 (1430–2019) | < 0.005 | 2212 (1057–3688)‡ |
| Left ventricular stroke work index (J/beat/m²) | 0.70 (0.40–1.16) | < 0.005 | 0.54 (0.43–0.64) | < 0.001 | 0.79 (0.48–1.27) |
| **Pulmonary circulation** | | | | | |
| Mean pulmonary arterial pressure (mmHg) | 12 (3–26) | < 0.05 | 9 (7–13) | < 0.01 | 13 (0.5–30) |
| Pulmonary capillary wedge pressure (mmHg) | 7 (–1–20) | NS | 5 (1–8) | < 0.05 | 7 (0–25) |
| Right atrial pressure (mmHg) | 2 (–4–10) | NS | 1 (0–2) | NS | 1 (–3–12) |
| Pulmonary vascular resistance index (dyn.s/cm⁵/m²) | 131 (47–379) | < 0.005 | 91 (63–128) | NS | 101 (8–317)‡ |
| Right ventricular stroke work index (J/beat/m²) | 0.06 (0.01–0.20) | NS | 0.05 (0.04–0.08) | < 0.05 | 0.08 (0.01–0.22)‡ |

* differences between untreated preeclamptic patients and normotensive controls; † differences between pharmacologically treated preeclamptic patients and normotensive controls; ‡ p < 0.05 versus untreated nulliparous patients

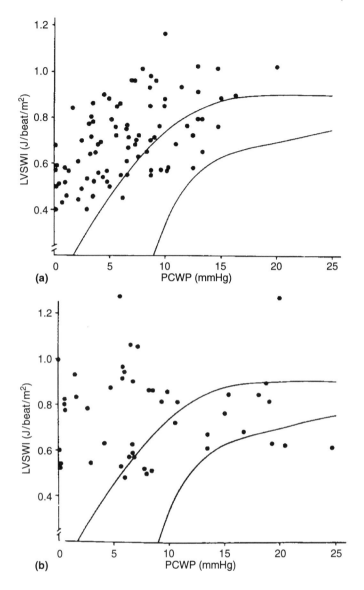

**Figure 5.3**  Left ventricular function in treated and untreated women with severe PIH – the Netherlands. Scatter plots show left ventricular stroke work index (LVSWI) in 87 treated (**a**) and 47 treated (**b**) preeclamptic patients plotted against pulmonary capillary wedge pressure (PCWP). Boundaries of normal non-pregnant left ventricular function are modified from Ross and Braunwald, 1964. (Redrawn by permission of the American Heart Association, Inc. from Visser and Wallenburg, 1991.)

instance the Memphis patients underwent right heart catheterization at a mean gestational age of 32.4 ± 0.5 weeks. By comparison, severe preeclamptic women at Baylor were studied an average of about 3 weeks later (mean 35.4 ± 0.6 weeks). This may account for the higher proportion of patients presenting with eclamptic seizures (31%) at Baylor compared to the Memphis population (8%). A third of the Memphis cases had received hydralazine and nearly half of their subjects were in early labor. However, no hydralazine had been administered prior to baseline measurements and only 29% of the Baylor cases were initially seen in early labor. Both study populations had received intravenous magnesium sulfate therapy. Magnesium sulfate has been found to cause a transient hypotensive effect from bolus administration but the hypotensive effect is not seen with continuous infusion in severely preeclamptic women (Cotton, Gonik and Dorman, 1984). Slightly higher cardiac values observed in the Memphis group led to mildly increased stroke volume measurements but these differences were minimal when indexed to body surface area.

The Dutch study appears to address an earlier stage of PIH with a mean gestational age of approximately 29–31 weeks (Visser and Wallenburg, 1991). Their diagnostic criteria for severe preeclampsia was defined by a diastolic blood pressure of 100 mmHg on more on two occasions at least 4 hours apart with proteinuria. By contrast, the American studies used a higher diastolic blood pressure criterion (greater than 110 mmHg) for the diagnosis of severe preeclampsia. Another important difference between the Dutch and American studies relates to administration of intravenous fluids. The Baylor and University of Tennessee investigations limited intravenous crystalloids to about 75–100 ml/h. The Erasmus University investigators stated that untreated severely preeclamptic patients received no more than 20–30 ml of saline for catheter flushing but implied that the untreated group may have been otherwise fluid restricted. Previous observations from their institution involved seven of ten women who were oliguric and on sodium-restricted diets (Groenendijk, Trimbos and Wallenburg, 1984). Therefore, the lower CI measurements from untreated preeclamptics in the Netherlands may be related to earlier gestational age, rela-

tive fluid restriction and lower blood pressure criteria for the diagnosis of severe PIH. Nonetheless, this study provides important information about the maternal circulatory system during the early stages of clinically evident and untreated preeclampsia. They were able to demonstrate that some of the hemodynamic variability seen with severe PIH could actually be attributed to medical therapy.

## 5.4 NON-INVASIVE STUDIES

Right heart catheterization studies have provided important perspectives about intracardiac pressures, left ventricular function and cardiac output for selected patients with severe preeclampsia. However, the potentially confounding variables of gestational age, labor and medical therapy, and the relatively small number of patients available for study, can limit our ability to accurately incorporate these observations into clinical practice. Doppler ultrasound has also been used to estimate maternal cardiac output values that correlate quite well with thermodilution methods (Easterling *et al.*, 1987; Robson *et al.*, 1987; Lee, Rokey and Cotton, 1988). This non-invasive technology has allowed study of more preeclamptic subjects that would have been possible with right heart catheterization alone.

Easterling *et al.* (1990) at the University of Washington longitudinally examined the hemodynamic profile of preeclampsia by Doppler ultrasound. All 179 nulliparous women were enrolled before 22 weeks. Subjects who had two diastolic blood pressures greater than 90 mmHg or were 15 mmHg above baseline in the first half of pregnancy were classified as being hypertensive. Hypertensive women with proteinuria were identified as preeclamptic ($n = 9$). Hypertensive women without proteinuria were classified as having gestational hypertension ($n = 81$). Cardiac output in preeclamptic women was elevated throughout pregnancy when compared to the normotensive group (Figure 5.4).

Cardiac output for preeclamptic women ranged from about 7–9.8 l/min compared to their normal range of about 6.2–7.2 l/min. This appeared to be primarily due to a slightly higher HR (7–17%) in the preeclamptic group. Cardiac output remained elevated after delivery in preeclamptic women, raising the possibility that hemodynamic abnormalities might have existed even before pregnancy. SVR estimations for the PIH group were generally not significantly different from the control group except at 23 weeks gestation and postpartum (Figure 5.5).

The University of Washington data provides some intriguing insight into the natural history of preeclampsia but these findings are not without controversy. It suggests that increased cardiac output and normal systemic vascular resistance are the fundamental hemo-dynamic changes, occurring in preeclamptic women as early as 20 weeks gestation when compared to normal pregnancy. This is contrary to other investigators, who have traditionally characterized PIH as a disease of increased vascular resistance (Cunningham, MacDonald and Gant, 1989; Roberts, 1984). The mean arterial pressure and cardiac output values taken from preeclamptic women were statistically different from normal controls as early as 11 weeks gestation. The association of elevated second trimester mean arterial blood pressure with the subsequent development of PIH has been previously reported but the increased cardiac output observations are new (Moutquin *et al.*, 1985; Ales, Norton and Druzin, 1989). It is unclear to what extent the omitted central venous pressure measurements from the systemic vascular resistance calculation may have affected the absolute values, although this should not have affected

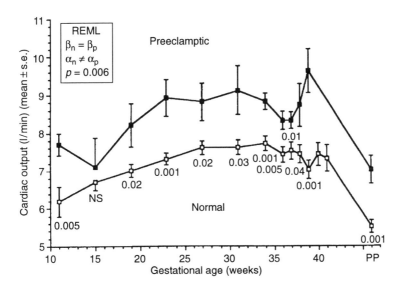

**Figure 5.4** Cardiac output in preeclamptic women by Doppler ultrasound. Mean ± s.e. cardiac output for the normotensive (normal) and preeclamptic groups plotted against gestational age. Levels of significance are indicated for each interval of gestational age. Restricted maximal likelihood (REML) analysis is reported where β indicates slope and α indicates intercept. NS = not significant; PP = postpartum. (Redrawn with permission from Easterling et al., with permission from The American College of Obstetricians and Gynecologists, *Obstet. Gynecol.*, 1990, **76**, 1061.)

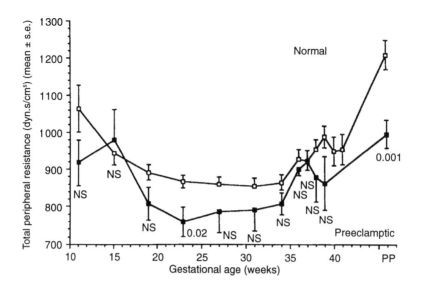

**Figure 5.5** Systemic vascular resistance in preeclamptic women by Doppler ultrasound. Mean ± s.e. total peripheral resistance for the normotensive (normal) and preeclamptic groups plotted against gestational age. Levels of significance are indicated for each interval of gestational age. NS = not significant; PP = postpartum. (Redrawn with permission from Easterling et al., with permission from The American College of Obstetricians and Gynecologists, *Obstet. Gynecol.*, 1990, **76**, 1061.)

relative comparisons between their preeclamptic women and normal controls.

Another controversial issue surrounding the Seattle study involves the extremely high incidence of gestational hypertension (45%) in their normal screening population. These investigators attribute the high proportion of hypertensive women to the strict use of the definition for gestational hypertension, in that every subject with a 15 mmHg rise in diastolic blood pressure was placed into this category This included women who had two elevated blood pressures during labor or women who originally had baseline diastolic readings of less than 60 mmHg. It is possible that a heterogeneous group of gestational hypertensive subjects may have actually consisted of clinically normal pregnancies that were essentially misclassified by these strict criteria (Easterling, personal communication).

Guyton (1989) has proposed a whole-body autoregulation model for chronic hyperten-sion and suggests that high cardiac output hypertension may progress into high systemic vascular resistance hypertension. This mechanism controls the total vascular resistance by regulating elevated cardiac output as a primary cause for hypertension. The subsequent elevation of systemic vascular resistance is a secondary result of hypertension rather than a primary cause in this model. The finding that early PIH is characterized by elevated cardiac output is consistent with the concept that women who clinically present with severe preeclampsia may experience a 'crossover' phenomenon from a high cardiac output to a high vascular resistance state.

This concept may also have important fetal consequences. Nisell, Lunell and Linde (1988) conducted an interesting study of 21 women with mild to moderate preeclampsia. All patients were studied by a dye-dilution technique (indocyanine-green indicator) and intra-arterial blood pressure measurements as well. Subjects were divided into two groups based upon actual birthweight. Five infants were classified as small for gestation age (SGA) with birthweight below the tenth percentile. The remaining 16 fetuses were classified as being appropriate for gestational age (AGA). Measurements were taken in the mothers for both SGA ($37.5 \pm 0.4$ weeks) and AGA fetuses ($36.2 \pm 1.4$ weeks) prior to delivery. Cardiac output and stroke volume were significantly lower in mothers with SGA fetuses ($5.8 \pm 0.2$ l/min, $76 \pm 7$ ml/beat) when compared to those with AGA infants ($8.2 \pm 0.3$ l/min, $100 \pm 5$ ml/beat). Heart rate was similar between the two groups. There was a tendency for SVR to be higher in SGA pregnancies but this was not statistically significant. A spectrum of hemodynamic findings ranged from a high-output, low-resistance state to a low-output, high-resistance condition; the latter condition was associated with low infant birthweight. These investigators suggested that increased systemic perfusion pressure in preeclamptic women may not be sufficient to overcome increased uteroplacental vascular resistance caused by structurally abnormal spiral arteries. This process could lead to compromised uteroplacental blood flow and IUGR.

The more recent application of Doppler ultrasound to a longitudinal pregnant population has also examined a possible hemodynamic crossover mechanisms for PIH. Easterling *et al.* (1991) studied 76 hypertensive pregnancies prior to 28 weeks gestation by Doppler ultrasound. High-resistance hypertension was defined as SVR of at least 1150 dyn.s.$^{-5}$. A total of 47% of these women demonstrated an increased cardiac output and low SVR. However, 42% were found to have elevated SVR. Eight subjects actually crossed over from a high-cardiac-output, low-vascular-resistance state to a low-cardiac-output, high-vascular-resistance condition during pregnancy (Figure 5.6).

The high-resistance group had lower birth percentile weights for gestational age (19th *versus* 3rd percentile) as well as a higher rate of intrauterine death (Figure 5.7). Therefore, this investigation confirmed the earlier work of Nissell, Lunell and Linde (1988) that low maternal cardiac output and high vascular resistance are unfavorable hemodynamic conditions that may lead to poor fetal growth.

An intriguing theme begins to collectively emerge from these hemodynamic studies. Early PIH appears to be characterized by none to elevated cardiac output but as the disease process advances these patients may eventually cross over into a high-resistance state. This high-resistance state is associated with varying degrees of normal to low cardiac output in the face of worsening hypertension. Increased uteroplacental vascular resistance with decreased uterine blood flow resulting from this process may lead to IUGR. Indeed, patients with high SVR and severe hypertension are the ones most likely to be selected by institutions studying invasive hemodynamics of severe PIH during later pregnancy. This could explain the apparent discrepancy between the invasive and non-invasive literature.

However, more studies will be required to confirm this evolutionary scenario and to further address several pertinent questions. For instance, could PIH-associated IUGR be reliably predicted by the detection of hemodynamic crossover from a normal-to-high-cardiac-output state to a normal-or-low-cardiac-output, high-resistance state? Could autoregulatory mechanisms compensate for decreased local uteroplacental circulation secondary to low maternal cardiac output? What is the practicality of treating low cardiac output or high vascular resistance with beta-blocking agents or afterload reduction with regard to maternal/fetal outcome (Easterling *et al.*, 1989)? Improved understanding of the pathophysiological processes underlying the development of preeclampsia will hopefully improve our understanding about how to better treat this condition.

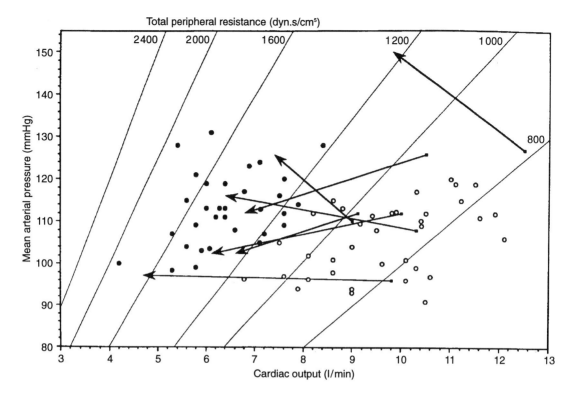

**Figure 5.6** Crossover phenomenon from high output to high resistance state with severe PIH. Mean arterial pressure of each subject is plotted against cardiac output. Isometric lines of vascular resistance are included so that all three parameters can be displayed on a single figure. Closed circles = High-resistance subjects; open circles = low-resistance subjects; closed square = subjects whose hemodynamics crossed over. Associated vector graphically displays change in hemodynamics associated with crossover. (Redrawn with permission from Easterling et al., 1991, The effect of maternal hemodynamics on fetal growth in hypertensive pregnancies. *Am. J. Ostet. Gynecol.*, **151**, 762-4.)

## 5.5 CLINICAL CONSIDERATIONS

Practical experience has demonstrated that most cases of severe preeclampsia can be successfully managed without invasive hemodynamic intervention (Pritchard, Cunningham and Pritchard, 1984; ACOG Technical Bulletin no. 128, 1988). However, occasional circumstances do occur where the critically ill gravida may benefit from information obtained by pulmonary artery catheterization. These conditions include severe hypertensive crisis that is refractory to medical therapy, treatment of pulmonary edema and PIH-related oliguria unresponsive to intravenous fluid therapy.

### 5.5.1 HYPERTENSIVE CRISIS

Medical therapy of hypertensive crisis is recommended for systolic blood pressures greater than 180 mmHg or diastolic blood pressures exceeding 110 mmHg to reduce the risk of maternal intracranial hemorrhage (Lubbe, 1987; Naden and Redman, 1985)). Intravenous hydralazine has been the drug of choice for treating diastolic blood pressures greater than 110 mmHg in preeclamptic patients. This agent reduces vascular resistance by direct relaxation of arteriolar smooth muscle (Koch-Weser, 1976). A useful regime has been to begin with 5 mg as an intra-

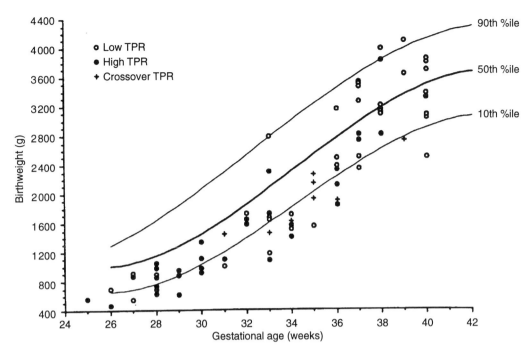

**Figure 5.7** Relationship between birthweight and systemic vascular resistance in women with PIH. Individual birthweights are plotted against gestational age. The 10th, 50th, and 90th percentiles of normal birth weight at sea level are included for reference. Closed circles = infants from high-resistance pregnancies; open circles = infants from low-resistance pregnancies; + = infants from crossover pregnancies. (Redrawn with permission from Easterling et al., 1991, The effect of maternal hemodynamics on fetal growth in hypertensive pregnancies. *Am. J. Ostet. Gynecol.*, **151**, 762-4.)

venous bolus followed by 5–10 mg every 20–30 min until the diastolic blood pressure has decreased to 90–100 mmHg (Pritchard, Cunningham and Pritchard, 1984).

Most preeclamptic women will respond to intermittent hydralazine boluses (total dosage of 30–40 mg). Cotton, Gonik and Dorman (1985a) found that the hemodynamic response to bolus hydralazine was quite unpredictable with a highly variable onset and duration of action. Unfortunately, continuous hydralazine infusion has not been found to be efficacious under these circumstances because of the high incidence of fetal distress (Sibai *et al.*, 1984; Kirshon, Wasserstrum and Cotton, 1991). We believe that hypertension refractory to the bolus hydralazine regime warrants further medical intervention by more potent pharmacological agents.

Central hemodynamic monitoring and an arterial line can be especially useful for guiding some types of intravenous antihypertensive therapy. This is especially true for potent vasodilatory agents such as sodium nitroprusside. Nitroprusside is very effective for rapid treatment of hypertensive crisis but its use is fraught with some potential disadvantages during pregnancy. For instance, the drug is light-sensitive and the intravenous tubing needs to be wrapped in foil to prevent deterioration. Nitroprusside has also been reported to be associated with abrupt hypotensive episodes and paradoxical bradycardia in severely preeclamptic women at doses as low as 0.35 mg/kg/min (Wasserstrum, 1991). Patients receiving nitroprusside also need to be carefully monitored for cyanide toxicity (methemoglobin levels, arterial oxygenation status, cyanosis). Cyanide toxicity related to nitroprusside has been described in the pregnant ewe but this has been poorly characterized in human fetuses (Naulty, Cafalo and Lewis, 1981). It is essential that patients should not be volume-depleted prior to nitroprusside administration. Pulmonary artery catheterization can provide valuable information about appropriate volume therapy prior to beginning infusion of this potent drug. At this time we can only cautiously recommend the use of nitroprusside for treatment of hypertensive crisis in severely preeclamptic women. However, the complexities associated with nitroprusside administration makes this agent less than ideal for routine use during pregnancy.

Nitroglycerin, labetalol, and verapamil are three other potent antihypertensive drugs that have been used to treat severe hypertension refractory to standard hydralazine therapy. All three agents have different mechanisms of action and their application to the severely preeclamptic patient is discussed below. Pulmonary artery catheterization is usually not required for intravenous labetalol or even for most cases of verapamil therapy. However, afterload reduction with potent vasodilators such as nitroglycerin or nitroprusside requires an accurate assessment of maternal volume status to avoid abrupt and poorly controlled blood pressure reduction that may also cause fetal bradycardia.

### (a) Nitroglycerin

Intravenous nitroglycerin is a potent antihypertensive agent with a rapid onset of action and a relatively short hemodynamic half-life (Opie, 1987; Fahmy, 1978; Armstrong, Armstrong and Marks, 1980). This drug induces both arterial hypotension and venous dilation (Ferrer *et al.*, 1966; Simon *et al.*, 1982; Herling, 1984)). Cotton *et al.* (1986) have examined the effect of intravenous nitroglycerin with and without volume expansion in severely preeclamptic women. Nitroglycerin

alone reduced mean arterial pressure by 28% without significant changes in heart rate, central venous pressure or stroke volume. Small decreases were also observed with PCWP, CI and oxygen delivery.

However, the combination of blood volume expansion and nitroglycerin led to a marked resistance to the hypotensive effect of nitroglycerin. Two of six patients on nitroglycerin without volume expansion experienced abrupt reduction of blood pressure with signs of fetal distress. In each case, nitroglycerin was discontinued, with return of blood pressure and normal fetal heart rate. Fetal bradycardia was not observed in these patients after the infusion was restarted at a lower dosing regimen. This propensity for abrupt and uncontrolled maternal blood pressure reductions may be due to sinoaortic baroreceptor reflex dysfunction in severe preeclampsia (Wasserstrum *et al.*, 1989). Another area of concern involved three cases of decreased fetal heart rate variability. However, there was no direct evidence for perinatal asphyxia on the basis of Apgar scores, umbilical cord gases or postnatal clinical condition. Volume expansion in these patients allowed a more precise control of afterload reduction without abrupt and profound reduction in arterial pressure. A similar benefit of volume expansion for preeclamptic women with low PCWP and CI values has been reported for dihydralazine infusion (Belfort *et al.*, 1989).

Intravenous nitroglycerin does appear to be a useful alternative agent for refractory hypertensive crisis but should be used cautiously in preeclamptic women with low pulmonary capillary wedge pressures or with signs of fetal compromise. Smoother blood pressure reduction will usually be achieved following volume expansion, although larger doses of nitroglycerin will be required to elicit a response when compared to the volume-depleted patient. It would be reasonable to correct a low PCWP (≤ 4 mmHg) with crystalloid infusion to a PCWP of at least 8–10 mmHg prior to nitroglycerin infusion. Nitroglycerin can be started at 0.1 μg/kg/min and titrated to a mean arterial pressure of approximately 106 mmHg or until fetal brady-cardia contraindicates further blood pressure reduction. Continuous monitoring of intra-arterial blood pressure and fetal heart rate patterns is essential. High levels of methemo-globinemia may result with high doses of intravenous nitroglycerin above 7 μg/kg/min. In this context, cyanotic patients with normal oxygen saturation should be evaluated for tox-icity (methemoglobin levels < 3%) (Gibson, 1982).

### (b) Labetalol

Labetalol is another potent antihypertensive drug that can be used for severe hypertension during pregnancy (Lamming and Symonds, 1979; Walker, Greer and Calder, 1983). It is a combined alpha and beta adrenergic receptor antagonist which may also possess intrinsic agonist activity at beta-2 receptors as well which accounts for vasodilator action (Rogers, Sibai and Whybrew, 1990). These pharmaco-logical properties allow this agent to decrease systemic vascular resistance and blood pres-sure without much effect on heart rate or car-diac output. Furthermore, uteroplacental blood flow studies suggest that a decrease in placental perfusion does not occur despite significant maternal blood pressure reduction (Nylund *et al.*, 1984). Others have reported its use for decreasing the hypertensive and tachycardia responses associated with laryn-goscopy and endotracheal intubation in preeclamptic women undergoing surgical procedures (Ramanathan *et al.*, 1988).

Mabie *et al.* (1987) compared the use of intravenous hydralazine and labetalol for blood pressure control of 60 preeclamptic women with diastolic blood pressures of at least 110 mmHg. There were four treatment failures in the labetalol group (*n* = 40) and none in the hydralazine group (*n* = 20) using a therapeutic goal of diastolic blood pressure

below 100 mmHg. Hydralazine lowered mean arterial pressure to a slightly greater degree but labetalol led to a more rapid effect. No significant fetal or neonatal compli-cations were associated with labetalol admin-istration in 13 cases prior to delivery but fetal distress was observed in two of six cases receiving hydralazine. Labetalol did not cause reflex maternal tachycardia. On the basis of this information, labetalol appears to be a reasonable alternative to hydralazine for treatment of severe PIH. The regimen usually consists of an initial 20 mg loading dose which is followed by subsequent doses of 20 mg every 10 min to a total of not more than 300 mg. An alternative intravenous regimen is one that starts at 1–2 mg/min until satisfactory blood pressure levels are obtained, after which time it can be decreased to 0.5 mg/min or completely stopped (Naden and Redman, 1985). Other investigators have found intravenous labetalol to provide better blood pressure control in preeclamptic pregnancies than either dihydralazine or diazoxide (Garden, Davey and Dommisse, 1982; Michael, 1986). However, occasional neonatal bradycardia has been observed following maternal labetalol exposure at birth (Garden, Davey and Dommisse, 1982). Additional clinical experience with labetalol will provide more specific guidelines for its use to treat severe preeclampsia

### (c) Verapamil

This calcium channel antagonist prevents influx of intracellular calcium into vascular smooth muscle and causes peripheral vasodi-latation (Bolton, 1979; Van Breeman, Aaronson and Loutzenhiser, 1978). However, it also has an effect upon blocking calcium influx into the cardiac conduction system and effectively minimizes the reflex tachycardia that may be seen with other calcium channel blockers such as nifedipine (Singh, Ellrodt and Peter, 1978). These pharmacological properties have promoted its possible application to preterm labor tocolysis, treatment for fetal supraventricular tachycardia and for severe PIH. The use of this agent for severely preeclamptic women is relatively limited but preliminary studies suggest that verapamil may be a useful antihypertensive agent under these circumstances (Serafini *et al.*, 1979; Belfort and Moore, 1988). Verapamil has a relatively short duration of antihypertensive activity that ranges from 10–20 min following IV infusion (Opie, 1980).

Belfort *et al.* (1990) studied the utility of intravenous verapamil for severe PIH following volume expansion with Dextran 70. The PCWP was raised to 14–16 mmHg. An intravenous solution (80 mg verapamil in 200 ml NaCl 0.9%) was begun at 5–10 mg/h and then titrated for a 20% maternal blood pressure reduction. After verapamil infusion, the heart rate was significantly higher than after volume expansion but not greatly increased over baseline measurements. There was a predictable maternal blood pressure reduction by 30–50 min after beginning the infusion. Three of nine patients developed peripartum complications. The first patient developed pulmonary edema following cesarean section due to a congestive cardiomyopathy. Another patient experienced a drop in cardiac output about 90 min after beginning verapamil. This was related to an interaction with an unintended simultaneous 4 g loading dose of magnesium sulfate. A first-degree heart block was subsequently diagnosed in this patient. A third pregnancy was complicated by placental abruption. Fetal outcome was favorable in all cases except for one that was associated with growth retardation, acidosis with elective cesarean delivery, low Apgar scores and cerebral leukomalacia.

The use of verapamil for blood pressure reduction in severe preeclampsia is encouraging but warrants further investigation about its safety and efficacy. Verapamil's short duration of action makes it especially suitable for intravenous infusion since its hypotensive

effect could be rapidly stopped shortly after discontinuation. Preliminary clinical experience suggests that verapamil therapy does not usually require pulmonary artery catheterization. However, afterload reduction by this agent should be carefully administered if there is a suspicion of volume depletion. Caution should also be taken when verapamil is started at the same time as magnesium sulfate because of their additive effect upon prolonging the PR interval. Verapamil should not be administered in close proximity to intravenous beta-adrenergic drugs that together may produce undesirable effects upon left ventricular function and atrioventricular conduction. Its use is contraindicated in patients with heart block, congestive heart failure or fetal bradycardia.

### 5.5.2 PULMONARY EDEMA

Cardiogenic pulmonary edema is the result of a imbalance between Starling forces that incorporate capillary pressure, colloid osmotic pressure interstitial fluid pressure, and tissue colloid osmotic pressure (Taylor, 1981). These variables define the net fluid movement across the pulmonary capillary wall. Outward forces that dominate these relationships favor the development of respiratory insufficiency reflected clinically by dyspnea, pulmonary rales, tachycardia, arterial oxygen desaturation and elevated PCWP measurements.

Pulmonary edema occurs infrequently as a complication of preeclampsia. Pulmonary edema was identified only twice among 91 eclamptic women (2.2%) at Parkland Memorial Hospital (Pritchard, Cunningham and Pritchard, 1984). One women was obese whose primary etiology for respiratory insufficiency was aspiration pneumonia. The other woman was also obese, with respiratory insufficiency developing 3 days after birth, presumably due to cardiomyopathy. The University of Tennessee at Memphis reported a 1.7% incidence of pulmonary edema among their preeclamptic population (Sibai *et al.*,

1984). Risk factors for pulmonary edema included iatrogenic fluid overload, advanced maternal age, multiparity, and patients with underlying chronic hypertension.

Mabie *et al.* (1988) also examined maternal obesity as another important risk factor for pulmonary edema in chronically hypertensive gravidas. Obese women were characterized by high PCWP, normal to high CI and normal SVR by right heart catheterization. Echocardiography revealed large chambers with increased left ventricular mass and abnormal diastolic function. The combination of intrinsic volume overload in the presence of impaired left ventricular relaxation was postulated to cause elevated filling pressure and pulmonary edema. On the basis of these findings, it would seem that obese chronic hypertensive women with severe preeclampsia are particularly prone to developing pulmonary edema.

The multifactorial nature of pulmonary edema was initially described by Benedetti, Kates and Williams (1985) who studied the hemodynamic presentation of ten preeclamptic women with respiratory insufficiency. All subjects underwent right heart catheterization. The majority (eight of ten) of these patients developed respiratory insufficiency during the postpartum period. The most common mechanism responsible for pulmonary edema ($n = 5$) was alteration in hydrostatic oncotic forces that typically occurred within 15 hours following delivery. This alteration was the net effect of a lowered colloid osmotic pressure (mean COP = 15.3 mmHg) and increased left ventricular filling pressure (mean 18.6 mmHg). Three patients had evidence of capillary leak, which was diagnosed when the ratio of pulmonary fluid protein concentration to serum protein exceeded 0.4. Two patients experienced depressed left ventricular function on the basis of decreased stroke work indices. These findings suggest that pulmonary edema with severe PIH can be caused by at least three different mechanisms that include capillary leakage, increased pulmonary capillary wedge pressure and decreased serum colloid osmotic pressure.

There are two additional points about pulmonary edema in PIH that have important clinical ramifications. The first involves a decreased COP–PCWP gradient which has been also observed in non-pregnant individuals with pulmonary edema (Fein *et al.*, 1979). Colloid osmotic pressure is an important reason why serum remains within the intravascular space by way of a delicate balance between Starling's forces. Pregnancy and preeclampsia both have an independent effect upon lowering serum COP (Wu *et al.*, 1983; Benedetti and Carlson, 1979). A small rise in PCWP can reverse the normal Starling forces that usually prevent pulmonary edema. Furthermore, peripartum hemorrhage, intravenous fluid, and even the supine position may also reduce serum COP to even lower levels (Cotton *et al.*, 1984). The association between a negative COP–PCWP gradient and pulmonary edema has been also established for severely preeclamptic women (Benedetti *et al.*, 1980; Strauss *et al.*, 1980; Benedetti, Kates and Williams, 1985). It is possible for a patient to develop pulmonary edema with a high normal PCWP measurement if the serum COP is low enough to make the COP–PCWP gradient negative. Unfortunately, efforts to routinely optimize serum COP by infusion of albumin have not been very effective for preventing pulmonary edema (Kirshon *et al.*, 1986).

The second point relates to the poor correlation that is often observed between CVP and PCWP in women with severe PIH (Benedetti, Kates and Williams, 1985; Strauss *et al.*, 1980; Cotton *et al.*, 1985) (Figure 5.8).

This disparity probably results from normal to high CO pumping from the left ventricle against an increased afterload. Under these circumstances, left ventricular filling pressures (PCWP) would be expected to be higher than right ventricular filling pressures (CVP). In this context CVP does not reliably

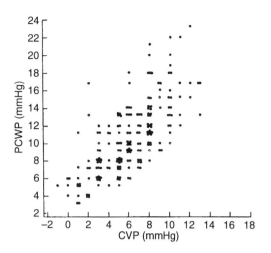

**Figure 5.8**  Correlation between CVP and PCWP in women with severe PIH The relationship of central venous pressure (CVP) to pulmonary capillary wedge pressure (PCWP) in 18 patients with severe pregnancy-induced hypertension is shown. (Redrawn with permission from Cotton *et al.*, 1985, Cardiovascular alterations in severe pregnancy-induced hypertension: relationship of central venais pressure to pulmonary capillary wedge pressure. *Am. J. Obstet. Gynecol.*, **151**, 762–4.)

reflect left ventricular filling pressure in severely preeclamptic women and its inappropriate use in these patients may be quite misleading. For instance, Benedetti, Kates and Williams (1985) reported that five of ten severely preeclamptic patients with pulmonary edema had CVP-PCWP differences ≥ 5 mmHg and two additional cases were found to have a difference ≥ 10 mmHg. These differences appear to be clinically insignificant as long as the CVP measurement is below 6 mmHg. On the other hand, it is very possible to have abnormally high PCWP measurements with a relatively low CVP value above 6 mmHg. For this reason, we recommend use of the PCWP to guide volume therapy or to assess left ventricular preload in cases of severe PIH.

Despite its infrequent occurrence, pulmonary edema usually develops in preeclamp-

tic women during the postpartum period. Hankins and colleagues (1984) further examined the peripartum hemodynamic changes that may contribute to the development of pulmonary edema in women with severe PIH. This investigation involved eight eclamptic women who were studied throughout the postpartum period by right heart catheterization. In some women, PCWP measurements became remarkably elevated (16–23 mmHg) despite normal left ventricular function and arterial oxygenation. Asymptomatic PCWP elevations eventually normalized when these women began spontaneous postpartum diuresis. This study identified yet another important risk factor – mobilization of extracellular extravascular fluid prior to postpartum diuresis – that will predispose eclamptic patients to respiratory insufficiency following delivery. Therefore, postpartum mobilization of extracellular fluid into the intravascular space also appears to be an important mechanism that may contribute to pulmonary insufficiency in preeclamptic women.

Treatment of pulmonary edema should optimize arterial oxygenation by careful manipulation of preload, afterload and cardiac output. Cardiogenic pulmonary edema with elevated PCWP usually responds well to oxygen supplementation, fluid restriction and preload reduction by furosemide. Intravenous furosemide can be administered in a 10–40 mg dose over 1–2 min. Congestive heart failure may also be caused by extremely high peripheral vascular resistance. In this case, afterload reduction with nitroglycerin would be a reasonable consideration especially due to its additional effect as a venodilator. Left ventricular function curves provide a convenient way to follow the progress of women who are given agents to improve hemodynamic performance – especially in cases where inotropic agents such as dopamine are required for depressed ventricular function.

Rarely, there will be instances where respiratory insufficiency with severe PIH occurs secondary to a capillary leak. Pulmonary artery catheterization can be used to establish this difficult diagnosis, which usually requires a longer treatment period. Finally, an occasional patient presents with uncertain etiology for her respiratory insufficiency or even does not respond to conventional medical therapy. This type of patient will be the most likely to benefit from hemodynamic assessment by pulmonary artery catheterization.

### 5.5.3 OLIGURIA

Preeclamptic women may also develop decreased urine output. One study reported that severe hypertension and oliguria were leading causes for admission into their obstetrical intensive care unit (Moller and Hartmann-Anderson, 1990). Grunfeld, Gameval and Bournerias (1980) observed that 12 of 57 patients with acute renal failure also had preeclampsia. Acute renal failure may also lead to acute tubular necrosis or bilateral renal cortical necrosis. Unfortunately, the precise relationship between oliguria and the development of acute renal failure in preeclamptic women is unclear (Smith *et al.*, 1965). Matlin and Gary (1974) have suggested that the hypercoagulable state of pregnancy combined with severe prolonged vasospasm may contribute to the development of acute tubular necrosis. This is supported by the finding that the urinary sediment in preeclamptic patients consist of numerous granular, hyaline, red cell and tubular casts (Leduc *et al.*, 1991). These findings uniformly reflect renal parenchymal damage but unfortunately do not correlate well with severity of disease. The Parkland Hospital experience suggests that azotemia seldom, if ever, progresses to renal failure requiring dialysis in eclamptic women (Pritchard, Cunningham and Pritchard, 1984). However, two cases of preeclampsia with untreated oliguria have been reported that progressed to acute tubular necrosis, with one patient requiring chronic dialysis (Clark *et al.*, 1986). Sibai and colleagues (1984) reported a 1% incidence of acute renal failure from their

series of 303 severely preeclamptic women. All three cases were associated with acute tubular necrosis, placental abruption and disseminated intravascular coagulation. Other than delivery, the need for aggressive medical therapy of severe PIH-associated oliguria remains controversial.

The hemodynamic profile of severely preeclamptic women can provide important clinical guidelines for treatment of oliguria. Clark *et al.* (1986) studied nine patients (mean gestational age 33 weeks) with severe preeclampsia and oliguria unresponsive to an initial intravenous fluid challenge. They defined oliguria as urine output of less than 30 ml per hour for three consecutive hours by indwelling catheter. These women did not respond to a 300–500 ml crystalloid infusion over 20 min.

Three hemodynamic groups were subsequently identified by pulmonary arterial catheterization. The first group ($n = 5$) exhibited hyperdynamic left ventricular function, low to low-normal PCWP and moderately increased SVR. Oliguria in this group resolved with simple volume expansion to remedy low left ventricular filling pressures. The second group ($n = 3$) was similar to the first group except for normal to high PCWP and slightly lower SVR. These patients responded to mild volume expansion on the basis of PCWP and arterial vasodilator therapy with hydralazine for probable renal vasospasm. Others have recommended low-dose intravenous dopamine as a selective renal vasodilator for this type of patient (Gerstner and Grunberger, 1980; Lee, Gonik and Cotton, 1987; Kirshon *et al.*, 1988). The third group ($n = 1$) was characterized by depressed left ventricular function, elevated PCWP and marked SVR elevation. This patient responded to afterload reduction with hydralazine and fluid restriction. Therefore, PIH-associated oliguria can be caused by a variety of etiological factors that include inadequate preload, renal vasospasm and left ventricular dysfunction.

The misconception that urinary output accurately reflects volume status and renal function was also examined by Lee, Gonik and Cotton (1987), who found a poor correlation between oliguria and volume status in seven preeclamptic women. Five of seven oliguric patients with normal volume status (PCWP = 8–14 mmHg) had urinary diagnostic indices consistent with prerenal hydration. Therefore, the clinician should be warned that low urine output alone does not necessarily reflect a volume-depleted state in preeclamptic women. Furthermore, traditional indices of renal function do not appear to be helpful for identification of the specific mechanism responsible for PIH-associated oliguria.

The treatment of PIH-associated oliguria remains controversial since most of time this condition will spontaneously resolve after delivery. However, occasional patients will develop azotemia, renal failure, acute tubular necrosis, and the subsequent need for dialysis. Pulmonary artery catheterization is recommended for either persistent oliguria (unresponsive to 1–2 liters of intravenous crystalloid replacement) or in patients with a worrisome rise in serum creatinine. Volume challenges should always be accompanied by monitoring of oxygenation status by pulse oximetry. Addition fluid therapy may be administered if the oxygen saturation remains above 95%. If this fluid challenge does not satisfactorily improve urine output (> 30 ml/h) or if maternal oxygen saturation falls below 95%, central hemodynamic monitoring allows one to more precisely evaluate volume status with identification of correctable etiological factors contributing to oliguria.

## 5.6 SUMMARY

Severe preeclampsia can present a formidable challenge to clinicians caring for pregnant women. It represents a broad spectrum of hemodynamic findings depending upon the severity and duration of disease. To date, the medical literature suggests that the hemodynamic profile of early PIH is characterized by normal to high cardiac output with mildly elevated systemic vascular resistance. Maternal cardiac output will progressively decrease with increasing systemic vascular resistance in the face of worsening hypertension. Increased uteroplacental vascular resistance with decreased uterine blood flow may lead to IUGR. The concept of hemodynamic crossover from a normal-to-high cardiac output state into a low-cardiac-output, high-vascular-resistance state requires further study. The role of beta-blockade or afterload reduction for the prevention of disease progression remains a provocative field of investigation. Most cases of severe PIH can be successfully managed without invasive hemodynamic monitoring. However, we feel that pulmonary artery catheterization can provide valuable information about severely preeclamptic patients who develop hypertensive crisis unresponsive to hydralazine, persistent oliguria despite adequate fluid challenge, pulmonary edema of uncertain etiology or respiratory insufficiency that does not respond to conventional therapy.

## REFERENCES

Armstrong, P. W., Armstrong, J. A., Marks, G. S. (1980) Pharmacokinetic–hemodynamic studies of intravenous nitroglycerin in congestive heart failure. *Circulation*, **62**, 160–166.

Ales, K. L., Norton, M. E. and Druzin, M. L. (1989) Early prediction of antepartum hypertension. *Obstet. Gynecol.*, **73**, 928–933.

Belfort, M. A. and Moore, P. J. (1988) Verapamil in the treatment of severe postpartum hypertension. *S. Afr. Med. J.*, **74**, 265–267.

Belfort, M., Uys, P., Dommisse, J. and Davey, D. A. (1989) Haemodynamic changes in gestational proteinuric hypertension: the effects of rapid volume expansion and vasodilator therapy. *Br. J. Obstet. Gynaecol.*, **96**, 634–641.

Belfort, M. A., Anthony, J., Buccimazza. A. and Davey, D. A. (1990) Hemodynamic changes associated with intravenous infusion of calcium antagonist verapamil in the treatment of severe gestational proteinuric hypertension. *Obstet. Gynecol.*, **75**, 970–974.

Benedetti, T. J. and Carlson, R. W. (1979) Studies of colloid osmotic pressure changes in pregnancy-induced hypertension. *Am. J. Obstet. Gynecol.*, **135**, 308–311.

Benedetti, T. J., Kates, R. and Williams, V. (1985) Hemodynamic observations in severe preeclampsia complicated by pulmonary edema. *Am. J. Obstet. Gynecol.*, **152**, 330–334.

Benedetti, T. J., Cotton, D. B., Read, J. A. and Miller, F. C. (1980) Hemodynamic observations in severe preeclampsia using a flow-directed pulmonary artery catheter. *Am. J. Obstet. Gynecol.*, **136**, 465–470.

Bolton, T. B. (1979) Mechanisms of action of transmitters and other substances on smooth muscle. *Physiol. Rev.*, **59**, 606–718.

Clark, S. L., Greenspoon, J. S., Aldahl, D. and Phelan, J. P. (1986) Severe preeclampsia with persistent oliguria: management of hemodynamic subsets, *Am. J. Obstet. Gynecol.*, **154**, 490–494.

Cotton, D. B., Gonik, G. and Dorman, K. F. (1984) Cardiovascular alterations in severe pregnancy-induced hypertension: acute effects of intravenous magnesium sulfate. *Am. J. Obstet. Gynecol.*, **148**, 162–165.

Cotton, D. B., Gonik, B. and Dorman, F. (1985) Cardiovascular alterations in severe pregnancy-induced hypertension seen with an intravenously given hydralazine bolus. *Surg. Gynecol. Obstet.*, **161**, 240–244.

Cotton, D. B., Gonik, G., Spillman, T. and Dorman, K. F. (1984) Intrapartum to postpartum changes in colloid osmotic pressure. *Am. J. Obstet. Gynecol.*, **149**, 174–177.

Cotton, D. B., Gonik, B., Dorman. K. and Harrist, R. (1985) Cardiovascular alterations in severe pregnancy-induced hypertension: relationship of central venous pressure to pulmonary capillary wedge pressure. *Am. J. Obstet. Gynecol.*, **151**, 762–764.

Cotton, D. B., Longmire, S., Jones, M. M. *et al.* (1986) Cardiovascular alterations in severe pregnancy-induced hypertension: effects of intravenous nitroglycerin coupled with blood volume expansion. *Am. J. Obstet. Gynecol.*, **154**, 1053–1059.

Cotton, D. B., Lee, W., Huhta, J. C. and Dorman, K. R. (1988) Hemodynamic profile of severe pregnancy induced hypertension. *Am. J. Obstet. Gynecol.*, **158**, 523–529.

Cunningham, F., MacDonald, P. and Gant, N. (1989) Hypertensive disorders in pregnancy, in *Williams Obstetrics*, 18th edn, (eds L. M. Hellman and J. A. Pritchard), Appleton & Lange, Norwalk, CT, p. 654–694.

Easterling, T. R., Watts, D. H., Schmucker, B. C. and Benedetti, T. J. (1987) Measurement of cardiac output during pregnancy: validation of Doppler technique and clinical observations in preeclampsia. *Obstet. Gynecol.*, **69**, 845–850.

Easterling, T. R., Benedetti, T. J., Schumcker, B. C. and Carlson, K. L. (1989) Antihypertensive therapy in pregnancy directed by non-invasive hemodynamic monitoring. *Am. J. Perinatol.*, **6**, 86–89.

Easterling, T. R., Benedetti, T. J., Schumcker, B. C. and Millard, S. P. (1990) Maternal hemodynamics in normal and preeclamptic pregnancies: a longitudinal study. *Obstet. Gynecol.*, **76**, 1061–1069.

Easterling, T. R., Benedetti, T. J., Carlson, K. C *et al.* (1991) The effect of maternal on fetal growth in hypertensive pregnancies. *Am. J. Obstet. Gynecol.*, **165**, 902–906.

Fahmy, N. R. (1978) Nitroglycerin as a hypotensive drug during general anesthesia. *Anesthesia*, **49**, 17–20.

Fein, A., Grossman, R. F., Jones, J. G. *et al.* (1979) The value of edema fluid protein measurement in patients with pulmonary edema. *Am. J. Med.*, **67**, 32–38.

Ferrer, M. I., Bradley, S. E., Wheeler, H. O. *et al.* (1966) Some effects of nitroglycerin upon the splanchnic, pulmonary, and systemic circulations. *Circulation*, **33**, 357–373.

Garden, A., Davey, D. A. and Dommisse, J. (1982) Intravenous labetalol and intravenous dihydralazine in severe hypertension in pregnancy. *Clin. Exp. Hypertension (B)*, **1**, 371–383.

Gerstner, G. and Grunberger, W. (1980) Dopamine treatment for prevention of renal failure in patients with severe preeclampsia. *Clin. Exp. Obstet. Gynecol.*, **7**, 219–222.

Groenendijk, R., Trimbos, J. B. M. J. and Wallenburg, H. C. S. (1984) Hemodynamic measurements in preeclampsia: preliminary observations. *Am. J. Obstet. Gynecol.*, **150**, 232–236.

Grunfeld, J. P., Ganeval, D. and Bournerias, F. (1980). Acute renal failure in pregnancy. *Kidney Int.*, **18**, 179–91.

Guyton, A. C. (1986) Dominant role of the kidneys and accessory role of wholebody autoregulation in the pathogenesis of hypertension. *Am. J. Hypertension*, **2**, 575–585.

Hankins, G. D. V., Wendel, G. D., Cunningham, F. G. and Leveno, K. J. (1984) Longitudinal evaluation of hemodynamic changes in eclampsia *Am. J. Obstet. Gynecol.*, **150**, 506–512.

Herling, I. M. (1984) Intravenous nitroglycerin. Clinical pharmacology and therapeutic considerations. *Am. Heart J.*, **108**, 141–149.

ACOG (1988) Invasive haemodynamic monitoring in obstetrics and gynecology, Technical Bulletin no. 128, American College of Obstetricians and Gynecologists, Washington, DC.

Kirshon, B., Moise, K. J., Cotton, D. B. *et al.* (1986) Role of volume expansion in severe pre-eclampsia. *Surg. Gynecol. Obstet.*, **167**, 367–371.

Kirshon, B., Lee, W., Mauer, M. B. and Cotton, D. B. (1988) Effects of low-dose dopamine therapy in the oliguric patient with preeclampsia. *Am. J. Obstet. Gynecol.*, **159**, 604–607.

Kirshon, B., Wasserstrum, N. and Cotton, D. B. (1991) Should continuous hydralazine infusions be utilized in severe pregnancy-induced hypertension? *Am. J. Perinatol.*, **8**, 206–208.

Koch-Weser, J. (1976) Hydralazine. *N. Engl. J. Med.*, **295**, 320–323.

Lamming, G. D. and Symonds, E. M. (1979) Use of labetalol and methyldopa in pregnancy-induced hypertension. *Br. J. Clin. Pharmacol.*, **8**, 217S–222S.

Leduc, L., Lederer, E., Lee, W. and Cotton, D. B. (1991) Urinary sediment changes in severe preeclampsia. *Obstet. Gynecol.*, **77**, 186–189.

Lee, W., Gonik, B. and Cotton, D. B. (1987) Urinary diagnostic indices in preeclampsia-associated oliguria: correlation with invasive hemodynamic monitoring. *Am. J. Obstet. Gynecol.*, **156**, 100–103.

Lee, W., Rokey, R. and Cotton, D. B. (1988) Noninvasive maternal stroke volume and cardiac output determination by pulsed Doppler echocardiography. *Am. J. Obstet. Gynecol.*, **158**, 505–510.

Lubbe, W. (1987) Hypertension in pregnancy: whom and how to treat. *Br. J. Clin. Pharmacol.*, **24**, 15S–20S.

Mabie, W. C., Gonzalez, A. R., Sibai, B. M. and Amon, E. (1987) A comparative trial of labetalol and hydralazine in the acute management of severe hypertension complicating pregnancy. *Obstet. Gynecol.*, **70**, 328–333.

Mabie, W. C., Ratts, T. E., Ramanathan, K. B. and Sibai, B. M. (1988) Circulatory congestion in obese hypertensive women: a subset of pulmonary edema in pregnancy. *Obstet. Gynecol.*, **72**, 553–558.

Mabie, W. C., Ratts, T. E. and Sibai, S. (1989) The central hemodynamics of severe preeclampsia. *Am. J. Obstet. Gynecol.*, **161**, 1443–1448 .Matlin, R. A. and Gary, N. E. (1974) Acute cortical necrosis. *Am. J. Med.*, **56**, 110–118.

Michael, C. A. (1986) Intravenous labetalol and intravenous diazoxide in severe hypertension complicating pregnancy. *Aust. NZ J. Obstet. Gynaecol.*, **26**, 26–29.

Moller, L. M. and Hartmann-Anderson, J. F. (1990) Treatment of women with severe pre-eclampsia in an intensive care unit during a 3-year period. *Ugeskr.-Laeger*, **152**, 2735–2737.

Moutquin, J. M., Rainvillie, R. N., Raynauld, P. *et al.* (1985) A prospective study of blood pressure in pregnancy: prediction of preeclampsia. *Am. J. Obstet. Gynecol.*, **151**, 191–196.

Naden, R. P. and Redman, C. W. G (1985) Antihypertensive drugs in pregnancy. *Clin. Perinatol.*, **12**, 521–538.

Naulty, J., Cefalo, R. C. and Lewis, P. E. (1981) Fetal toxicity of nitroprusside in the pregnant ewe. *Am. J. Obstet. Gynecol.*, **139**, 708–711.

Nisell, H., Lunell, N. and Linde, B. (1988) Maternal hemodynamics and impaired fetal growth in pregnancy of hypertension. *Obstet. Gynecol.*, **71**, 163–166.

Nylund, L., Lunell, N. O., Lewander, R. *et al.* (1984) Labetalol for the treatment of hypertension in pregnancy. *Acta Obstet. Gynecol. Scand.*, **118**, 71–73.

Opie, L. H. (1980) Drugs and the heart. III. Calcium antagonists. *Lancet*, **i**, 806–810.

Opie, L. H. (1987) Nitrates: myocardial infarction; heart failure, in *Drug for the Heart*, 2nd edn, Grune & Stratton, Orlando, FL, p. 27.

Pritchard, J. A., Cunningham, F. G. and Pritchard, S. A. (1984) The Parkland Memorial Hospital protocol for the treatment of eclampsia: evaluation of 245 cases. *Am. J. Obstet. Gynecol.*, **148**, 951–963.

Ramanathan, J., Sibai, B. M., Mabie, W. C. *et al.* (1988) The use of labetalol for attenuation of the hypertensive response to endotracheal intubation in preeclampsia. *Am. J. Obstet. Gynecol.*,**159**, 650–654.

Roberts, J. (1984) Pregnancy-related hypertension, in *Maternal–Fetal Medicine: Principles and Practice* (eds R. Creasy and R. Resnik), W. B. Saunders, Philadelphia, PA, p. 703–752.

Robson, S. C., Dunlop, W., Moore, M. and Hunter, S. (1987) Combined Doppler and echocardiographic measurements of cardiac output. Theory and application in pregnancy. *Br. J. Obstet. Gynaecol.*, **94**, 1014–1027.

Rogers, R. C., Sibai, B. M. and Whybrew, W. D. (1990). Clinical articles: labetalol pharmacokinetics in pregnancy-induced hypertension. *Am. J. Obstet. Gynecol.*, **162**, 362–366.

Ross and Braunwald (1964) *Circulation*, **29**, 1439–1442.

Serafini, P. C., Petracco, A., Vicosa, H. M. and Costa, L. P. (1979) Efeito hipotensor arterial do verapamil na pre-eclampsia grave. Estudo preliminar. *Arq. Bras. Cardiol.*, **32**, 57–61.

Sibai, B. M., Spinnato, J. A., Watson, D. L. *et al.* (1984). Pregnancy outcome in 303 cases with severe preeclampsia. *Obstet. Gynecol.*, **64**, 319–325.

Simon, A. C., Levenson, J. A., Levy, B. Y. *et al.* (1982) Effect of nitroglycerin on peripheral large arteries in hypertension. *Br. J. Clin. Pharmacol.*, **14**, 241–246.

Singh, B. N., Ellrodt, G. and Peter, C. T. (1978) Verapamil: a review of its pharmacological properties and therapeutic use. *Drugs*, **15**, 169–197.

Smith, K., Browne, J. C. M., Shackman, R. *et al.* (1965) Acute renal failure of obstetric origins. *Lancet*, **ii**, 351–354.Strauss, R. G., Keefer, J. R., Burke, T. and Civett, J. M. (1980) Hemodynamic monitoring of cardiogenic pulmonary edema complicating toxemia of pregnancy. *Obstet. Gynecol.*, **55**, 170–174.

Taylor, A. E. (1981) Capillary fluid filtration: Starling forces and lymph flow. *Circ. Res.*, **49**, 557–575.

Van Breemen, C., Aaronson, P. and Loutzenhiser, R. (1978) Sodium–calcium interactions in mammalian smooth muscle. *Pharmacol. Rev.*, **30**, 167–208.

Visser, W. and Wallenburg, H. C. S. (1991) Central hemodynamic observations in untreated preeclamptic patients. *Hypertension*, **17**, 1072–1077.

Walker, J. J., Greer, I. and Calder, A. A. (1983) Treatment of acute pregnancy-related hypertension: labetalol and hydralazine compared. *Postgrad. Med. J.*, **59**, 168–170.

Wasserstrum, N. (1991) Nitroprusside in preeclampsia. Circulatory distress and paradoxical bradycardia. *Hypertension*, **18**, 79–84.

Wasserstrum, N., Kirshon, B., Rossavik, I. K. *et al.* (1989) Implications of sino-aortic baroreceptor reflex dysfunction in severe preeclampsia. *Obstet. Gynecol.*, **74**, 34–39.

Wu, P. Y., Udani, V., Chan, L. *et al.* (1983) Colloid osmotic pressure: variations in normal pregnancy. *J. Perinat. Med.*, **11**, 193.

# A PRACTICAL APPROACH TO THE MANAGEMENT OF PREGNANCY HYPERTENSION

*James J. Walker and Norman F. Gant*

## 6.1 INTRODUCTION

Hypertension in pregnancy is a major contributor to the workload and anxiety in the practice of obstetrics. It produces a management dilemma and is responsible for a large percentage of the admissions. It is not a disease in itself but a reflection of a maternal response to an underlying pathology. It can be used as a marker of risk for the mother or the baby. However, since preeclampsia is a multisystem disorder, blood pressure alone may be inadequate for assessing absolute risk. The disease affects different organs in different ways and to different degrees. Some mothers who have severe complications of preeclampsia, such as eclampsia and HELLP syndrome, may have little or no elevation of blood pressure. The risks to the mother and baby depend on how the disease affects the patient and which organs are involved. Not all patients with the same abnormalities of disease parameters will necessarily have the same risks and need to be managed in the same way. The approach that any center will take will depend on what the perceived risk to the mother and baby is. Since these problems are different, they should be treated separately.

## 6.2 RISKS TO THE MOTHER

The figures from the *Confidential Enquiries into Maternal Deaths in the United Kingdom* show that hypertension in pregnancy remains the biggest killer of pregnant women, with 20.5% of maternal deaths associated with pregnancy-induced hypertension and another 8.3% related to other hypertension-related factors. A look at the rates over the last four reports show that there has been little change over the last 30 years (Table 6.1).

**Table 6.1** Number of women who died from hypertensive diseases of pregnancy and the death rate per million maternities, 1970–90 in England and Wales. There had been no fall in the rate of maternal death between 1970 and 1981. The fall seen in the last two triennia is encouraging.

| Triennium | n | Preeclampsia | | Eclampsia | | | |
|---|---|---|---|---|---|---|---|
| | | Rate | n | Rate | n | | Rate |
| 1970–72 | 43 | 18.7 | 14 | 6.1 | 29 | | 12.6 |
| 1973–75 | 34 | 17.7 | 15 | 7.8 | 19 | | 9.9 |
| 1976–78 | 29 | 16.6 | 16 | 9.1 | 13 | | 7.4 |
| 1979–81 | 36 | 18.7 | 16 | 8.3 | 20 | | 10.4 |
| 1982–84 | 25 | 13.3 | 11 | 5.8 | 14 | | 7.4 |
| 1985–87 | 25 | 12.6 | 13 | 6.5 | 12 | | 6.0 |
| 1988–90 | 24 | 11.5 | 10 | 4.8 | 14 | | 6.7 |

*Hypertension in Pregnancy*
Edited by J.J. Walker and N.F. Gant. Published by Chapman & Hall, 1997 ISBN 0 412 30910 6

If the cause of death within the hypertensive group is studied, it can be seen that the main cause of death was cerebral hemorrhage and other types of cerebral damage (Table 6.2).

Respiratory problems, mostly pulmonary edema are the next most common. Renal failure was not a common cause of death, being responsible for less then 5% of cases of maternal mortality. If it does occur, it is usually due to acute tubular necrosis and can be easily managed. These findings are similar to those quoted in 1961 by Govan. If CVA does occur, it is generally early in the disease presentation. When cardiac failure occurs, it is most common between 24 and 48 hours postdelivery. It is not due to modern fluid management but a risk of the disease itself. Obviously, excessive fluid replacement can contribute to the problem. Although there may be depletion of the plasma volume, the vascular tree is contracted, reducing the capacity for fluid replacement.

Even if patients with eclampsia are studied, cerebral hemorrhage still appears to be the main cause of mortality rather than the convulsion itself. The risk to both mother and baby appears to relate to the degree of preeclampsia preceding the seizure, rather

**Table 6.2** The causes of the 78 maternal deaths associated with eclampsia or preeclampsia in England and Wales 1982–90. One of the patients with preeclampsia in the triennium 1982–84 did not have a postmortem and is not included in the figures. Of the 78 patients, 46 had evidence of cerebral lesions.

| Causes | n |
| --- | --- |
| Cerebral hemorrhage | 36 |
| Cerebral edema | 5 |
| Cerebral infarction | 3 |
| Cerebral cortical necrosis | 1 |
| Cerebral softening | 1 |
| Pulmonary complication | 24 |
| Hepatic necrosis | 3 |
| Other | 5 |
| Total | 78 |

than the seizure itself. Therefore, in the United Kingdom CVA is seen as the main maternal risk of hypertension in pregnancy, not eclampsia. In most studies, about 30% of the patients who suffered seizures had diastolic blood pressures of less than 90 mmHg. The chances of eclampsia occurring may be related more to the patient's seizure threshold than to the level of blood pressure. The risk of vascular damage with hypertension correlates with the animal studies that showed vessels are damaged when the diastolic blood pressure rises above 110 mmHg. Therefore, the main risks to the mother would appear to occur only after the blood pressure has reached 110 mmHg diastolic. Although convulsions may occur below this level, the maternal mortality and morbidity are related to the vascular damage associated with the hypertension, rather than to the convulsions, unless repeated convulsions occur.

Because of the dramatic presentation, it was eclampsia that was recognized before the hypertension. Even with modern methods of blood pressure measurement, it is often eclampsia that brings the patient to the attention of medical care. This is particularly true in the Third World, where there is less antenatal care available. This has led to the prevention and treatment of eclampsia being the first line of management in many parts of the world. In North America, many centers still see a high level of eclampsia and anticonvulsant therapy is the mainstay of their therapeutic protocols (Chapter 15). However, the role of prophylactic anticonvulsants has been questioned (Chapters 14 and 16). The risk of seizures in a hypertensive patient may be overrated, but there is little good evidence of the true risk. In the Johns Hopkins Hospital, Baltimore, MD, in the 1930s, fewer than 1 in 300 preeclamptics became eclamptic. There were similar figures from Guy's Hospital, London at the same time. In Scotland, the incidence of eclampsia is 1 in 300 of the total preeclamptic/eclamptic patients. Since many of the eclamptic patients show acute onset or are intrapartum/postpartum with no prodromal preeclampsia, the incidence of eclampsia occurring in any hypertensive patient must be even lower than 1/300. Therefore the risk of eclampsia for the average hypertensive patient is low, and the main risk of mortality is from the hypertension itself, leading to CVA.

A common belief is that delivery cures the patient with preeclampsia. If the Scottish figures are reviewed, it can be seen that all the patients who died did so after delivery. Therefore, although the removal of the trophoblast will eventually remove the stimulus to the disease, this is not immediate and continued vigilance is required after delivery. Eclampsia can occur some days after delivery.

Delivery in the unstable patient is probably more dangerous than a delay in order to stabilize the situation. Intubation causes a further rise in blood pressure of between 20 and 30 mmHg in both systolic and diastolic pressures. This is associated with CVAs occurring under anesthetic, leading to postpartum death. Adequate therapy with antihypertensives and/or narcotics prior to intubation reduces this risk. Pulmonary edema is the next major cause of maternal mortality. This is often due to fluid overload, partly caused by overenthusiastic replacement. Plasma protein solutions are particularly dangerous. Although there may be depletion of the plasma volume, the vascular tree is contracted, reducing the capacity for fluid replacement. Some workers suggest that Swan–Ganz catheters are required to monitor the fluid replacement in order to reduce this iatrogenic cause of maternal mortality and morbidity (Chapter 5). The classical risks of renal and liver damage are rarely seen in present day practice in the United Kingdom, although they are still encountered in other parts of the world and in association with abruption (Chapter 16).

The reason for the reduction in renal risk is partly due to the availability of renal dialysis but, with adequate attention to the fluid balance and the careful monitoring of the urine output, renal failure should not occur. Coagulation abnormalities associated with elevated liver enzymes and hemolysis (HELLP syndrome) is a serious but not new phenomenon as low platelets, liver problems and hemolysis are well recognized complications of preeclampsia. The realization that these signs identify a high-risk patient is important, however, as the assessment of risk in preeclampsia has often been arbitrary in the past.

Despite these well accepted risks to the mother, it should be remembered that the vast majority of these patients do well, with little or no morbidity. This implies that proper assessment of the mother is required (Chapter 7), and properly targeted monitoring and care (Chapters 8–17) may help to further reduce the maternal mortality statistics.

## 6.3 RISKS TO THE FETUS AND NEONATE

The effects of hypertension on the fetus depend on the degree of involvement of the placenta, acute occurrences such as abruption and the gestation at delivery.

Although preeclampsia is thought by many to be a placental disease, it is plain that not all the pregnancies are equally badly affected. The incidence of intrauterine growth retardation is not absolute and many babies are well-grown with no apparent placental insufficiency.

The classic pathology seen with preeclampsia consists of two parts. First, there is the failure of the spiral arteries to dilate and lose their muscular coat and then there are secondary changes of infarction and thrombosis (Chapter 4). The first changes are probably present in most if not all of the true preeclamptic patients, but the secondary changes are not universal and may not be present in all parts of the placenta in the same patient. It is at the secondary changes that therapies such as low-dose aspirin have been directed, in an attempt to reduce the effects of the disease. Many workers believe that it is the placental damage that leads to ischemia. Such damage stimulates the release of a factor X that produces the vasoconstriction and hypertension found in preeclampsia (Chapter 4). The secondary changes are similar in essential hypertension and may be partly an effect of hypertension. The primary changes in the spiral arteries are absent in essential hypertension but present in cases of IUGR even though signs of preeclampsia are absent.

Therefore, the effect on the baby depends not only on the presence of the disease but on the degree of placental involvement. Although diastolic blood pressure above 95 mmHg is associated with an increased perinatal mortality, the level of blood pressure does not appear to be a good marker in clinical practice.

So, if blood pressure does not necessarily help in the prediction of perinatal outcome, is there anything that is better? Redman showed that uric acid was a better predictor of poor perinatal outcome than blood pressure. An increasing uric acid level is thought to be a sign of renal involvement in the disease. The platelet count also falls in patients with progressive disease before the increasing severity becomes apparent. Platelet consumption is thought to be associated with placental deposition and fibrin formation. This could be a sign of impending placental insufficiency. There is a higher incidence of IUGR in cases of perinatal mortality associated with hypertension compared to the other causes of perinatal mortality. Therefore the risks to the fetus are associated with changes found in placental insufficiency. This makes the assessment of fetal wellbeing paramount in the assessment of the hypertensive pregnancy (Chapter 8).

In the presence of a normally functioning placenta, is hypertension any problem to the fetus at all? If the hypertension remains mild or moderate, the risk to the fetus appears to be less than normal.

In cases of eclampsia, the risk to the fetus relates to the degree of preeclampsia that existed prior to the convulsion rather than the convulsion itself. There is a small increase in the incidence of abruption, but the risk only appears to rise when the systolic blood pressures is above 200 mmHg.

One of the significant causes of perinatal mortality in pregnancies complicated by pregnancy hypertension is prematurity. Many workers have shown the poor outcome of hypertensive pregnancies in the second and early third trimesters. Some have suggested that it is a different disease.

The reason for this is obvious. If the patient has severe disease in early gestation, delivery of the fetus carries a poor outcome, whereas severe preeclampsia occurring at 34 weeks can easily be treated by delivery with an excellent prospect of a satisfactory fetal outcome. In later pregnancy, the presence of placental insufficiency increases the risk of fetal mortality and morbidity irrespective of the degree of blood pressure rise.

Therefore, the need to deliver the baby in the maternal interest is only a risk to the fetus in the earlier trimesters when, despite good growth and wellbeing, the fetus may well die because of prematurity. The other risk is of placental insufficiency and IUGR, which can cause problems at any gestation and with any severity of hypertension. This can be seen in the Scottish perinatal mortality figures, which show that the perinatal loss associated with PIH is mostly postnatal prior to 32 weeks and antenatal after 32 weeks.

As the risk to the fetus varies with gestation, in order to reduce this loss a two-pronged approach is required: attempt to prolong the pregnancies to allow improved fetal viability in early gestation; and increase fetal monitoring to reduce intrauterine death in later pregnancy. The chapters in this book will describe how many attempt to tackle these problems. Chapter 17 tackles the long-term problems associated with babies born from mothers with preeclampsia.

## 6.4 A PRACTICAL APPROACH TO THE MANAGEMENT OF HYPERTENSION IN PREGNANCY

Maternal mortality is associated with poor antenatal care and unbooked patients. It is through the antenatal screening process that most of the hypertensive patients will be found. Therefore, the basis of management of hypertensive diseases is comprehensive antenatal care.

The hypertensive patient can present in various ways. The hypertension may be an incidental finding at routine antenatal examination. There may be no symptoms and the diagnosis of a 'disease' with serious implications is difficult for the patient to accept. Many obstetricians would favor admission for assessment and/or observation once hypertension has been found. The patient may find this unacceptable and it may invoke a conflict between her and her doctor. In many parts of the world, the first contact with the hospital is made when she presents herself at the hospital with headache, increasing edema or convulsion.

Assessment of the risk for the mother and baby is the initial stage of the management process and the following chapters cover the methodology of this and how workers in different parts of the world manage this serious problem. Management should be targeted at the main problems that are seen. If convulsion is the main risk, then prevention of convulsion is the mainstay of the approach.

Delivery will lead to resolution of the symptoms over time. It is the only ultimate cure of the condition. However, it is important to remember that many of the maternal deaths occur after delivery. Continuing vigilance is required. Delivery is not always a simple solution and can be a procedure of great risk. It should be carried out on the best day, in the best place, in the best way, by the best team available.

The timing of the delivery will affect the outcome for both mother and baby. If the mother is unstable, a rushed delivery may add to her risk, but delay in delivery can be equally treacherous. As far as the mother is concerned, it is stabilization of her blood pressure and/or convulsions that is paramount. Once this is achieved, a decision of when to deliver can be made in a calm and considered way.

All these factors are approached in different ways in different parts of the world. These are outlined in the management chapters.

# MATERNAL ASSESSMENT IN PREGNANCY-INDUCED HYPERTENSIVE DISORDERS: SPECIAL INVESTIGATIONS AND THEIR PATHOPHYSIOLOGICAL BASIS

*Gustaaf A. Dekker and James J. Walker*

## 7.1 INTRODUCTION

According to the World Health Organization, hypertensive disease during pregnancy is the main cause of maternal and perinatal mortality and morbidity. It has always been assumed that pregnancy-induced hypertensive diseases are a pathological response. However, in developed countries approximately 10% of all nulliparous women will become hypertensive during pregnancy and it seems improbable that a totally harmful process should be present at such high incidence in the population. Non-proteinuric hypertension arising late in pregnancy is associated neither with any increase in perinatal mortality or morbidity nor with a decreased birthweight (Consensus Report, 1990). In the rarer, severe form of the disease, usually arising late in the second trimester and usually accompanied by significant proteinuria, there is a significant increase in perinatal mortality and morbidity (Sibai, 1988a; Friedman and Neff, 1977). Arguing teleologically, it appears that an increase in blood pressure is in some way an adaptive phenomenon, of intrinsic survival value, which in some women breaks down, converting a physiological process into one of pathology (Broughton Pipkin, 1985).

Proper definitions and classifications of the hypertensive disorders of pregnancy should await the finding of either a marker for or the cause of preeclampsia (Sibai, 1990a). Presently, clinicians have to rely on clinical signs and symptoms to classify these disorders. Numerous attempts have been made to classify the hypertensive disorders of pregnancy. Most of these classifications are cumbersome and have no value for the obstetrician. For clinical purposes the classification given in Table 7.1 is used.

This pragmatic classification is based on the premise that, in clinical obstetrics, preeclampsia should be overdiagnosed. The selection of cases for research on preeclampsia demands that far more stringent criteria must be met. In clinical research preeclampsia should be defined as a disorder in a nulliparous woman with pregnancy-induced hypertension, pro-

*Hypertension in Pregnancy*
Edited by J.J. Walker and N.F. Gant. Published by Chapman & Hall, 1997 ISBN 0 412 30910 6

---

**Table 7.1**   Pragmatic classification of pregnancy-induced hypertensive disorders

1. **Pregnancy-induced hypertensive disease**: hypertension without any sign of circulatory compromise and organ dysfunction
2. **Preeclampsia**: pregnancy-induced vasospasm, resulting in manifestations of circulatory compromise and/or organ dysfunction

Apart from hypertension the following manifestations may represent vasospasm and thus potential danger to mother and/or fetus:

- Proteinuria
- Hemoconcentration
- Thrombocytopenia
- Elevated liver enzymes
- Hyperuricemia
- Abnormal coagulation/fibrinolysis criteria
- Fetal growth retardation
- Abnormal uteroplacental and/or umbilical Doppler flow velocity wave forms

(Hypertension induced by pregnancy = diastolic blood pressure increase of 20 mmHg or greater from average of values before 20 weeks gestation)

---

teinuria and hyperuricemia. Furthermore, all abnormalities must have resolved by 12 weeks postpartum (Chesley, 1985; Consensus Report, 1990). This chapter presents a review on clinical and laboratory methods used for maternal surveillance in established pregnancy-induced hypertensive disorders. Emphasis is placed on the differentiation between hypertension as an 'adaptive' phenomenon and the 'real' disease, preeclampsia. In the discussion of results of published studies, the classifications of hypertensive disorders of pregnancy found in these original articles are maintained in this chapter as far as possible. On the whole, the term 'pregnancy-induced hypertensive disease' will be used to indicate the presence of non-proteinuric hypertensive disease of pregnancy, not associated with adverse perinatal outcome and/or serious maternal morbidity or mortality. The term 'preeclampsia' will be used to designate the 'real' disease, associated with significant proteinuria and/or hemostatic changes and/or signs of liver and renal involvement and/or adverse perinatal outcome. The general term 'pregnancy-induced hypertensive disorder(s)' will be used as a denomination for all hyper-

tensive disorders, with or without proteinuria, induced by the pregnant state. This chapter will not focus on prediction of pregnancy-induced hypertensive disorders (Dekker and Sibai, 1991). However, predictive aspects of several maternal assessment methods will be mentioned briefly where it is deemed appropriate.

## 7.2. CLINICAL ASSESSMENT

Most patients with a pregnancy-induced hypertensive disorder have no clinical symptoms, so it can only be reliably detected by repetitive searches (screening) for the early signs and symptoms in the second half of pregnancy. The standard pattern of antenatal care (monthly visits at 20, 24 and 28 weeks) leaves two dangerous gaps where severe early-onset preeclampsia can evolve undetected, i.e. the months before and after 24 weeks. In the Oxford region 50% of antenatal eclampsia occurs at this time. To identify all cases of preeclampsia, women would need to be screened at weekly intervals from 20 weeks. Because this is impossible, a compromise is needed. Redman advocated assessing the individual risk of a pregnant woman at the end of the first trimester. Further antenatal care and the frequency of the antenatal visits can than be individualized to the risk of the individual woman. In pregnant women with an above-average risk, the two gaps in antenatal care (20–24 weeks/24–28 weeks) should be closed (Redman, 1989a).

## 7.3 HEMODYNAMIC ASSESSMENT

### 7.3.1 BLOOD PRESSURE

Hypertension is the most common sign and potentially the most dangerous clinical manifestation of pregnancy-induced hypertensive disorders, and is implicated in a large number of fatal cases. The increase in blood pressure in pregnancy-induced hypertensive disorders is caused by an increase in systemic peripheral resistance and is a rather early feature of the disease. The most widely used technique for measuring blood pressure by the indirect method involves the use of the mercury sphygmomanometer. Oscillometric techniques are increasingly used in clinical obstetrics. The oscillations of pressure in a sphygmomanometer cuff begin above systolic pressure and continue below diastolic pressure, so that systolic and diastolic pressure can only be estimated indirectly according to some empirically derived algorithm. The point of maximum oscillation corresponds with the mean intra-arterial pressure. The method works reasonably well in general, but it may be seriously in error in some patients (Ramsey, 1979). Ultrasound techniques use an ultrasound transmitter and receiver placed over the brachial artery under a sphygmomanometer cuff. As the cuff is deflated, the movement of the arterial wall at systolic pressure causes a Doppler phase shift in the reflected ultrasound waves, and diastolic pressure is recorded at the point at which diminution of arterial motion occurs. The accuracy of such devices for measuring diastolic blood pressure has been questioned, and

further studies are indicated before this technique is introduced in clinical obstetrics (Pickering and Blank, 1990).

A new device is the Finapress recorder, a method based on the finger-cuff method of Penaz (1973). Arterial pulsation in a finger is detected by a photoplethysmograph under a pressure cuff. This method gives an accurate estimate of systolic and diastolic pressure, although both may be underestimated when compared to intra-arterial brachial artery pressures, especially in case of hypertension (Pickering and Blank, 1990). The device can accurately monitor changes in blood pressure. Its application in clinical obstetrics is likely to be greatest in situations where short-term circulatory changes and changes in peripheral perfusion are expected to occur, e.g. during cesarean section in a preeclamptic patient.

A recently described technique is the Korotkoff Signal Technique (the K2 method). This method is based on waveform analysis of the Korotkoff signal, using a specially designed transducer called a foil electric sensor (West *et al.*, 1983). As cuff pressure is reduced, a high-frequency component (K2) develops, corresponding to systolic blood pressure. K2 disappears at diastolic blood pressure. The appearance and disappearance of the K2 signal has been demonstrated to be closer to true systolic and diastolic intra-arterial blood pressures than those given by the auscultatory method.

In conclusion, a large number of devices that monitor blood pressure more or less automatically are now available. Presently, there is no (semi)automatic blood pressure recording device that is universally reliable. Every time such a device is used it should be calibrated against a standard method, which, for practical reasons, means a mercury sphygmomanometer.

### (a) Korotkoff sounds

At the present time, the auscultatory technique, based on the Korotkoff sounds, remains the standard method for recording blood pressure. However, there is still no universal agreement as to which phase of the Korotkoff sounds should be used for recording diastolic blood pressure. In non-pregnant patients phase IV (muffling) is about 8 mmHg higher than the intra-arterial diastolic blood pressure and is more subject to interobserver error. Phase V of the Korotkoff sounds (disappearance) corresponds most closely with intra-arterial diastolic pressure (on average 2 mmHg lower than the true diastolic pressure (Pickering and Blank, 1990), and is widely used in non-obstetric practice. However, due to the hyperkinetic circulation of pregnancy the Korotkoff sounds are often (15% of pregnant women) audible to very low or even zero diastolic blood pressure. Indeed, the problem with the use of many automatic sphygmomanometers in pregnancy is that, because Korotkoff phase V is measured, diastolic blood pressure can appear very low (MacGillivray, 1983).

It is essential that the technique and conditions of measurement should be standardized if consistent results are to be obtained (Davey, 1985). Measuring blood pressure with the cuff on the superior arm in a patient in lateral recumbent position will result in a predictable decrease in diastolic blood pressure of approximately 10–14 mmHg due to a decrease in hydrostatic pressure relative to the level of the heart (each centimeter above or below the heart translates to an 0.8 mmHg change). The same mechanism is the major cause of the pressor response when performing the rollover test (Wichman, Ryden and Wichman, 1984; Dekker, Makovitz and Wallenburg, 1990). In addition, if blood pressure is measured in the supine position then, as the result of the decreased venous return secondary to compression of the vena cava, supine hypotension may occur.

During pregnancy blood pressure should be measured with the woman in a sitting (ambulatory patient) or semi-reclining position (hospitalized patient), the right arm should be used consistently and the arm should be in a roughly horizontal position at heart level. For diastolic blood pressure measurement, both Korotkoff phase IV and V should be recorded, but phase IV should be used for diagnosis (Sibai, 1988b). The size of the cuff relative to the diameter of the arm is critical. In general, the error can be reduced by using a large adult sized cuff for all except the skinniest arms (Pickering and Blank, 1990). For the diagnosis of hypertension during pregnancy, it is accepted practice to require two consecutively abnormally high measurements made at least 4–6 hours apart (Consensus Report, 1990).

Although measurement of intra-arterial blood pressure is generally accepted as being the most accurate method of blood pressure recording, its clinical use is limited by virtue of its invasiveness. Therefore, this method is usually reserved for severely ill patients. The sites most commonly used for intra-arterial pressure recording are the brachial and radial arteries. In pregnant women, diastolic blood pressure values obtained by indirect sphygmomanometry are about 15 mmHg higher than diastolic pressures measured with an intra-arterial catheter (Wallenburg, 1988). In the management of a severely ill patient the individual difference between direct and indirect measurements of diastolic blood pressure should be obtained and taken into account for management and treatment purposes.

### (b) Self-monitoring

Approximately 20% of an average non-pregnant population have 'white coat' hypertension: blood pressures recorded by a physician can be as much as 30 mmHg higher than pressures taken by the patient at home (Pickering and Blank, 1990). Zuspan and Rayburn (1991) stated that self-monitoring of blood pressure should antedate and accompany therapy for pregnancy-induced hypertensive disorders. Home recordings can give a more accurate picture of the patient's dynamic blood pressure. Blood pressures in pregnant women are usually lower outside the physician's office. From a theoretical point of view, the lower blood pressures at home may be a drawback of this method. The obstetrician may forget that all maternal and perinatal morbidity and mortality studies are based on measurements done in physician's offices, and may feel reassured by the 'decreased' blood pressure levels at home.

An alternative method of assessment is the use of antenatal daycare units, as described in Chapter 9. This has the advantage of being a relaxed surrounding where several blood pressure readings can be taken over time and the average assessed. This allows the error of individual readings to be overcome.

### 7.3.2 INVASIVE HEMODYNAMIC MONITORING

Since 1980 the pulmonary artery (PA) catheter has been used for critically ill obstetric patients. The Swan–Ganz catheter is a flow-directed balloon-tipped multilumen PA catheter named after its inventors. A review of invasive hemodynamic monitoring in severe preeclampsia is given in Chapter 5. Invasive hemodynamic monitoring provides the obstetrician with the following direct and calculated hemodynamic variables: cardiac output (CO), central venous pressure (CVP), pulmonary capillary wedge pressure (PCWP) and systemic vascular resistance (SVR). Measurements of CO are performed with a triple-lumen catheter that has a thermistor on the tip. In addition to lumens for the balloon and the catheter tip, these devices have a lumen leading to a proximal port opening into the right atrium. The principle employed by this catheter is that net blood flow can be calculated when a known quantity of cold solution is adequately mixed with the circulation and a cooling curve is registered at the thermistor placed at the tip of the catheter. A bedside computer integrates the area under the cooling curve generated and calculates the CO. This thermodilution method has been proved to be simple, efficient and accurate (Clark and Harman, 1988).

The CVP has been used for many years to monitor the relative relationship of blood volume to vascular capacity. The CVP reflects right ventricular function and systemic vascular compliance. However, LV failure and pulmonary congestion may occur without an elevation of the CVP.

The PCWP is an important variable for two basic parameters of cardiopulmonary function.

1. It reflects pulmonary venous pressure and consequently capillary hydrostatic pressure, which is a critical factor in the development of pulmonary edema.
2. The PCWP is closely related to left atrial pressure, which, in absence of significant mitral valve disease, reflects left ventricular end-diastolic pressure (LVEDP).

The PCWP therefore provides considerable insight into the functional status of the left ventricle.

The data obtained with the catheter enable the clinician to calculate the SVR, a parameter of obvious importance in the management of a vasoconstrictive disease process such as severe preeclampsia. The equation for calculating SVR is: SVR = (MAP – RAP/CO) × 80 dyn.s/cm$^5$, where MAP = mean arterial pressure in mmHg, RAP = right atrial pressure in mmHg and CO = cardiac output in l/min.

The use of these techniques should be limited and invasive hemodynamic monitoring should be used in:

1. severe early-onset (24–32 weeks gestational age) preeclampsia (including HELLP syndrome) if fetoplacental reserve appears to be more or less adequate;
2. severe preeclampsia–eclampsia associated with persistent oliguria/anuria and/or pulmonary edema;
3. extreme hypertension unresponsive to conventional antihypertensive treatment

The use of invasive hemodynamic monitoring for these indications will greatly help the obstetrician in a judicious assessment of the maternal condition and thus in providing a careful, individualized management strategy. The treatment of a patient with severe early-onset preeclampsia, referred because of persistent oliguria and severe hypertension, is extremely difficult without these hemodynamic data. The PA catheter will tell the obstetrician if oliguria is caused by intravascular volume depletion, systemic vasospasm, intrarenal vasospasm or even cardiac failure (Clark *et al.*, 1986). Plasma volume expansion is easily guided on the basis of these variables. An increase in CO or a rise in SVR, or both, may increase systemic blood pressure. Invasive hemodynamic monitoring will reveal the exact cause of the increase in blood pressure and, with the help of the PA catheter, antihypertensive therapy may be adapted for the individual patient (Wallenburg, 1988; Ackerman *et al.*, 1990).

There are risks of invasive hemodynamic monitoring. Complications of PA catheter placement range from 0.4–9.9% depending on the experience of the practitioner and the severity of the illness of the patient. Certainly the list of complications attributable to PA catheterization is longer than that of complications attributable to obtaining central venous access. Complications include pneumothorax, hemothorax, injury to vascular and neurological structures, cardiac arrhythmias, pulmonary hemorrhage and pulmonary infarction. With the exception of cardiac arrhythmias, pulmonary hemorrhage and pulmonary infarction, these complications are essentially the same as have been encountered after placing a central venous pressure catheter. Serious cardiac arrhythmias and pulmonary hemorrhage are very rare, and pulmonary infarction can be prevented by meticulous care in handling the catheter and removing the catheter after a maximum period of 48–72 hours. Therefore, if there is a clear indication for invasive hemodynamic monitoring, place a PA catheter instead of a central venous pressure catheter. The risks in a young

woman without intrinsic cardiac disease are nearly the same. The vast amount of additional information obtainable with the PA catheter far outweighs the slight additional increase in risk attributable to PA catheter insertion and is nearly always preferable (Easterling and Benedetti, 1991a).

The safest access for catheter placement is via the internal jugular vein or a large peripheral vein, especially in patients with a bleeding tendency. Insertion via the right internal jugular vein has the following advantages over the subclavian approach (Clark, 1991).

1. Pneumothorax, the principal complication of subclavian puncture, is far less likely when using the internal jugular approach.
2. Should inadvertent arterial puncture occur the carotid artery is much more accessible to direct pressure hemostasis than the subclavian artery.
3. Insertion of the PA catheter and advancement into the right ventricle is facilitated with the right jugular approach because the ventricle lies directly below the jugular vein.

After placement of the PA catheter, a chest X-ray should be obtained to rule out pneumothorax and to confirm the position of the catheter. In the hands of an experienced operator PA catheterization is surprisingly free from risk; withdrawal of the catheter within 48 hours largely eliminates the thrombotic and infective hazards.

### 7.3.3 NON-INVASIVE HEMODYNAMIC MONITORING

Three techniques are currently used to assess cardiac output non-invasively:

1. **Echocardiographic methods** measure stroke volume by estimating end-systolic and end-diastolic left ventricular volumes from long and short axis dimensions of the ventricle. The corresponding volumes are than calculated from a single measurement using

various stereometric assumptions. Validations of this echo technique in non-pregnant subjects are limited, and no validation studies have been done in pregnancy. Given the remodeling of the heart during pregnancy, this kind of validation study is certainly needed before this method can be adopted for clinical purposes (Easterling, 1992).

2. **Doppler techniques** measure blood flow velocity in the aorta or left ventricular outflow tract. The cross-sectional area of the aorta or outflow tract is measured. The product of this cross-sectional area and the calculated time–velocity integral gives an estimation of stroke volume. The hardware to make the required measurements and the software to make the calculations are commercially available. In experienced hands this technique has been demonstrated to be associated with an intraindividual/intraobserver variability of less than 5% (Robson *et al.*, 1987). Several studies validated this method against PA catheter data and found a close correlation between the results of both techniques in normotensive and hypertensive pregnant women (Easterling *et al.*, 1987; Lee, Rokey and Cotton, 1988; Lee and Pivarnik, 1992). Easterling and Benedetti (1991b) state 'where labs have demonstrated their expertise with the methodology, measurements of cardiac output with the Doppler technique may be assumed to be equivalent to those made by thermodilution'. An important aspect, and at the same time a major drawback is the expertise of the operator that is essential for this assessment method. Measuring CO with invasive techniques is much easier, and can be done by intensive care nurses on a 24-hour base. Also, the PA catheter will provide the clinician with the PCWP, a parameter that can not be obtained with non-invasive techniques.

3. **Impedance cardiography** is based on the fact that the ability of blood to transmit an electrical current is increased when the blood is flowing. Stroke volume is estimated by measuring transthoracic impedance from electrodes on the chest. Kubicek *et al.* (1966) introduced the method in 1966. However, their equation to calculate stroke volume was inaccurate. Later on, Smarek and Bernstein proposed an new equation (Bernstein, 1986a; Banner and Banner, 1988), and this equation has been incorporated into the software of a microprocessor and is commercially available. Using this instrument agreement between impedance and thermodilution techniques has been demonstrated in non-pregnant subjects. However, in high-flow states such as septic shock the impedance may underestimate cardiac output by more than 50% (Bernstein, 1986b; Banner and Banner, 1988). Several studies compared the impedance technique with data obtained by PA catheterization. The conclusion of the majority of these studies is that the impedance technique consistently underestimates cardiac output in normotensive and preeclamptic pregnancy (de Swiet and Talbert, 1986; Easterling *et al.*, 1989). In contrast, Masaki, Greenspoon and Ouzounian (1989) reported good correlation between electrical impedance and thermodilution CO in 11 critically ill pregnant patients with a variety of diseases. The impedance technique may be an accurate method for assessing acute, relative changes in cardiac output. However, absolute values do not correspond with results obtained by the other techniques. In a recent review Easterling (1992) advocates against the use of this method in the management of preeclamptic patients.

### 7.3.4 HEMODYNAMICS IN PREECLAMPSIA

In preeclampsia, CO, as measured with the thermodilution method, has been described as decreased, unchanged and increased, and likewise there are conflicting data regarding alterations in PCWP. This controversy is caused by the fact that investigators have combined results from heterogeneous populations, often neglecting to distinguish between preeclampsia and chronic hypertension. Measurements were often made after therapeutic interventions such as volume loading and magnesium sulfate administration (Sibai, 1990a). Easterling *et al.* (1990), studied CO with Doppler technique in obese women that develop late-onset mild 'preeclampsia'. In these women CO was found to be elevated, and Easterling *et al.* (1990) hypothesized that elevated cardiac output is the fundamental hemodynamic alteration in preeclampsia. Others do not agree with this hypothesis (Dekker and van Geijn, 1992). The elevated CO in these patients is probably associated with their obesity and not an expression of 'preeclampsia'. All authors that studied untreated, primigravid proteinuric hypertensive pregnant women all found a decreased cardiac output, elevated systemic peripheral vascular resistance and low PCWPs (Hankins *et al.*, 1984; Wallenburg, 1988). The 'real' disease preeclampsia is primarily characterized by vasoconstriction caused by endothelial damage, resulting in increased cardiac afterload, decreased cardiac output and hypovolemia (De Jong, Dekker and Sibai, 1991; Zeeman and Dekker, 1992).

## 7.4 EDEMA AND WEIGHT GAIN

The one visible sign of pregnancy-induced hypertensive disorders is swelling, but this is not a reliable sign. Moderate edema can be detected in 60–80% of normotensive pregnancies, and pedal edema, even extending to the lower tibia, is a common finding in normal pregnant women (Chesley, 1978). Although, the classic sequence of signs is edema, increased blood pressure and proteinuria, any order of appearance may occur, and edema is not a prerequisite for diagnosing pregnancy-induced hypertensive disorders (Chesley, 1978; Consensus Report, 1990). Weight gain cannot be used to predict the development of

pregnancy-induced hypertensive disorders (Dekker and Sibai, 1991), and excess weight gain alone imparts no adverse prognosis to perinatal outcome. In fact, weight gain in pregnancy is known to be correlated with birthweight. Pathological edema affects 85% of women with a pregnancy-induced hypertensive disorder (Thomson, Hytten and Billewicz, 1967). Pathological edema appears suddenly and is associated with an accelerated rate of weight gain. Chesley (1978) stated that if pedal edema does not regress overnight, the pregnant woman bears careful watching. A woman with established preeclampsia will often have facial and particularly periorbital edema, in contrast to the physiological pedal edema.

It is probably fair to say that sudden swelling linked with a gain of more than 1 kg per week over 2 or 3 weeks, or more than 2 kg in 1 week should warn the clinician and indicate the need for an accurate search for other clues of the presence of the disease. Fluid retention can be assessed accurately by keeping record of a detailed fluid balance and daily weight measuring. In most patients with mild to moderate disease a decrease in edema is noted during the first days of bed rest. If a rapid daily increase in weight and/or edema occurs the disease has reached its preterminal phase. In the majority of these cases the obstetrician will be forced to induce labor or perform a cesarean section. Massive edema is associated with an increased risk of pulmonary edema, especially in the postpartum period. In 15–39% of cases of severe preeclampsia–eclampsia there is no edema (Sibai, 1990c). This so called dry preeclampsia has been reported to be particularly dangerous (Eden, 1922). In conclusion, edema is an early and common sign of preeclampsia but it is not diagnostic. In the near future new noninvasive methods such as segmental multiple frequency conductivity measurements may provide us with more accurate data on dynamic changes in intra- and extracellular volume in pregnancy (Segal *et al.*, 1991).

## 7.5 URINE OUTPUT

The range of normal daily volume of urine is 600–2000 ml (mean 1400 ml). In the non-pregnant adult the night urine is generally not in excess of 400 ml. Diuresis has been described as the best test of renal function. However, in pregnancy this can be misleading, for what passes as oliguria by non-pregnant standards may be quite normal in pregnancy; it is not uncommon for healthy pregnant women to excrete urine at 25–35 ml per hour for days on end (Wood, 1977). In normal pregnancy, the usual diurnal variation is reversed, causing nocturia and the excretion of dilute urine. This is probably caused by the accumulation of water in the form of dependent edema during the day. At night, while recumbent, this fluid is mobilized and excreted via the kidneys.

MacGillivray (1983) stated that 'oliguria or anuria is a most important sign to look for in established cases of pre-eclampsia, as it is an indication that the baby and placenta should be delivered promptly'. Although oliguria is indeed a serious sign, it is not as such an indication for immediate delivery. Oliguria/anuria may be classified as prerenal, renal and postrenal. In preeclampsia–eclampsia hypovolemia, without serious intrarenal vasoconstriction, may be the cause of oliguria. However, in most patients oliguria/anuria is a consequence of a combination of glomerular endotheliosis, intrarenal vasoconstriction and hypovolemia. Although acute renal failure is a rare complication of preeclampsia–eclampsia, preeclampsia–eclampsia is a major cause of obstetric acute renal failure. Usually acute renal failure in preeclampsia–eclampsia is of the tubular necrosis variety, but sometimes it is caused by the more ominous bilateral cortical necrosis. Sibai, Villar and Mabie (1990) described 31 cases of acute renal failure occurring with hypertensive disorders of pregnancy. In 50% of these cases the hypertensive pregnancies were complicated by disseminated intravascular coagulation caused by abruptio placentae. In established preeclampsia it is obligatory to monitor daily fluid intake and output. In severe preeclampsia urine output should be measured on an hourly basis with a urinary catheter. In these patients kidney function should be assessed at least twice daily. Most patients with acute renal failure have a marked decrease in urine flow (< 600 ml/24 h). Total anuria is rare in intrinsic renal failure but if observed suggests cortical necrosis as a possible diagnosis, although postrenal (obstructive) failure must always be considered. Persistent oliguria/anuria unresponsive to fluid challenge is considered an indication for invasive hemodynamic monitoring (Clark *et al.*, 1986).

## 7.6 CENTRAL NERVOUS SYSTEM

### 7.6.1 SIGNS AND SYMPTOMS

Most obstetric textbooks suggest that the clinical course in eclampsia is characterized by a chronic, gradual process that begins with progressive weight gain followed by hypertension and proteinuria. However, a recent report revealed that at the onset of convulsions 23% had minimal or absent hypertension, 19% did not have proteinuria and in 32% edema was absent (Sibai, 1990b). In some series, up to 41% of cases have been reported to have little or no proteinuria (Eden, 1922; Porapakkham, 1979; Sibai *et al.*, 1981), only a minority (30%) are thrombocytopenic (Pritchard, Cunningham and Mason, 1976) and in 15-20% of eclamptic patients a prodromal phase appears to be completely absent (Campbell and Templeton, 1980; Moller and Lindmark, 1986; Sibai *et al.*, 1986). This said, eclampsia occurs seven to eight times more commonly in the context of proteinuric than of non-proteinuric pregnancy-induced hypertensive disease and the average blood pressures of women with eclampsia are higher than those with severe preeclampsia (Redman, 1989b). Eclamptic seizures continue to occur occasionally during the puerperium. In general eclamptic seizures are grand mal in character with tonic/clonic phases, focal seizures have been described occasionally. Cerebral signs and symptoms of preeclampsia–eclampsia are headache, dizziness, tinnitus, hyperreflexia, clonus, drowsiness, mental changes, visual disturbances, paresthesias and seizures. Severe cerebral signs such as cortical blindness and coma can occur without convulsion even though the pathology is identical to the lesions causing convulsions (Donaldson, 1989). Deep tendon reflexes are increased in many women prior to seizures and hyperreflexia and clonus are used as a diagnostic signs. However, seizures may occur in the absence of hyperreflexia (Sibai *et al.*, 1981), and many young subjects have a consistent physiological hyperreflexia. Clonus is 'always' a pathological sign, and thus must warn the obstetrician of impending eclampsia. Severe and persistent headache, visual disturbances, irritability, transient mental changes, epigastric or right upper-quadrant pain, nausea and vomiting are important warning signals. The headache is unrelieved by salicylates or phenacetin and is frequently described as throbbing. The most frequent symptoms preceding convulsions are headache (82.5%), visual disturbances (44.4%) and upper abdominal pain (19%) (Sibai *et al.*, 1981).

Visual disturbances in severe preeclampsia may be similar to the 'aura' preceding migraine attacks, may include flashing or multicolored lights and may range from blurring to scotomata and temporary blindness. Retinal arteriolar spasm, ischemia and edema are believed to produce these visual disturbances (Dieckman, 1952). Blindness is uncommon (1–3% incidence in eclampsia). Chesley reported an incidence of amaurosis of 4.3% among 330 eclamptic women at the Margaret Hague Hospital (Chesley, 1978). Women with amaurosis usually recover completely within 1 week. Retinal detachment also may cause altered vision, although it is usually one-sided and seldom causes total loss of vision. Without surgical treatment, vision returns to normal within approximately 1 week

(Consensus Report, 1990). Magnesium intravenously is known to cause neuro-ophthalmological effects, which may thus cause a differential diagnostic problem. However, there are significant differences between preeclamptic visual complaints and those induced by magnesium (Digre, Varner and Schiffman, 1990). Preeclampsia–eclampsia is associated with positive and negative scotomata and/or segmental visual blurring; use of magnesium intravenously is associated with blurred vision and diplopia.

An examination of the retina may be helpful in differentiating pregnancy-induced hypertensive disorders from chronic hypertension. If chronic hypertension has existed for long enough, the arterioles are likely to show angiosclerosis and tortuosity. In pregnancy-induced hypertensive disorders, retinal changes are often undetectable or minimal unless the blood pressure exceeds about 150/100 (Hallum, 1936). In women with blood pressures exceeding 150/100 the initial change in optic fundi is arteriolar narrowing without arteriovenous crossing compression. Localized or generalized changes occur in retinal arterioles in at least 50% of preeclamptic women with this degree of elevated blood pressure. Arteriolar vasospasm is indicated by a decrease in the ratio of arteriolar:venous diameter from the usual 3:5 to 1:2 or even 1:3. It may occur in all vessels or, in early stages, in single vessels. Angiospasm may be severe enough to cause central retinal arterial occlusion. These retinal vascular changes correlate with renal biopsy changes (Pollak and Nettles, 1960) and adverse perinatal outcome (Chesley, 1978; Hazoff *et al.*, 1987). Retinal edema, not papilledema, is the next change. Retinal edema, as indicated by an inability to focus clearly upon the retina, begins in the periphery and may not be seen until the posterior pole is involved. By that time retinal hemorrhages and exudates are common. Serious retinal detachment in eclampsia occurs in about 1–2% of cases (Donaldson, 1989; Chesley, 1978).

Cortical blindness in preeclampsia–eclampsia is caused by multiple microinfarctions and microhemorrhages, with edema in the occipital gray matter. Each flash or streak of light experienced in cases of severe preeclampsia could signal the occurrence of another small lesion. The pupils continue to react to light (a midbrain reflex), but the ability to blink in response to a threat is lost. If the lesion is complete, optokinetic nystagmus is absent and the patient is indifferent to her blindness (Anton's symptom; Donaldson, 1989). Cortical blindness should have the same clinical significance as eclamptic seizures, because the pathology is identical. Papilledema in eclampsia signifies cerebral edema.

Tightness of hands and feet and paresthesias secondary to medial or ulnar nerve compression are caused by fluid retention. Although these are of concern to the patient, who may be quite uncomfortable, they are not of prognostic significance and are also common in normal pregnancy.

### 7.6.2 COMPUTED AXIAL TOMOGRAPHY SCAN (CT SCAN)

In earlier years cranial CT scans were reported to be normal in women with otherwise uncomplicated eclampsia. With the introduction of high-resolution CT-scan equipment (fourth generation), nearly half of women with eclampsia have abnormal radiographic findings (Consensus Report, 1990; Brown, Purdy and Cunningham, 1988). CT scanning can not detect petechial hemorrhages in cortical gray matter. Table 7.2 summarizes the reported findings in the literature on CT-scanning in eclampsia (Sibai and Fairlie, 1992).

The most common findings are large hematomas, subarachnoid and intraventricular bleeding and unusual arcuate bands of edema in the end-distribution of the lenticular striate vessels. Hypodense bands of cerebral cortex bespeak vasogenic cerebral edema. This has been demonstrated in wedge in a region presumed to be a watershed. Both occipital lobes are symmetrically edematous in cases of cortical blindness.

### 7.6.3 MAGNETIC RESONANCE IMAGING

Magnetic resonance imaging (MRI) provides images in multiple planes, avoids the use of ionizing radiation and, except for selected contraindications (some aneurysm clips, pacemakers), there are no significant health risks associated with its use. MRI has been demonstrated to be a better way to visualize cortical lesions than CT scanning in the non-pregnant

---

**Table 7.2**   Reported CT findings in eclampsia

**Cerebral edema**
- Low-density pattern diffusely distributed throughout the white matter
- Patchy areas of low density
- Occipital white matter edema
- Loss of normal cortical sulci
- Reduced ventricular size
- Acute hydrocephalus

**Cerebral hemorrhage**
- Intraventricular hemorrhage
- Parenchymal hemorrhage (high density)

**Cerebral infarction**
- Low attenuation areas
- Basal ganglia infarcts

population (Donaldson, 1989). MRI changes have been demonstrated to correlate cortical petechiae and other forms of cerebral pathology in eclampsia (Crawford *et al.*, 1987). Further studies are necessary to assess the definite value of MRI scanning in the (early?) diagnosis and management of eclampsia.

### 7.6.4 ANGIOGRAPHY

The use of cerebral angiography in the evaluation of eclampsia is limited. Studies reported so far all demonstrate widespread vasoconstriction of the intracranial arterial circulation (Will *et al.*, 1987). Neuroradiodiagnostic tests are of no use in uncomplicated cases of eclampsia, which show prompt response to standard treatment. In these patients CT scan findings, which may disappear in a matter of days, will not alter clinical management (Brown, Purdy and Cunningham, 1988). Neuroradiodiagnostic tests should be restricted to evaluation of patients with focal neurological deficits or late postpartum eclampsia to rule out the presence of potential cerebrovascular pathology (Sibai, 1988a).

### 7.6.5 ELECTROENCEPHALOGRAM

Eclamptic patients almost uniformly have an abnormal electroencephalogram (EEG) (Jost, 1948; Kolstad, 1961; Barton and Sibai, 1991). The EEG during eclampsia is predictable – diffusely slow (theta or delta waves) with intermittent general seizure activity, which may have focal or multifocal features. Some preeclamptic patients (15–35%) also have slow activity. None of these EEG findings is pathognomonic of eclampsia, because similar patterns can be found in case of hypoxia, renal encephalopathy, polycythemia, hypocalcemia and water intoxication. Some investigators reported that EEG recordings in eclampsia correlate with the severity of maternal hypertension and improve after initiation of adequate antihypertensive therapy (Jost, 1948). Most investigators, however, find no

correlation between the degree of blood pressure elevation and EEG abnormalities (Kolstad, 1961; Sibai *et al.*, 1984). After the occurrence of eclampsia posterior slowing can persist for at least 6 months (Donaldson, 1989).

### 7.6.6 INTRACRANIAL PRESSURE

Increased intracranial pressure is a severe complication of eclampsia and should be considered in patients who remain persistently comatose after their seizure or those with oval pupils and/or papilledema. If increased intracranial pressure is suspected, a cranial CT scan is indicated to assess for intracranial hematomata or other lesions (Barton and Sibai, 1992). Intracranial pressure (normal < 10 mmHg) can be measured directly with a subarachnoid monitor, epidural monitor, intraparenchymal fiberoptic transducer or through an intraventricular catheter. The intraventricular catheter offers the advantage of serving as a port for withdrawal of cerebrospinal fluid. Tissue ischemia may occur at intracranial pressures above 40 mmHg (Barton and Sibai, 1991, 1992).

## 7.7 LIVER AND GASTROINTESTINAL TRACT

Upper abdominal pain associated with liver involvement is a particularly ominous sign. This type of pain, often accompanied by nausea and/or vomiting, is frequently misdiagnosed or overlooked. Sibai (1990c) noted that 90% of HELLP syndrome patients complain of epigastric or right upper quadrant pain, 50% have nausea and/or vomiting and others have non-specific viral-syndrome-like symptoms. The majority of patients (90%) will have a history of malaise for the past few days prior to presentation. Upon physical examination 80% of patients will have right upper quadrant tenderness and 60% significant weight gain with generalized edema. Hypertension may be absent (20%), mild (30%) or severe (50%), depending on the duration of signs and symptoms. In some cases, the patient may present with gastrointestinal bleeding, hematuria, flank or shoulder pain and jaundice. As a result, these patients are often misdiagnosed as having various medical and surgical disorders. Cholelithiasis, cholecystitis, hepatitis, acute fatty liver of pregnancy, pancreatitis, perforated peptic ulcer, severe hiatus hernia, pyelonephritis and even Budd–Chiari syndrome should be included in the differential diagnosis of epigastric or right upper quadrant pain during pregnancy, and thus in the differential diagnosis of HELLP syndrome. If a clinician is confronted with these aspecific complaints laboratory tests are obligatory to confirm or exclude the diagnosis HELLP syndrome. Subcapsular hematoma and liver rupture are further extensions of the HELLP syndrome. Patients presenting with severe epigastric pain, shoulder pain, shock, evidence of massive ascites (hemoperitoneum), respiratory difficulties or pleural effusions should have ultrasound examination of the liver to rule out subcapsular hematomata of the liver. When the rupture is contained within the capsule, the patient experiences severe pain but is hemodynamically stable. Subcapsular hematomata are clearly visible by ultrasonography and CT scanning.

The CT scan is probably more useful, since it is less operator-dependent and can visualize the entire abdomen. Ultrasonography, however, is more practical to perform, since the equipment is often on hand in an obstetric unit. Most often the hematoma is on the surface of the right lobe of the liver, on either the anterior or the inferior surface. The left lobe is involved in less than 11%. A right pleural effusion may occur in some cases. A peritoneal tap may be used to differentiate between ascites and peritoneal blood. The differential diagnosis of a patient presenting with hypovolemic shock, generalized abdominal pain and a dead fetus in the second half of pregnancy should include not only abruptio placentae but also liver rupture as a complica-

tion of severe HELLP syndrome. Acute fatty liver of pregnancy (AFLP) may be difficult to differentiate from HELLP syndrome. The clinical characteristics typical of AFLP include presentation late in the third trimester, with signs and symptoms typical of both acute hepatitis and preeclampsia. The fetus involved in fatty liver of pregnancy is male in more than 75% of cases, and multiple pregnancies are noted in more than 14% of involved pregnancies (Latham, 1992). Patients often have nausea, vomiting, severe malaise, abdominal pain and fatigue. Jaundice occurs frequently (> 70%), but not invariably. Other symptoms and signs may include pyrexia and tachycardia in approximately 50%, oliguria in approximately 40% and gastrointestinal bleeding in 60%. Further laboratory tests are needed to differentiate between HELLP syndrome and AFLP.

## 7.8 BIOCHEMICAL MARKERS

It is important to emphasize that the majority of women with a pregnancy-induced disorder are asymptomatic. This lack of symptoms is in fact an important part of the rationale for the frequent antenatal care visits in late pregnancy. Laboratory tests have been used for prediction, diagnosis and monitoring of disease progress. The diagnosis 'preeclampsia' is even based on a laboratory test.

### 7.8.1 URIC ACID

Williams (1921) was one of the first authors to describe a clear correlation between the increase in urate levels and clinical symptoms in patients with 'toxemia of pregnancy'. Since Williams, increments in urate levels have been demonstrated to correlate with the severity of the preeclamptic lesion in renal biopsies, the degree of uteroplacental vascular pathology, and with poor fetal outcome (Pollak and Nettles, 1960; Redman, Beilin and Bonnar, 1976; Redman *et al.*, 1976). Redman *et al.* (1976) clearly demonstrated that hyperuricemia (> 350 μmol/l) was associated with a significant increase in perinatal mortality. Redman *et al.* (1976) performed a prospective but not blinded study in 332 hypertensive pregnant patients with mixed parity. Redman used mean uric acid level plus twice standard deviation at 16, 28, 32 and 36 weeks gestational age (0.28/0.29/0.34/0.39 μmol/l), and concluded that the degree of hyperuricemia is a better predictor for adverse perinatal outcome than blood pressure. Sibai, Anderson and McCubbin (1982) did not confirm these findings. The results of many studies, but not of others (recently reviewed by Dekker and Sibai, 1991), suggest that serum uric acid levels may begin to rise before the appearance of proteinuric hypertension. In most patients the increase in urate levels appears to coincide with the increase in blood pressure and precedes the development of the proteinuric stage of the disease. As such, uric acid levels have been used for the early diagnosis of preeclampsia. In conclusion, uric acid is one of the most sensitive indicators of disease severity in pregnancy-induced hypertensive disorders and can be of great help in monitoring the course of the disease process. Significant hyperuricemia (actual value ≥ 2 × baseline value) in a pregnant woman is an indication for intensive maternal and fetal monitoring. In the near-term period labor should be induced in case of hypertension associated with significant hyperuricemia.

## 7.8.2 RENAL FUNCTION TESTS

In clinical practice creatinine clearance is generally taken as a satisfactory index of GFR. Creatinine is derived from muscle metabolism. The amount of creatinine formed is proportional to the muscle mass and is relatively constant, with a variation of about 10–15% from the mean value from day to day. Therefore, most patients produce and excrete a fixed amount in a 24-hour period, no matter what their level of stable kidney function. A 24-hour collection is complete if total creatinine is 0.12–0.19 mmol/kg bodyweight per day. Consequently, alterations in GFR bring about the majority of changes in the serum creatinine level. Single measurements of creatinine are of no use, and serial measurements should be used to follow the course of a renal disease process. Elevated serum creatinine is not an early sign of acute renal insufficiency. In general, serum creatinine is unlikely to be elevated until GFR has fallen by at least 50% below normal values. If renal function is more severely compromised a small further decrement in GFR causes a marked rise in serum creatinine.

Normal ranges for creatinine clearance in pregnancy are 120–150 ml/min, compared with approximately 100 ml/min in the nonpregnant state. During normal pregnancy creatinine clearance increases by 25% in the first two weeks after conception, and by 45% at 9 weeks gestation. In the near-term period there is a reduction of about 15% and some authors report that creatinine clearance may even decrease to non-pregnant values. Plasma creatinine levels decrease from a nonpregnant value of 73 μmol/l to 65, 51 and 47 μmol/l, respectively in successive trimesters. Familiarity with these changes is vital, because values considered normal in nonpregnant women may signify decreased renal function in pregnancy.

Because creatinine clearance is a glomerular function, measuring serum creatinine or creatinine clearance is certainly not useful for early diagnosis of pregnancy-induced hypertensive disorders. A decrease in creatinine clearance and elevated creatinine levels are late features of preeclampsia, more or less coinciding with the appearance of proteinuria, and are often discerned only in the range that would be considered healthy for non-pregnant women (Chesley and Williams, 1945). Serum creatinine determinations, if obtained serially, may reflect the decrease in creatinine clearance but, unless very elevated, are not helpful because of the wide range of normal single values. Smaller changes in glomerular filtration are best determined by measurement of creatinine clearance. Measuring creatinine is essential not for diagnosis but to anticipate increasing renal impairment, which might precede acute renal failure. Hallmark clinical features of acute renal failure include a near-linear increase in serum creatinine at a rate of 45–130 μmol/l/d, and usually a fall in urine flow to less than 400–500 ml/d.

Measurement of urea is far less precise than that of creatinine. Urea, the primary end product of hepatic protein catabolism, is excreted primarily, but not exclusively, by the kidneys. Urea is freely filtered by the glomeruli. In normal pregnancy plasma urea levels fall from non-pregnancy values of 4.3 mmol/l to pregnancy values of 3.5, 3.3 and 3.1 mmol/l, respectively in successive trimesters. Depending on the state of hydration and therefore the rate of urine flow, 40–80% of the filtered urea is passively reabsorbed with water, mostly in the proximal tubules. Measuring urea is a fickle test greatly influenced by protein metabolism and intake, and the state of hydration. However, in patients with severely impaired renal function, urea is better correlated with the symptoms of uremia than with the creatinine level. Urea is particularly elevated in patients with severe prerenal azotemia, since greatly increased reabsorption of filtered urea by the renal tubules occurs. Any situation that increases tissue break down, such as gastrointestinal bleeding, fever, and stress similarly results in an inordinately high urea level. High protein feeds, either intravenously or by mouth, also can overwhelm the kidney's ability to excrete urea. There is some advantage in terms of clinical interpretation to determine both the serum urea and creatinine concentrations. Creatinine is affected very little by diet and minimally if at all by the state of hydration. Circumstances that lead to a relative marked increase of urea as compared to the increase in creatinine include prerenal conditions with loss of intravascular volume, hypoalbumine-

mia and decreased left ventricular function. Catabolic states, gastrointestinal bleeding, with the digestion and absorption of blood protein, and steroid therapy may also increase it. Also, postrenal azotemia typically results in a greater increase of urea.

The (U/P)urea and (U/P)creatinine ratios may also be useful in order to distinguish prerenal failure from acute tubular necrosis. (U/P)urea usually is greater than 20 in prerenal failure but below 3 in tubular necrosis, and (U/P)creatinine is often about 40 (at least > 10) in case of prerenal failure and always below 15 in acute tubular necrosis.

### 7.8.3 URINARY DIAGNOSTIC INDICES

The specific gravity of the protein-free glomerular filtrate is 1.007. Urine specific gravity varies from 1.003–1.035, reflecting either dilution or concentration of the glomerular filtrate. Urine specific gravity is measured with a calibrated hydrometer, called a urinometer, or more commonly a temperature compensated refractometer calibrated in specific gravity units. Normal adults with normal diets and normal fluid intake will produce urine of specific gravity 1.016–1.022 during a 24-hour period. If a random specimen of urine has a specific gravity of 1.023 or more, concentrating ability can be considered normal. If oliguria is based on prerenal renal failure, as may be the case in severe preeclampsia, urinary specific gravity is elevated to about 1.030. Also renal ischemia is associated with the production of urine with a high specific gravity. Intrinsic renal disease is associated with low urinary specific gravity.

The fractional sodium excretion (FE Na⁺) can be used to assess the integrity of the renal tubules. If the value is less than 1%, tubular function is excellent. Azotemia in a patient with such a low fractional Na⁺ excretion must be due to a prerenal cause (impaired renal perfusion), such as hypotension, preglomerular vasoconstriction, decreased circulating plasma volume, or a decreased cardiac output. Common causes of renal hypoperfusion in pregnancy are hyperemesis gravidarum, septic shock and preeclampsia. FE $Na^+$ between 1% and 3% is difficult to interpret; only when this value is greater than 3% is the azotemia unequivocally due to renal parenchymal damage (Murphy, Preuss and Henry, 1984). The renal failure index can be calculated by dividing urinary sodium concentration (mEq/l) by UCr/PCr.

In the presence of oliguria, urinary diagnostic indices have been used in non-pregnant patients to differentiate between prerenal and renal etiologies. Lee, Gonik and Cotton (1987) compared urinary diagnostic indices to wedge pressure in seven oliguric preeclamptic patients. Although urine sodium was high in six patients, indicating intrinsic renal disease, most of the other parameters indicated a prerenal causation of their oliguria. PA catheter readings showed predominantly normal wedge pressures. They concluded that oliguria is a poor index of volume status in preeclampsia and that urinary diagnostic indices may be misleading if used to guide fluid management in these patients. This incorrectness is caused by the fact that preeclampsia oliguria is related not only to volume depletion but also to regional (intrarenal) vasoconstriction.

In conclusion, renal function tests, including urinary diagnostic indices, must be interpreted with caution in severe preeclampsia. Prerenal findings (urine sodium < 20 mEq/l, urine osmolality > 500 mosmol/kg, (U/P)urea nitrogen > 8, (U/P)creatinine > 40, renal failure index < 1 and FE $Na^+$ <1) suggest the need for volume expansion. A fluid challenge (500 ml of normal saline in 30 min) may be given, after which at least 1 hour should be allowed to see a response in the urine output. If a patient does not respond, fluid management cannot be guided any more with the help of urinary diagnostic indices. Invasive hemodynamic monitoring remains invaluable

for the optimum management of these severely sick patients.

All patients with severe preeclampsia–eclampsia, especially if complicated by DIC, must be watched carefully for the development of renal failure. The best overall screening procedures include serial determinations of serum creatinine (at least daily), and a careful measurement of all fluid intake and output. Renal parenchymal injury may be acute tubular necrosis or cortical necrosis. In contrast to prerenal failure, tubular function in acute tubular necrosis is markedly impaired, which results in FE $Na^+$ > 1% and impaired concentrating ability (< 400 mosmol /kg $H_2O$). Restoration of renal function usually becomes clinically evident within 5–35 days of onset and requires another 1–2 weeks to return to normal. The cause and clinical features of cortical necrosis are similar to those encountered in acute tubular necrosis, except for the lack of functional recovery.

### 7.8.4 URINARY MICROSCOPY

In most cases of severe preeclampsia the urinary sediment demonstrates red blood cells, granular casts, hyaline casts and tubular cells, presenting singly, in clumps or in casts (Leduc *et al.*,1991). However, the sediment may equally be completely normal (Pollak and Nettles, 1960). The sediment changes do not correlate with or predict the clinical course of the disease. Thus, patients with pregnancy-induced hypertensive disorders may represent with a normal or an abnormal sediment; examination of the urine may help in the differentiation from renal diseases presenting with more 'active' sediments, only when the sediment is benign.

### 7.8.5 ASYMPTOMATIC BACTERIURIA

Hill, Devoe and Bryans (1986) found a significant difference in the rate of asymptomatic bacteriuria (urine sample obtained by bladder catheterization) between patients with preeclampsia (19%) and normotensive pregnant patients (3–6%). Preeclamptic patients with significant bacteriuria had significantly lower total serum protein and albumin levels than preeclamptic patients without proteinuria. The results of this carefully conducted study and of earlier studies (Kincaid-Smith, 1985) suggest that it is appropriate to check all preeclamptic patients for the presence of significant bacteriuria.

## 7.8.6 PROTEINURIA

Normal non-pregnant urinary protein excretion is less than 150 mg/24 h. Physiological proteinuria may increase during exercise or with dehydration. Proteinuria can occur in the absence of renal tract disease in patients with hemorrhage, salt depletion and febrile illnesses, probably by causing relative renal ischemia. To detect the kinds of protein present in the urine requires electrophoretic separation of serum and urine proteins. Based on nephelometric findings, proteinuria may be separated into a glomerular pattern and tubular pattern indicating which part of the nephron is primarily affected. However, these anatomical entities tend to merge as the renal disease processes progress. A third type of proteinuria has been designated 'overflow proteinuria' because the protein material initially results from disease elsewhere, e.g. hemoglobin following intravascular hemolysis, or from exogenic sources e.g. plasma volume expanders such as polygeline (Haemaccel).

In normal pregnancy the urinary excretion of protein may increase as pregnancy progresses, from approximately 5 mg/dl in the first and second trimester to 15 mg/dl in late pregnancy. In normal pregnant women the degree of proteinuria is influenced by several factors, including urine specific gravity, urine pH, postural proteinuria and contamination with vaginal secretions, blood or bacteria. Furthermore, pregnant women are in the age range where women may have postural proteinuria, which may be detected initially or be present only during pregnancy. Postural proteinuria is more frequent near term, since during this period women tend to assume a more lordotic posture, which augments excretion (Lindheimer and Katz, 1991).

The practice of periodic urinalyses and in fact the beginning of prenatal care stems from Lever's observation (1843) of the association between eclampsia and proteinuria. Obstetricians recognized the 'albuminuria of pregnancy' as a 'precursor of puerperal convulsions' (Lever's words). Preeclamptic proteinuria is caused by altered transglomerular passage of proteins as a consequence of glomerular damage. It is a familiar clinical observation that the degree of preeclamptic proteinuria may vary greatly from day to day, or even from hour to hour (Chesley, 1939). Because structural glomerular changes are obviously more or less constant, preeclamptic proteinuria must depend at least in part on the intensity of intrarenal vasospasm (vasoactive proteinuria). In preeclampsia the glomerulus is damaged by a combination of glomerular endothelial cell dysfunction, vasospasm, platelet deposition and secondary localized intravascular coagulation.

Proteinuria is a late sign of pregnancy-induced hypertensive disorders and is a reflection of advanced disease. The occurrence of proteinuria is an expression of glomerular dysfunction and coincides more or less with a decrease in creatinine clearance. Proteinuria is associated with a poorer perinatal outcome and a poorer prognosis for the mother. On average proteinuria appears about 3 weeks before intrauterine demise or mandatory delivery (Friedman and Neff, 1977; Naeye and Friedman, 1979). Hypertension plus proteinuria is associated with a twofold increased risk of perinatal death as compared to normotensive pregnancy and hypertension without proteinuria. Proteinuria is obligatory for the classic diagnosis of preeclampsia. However, proteinuria is only one sign of vessel wall damage, and it would be unreasonable to consider a hypertensive patient with a hemoglobin level of 9.4 mmol/l and a platelet count of 105 × 109/l as a case of 'innocent' pregnancy-induced hypertensive disease. HELLP syndrome and eclampsia may occur in the absence of proteinuria prior to the event.

Various methods are used for diagnosing the presence of proteinuria. Dipstick tests are based on the principle of protein-error of pH indicators. The test area is buffered to a constant pH of 3, so that color changes reflect the presence and concentration of proteins. Dipsticks may give false-positive results if the urine has a pH greater than of 7.0, for instance if urine pH is elevated by quaternary ammonium compounds such as chlorhexidine (skin cleanser), and if it is highly concentrated (specific gravity > 1030), and false-negative results if it is highly diluted (specific gravity < 1010) or contains proteins other than albumin, because the method is relatively insensitive to positively charged proteins such as some immunoglobulins. False-positive readings can also occur if urine is contaminated with blood or in case of bacteriuria. The commonly used qualitative dipstick test (Albustix) can only detect albumin concentrations above 200 mg/l and will not identify the physiological gestational increase in proteinuria (Murphy, Preuss and Henry, 1984). Any positive (> 1+) must be immediately evaluated in a midstream sample of urine while a vaginal tampon excludes contamination. Urinary infection should be ruled out. Because the development of proteinuria is a late feature of the disease, routine use of dipsticks in a normotensive low-risk population is probably just as ineffective as measuring maternal weight gain (Dawes and Grudzinskas, 1991).

The urinary albumin excretion within the range from the normal level to the detection limit for Albustix is referred to as microalbuminuria (approximately 30–300 mg/24 h). It can be detected by a rapid qualitative latex agglutination test, which has a sensitivity of 25 mg/l. Microalbuminuria tests have been tried in order to predict preeclampsia. Lopez-Espinoza *et al.* (1986) studied microalbuminuria using a sensitive radioimmunoassay and found no evidence that gross proteinuria is preceded by a gradual increase in microalbuminuria. Rodriguez *et al.* (1988) using an urine albumin concentration ≥ 11 µg/ml as a positive test, reported a sensitivity of 50%, a specificity of 82%, a positive predictive value of just 26% and a negative predictive value of 93% (11.4% incidence of preeclampsia), and concluded that measuring microalbuminuria is of little or no use for the early diagnosis of preeclampsia. However, Nakamura *et al.* (1992) studied 199 normotensive pregnant women at 20–30 weeks gestation. A fasting urinary albumin/creatinine ratio (FU Alb/Cr) was evaluated to predict pregnancy-induced hypertensive disorders. When FU Alb/Cr > 16 was considered to represent a positive test result, the positive and negative predictive values were 94% and 96% respectively. The authors concluded that FU Alb/Cr is a useful screening tool for the early diagnosis of pregnancy-induced hypertensive disorders. Thong *et al.* (1991a) found that an elevated albumin/creatinine ratio (> 3.5 mg/mmol) preceded preeclampsia in 89% of the cases, but only 20% of the cases of pregnancy-induced hypertensive disease. The ratio did not predict adverse pregnancy outcome and did not correlate with platelet count, uric acid level and liver function tests. On the whole there appears to be little value in using precise techniques of detecting proteinuria in the early diagnosis of preeclampsia. Other signs such as an increase in blood pressure, a fall in the number of platelets and a rise in plasma uric acid levels appear to antedate the occurrence of detectable microalbuminuria (Dekker and Sibai, 1991). Irgens-Moller, Hemmingsen and Holm (1986) advocated the use of the relative albumin clearance (immunonephelometric method) as a valuable quantitative and objective measurement for the follow-up of the progression of renal damage in preeclampsia.

Because protein levels fluctuate widely, the final diagnosis of significant proteinuria should be based on a quantitative measurement of total urinary protein excretion over a 24-hour period. Significant proteinuria is defined as more than 300 mg in a 24-hour urine sample. For making a diagnosis of severe preeclampsia based on proteinuria, it is recommended that a 24-hour excretion of protein above 5 g be documented (Sibai, 1988b; Consensus Report, 1990).

Recently, untimed urine samples have been used to estimate total protein excretion over 24 hours. Because the urinary excretion of creatinine in a single person is reasonably constant it has been proposed that the protein/creatinine ratio provides a satisfactory estimation of the 24-hour urinary excretion of proteins. In addition, the creatinine correction introduces a correction for body size. In nonpregnant patients the protein/creatinine ratio appears to be an acceptable method to assess the 24-hour urinary protein excretion. In uncomplicated pregnancy Uttendorfsky *et al.* (1988) found an excellent correlation between the protein/creatinine ratio and 24-hour urinary protein excretion. In contrast, Combs, Wheeler and Kitzmiller (1991) demonstrated that large errors can occur when the protein/creatinine ratio is used to estimate 24-hour urine protein excretion in pregnant women with diabetes. The positive results from Uttendorfsky *et al.* (1988) may be explained by the fact that they studied pregnant women with an urinary protein excretion in the physiological range. Although this method has obvious advantages for patients and physicians alike, it has also limitations. First, urine collected during the night or upon arising should not be used, because the ratio of protein to creatinine does not correlate as well with the 24-hour urine collection as does the ratio in urine samples collected during the day. Second, the ratio is influenced by the urinary creatinine excretion, which may vary more than fourfold among individuals. In conclusion, serial measurements of the protein/creatinine ratio in untimed urine samples may be of use in the follow-up of an individual woman with established preeclampsia, and in circumstances when 24-hour urine samples are difficult to obtain.

Renal biopsies show that the urinary protein selectivity decreases in rough proportion to increasing degrees of anatomical change in the glomeruli. On the whole, the protein selectivity in preeclamptic proteinuria falls within the intermediate range (Simanowitz, MacGregor and Hobbs, 1973). Initially, preeclamptic proteinuria is mainly vasoactive glomerular proteinuria, resulting in the urinary excretion of albumin and also some transferrin (Murphy, Preuss and Henry, 1984). This predominantly vasoactive highly specific proteinuria seen in the early stages of the disease process changes into a less specific proteinuria in the later stages of the disease. The degree of immunoglobulinuria increases with progression of disease severity, and significant immunoglobulinuria is associated with poor perinatal outcome and significant maternal morbidity. Significant immunoglobulinuria develops prior to the development of azotemia, significant decreases in creatinine clearance, significant proteinuria ($> 5$ g/24 h) or oliguria. The use of nephelometric measurement of urine IgG concentration has been advocated as a rapid and accurate method for the assessment of disease severity, the degree of renal involvement and the likelihood of serious maternal morbidity (Eden *et al.*, 1984). A simple index to the selectivity of proteinuria is the ratio of clearances (not merely excretory rates) of IgG and transferrin (CIgG/CT). In case of selective proteinuria the CIgG/CT is less than 0.1. The CIgG/CT ratio in preeclampsia has been reported to be 0.2–0.5, and preeclampsia can be excluded as the cause of proteinuria during pregnancy if the CIgG/CT is less than 0.15, because that degree of selectivity is not encountered in preeclampsia. On the other hand a CIgG/CT of more than 0.15 is certainly not diagnostic for preeclampsia (Studd, 1971).

### 7.8.7 URINARY CALCIUM EXCRETION

Women who develop preeclampsia during pregnancy excrete less calcium than healthy pregnant women (Taufield *et al.*, 1987; Sanchez-Ramos *et al.*, 1991). The mechanism of hypocalciuria in preeclampsia is independent of the parathyroid-hormone–calcitriol axis and is probably due to intrinsic renal tubular dysfunction based on a disturbance of renal prostaglandin $E_2$ synthesis (Frenkel *et al.*, 1991; Covi *et al.*, 1990). The results of several other studies (Huikeshoven and Zuijderhoudt, 1990), but not Roelofsen *et al.*, 1988, confirmed Taufield's original findings. These differences are probably caused by the fact that some authors studied a very heterogeneous population (Roelofsen *et al.*, 1988). Sanchez-Ramos *et al.* (1991) studied the value of urinary calcium as an early marker for preeclampsia in 103 consecutive nulliparous women. At 10–24 weeks gestation patients who later developed preeclampsia excreted significantly less urinary calcium than those who remained normotensive. This reduction persisted throughout gestation. Using a receiver operator curve a predictive threshold calcium value for hypertension of 195 mg/24 h was calculated. The difference in the incidence of preeclampsia between pregnant women with calcium excretion values at or below this threshold (87%) and those with values above that level (2%) was highly significant. In contrast, Hutchesson *et al.* (1990) were unable to demonstrate a reduction in urinary calcium excretion in preeclamptic women prior to the onset of hypertension and renal involvement.

Huikeshoven and Zuijderhoudt (1990) reported an excellent correlation between the 24-hour urinary calcium excretion and the calcium/creatinine ($U_{ca}/U_{cr}$) ratio of a single voided urine sample in normotensive and hypertensive pregnant women. The $U_{ca}/U_{cr}$ ratio is a method for assessment of renal function very similar to the use of the urinary-urate/creatinine ratio. Both ratios compare a tubular function with a glomerular function. Because tubular function is impaired at an earlier stage of the preeclamptic disease process than glomerular function (Chesley and Williams, 1945) the $U_{ca}/U_{cr}$ ratio have been used for the early diagnosis of preeclampsia. Rodriguez *et al.* (1988) assessed the value of the $U_{ca}/U_{cr}$ ratio between 24 and 34 weeks gestation. A $U_{ca}/U_{cr}$ ration < 0.04 was reported to have a sensitivity of 70%, a specificity of 95%, a positive predictive value of 64% and a negative predictive value of 96% (11.4% incidence of preeclampsia). Thong *et al.* (1991b) confirmed the presence of a significantly lower $U_{ca}/U_{cr}$ ratio in preeclampsia as compared to normotensive pregnant women and women with pregnancy-induced hypertensive disease. In this study the $U_{ca}/U_{cr}$ ratio correlated negatively ($r = -0.33$; $p\ 0.01$) with the albumin/creatinine ratio. However, there was no correlation between the $U_{ca}/U_{cr}$ ratio and the platelet count, uric acid levels or birthweight centile.

In conclusion, hypocalciuria is certainly present in the moderate to severe stage of the disease and not in chronic hypertension. Assessment of urinary calcium excretion can be useful in the differential diagnosis of hypertensive disorders during pregnancy. Further studies are necessary to assess the actual clinical value of urinary calcium excretion for monitoring pregnancy-induced hypertensive disorders in comparison with other tubular tests such as measuring plasma uric acid.

### 7.8.8 COLLOID ONCOTIC PRESSURE

Plasma and interstitial colloid oncotic pressure (COP), and hydrostatic pressures, are important factors in edema formation. Albumin is responsible for at least 70% of plasma COP ($COP_p$), whereas globulins and fibrinogen are responsible for most of the remaining pressure.

In pregnancy the Landis and Pappenheimer equation for calculating $COP_p$, gives a result that correlates poorly with the measured $COP_p$. New equations have been introduced for the calculation of $COP_p$ during pregnancy:

$COP_p$ (mmHg) = 5.21 × total serum protein (g/dl) −11.4

and/or

$COP_p$ (mmHg) = 8.1 × serum albumin (g/dl) −8.2

These two equations are thought to be reasonably accurate, with a 10% range of error in 75% and 80% of cases respectively (Moise and Cotton, 1991). The $COP_p$ can be measured directly and more reliable with a commercially available transducer membrane system (colloid osmometer). In this instrument two chambers are separated by a semipermeable membrane, which is impermeable to molecules with molecular weights > 30,000. One chamber is filled with a colloid-free isotonic saline solution and connected to a pressure transducer. The other chamber is filled with the sample to be measured. The pressure is expressed in mmHg.

The $COP_p$ decreases about 15% in normal pregnancy. This decrease is mainly caused by the physiological fall in albumin concentration. Normal $COP_p$ in pregnancy at term is about 22 mmHg, and decreases to about 16 mmHg in the postpartum period as a result of blood loss and/or crystalloid infusions during labor (Gonik *et al.*, 1985). The $COP_p$ is noted to decrease by about 15% when measured in patients in the supine position for several hours. A significant lowering (about 50%) of the interstitial COP is of major importance in preventing edema in normal pregnancy (Oian *et al.*, 1985).

$COP_p$ is significantly lower in preeclampsia than in uncomplicated pregnancy. This pathological decrease in $COP_p$ is mainly caused by endothelial damage and the subsequent loss of albumin and other proteins across capillaries. In preeclampsia, serum protein content is also reduced as a result of proteinuria. The degree of lowering of $COP_p$ is dependent on the severity of the disease process, type and amount of infused fluid, as well as amount of blood loss at delivery. Reported values have ranged from 15–17 mmHg before delivery to 13–14 mmHg in the immediate postpartum period (Zinaman, Rubin and Lindheimer, 1985). In preeclampsia–eclampsia $COP_p$ is lowest 6–18 h postpartum (Zinaman, Rubin and Lindheimer, 1985; Gonik *et al.*, 1985; Chesley and Lindheimer, 1988; Moise and Cotton, 1991). Interstitial COP is increased in preeclampsia because of the increased capillary permeability to proteins (Oian *et al.*, 1986). Low $COP_p$ values, increased interstitial COP values and narrowing of the $COP_p$–wedge gradient is one of the major causes of pulmonary edema in severe preeclampsia–eclampsia. The $COP_p$–wedge gradient can be calculated by simply subtracting the PCWP from the $COP_p$. The normal gradient during pregnancy in the third trimester is approximately 14 mmHg. Reduction of this gradient to less than 4 mmHg is associated with an increased risk of pulmonary edema. This explanation for the pathogenesis of pulmonary edema is of course an oversimplification of the complex Starling forces in the lung. Other mechanisms involved in the causation of pulmonary edema in preeclampsia–eclampsia are alveolar–capillary membrane injury, COP and hydrostatic pressure in the pulmonary interstitium, pulmonary lymph flow and surfactant (Moise and Cotton, 1991). However, the $COP_p$–PCWP gradient is the closest approximation of the net Starling interactions in the lung available and is a very useful parameter in the management of the severely sick preeclamptic patient. Most (70–80%) cases of pulmonary edema associated with severe preeclampsia–eclampsia occur postpartum (Sibai *et al.*, 1987). In this period $COP_p$ is at its lowest. In addition, wedge pressure increases due to delayed mobilization of extravascular fluid, i.e. beginning 24–72 h postpartum. Edema fluid is mobilized and may be returned to the intravascular space faster than the diseased kidneys can excrete it (Hankins *et al.*, 1984). Iatrogenic fluid overload may also contribute to raising the wedge pressure, and when crystalloid solutions are used, to a further decrease of the $COP_p$ value.

In conclusion, $COP_p$ can be measured with relative ease. The measurement of $COP_p$ appears is an useful clinical tool in conjunction with the use of PA catheters in critically ill preeclamptic patients (Moise and Cotton, 1986).

### 7.8.9 ELECTROLYTE CHANGES

There have been few studies reported in the literature on the electrolytes in blood in normal and hypertensive pregnancy. Sodium levels decrease in normal pregnant women to about 139 mEq/l in the first trimester, and this level is maintained throughout pregnancy. Similarly, potassium levels fall about 4 mEq/l in the first trimester, and this level is also maintained throughout pregnancy (Newman, 1957).

In general, the concentrations of electrolytes in the blood in pregnancy-induced hypertensive disorders, including severe preeclampsia, do not show any significant change from normal pregnancy (Bonsnes, 1956; Chesley, 1978). However, Tatum and Mule (1956) reported that preeclamptic women in New Orleans show consistent diminutions in plasma sodium. Tatum and Mule (1956) and Kalur *et al.* (1991) described 11 cases of postpartum vascular collapse, associated with severe pre-eclampsia–eclampsia and extremely low sodium levels (mean 125.9 mEq/l). This appears to be a rare clinical entity, but a high index of suspicion will allow the obstetrician to measure sodium and perhaps cortisol levels in postpartum preeclamptic patients with signs of vascular collapse.

### 7.8.10 IRON, CARBOXYHEMOGLOBIN AND FERRITIN

Entman *et al.* (1982a) found serum iron concentrations of 135.3 μg/dl in intrapartum preeclamptic patients, compared with intra-partum values of 61.6 μg/dl and 72.5 μg/dl for normotensive and chronically hypertensive gravidas. This increase is caused by increased red cell destruction, which occurs in pregnancy-induced hypertensive disorders. Entman and Richardson (1983) compared serum iron levels with other laboratory tests and reported that results expressed as serum iron (> 100 μg/dl or an increase of more than 70% above baseline values) achieved a sensitivity of 83% and a specificity of 87% in identifying preeclamptic patients. These results exceeded those obtained with renal, hematological and coagulation tests. Although serum ferritin levels are also elevated, the measurement of serum iron is superior within the context of diagnosing and monitoring pregnancy-induced hypertensive disorders (Entman *et al.*, 1982b). The increase in serum iron may antedate more regular methods for detecting hemolysis, such as LDH, red blood cell morphology, haptoglobin, etc. An increased extravascular turnover of red cells in preeclampsia probably accounts for this. Hemolysis, as evidenced by an increase in serum iron may already exist in mild pregnancy-induced hypertensive disease (Entman *et al.*, 1982a, 1987; Samuels *et al.* (1987). In conclusion, serum iron measurements are of use in the differential diagnosis of hypertension in the second half of pregnancy and the management of patients with pregnancy-induced hypertensive disorders. Changes in serum iron reflect the course of the disease (Entman and Richardson, 1983; Entman *et al.*, 1987). Further studies are indicated to assess the value of serum iron as a predictive test.

### 7.8.11 ASSESSMENT OF HEPATIC INVOLVEMENT

Clinicians tend to refer to all biochemical determinations that reflect hepatic disease as 'liver function tests'. In fact, routine biochemical determinations of 'liver function' are of great help in the recognition of hepatic disease but do not measure liver function.

Serum activity of the aminotransferases (transaminases), aspartate aminotransferase (AST, ASAT, glutamate oxaloacetic transaminase, GOT, SGOT) and alanine aminotransferase (ALT, ALAT, glutamate pyruvate transaminase, GPT, SGPT) are elevated in patients with hepatocellular disease, to a degree that may assist in diagnosis. In humans, ASAT has been found in cardiac, hepatic, skeletal muscle, renal and cerebral tissue in decreasing concentrations. Abnormal levels of ASAT are seen in patients with hepatocellular disease, and myocardial and skeletal muscle necrosis. Acute pancreatitis, renal necrosis and cerebral necrosis may also cause an elevation of ASAT levels. Hemolysis may cause a mild increase in ASAT levels. ALAT elevations are absent or slight in diseases that do not involve the liver (Zimmerman, 1984).

Lactic dehydrogenase (LDH), the enzyme that catalyzes the reversible oxidation of lactate to pyruvate, is widely distributed in mammalian tissues, being rich in myocardium, kidney, liver, erythrocytes and muscle. The serum LDH does not provide a sensitive measure of hepatic disease. Patients with viral hepatitis have slightly elevated (one- to twofold) values. Hemolytic anaemias yield slightly elevated levels unless the hemolysis is acute and severe (Zimmerman and Henry, 1984). Tissue LDH consists of five isoenzymes in varying proportions and the LDH activity of each tissue has a characteristic isoenzyme composition.

Most standard liver 'function tests' are essentially unchanged during normal pregnancy and thus retain their diagnostic usefulness. Serum transaminases, γ-glutamyl transpeptidase (tGT), LDH and total, indirect and direct bilirubin levels are unchanged during normal pregnancy.

Albumin concentration falls, usually quite abruptly in early pregnancy and then more slowly until late pregnancy. The overall fall is about 1 g/dl, typically from 3.5–2.5 g/dl, and it is this fall which is largely responsible for the fall in total protein concentration. This decrease is caused by the expansion of the circulating plasma volume and a decreased gene expression. In normotensive pregnancy, markedly decreased albumin levels do not necessarily indicate impaired synthetic reserve of the liver, particularly in the absence of a lengthened prothrombin time (Galbraith, 1992).

Hepatic involvement in preeclampsia is increasingly recognized to be common and to have serious implications for the severity of the disease process. The preeclamptic spectrum of liver disease may range from subclinical involvement, with the only manifestation of liver disease being deposition of fibrinogen along the hepatic sinusoids, to rupture of the liver. Within these extremes fall the HELLP syndrome and hepatic infarction.

Chesley (1978) reviewed the literature on the frequency and severity of abnormal ASAT and ALAT levels in mild pregnancy-induced hypertensive disorders, severe preeclampsia and eclampsia. This review demonstrated that about one-fifth of women thought to have mild disease had increased enzymatic activities, with a considerably higher frequency of especially ASAT (50.3%) in severe preeclampsia, and increased activity of ASAT and ALAT in most women with eclampsia. An increment in ASAT and ALAT is essential for the diagnosis of HELLP syndrome. In a series of 158 HELLP syndrome patients, Martin *et al.* (1991) found ASAT levels to be higher than ALAT levels during the acute phase of the disease. Around delivery the largest difference between the two values was apparent. The dominance of ASAT relative to ALAT levels is of use in the recognition of the acute, progressive phase of HELLP syndrome. During recovery the ASAT/ALAT ratio decreases and eventually reverses or reaches parity. The transaminase elevations may be modest or may exceed 1000–2000 units. Marked increases in ASAT/ALAT are associated with potential hepatic capsule rupture. In most patients the increment in ASAT/ALAT precedes the appearance of epigastric pain. Occasionally, elevated transaminases after 20 weeks gestation can presage the onset of preeclampsia.

Exaggerated increases in alkaline phosphatase activity in preeclampsia may point to placental as well as to hepatic damage. In daily clinical obstetrics, subtyping of ALP isoenzymes (or measuring 5'-nucleotidase) is not indicated in managing a patient with severe preeclampsia. Only in the differential diagnosis of unexplained hepatic dysfunction is there a place for these laboratory tests.

Lactic dehydrogenase may increase in preeclampsia as a sign of hepatic damage, but more often as a sign of hemolysis. A disproportional rise in LDH, as compared to the increase in ASAT/ALAT points, indicates hemolysis. Martin *et al.* (1991) found that individual peak values of LDH levels ranged from 581–2380 IU/l with a mean of 1369 IU/l. In seven out of ten patients LDH values exceeded 900 IU/l. Of all the potentially commonly available tests of liver dysfunction for the assessment and management of patients with severe preeclampsia and/or HELLP syndrome, LDH reliably demonstrates the most dramatic rise in serum levels. As a reflector of the degree of hemolysis, as well as hepatic dysfunction, measuring LDH levels is an easy and very useful parameter in the management of these patients. In most HELLP syndrome patients LDH levels usually peak 24–48 h postpartum (Martin *et al.*, 1991).

Severe hyperbilirubinemia is uncommon in pregnancy-induced hypertensive disorders. In eclampsia, significant hyperbilirubinemia has been reported to occur in 4–20%. An elevation of bilirubin is usually mild and rarely exceeds a fivefold elevation (Combes and Adams, 1972; Latham, 1992). On the other hand, icterus has been reported to occur in 10–15% of fatal cases of eclampsia (Chesley, 1978). Unconjugated hyperbilirubinemia indicates intravascular hemolysis, or the presence of an extensive hematoma. Conjugated hyperbilirubinemia indicates hepatic parenchymal cell necrosis or cholestasis (intra- or extrahepatic).

In preeclampsia, capillary leakage and heavy proteinuria may cause very low albumin. Impairment of hepatic albumin synthesis is only involved in extremely severe disease (Honger, 1968).

Some patients with severe preeclampsia and normal to moderately increased ASAT/ALAT levels, may suddenly develop agonizing epigastric pain and in the following hours demonstrate an enormous increase in ASAT/ALAT. This sequence of events is suspect for liver infarction. The transaminase elevations in case of liver infarction are beyond the range of those seen in acute fatty liver of pregnancy. The further course of these patients is characterized by anemia, without a proved source, and protracted fever (Riely *et al.*, 1987). These infarcts are best visualized on CT scanning or MRI. Ultrasonography may fail to reveal even extensive areas of infarction. Severely affected women may have enough hepatic injury to develop the full syndrome of hepatic failure, with coagulopathy, encephalopathy and jaundice.

Acute fatty liver of pregnancy may be associated with preeclampsia. HELLP syndrome and AFLP are both characterized by elevated liver enzymes. In AFLP, transaminase levels average less than 300–500 IU, and rarely increase to values of more than 1000 units, as is common in acute viral hepatitis. In contrast to most cases of HELLP syndrome, laboratory tests in AFLP usually confirm the existence of some degree of hepatic failure such as prolonged PT and aPTT, decreased fibrinogen levels, hypoglycemia and hyperammonemia. Bilirubin levels typically rise to levels much higher than the values normally recorded even in patients with severe HELLP syndrome; bilirubin levels in AFLP are usually á 170 μmol/l but may be as high as 500 μmol/l.

On average, ATIII deficiency is more obvious in AFLP than in HELLP syndrome. Because most AFLP patients also have preeclampsia, most patients with AFLP have hyperuricemia. Other characteristic laboratory results include an elevated white blood count in the range of 20 000–30 000. Clinical signs of diabetes insipidus (nephrogenic type) have been reported to occur in some cases of AFLP, but also in case of severe HELLP syndrome (Mabie and Sibai, 1990; Latham, 1992). For the differential diagnosis, AFLP *versus* HELLP syndrome, it is important to emphasize that in AFLP patients disseminated intravascular coagulation (DIC) precedes and exceeds laboratory studies suggestive of microangiopathic hemolytic anemia (MAHA) (Watson and Seeds, 1990; Martin and Stedman, 1991). However, there may well be an overlap between these disorders, and patients with both HELLP syndrome and acute fatty liver of pregnancy have been reported. Microscopic examination of liver biopsy samples will provide the definitive diagnostic test. Liver biopsy in AFLP shows diffuse, low-grade panlobular microvascular fatty changes (steatosis), and in HELLP syndrome fibrin deposition (Shaffer, 1987).

## 7.8.12 ASSESSMENT OF PANCREATIC INVOLVEMENT

Genuine preeclampsia may be associated with injury of the pancreas (Schmorl, 1901). Haukland *et al.* (1987) found significantly higher mean levels of cationic trypsinogen and amylase in severe preeclampsia (64 ng/ml and 1.6 µmol/l) than the corresponding mean values in uncomplicated pregnancies (22 ng/ml and 1.1 µmol/l). In case of upper abdominal pain in a preeclamptic patient it is prudent to include an assessment of pancreatic injury in the laboratory analysis of such a patient.

## 7.9 ENZYMES AND HORMONES

### 7.9.1 ESTROGENS

Adequate formation of estriol depends on the integrate function of the fetoplacental unit. Measurement of urinary estriol became a widely used test for evaluation of the feto-placental unit in pregnancy-induced hypertensive disorders and other conditions following the report of Greene and Touchstone (1963). In case of mild pregnancy-induced hypertensive disease estriol values seldom fall below the normal range, but most values are less than average. In severe preeclampsia the excretion of estriol is diminished, although occasional values still fall inside the normal range. In general, a day-to-day decrease of 35–50% is considered a significant fall in plasma or urinary estriol measurements. However, measuring estriol in blood or urine only reflects fetoplacental function (Kunzig and Geiger, 1976) and is of no use in assessing the maternal condition. As a method for ascertaining fetal wellbeing measuring estriol has been completely replaced by biophysical methods. In 1976 Duenhoelter, Whalley and MacDonald (1976): stated 'measurement of estrogen levels is of little value in management of women with a fetus at risk; it may even lead to erroneous premature delivery'.

### 7.9.2 HUMAN PLACENTAL LACTOGEN (HPL)

The major putative role of hPL is control of maternal carbohydrate and lipid metabolism in late pregnancy and immunosuppression. The normal rate of synthesis in late pregnancy has been estimated at 1–2 g/d, and is related to the mass of functioning placenta, and thereby secondarily to fetal weight (Chard, 1982; Grudzinskas and Chard, 1991). Patients with pregnancy-induced hypertensive disease, without associated fetal growth retardation have normal or even elevated hPL levels (Obiekwe *et al.*, 1984). Spellacy *et al.* (1971) defined a 'fetal danger zone' for hypertensive pregnant women; in this analysis hPL levels less than 4 µg/ml after the 30th week indicated a fetal mortality of 24%. In conclusion, hPL levels are reduced in case of moderate to severe pregnancy-induced hypertensive disorders, the lowest levels being found in case of severe preeclampsia, associated with fetal growth retardation, but measuring hPL is of no value in assessing the maternal condition (Letchworth, 1976).

### 7.9.3 HUMAN CHORIONIC GONADOTROPHIN (HCG)

Some studies found elevated levels of β-hCG in pregnancy-induced hypertensive disorders, and it has been suggested that β-hCG determination may have value for the early diagnosis of preeclampsia (Said *et al.*, 1984). However, levels of β-hCG in normotensive and hypertensive pregnancies appear to overlap considerably, also levels show a large scatter. Therefore, the clinical value of (β)-hCG measurements for predicting or monitoring pregnancy-induced hypertensive disorders seems limited at the most (Teph and Sivasamboo, 1968; Crosignani *et al.*, 1974; Keller, 1976).

### 7.9.4 PREGNANCY-ASSOCIATED PLASMA PROTEIN A (PAPP-A)

PAPP-A does not fit the picture of a typical placental protein. Indeed, there have been doubts whether it is purely a placental protein or whether the decidua might be contributing to its biosynthesis. PAPP-A appears to exercise its function at the trophoblast–maternal interface, that is the apical border of the syncytiotrophoblast (Bischof and Klopper, 1983; Stabile, Grudzinskas and Chard, 1988). Bischof and Klopper (1983) have stated: 'if this is true, the concentration of PAPP-A in the peripheral circulation may be irrelevant; merely smoke blowing from the fire at the placental level'. The most fruitful area of clinical research, with respect to PAPP-A levels, turned out to be the pregnancy-induced hypertensive disorders. The surprising feature about PAPP-A in pregnancy-induced hypertensive disorders is that it is raised, not lowered. The increase in PAPP-A levels is most marked in severe preeclampsia. Some investigators have reported that the rise in PAPP-A may precede the onset of overt clinical signs of pregnancy-induced hypertensive disease (Toop and Klopper, 1981; Klopper,

1982; Bischof and Klopper, 1983). However, the results of the Odense study, in which the diagnostic criteria for hypertensive disorders during pregnancy were rigidly defined, clearly demonstrated that it is impossible to predict the occurrence of pregnancy-induced hypertensive disorders by the measurement of fetoplacental steroids or proteins (PAPP-A, hPL, SP1; Westergaard *et al.*, 1984). The difference between the Odense study and the other, more positive studies is probably caused by the presence of heparin in the test tubes that were used in the earlier studies. Presently, it is clear that anticoagulants should be avoided in sample collection and that only serum should be used for measurements of PAPP-A. The potential value of PAPP-A levels in monitoring of high-risk pregnancies will only become clear after the real functional importance of this 'placental protein' has been elucidated.

### 7.9.5 PLACENTAL PROTEIN 12 (PP12)

Several investigators reported elevated PP12 levels in patients with hypertensive disorders of pregnancy, as compared to patients with an uncomplicated pregnancy (Iino, Sjoberg and Seppala, 1986; Howell *et al.*, 1985; Than *et al.*, 1984). Howell *et al.* (1985) found a significant negative association between PP12 levels and infant birthweight. The clinical efficiency of elevated PP12 levels in the prediction of low-birthweight infants compared favorably with that of reduced hPL levels. Because PP12 has recently been found to be synthesized by decidua and not by trophoblast, these results support the concept that the decidua is primarily affected in preeclampsia. Further studies are needed to assess if PP12 is useful for early diagnosis or to monitor the course of the disease.

### 7.9.6 PREGNANCY-SPECIFIC BETA-1 GLYCOPROTEIN/ *SCHWANGERSCHAFTSPROTEIN* 1 (SP1)

SP1 is synthesized in the syncytiotrophoblast but has also been found in non-pregnancy serum, fibroblast cultures and brain cells. The physiological importance of SP1 is uncertain: claims have been made that it is concerned with maternal carbohydrate metabolism. The clinical information provided by the measurement of serum SP1 is equivalent to that of hCG in early pregnancy and hPL in late pregnancy. There is an association between decreased levels of SP1 and fetal growth retardation, in both the presence and the absence of maternal hypertension (Grudzinskas and Sinosich, 1982). The change in SP1 levels in pregnancy-induced hypertensive disorders appears to be small and inconsistent (Weber, Heller and Seulen, 1980; Bischof and Klopper,1983).

### 7.9.7 PLACENTAL PROTEIN 5 (PP5)

There are some curious similarities between PAPP-A and PP5. Both proteins complex with heparin and both appear to act as a serine protease inhibitor. Salem, Seppala and Chard (1981) have proposed that PP5 is the placental equivalent of ATIII. Neither PAPP-A nor PP5 is affected by fetal growth and neither is correlated with placental weight. Both are raised in pregnancy-induced hypertensive disorders, abruptio placentae and premature labor. Their association with these apparently different disease entities may be part of the same story. Future studies are needed in order to get a better understanding of the exact involvement of PAPP-A and PP5 in coagulation processes and in the complement cascade during pregnancy (Lee *et al.*, 1981; Salem, Seppala and Chard, 1981; Bischof and Klopper, 1983; Stabile, Grudzinskas and Chard, 1988).

In conclusion, the studies reported in the literature demonstrate that measuring 'placental proteins' is of no use in predicting pregnancy-induced hypertensive disorders. The availability of biophysical tests for fetal surveillance in the hour-to-hour and day-to-day care of high-risk pregnant women has rendered these biochemical tests obsolete;

they are also of no use in the assessment of the maternal condition.

### 7.9.8 MATERNAL SERUM ALPHA-FETOPROTEIN (MSAFP)

In recent years it has been reported that mothers with elevated MSAFP but normal amniotic fluid AFP concentrations constitute a group of gravidas at high risk of later spontaneous abortion, stillbirth, prematurity, fetal growth retardation, preeclampsia, abruptio placentae, intrapartum fetal distress and neonatal death (Milunsky *et al.*, 1989; Martin and Cowan, 1990; Thomas and Blakemore, 1990; Crandall, Robinson and Grau, 1991). It has been assumed that in these pregnancies abnormalities in placental structure may cause an increased direct transport of this typical fetal protein from the fetal to the maternal compartment. A recent major study demonstrated that unexplained elevated MSAFPs offer little if any additional predictive value for adverse perinatal outcome in populations already at high risk for such outcomes on the basis of obstetric or socioeconomic criteria (Philips *et al.*, 1992). One group of investigators noted significantly lower MSAFP concentrations in pregnancies that later developed preeclampsia (Gupta and Srivastava, 1987), and hypothesized that the impaired trophoblast invasion is the mechanism behind these lowered MSAFPs in future preeclamptic women. In conclusion, MSAFP levels may be of some use to identify 'a high-risk pregnancy' but further studies are needed to clarify this issue. MSAFP is of no value in the diagnosis and management of established hypertensive disease.

### 7.9.9 DEOXYCYTIDYLATE DEAMINASE AND CYTIDINE DEAMINASE

The enzyme deoxycytidylate deaminase catalyzes the conversion of deoxycytidylate monophosphate to deoxyuridylate and ammonia. The production of ammonia is the basis for assessment of enzymatic activity (µmol/min/ml). Increased enzymatic activity is encountered in most acute liver diseases, acute infectious diseases, systemic lupus erythematosus, and after surgery. In pregnancy-induced hypertensive disorders, serum levels of deoxycytidylate deaminase are elevated, as compared to normotensive pregnancy and pregnancies complicated by preexisting hypertension. Enzymatic activity is similar in non-pregnant women, normal pregnant women and pregnant women with chronic hypertension (Williams and Jones, 1975, 1982; Redman *et al.*, 1977; Jones *et al.*, 1982). In their first report Williams and Jones (1975) defined ammonia production of more than $4.8 \times 10^{-4}$ µmol/min/ml as pathological. These values were found in all preeclamptic patients, in all cases of fetal demise and in all twin pregnancies of more than 36 weeks gestational age. In pregnancy-induced hypertensive disorders these abnormally elevated levels of enzymatic activity were only reached in established disease, and the authors concluded that this method was not useful for early diagnosis. The enzyme deoxycytidylate deaminase exists in an A and a B form. The A form has been found in large quantities in the placenta; the B form has been found in the kidneys and the heart. The B type of the enzyme is the fraction that is increased in preeclampsia. Redman *et al.* (1977) demonstrated that the increase in enzymatic activity runs parallel with the increase in uric acid levels, and stated that the increase in deoxycytidylate deaminase activity has a similar predictive value for adverse perinatal outcome as serum urate levels. Assessment of deoxycytidylate deaminase activity has been evaluated as a test for early diagnosis. A large prospective study demonstrated that the increase in enzymatic activity just precedes the onset of proteinuria (Williams and Jones, 1982). In 1982 Jones *et al.* reported on their results in measuring cytidine deaminase. This enzyme catalyzes the conversion of cytidine to uridine and ammonia. Enzymatic activity of cytidine deaminase

is also expressed as µmol/min/ml ammonia formed. Cytidine deaminase also exists in an A and a B form (kidney). This study demonstrated a near perfect correlation between deoxycytidylate deaminase activity and cytidine deaminase activity. As a predictor for adverse perinatal outcome the clinical value of both enzymatic activities is similar, but the cytidine deaminase assay is much simpler. Measuring cytidine deaminase is a simple method that can be used as a routine laboratory test, but determination of serum uric acid levels appears to be at least as good for monitoring the course of the disease.

## 7.10 HEMATOLOGICAL MARKERS

### 7.10.1 ROUTINE CLOTTING TESTS

The activated partial thromboplastin time (aPTT) evaluates the intrinsic and common coagulation pathways – factors XII, XI, IX, VIIIc, X, V, II and fibrinogen – but is designed to detect abnormalities in the intrinsic pathway. The aPTT is most sensitive to deficiencies in the early stages of the coagulation cascade; in contrast, fibrinogen levels of 0.5–1 g/l are necessary to alter the test. The prothrombin time (PT) evaluates the extrinsic and common coagulation pathways, but is designed to detect abnormalities in the extrinsic pathway. It is most sensitive to deficiencies of factors VII, X and V. The PT is unaltered by hypofibrinogemia until the fibrinogen level is very low (< 0.1–0.5 g/l). The thrombin time (TT) evaluates the final common pathway of the extrinsic and extrinsic coagulation systems. A deficiency (or abnormality) of fibrinogen, the presence of heparin and fibrin(ogen) degradation products are the most common causes of a prolonged TT.

The aPTT, PT and TT are normal in preeclampsia, with the exception of terminal-stage preeclampsia–eclampsia complicated by DIC. Occasionally a prolonged aPTT is encountered in a patient with severe early-onset preeclampsia, as a manifestation of the lupus anticoagulant syndrome.

## 7.10.2 FIBRINOGEN/FIBRIN DEGRADATION PRODUCTS

When fibrinogen or fibrin is broken down by plasmin, fibrin(ogen) degradation products (FDPs) are formed; these comprise the high-molecular-weight split products X and Y, and smaller fragments, A, B, C, D and E. When a fibrin clot is formed, 70% of fragment X is retained in the clot, Y, D and E being retained to a somewhat lesser extent. FDPs are removed from the circulation by the reticuloendothelial system and have a half-life of about 9 hours. FDPs can inhibit normal fibrin monomer polymerization and platelet aggregation (by blocking the platelet fibrinogen receptor). These effects can aggravate the coagulation defects that are already present in DIC (Letsky, 1989). Blood should be taken for estimation of FDPs by clean venepuncture. The tourniquet should not be left too long, since venous stasis also stimulates fibrinolytic activity. Simple immunological tests such as agglutination reactions can be used as a rapid assay for the presence of these FDPs.

A newer monoclonal antibody assay has been developed, which measures the degradation product of cross-linked fibrin (D-dimer). In contrast to FDPs, which represent the breakdown of both fibrin and fibrinogen, D-dimer is released during lysis of the fibrin polymer. The generation of D-dimer results from thrombin generation in excess of that neutralized by ATIII and hence its measurement is specific for lysis of the fibrin polymer (Wilde *et al.*, 1989).

Measurement of FDPs has proved to be useful for the detection of overt disseminated intravascular coagulation. However, there is a considerable overlap in the levels found between patients with and without thromboembolic disease. Therefore, measurement of serum FDPs is of very limited practical value for predicting or detecting silent thromboembolic disease in high-risk patients (Hirsch, 1987).

Overall, fibrinolytic activity appears to be impaired during pregnancy, although it returns rapidly to normal following delivery. This appears to be the result of placentally derived plasminogen activator inhibitor type 2 (PAI-2). It has also been shown that the endothelium-derived PAI-1 increases by around threefold, and PAI-1 has been demonstrated to be the primary inhibitor of tPA during pregnancy (Wiman *et al.*, 1984; Kruithof *et al.*, 1987; Jorgensen *et al.*, 1987; Forbes and Greer, 1992). In normal pregnancy, tPA measurements have produced controversial results. Kruithof *et al.* reported increased levels (1987), and Ballegeer *et al.* (1987) found tPA release to be significantly reduced throughout normal pregnancy. The fibrinolytic response after stimulation by venous occlusion has been demonstrated to be impaired (Ballegeer *et al.*, 1987). However, despite this impairment in the response to venous occlusion, D-dimers are substantially increased in the first, second and third trimesters as compared to non-pregnant women. This indicates that fibrinolysis is still occurring and is clearly not impaired to the extend suggested by the reduced levels of tPA and increased PAI-1 and PAI-2 levels (Ballegeer *et al.*, 1987; Wilde *et al.*, 1989).

Studies on the fibrinolytic system in preeclampsia have provided conflicting data. Most studies, however, reported that overall activator activity was normal or only slightly reduced in preeclampsia as compared to uncomplicated pregnancy (Howie, Prentice and McNicol, 1971; Wallmo, Karlsson and Teger-Nilsson, 1984). Plasminogen levels, as determined by various methods, appear to be somewhat lower in some patients with severe preeclampsia (Maki, 1983).

In contrast, other fibrinolytic parameters are indicative of enhanced fibrinolytic activity in preeclampsia. These parameters include serum FDP and fragment D-dimers raised to levels exceeding those observed in normal pregnancy. The levels of FDPs have been studied extensively in preeclampsia. The results are largely inconclusive: some groups have reported elevated FDPs, others found normal or near normal levels (Bonnar, McNicol and Douglas, 1971; Howie, Prentice and McNicol, 1971; Chesley, 1978; Gibson *et al.*, 1982; Maki, 1983; Ballegeer *et al.*, 1987; Wilde *et al.*, 1989; Trofatter *et al.*, 1989). There is certainly no value in measuring FDPs for early diagnosis of pregnancy-induced hypertensive disorders. In fact, Pritchard, Cunningham and Mason (1976) found no detectable FDPs in 51 out of 59 eclamptic women. In general the highest levels of FDPs are found in the period after eclamptic seizures. Monoclonal antibodies to D-dimers are increasingly being used to screen for coagulation abnormalities in preeclampsia (Dimertest) (Wilde *et al.*, 1989). Preeclamptic women with detectable D-dimer have a more severe disease and a greater risk on adverse outcome than preeclamptic women without detectable D-dimer. The presence of D-dimer correlates strongly with elevated FDPs and a platelet count of less than $10^9/l$ (Trofatter *et al.*, 1989; Terao *et al.*, 1991). The Dimertest is a sensitive and simple means of detecting fibrinolysis, and is very useful in early screening and follow-up for preeclamptic coagulopathy. In addition, the Dimertest is of great help in defining the subset of patients with severe disease and a high risk of maternal morbidity/mortality.

The endothelial release of tPA is increased in preeclampsia (Estelles *et al.*, 1987; Gilabert *et al.*, 1990), as compared to uncomplicated pregnancy. The increased release of tPA in preeclampsia is an expression of endothelial cell damage (Zeeman and Dekker, 1992). In theory, the release of tPA in preeclampsia may induce a fibrinolytic response (Perry and Martin, 1992). However, the increase in tPA is overshadowed by the increase in plasminogen activator inhibitor activity (PAI) (Gilabert *et al.*, 1990). In preeclampsia, as compared to uncomplicated pregnancy, PAI-1 levels

increase. The increase in PAI-1 levels is also an expression of endothelial cell damage (Estelles *et al.*, 1987; Gilabert *et al.*, 1990; Zeeman and Dekker, 1992). In preeclampsia, especially if complicated by fetal growth retardation, PAI-2 levels decrease. Because PAI-2 is synthesized by the placenta, this decrease is probably an expression of placental damage. In this way the PAI-2 level can be considered as a marker of placental function (Aznar *et al.*, 1986; de Boer *et al.*, 1988; Gilabert *et al.*, 1990; Estelles *et al.*, 1991). Ballegeer *et al.* (1989) studied fibronectin and PAI-1 levels in 120 normotensive primigravid women throughout pregnancy. Of these women, 32 eventually developed preeclampsia. Ballegeer *et al.* found increased levels of PAI-1 (> 280 ng/ml) at 25–32 weeks gestation in 16 of the 32 women (sensitivity 50%, specificity 95%). In this study plasma fibronectin measurements were demonstrated to be a better predictor. The imbalance between tPA and the high level of PAI-1 levels in preeclampsia may cause a decreased fibrinolytic activity and thus contribute to the persistence of microthrombi in the microcirculation. Although most hospital laboratories can measure tPA and PAI-1, further studies are necessary to assess if there is a need for these measurements in monitoring the course of the disease.

### 7.10.3 FIBRONECTIN

Measuring fibronectin levels may be of great help in the early diagnosis of preeclampsia (Ballegeer *et al.*, 1989; Dekker and Sibai, 1991). Ballegeer *et al.* (1989) compared plasma fibronectin, PAI-1, fVIIIrag and uric acid, and concluded that fibronectin is the best predictor of preeclampsia. Ballegeer *et al.* (1989), evaluated the presence of increased fibronectin levels (mean + 2 s.d.) at 25–32 weeks gestation in the early diagnosis of preeclampsia and found a sensitivity of 96% and a specificity of 94%.

The increase in plasma fibronectin antedates the increase in blood pressure by 4–6 weeks on average. Ballegeer *et al.* (1992) also performed a detailed longitudinal study on platelet activation, vascular damage and coagulation changes, and demonstrated that at least 4 weeks before the development of hypertension fibronectin levels increased to levels above 450 µg/ml (> 2 s.d. above mean). These patients demonstrated a simultaneous significant increase in β-thromboglobulin and, to a lesser degree, of platelet factor 4. The earliest signs of fibrin formation occurred later; there was a significant rise in TAT complexes and a steady, but not significant, rise in fibrinopeptide A levels from 2 weeks before the development of hypertension. The recent studies on ED 1+ fibronectin demonstrating an increase in ED 1+ fibronectin already occurring in the first and second trimesters, long before the appearance of any clinical evidence of pregnancy-induced hypertensive disorders, is extremely promising (Lockwood and Peters, 1990; Taylor *et al.*, 1991).

### 7.10.4 PLATELET COUNT, PLATELET VOLUME, PLATELET FUNCTION, BLEEDING TIME AND PRODUCTS RELEASED BY AGGREGATING PLATELETS

Trudinger (1976) showed that the fall in the number of platelets is related to clinical severity and perinatal outcome. Thrombocytopenia may occur as an early feature of the disorder (Redman, Bonnar and Beilin, 1978). In a longitudinal study on pregnant women with chronic hypertension and the subsequent development of superimposed preeclampsia, a rise in plasma urate preceded the development of proteinuria by three weeks and a fall in the platelet count was observed at the same time (Redman, Beilin and Bonnar, 1976; Redman *et al.*, 1976). Although the standard deviations in the normotensive and hypertensive pregnant women preclude the use of platelet counts as an effective method for early detection (Dekker and Sibai, 1991), prospective serial counts in selected high-risk patients are certainly useful when the patient's own baseline is established in early pregnancy.

In established preeclampsia platelet counts may vary greatly but, on the whole, thrombocytopenia is the most frequent hemostatic abnormality (Gibson *et al.*, 1982). The results of various large studies demonstrate that approximately 20% of all patients with a pregnancy-induced hypertensive disorder develop mild thrombocytopenia, defined as a platelet count of less than $150 \times 10^9$/l, varying between 7% in mild pregnancy-induced hypertensive disease and 50% in severe preeclampsia (Giles and Inglis, 1981; Gibson *et al.*, 1982). Low platelet counts are not even found in all cases of eclampsia (Pritchard, Cunningham and Mason, 1976; Giles and Inglis, 1981; Chesley, 1978). Pritchard, Cunningham and Mason (1976), studying 95 eclamptics, found the platelet count to be less than $150 \times 10^9$/l in 28 patients, less than $100 \times 10^9$/l in 16 patients and less than $50 \times 10^9$/l in only 3 patients. Preeclamptic patients, especially when fetal growth retardation is present, may show a marked day-to-day variability in platelet counts as well as in platelet volume distribution (Wallenburg, 1987). Thrombocytopenia does not occur in pregnant women with pre-existing hypertension.

A typical constellation of abnormalities consisting of hemolysis, elevated liver enzymes and low platelets was given the acronym HELLP syndrome by Weinstein in 1982. However, the first thrombocytopenic preeclamptic patient with hemolysis was described by Stahnke in 1922. The University of Tennessee, criteria for HELLP syndrome are presented in Table 7.3.

---

**Table 7.3** University of Tennessee, Memphis, criteria for HELLP syndrome

- Abnormal peripheral blood smear
- Hemolysis – total bilirubin $> 20\,\mu$mol/l
- LDH $> 600$ U/l
- Elevated ASAT $> 70$ U/l
- Liver enzymes – LDH $> 600$ U/l
- Low platelets – platelet count $< 10 \times 10^9$/l

Martin *et al.* (1990) have proposed the following simple classification of subpopulations based on platelet count nadir:

1. Class 1 HELLP syndrome – platelet nadir less than $50 \times 10^9/l$;
2. Class 2 HELLP syndrome – platelet nadir $50–100 \times 10^9/l$;
3. Class 3 HELLP syndrome – platelet nadir more than $100 \times 10^9/l$.

These classes were used to predict the rapidity of postpartum disease recovery, risk of recurrence of HELLP syndrome, perinatal outcome and the need for plasmapheresis. Most patients with HELLP syndrome show decreasing platelet counts until 24–48 h after delivery. Although most cases of thrombocytopenia associated with preeclampsia should resolve by the fourth postpartum day, women with class I HELLP syndrome require as long as 11 days to achieve a platelet count above $100 \times 10^9/l$ (Martin *et al.*, 1990). A low platelet count should always be confirmed by a manual count, because the anticoagulant EDTA does not always prevent platelet clumping. These clumps are not recognized by the automated counters, which then erroneously report a low platelet count (pseudothrombocytopenia) (Jackson, 1978). Pseudothrombo-cytopenia can also be excluded by reviewing the stained blood film, which shows clumped platelets.

In established preeclampsia the platelet count should be checked at least twice a week. In case of a declining number of platelets, the platelet count should be repeated at least daily. During the treatment of patients with HELLP syndrome with plasma volume expansion and vasodilator drugs, most patients demonstrate a normalization of liver enzymes and platelet count. However, we have seen some patients in which the platelet count only demonstrated a partial recovery, while at the same time the clinical condition improved and the liver enzymes normalized completely. The further clinical course of these patients was complicated with liver infarction, beginning with sudden, agonizing upper abdominal pain.

The differential diagnosis for thrombocytopenia in a pregnant woman should always include preeclampsia. However, other causes should not be disregarded. If there are no other signs of uteroplacental insufficiency the differential diagnosis includes autoimmune thrombocytopenia, hematological malignant diseases, severe folate deficiency, antiphospholipid syndrome and pseudothrombocytopenia. It is important to remember that about 10% of patients with immune thrombocytopenia (ITP) are positive for anticardiolipin antibodies and/or lupus anticoagulant. Because the antiphospholipid syndrome may also be associated with severe preeclampsia, the differential diagnosis in a pregnant woman with a low platelet count may be difficult.

Mean platelet volume and, in particular, platelet volume distribution and the percentage of circulating large platelets are indices that are considered to reflect thrombocytopoietic activity. In case of increased platelet turnover, changes in these indices may precede changes in the number of circulating platelets. The increase in mean platelet volume and volume distribution width confirms the compensated state of platelet destruction in the late second and third trimester of pregnancy (Fay, Hughes and Farron, 1983; Sill, Lind and Walker, 1985; Tygart *et al.*, 1986). However, there is no difference in the percentage of large platelets (volume 15.9–30.1 $\mu m^3$) between non-pregnant women and normotensive pregnant women in the third trimester (Wallenburg, 1987). Platelet volume is increased in pregnancy-induced hypertensive disorders (Giles and Inglis, 1981; Stubbs *et al.*, 1986). Macrothrombocytosis is found in about 50% of patients with fully developed preeclampsia (Giles, 1982). Measurement of platelet volume is not useful as a screening test in a low-risk population. However, increasing platelet size can predict which patients with essential hypertension or established mild pregnancy-induced hypertensive disease are likely to progress to severe disease. A significant increase in platelet size occurs at least 1 week before the development of severe hypertension and/or preeclampsia (Walker *et al.*, 1989).

In general a platelet count of more than 50 $\times 10^9/l$ is usually associated with normal platelet hemostasis. Spontaneous bleeding may be associated with platelet counts of less than $20 \times 10^9/l$. Intracranial hemorrhage is the leading cause of death in severe thrombocytopenia and is particularly likely with platelet counts of less than $5 \times 10^9/l$. No currently available laboratory test faithfully reflects the platelets' ability to accomplish their enormously complex series of functions in a manner consistent with normal hemostasis. Whether the platelet count is normal or low, the bleeding time is the most important functional test of the *in vivo* role of platelets in hemostasis. All of the other 'function' tests are *in vitro* assays designed to reflect the physiological role of the platelet, but there may not always be a good correlation between an abnormal test result and clinical bleeding (White *et al.*, 1987). Measurement of template bleeding time provides a sensitive but nonspecific overall assessment of primary hemostasis. The bleeding time evaluates overall primary hemostatic competence and therefore reflects both platelet number and function. The modified Ivy technique is probably the most sensitive available. Marked thrombocytopenia, qualitative defects in platelet function, FDPs, von Willebrand factor deficiency (fVIIIrag), marked anemia and abnormalities in vascular collagen can all result in an abnormally prolonged bleeding time (> 10 min). Prolongation of the bleeding time from a normal of 4–7 min usually occurs at a platelet count of $35–50 \times 10^9/l$, with progressive prolongation noted with more significant decreases in number. At counts less than $10 \times 10^9/l$ the bleeding time is often 15 min or longer.

*In vitro* platelet aggregation, in response to various agents, has been reported to be decreased in a considerable portion of women with severe preeclampsia (Whigham *et al.*, 1978; Maki, 1983). This finding may be explained by the return of 'used' platelets into the circulation. A 'used' platelet means that a platelet has released some of its vasoactive, platelet aggregation and coagulation-stimulating contents somewhere in the microcirculation, before it reentered the 'major' circulation. Thus, a mild decrease in platelets is no proof of the existence of an adequate hemostasis, as far as the platelets are concerned. The prolongation of the bleeding time in preeclampsia, in non-thrombocytopenic and thrombocytopenic patients, may be out of order with the platelet number (Ramanathan *et al.*, 1989). In contrast, in the case of ITP all circulating platelets are very young and active, and hemostasis is often more or less normal even at rather low platelet counts.

Episodes of platelet activation and consumption may also be assessed by measuring plasma β-thromboglobulin and platelet factor IV levels. These proteins are localized in the α-granules of platelets, and approximately 70% are released during the platelet release reaction (Hirsch, 1987). β-thromboglobulin has a half-life in plasma of approximately 100 min; platelet factor IV has a lifespan of less than 10 min (Firkin, 1984). In non-pregnant patients Ludlam (1979) clearly showed a strong negative correlation between β-thromboglobulin and platelet lifespan. In the first trimester of uncomplicated pregnancy β-thromboglobulin levels are equal to non-pregnant levels; in the second and third trimester there appears to be a significant increase (although with considerable overlap), supporting the concept of *in vivo* platelet activation in late pregnancy (Maki, 1983; Douglas *et al.*, 1982). In preeclampsia platelet release is evidenced by the finding of elevated plasma levels of β-thromboglobulin and platelet factor IV, as compared to normotensive pregnant women or pregnant patients with essential hypertension (Inglis *et al.*, 1982; Maki, 1983; Douglas *et al.*, 1982; de Vries, Vellenga and Aarnoudse, 1983; Borok *et*

*al.*, 1984). Borok *et al.* (1984) found a dispropor-
tionate increase in β-thromboglobulin and
platelet factor IV as compared to the increase
in fibrinopeptide A. This finding, once again,
is evidence for the non-thrombin-mediated
platelet release reaction in preeclampsia.
Boneu *et al.* (1980) found an excellent correlation between platelet life-span, β-thromboglobulin and the fVIIIrag/fVIIIc ratio. The
increase in β-thromboglobulin has been
shown to correlate with proteinuria and
serum creatinine (Socol *et al.*, 1985).

7.10.5 OVERVIEW OF HEMOSTATIC CHANGES
IN PREGNANCY-INDUCED HYPERTENSIVE
DISORDERS

With regard to platelets, preeclampsia is a
compensated thrombocytolytic state, a condition that has been demonstrated in a variety
of disorders, characterized by increased
peripheral platelet consumption due to non-
immune, surface-mediated platelet activation.
Thornton *et al.* (1986) found no differences in
platelet counts, β-thromboglobulin levels,
thrombin time, FDPs, platelet factor IV and
fibrinopeptide A at 28 weeks gestational age
between 20 normotensive pregnant women
and 20 normotensive pregnant women, who
later on developed preeclampsia. Thus, even
sophisticated hemostatic parameters are of no
use in the early detection of preeclampsia.
Markers for endothelial damage appear to be
superior in this respect (Dekker and Sibai,
1991).

According to most clinicians and investigators HELLP syndrome is not a form of DIC. In
contrast Sibai (1990c) found DIC (defined as
platelets less than $10 \times 10^9/l$, plasma fibrinogen less than 3 g/l, and FDPs moe than 40
mg/l) in 38% of patients with HELLP syndrome. Van Dam *et al.* (1989) advocate the use
of the coagulation scoring system, introduced
by Hellgren, Egberg and Eklund in 1984, in
the classification and management of HELLP
syndrome patients. This system is based on
platelet count less than $10 \times 10^9/l$, PT less than

70%, ATIII activity less than 80%, FDPs more
than 40 mg/l and fibrinogen less than 3 g/l.
DIC was diagnosed if three or more of these
tests were pathological. If only two tests were
abnormal, a diagnosis of suspected DIC was
made. Van Dam *et al.* (1989) demonstrated
that HELLP patients with DIC developed significantly more life-threatening complications
than HELLP patients without DIC, as defined
in this study. All patients with DIC showed
rapidly deteriorating maternal and fetal condition and these pregnancies could not be
managed conservatively. De Boer *et al.* (1991)
found evidence of compensated intravascular
coagulation in most patients with HELLP syndrome and a small percentage of preeclamptic
patients. Real decompensated intravascular
coagulation (DIC) was not found in this
series. These studies demonstrate the presence of a localized increase in intravascular
coagulation (uteroplacental vascular bed, kidney and liver). The localized increase in
intravascular coagulation is secondary to
endothelial cell injury. The high incidence of
DIC reported by some authors is probably
caused by the fact that the patients in these
studies are already in the (pre)terminal stage
of their disease process. In general, it is only
when a patient's platelet count falls consistently below $80 \times 10^9/l$ that an increasing percentage of those with HELLP syndrome show
evidence of increased intravascular thrombin
production and accelerated fibrin consumption, measured by coagulation studies such as
ATIII, TAT complexes, fibrininopeptide A and
D-dimer measurements. Only in well-
advanced cases of HELLP syndrome with
platelets less than $50 \times 10^9/l$ and LDH levels
more than 600 IU/l do routinely available clinical laboratory tests of fibrinogen and FDPs
become abnormal, occasionally with some
prolongation of the PT and aPTT. The semiquantitative scoring system of Hellgren,
Egberg and Eklund (1984), advocated by van
Dam *et al.* (1989), is very useful to detect deteriorating maternal and fetal condition in
HELLP syndrome. Importantly, in cases of

HELLP syndrome, MAHA and severe thrombocytopenia precede the appearance of fibrin consumption and DIC and not the reverse, as seen, for instance, in patients with placental abruption and AFLP (Martin and Stedman, 1991). Endothelial cell injury can be evidenced and followed in daily clinical practice by measuring fibronectin and the fVIIIrag/fVIIIc ratio. Fibronectin levels, ATIII activity and the presence or absence of D-dimer are invaluable parameters to monitor the course of the disease and to predict the development of overt DIC.

## 7.10.6 ASSESSMENT OF RED BLOOD CELL INVOLVEMENT

The woman of average size usually has a blood volume of nearly 5000 ml in the near-term period, compared with about 3500 ml when not pregnant. In case of pregnancy-induced hypertensive disorders this increment in plasma volume is smaller or may even not exist. Reduced blood volume and consequent hemoconcentration have been viewed as ominous signs in the development of preeclampsia since the time of Zangmeister (1903). Chesley (1972) reviewed the literature and concluded that the average plasma volume in women with pregnancy-induced hypertensive disease was 9% below expected values, and as much as 30–40% below normal in cases of severe preeclampsia. Several studies have demonstrated that significant hypovolemia is only present in pregnancy-induced hypertensive disorders associated with fetal growth retardation (Sibai *et al.*, 1983). Inadequate plasma volume expansion has been associated with a high risk of fetal growth retardation, premature labor, oligohydramnios, chronic hypertension and pregnancy-induced hypertensive disorders (Soffronoff, Kaufmann and Connaughton, 1977; Chesley, 1978; Hays, Cruickshank and Dunn, 1985). It has been demonstrated that there is a relationship between maternal plasma volume and birthweight, both before and after the development

of pregnancy-induced hypertensive disease/preeclampsia (MacGillivray and Campbell, 1980). The fact that a reduction in plasma volume may antedate the appearance of hypertension (Bletka *et al.*, 1970; Gallery, Hunyor and Gyory, 1979; MacGillivray and Campbell, 1980) made some investigators believe that the reduction in plasma volume is the primary feature of preeclampsia, and thus the cause of the vasoconstriction and hypertension. However, the development of preeclampsia begins with a loss of vascular refractoriness to vasoactive agents, followed by vasoconstriction. The increased vascular sensitivity and subsequent vasoconstriction results in a decrease in intravascular volume, and intravascular volume is shunted, across the 'leaky' capillaries, to extravascular spaces (Assali, 1977; Assali and Prystowsky, 1952; Gant *et al.*, 1973; Dekker, 1989).

The methods used for estimating plasma volume are subject to serious criticism, and they are too complicated to be used in a clinical setting. Because red cell volume in preeclampsia is not significantly different from normotensive pregnancy, measuring hemoglobin levels (Hb) and/or hematocrit (Ht) is a convenient way to get an impression of the plasma volume (Bletka *et al.*, 1970; Chesley, 1972). Abnormal high Hb/Ht levels are a better predictor of adverse perinatal outcome than abnormally low estriol or hPL levels (Koller, 1982; Sagen *et al.*, 1984). High maternal Hb/Ht levels are associated with low birthweight and placental weight, increased incidence of prematurity and perinatal mortality, as well as with peripheral vascular resistance and the degree of maternal hypertension (Mau, 1977; Curzen, Lloyd and Thomas 1980; Garn *et al.*, 1981; Heilmann *et al.*, 1981; Koller, 1982; Sagen, Koller and Haran, 1982; Sagen *et al.*, 1984; Huisman and Aarnoudse, 1986; Murphy *et al.*, 1986; Meng Lu *et al.*, 1991). The number of infarcts and syncytial knots is markedly elevated in patients with high Hb/Ht levels (Nordenvall and Sandstedt, 1990).

Hemorheological features of pregnancy-induced hypertensive disorders were recently reviewed in detail by Lowe (1992). This paragraph will be restricted to some short comments. In preeclampsia whole blood viscosity at low and high shear rate is raised compared to normotensive uncomplicated pregnancies. After correction for the increased hematocrit these differences can no longer be found, thus demonstrating that preeclamptic hypovolemia and hemoconcentration are of primary importance in the causation of these hemorheological changes (Lowe, 1992). The reduced flow qualities of the blood in severe preeclampsia may be of pathophysiological importance in causing, in concert with a disturbed platelet–vessel-wall interaction, thrombosis in the uteroplacental arteries and the microcirculation of vital organs. In the management of preeclampsia sophisticated hemorheological studies are not needed. Measuring Hb/Ht levels is a rough but usable method for assessing the degree of plasma volume contraction. In addition, hemoconcentration is the major compounding factor in the increase of whole blood viscosity in preeclampsia. Because hemoconcentration means hypovolemia and impaired flow qualities of the blood, and is associated with an increased incidence of adverse perinatal outcome, pregnancy-induced hypertension associated with significant hemoconcentration is not a phenomenon indicating 'benign' adaptation, but is pathological, indicating preeclampsia (Broughton Pipkin, 1985). There is no exact Hb/Ht level to define significant hemoconcentration. Hemoglobin levels vary with altitude, smoking habits and deficiency of iron, etc. Thus trend detection is indispensable. Serial measurements of Hb/Ht are of definite use to monitor pregnancies at high risk of developing uteroplacental insufficiency, and to monitor the course of disease in established pregnancy-induced hypertensive disorders and/or pregnancies complicated by fetal growth retardation. Marked elevation of hemoglobin levels in the second trimester

have been shown to precede the development of pregnancy-induced hypertensive disorders and to be useful as a predictor. However, the predictive value of less pronounced hemoglobin levels is low (Murphy *et al.*, 1986; Huisman and Aarnoudse, 1986).

Microangiopathic hemolysis, present in severe preeclampsia and an essential feature for the diagnosis of HELLP syndrome, can be recognized by the presence of burr cells, triangular cells, schistocytes, echinocytes or polychromasia on a peripheral smear. Whereas schistocytes are characteristic of microangiopathic hemolysis, echinocytes are characteristic of aberrations in the red cell membrane. The echinocytosis appears to be, like the increased red cell rigidity, another feature of intrinsic erythrocyte changes in preeclampsia (Cunningham *et al.*, 1985).

It is not usually necessary to perform a complete blood smear to diagnose hemolysis. An increase in LDH levels out of proportion with the increase in liver enzymes, an increase in heat-stable LDH, an increase in LDH1 and LDH2 (Zimmerman and Henry, 1984) and a decrease in haptoglobin levels are alternative, more convenient methods of assessing the degree of hemolysis. The plasma level of haptoglobin appears to be related inversely to the activity of the hemolytic process. Plasma haptoglobin is absent when the hemolysis is severe enough to produce an apparent red-cell life of 17 days. Measuring indirect bilirubin levels or waiting for a decrease in Hb levels are insensitive methods of establishing the presence of hemolysis. However, the clinician should be warned if a preeclamptic patient who has demonstrated a significant hemoconcentration on an earlier occasion suddenly has a normal Hb. Hemoglobinuria is a more common finding in HELLP syndrome than jaundice, especially in severe HELLP syndrome complicated by the occurrence of DIC.

A great number of other conditions should be considered by the clinician in the differential diagnosis of a pregnant woman with manifestations of MAHA and other manifestations of severe preeclampsia and/or HELLP syndrome. Martin and Stedman (1991) stated that at least five categories of disease with primary or secondary hematological features should be taken into consideration in the hematological differential diagnosis of HELLP syndrome. Diagnostic confusion can arise in relation to the following.

### (a) A thrombotic microangiopathy similar to HELLP syndrome but secondary to other causes

The term microangiopathic hemolytic anemia (MAHA), as proposed by Symmers (1952) describes the spectrum of disease in patients that includes TTP, HUS, connective tissue disorders and HELLP syndrome. All these disease entities are characterized by an abnormal platelet–endothelium relationship. The most frequent clinical presentation of TTP consists of neurological and/or hemorrhagic symptoms, often in combination with fever (> 38.30°C). Hypertension is not a feature of TTP. Fibronectin levels are not elevated and ATIII activity not depressed in TTP, as they are in severe preeclampsia. Most patients with TTP have only mild elevations of transaminases, because there is no widespread hepatic dysfunction, in contrast to HELLP syndrome. Fractionation of the LDH increase in TTP reveals minimal to absent contribution from liver parenchymal cells (LDH5), and almost all from hemolysis (LDH1 and LDH2). Ordinarily, patients with TTP exhibit only moderate elevations of plasma creatinine and urea levels, and are not oliguric unless volume-depleted. Although HUS may occur in every trimester of pregnancy, as does TTP, this dangerous condition is most often (95%) encountered by obstetricians in the puerperium. Hence, it is often called postpartum HUS or postpartum renal failure. Typically, an adult patient with HUS develops acute renal failure associated with anuria, hypertension, MAHA and thrombocytopenia following a symptom-free interval devoid of any clinical suggestion of preeclampsia. In addition to renal damage, the gastrointestinal tract may be injured, with resultant symptoms of nausea, vomiting and pain in many patients. No evidence of hepatic dysfunction is typically seen on laboratory examinations; ATIII activity level and plasma fibronectin levels are usually normal (Sipes and Weiner, 1992). MAHA features, including severe thrombocytopenia, have also been described as occurring in association with several drugs, toxins and certain rare medical conditions (Barton, Riely and Sibai, 1992).

### (b) DIC secondary to obstetric or rarely other causes

DIC, primarily a thrombin-driven disorder, can mimic HELLP syndrome. DIC is characterized by an increased intravascular production of thrombin, an increased turnover of fibrinogen and platelets and a secondary fibrinolytic response. Because DIC is a disease of the coagulation system, the coagulation profile is grossly abnormal relative to milder decreases in platelet count. In contrast, the thrombotic microangiopathy disorders are platelet-driven processes in which there is increased platelet consumption, normal fibrinogen turnover and no coagulopathy, although FDPs are mildly increased in some patients secondary to platelet-derived fibrinogen degradation. Sepsis may cause a combination of thrombin-driven and platelet-driven hemostatic changes. AFLP is frequently complicated by a coagulopathy that probably results from a combination of impaired hepatic production of coagulation factors and increased peripheral consumption of these factors. Unlike gravidas with TTP, these patients are usually afebrile. In AFLP patients the evidence of DIC precedes and exceeds laboratory studies suggestive of MAHA. Abnormally prolonged clotting tests and very low fibrinogen levels are detected earlier, and in excess of the degree of thrombocytopenia. Hypoglycemia, impaired renal function, hyperuricemia, hyperlipidemia, elevated amylase, extreme leukocytosis and extreme polydipsia are often present. Bilirubin levels, in particular, rise much higher than the values normally recorded, even in class I HELLP syndrome (Martin and Stedman, 1991).

### (c) Autoimmune disorders/vasculitis

The differential diagnosis between active SLE and severe preeclampsia can be a frustrating exercise. In general, serum complement is an unreliable indicator of lupus activity in pregnancy. When a high-titer antinuclear antibody is coupled with hypocomplementemia (CH50, C3, C4 and C5), the diagnosis can usually be made. C3 and C4 levels are significantly lower in women with active SLE than in women with preeclampsia (Buyon *et al.*, 1986). In addition, ATIII activity is not significantly reduced in active lupus. Thrombocytopenia occurs in about one-third of SLE patients; however, the platelet count rarely drops below $100 \times 10^9/l$. Antiphospholipid antibodies and lupus anticoagulant should be sought routinely in every patient with a thrombotic microangiopathy (Martin and Stedman, 1991).

### (d) Severe primary renal disease

Patients with severe primary renal disease may develop malignant hypertension and renal failure, but also severe superimposed preeclampsia and/or HELLP syndrome.

### (e) Miscellaneous conditions

An array of other diagnoses should be considered in any complete differential diagnosis of severe preeclampsia/HELLP syndrome, including (among others) ITP, post-transfusion purpura and severe folate deficiency. The order of consideration is critically important: HELLP syndrome first, all other diseases second (Martin and Stedman, 1991).

## 7.11 DOPPLER ULTRASOUND ASSESSMENT OF THE UTEROPLACENTAL CIRCULATION

### 7.11.1 UTEROPLACENTAL CIRCULATION

In normotensive pregnancy endovascular trophoblast results in the conversion of approximately 100–150 spiral arteries into uteroplacental arteries, distended, tortuous and funnel-shaped vessels that communicate through multiple openings into the intervillous space (Zuspan, 1990; Redman, 1991). The timing and extent of the trophoblastic invasion may be more variable than is usually assumed, and is not confined to the first two trimesters. A recent Doppler-flow study of the uterine arteries demonstrated that the secondary trophoblast invasion into the muscular portion of the spiral arteries begins between 8 and 13 weeks gestation (Den Ouden, Cohen-Overbeek and Wladimiroff, 1990). In normal pregnancy about 32% of spiral arteries have undergone physiological changes by 16–18 weeks, but almost all the 100–150 arteries show physiological changes by term (Pijnenborg *et al.* (1991). In preeclamptic women physiological changes are confined to the decidual portions of the arteries; the myometrial segments remain intact and do not dilate (Zuspan, 1990; Redman, 1991; Pijnenborg *et al.*, 1991). About one-third to one-half of the spiral arteries in the placental bed escape entirely from the endovascular invasion of trophoblast. In addition, many vessels are occluded by fibrinoid material and exhibit adjacent foam cell invasion (atherosis). The absence or presence of physiological changes in the uteroplacental vessels is the pathophysiological basis for the use of Doppler-flow studies in the early diagnosis of preeclampsia. The increase of the uteroplacental flow velocity waveform resistance indices has been found to correlate with the results of pathological examination of the placental bed and placentas. The best correlation between resistance index and depth of endovascular trophoblast invasion has been found at the placental side of the uterus (Khong and Pearce, 1987). It is important to note that these pathological vascular changes have been demonstrated to exist in a significant proportion of normotensive pregnancies complicated by fetal growth retardation (Sheppard and Bonnar, 1976).

## 7.11.2 DOPPLER VELOCIMETRY OF THE UTEROPLACENTAL CIRCULATION

There are inherent difficulties in insonating the uteroplacental circulation (Bewley and Bower, 1992). First of all, the uteroplacental vascular bed is a complicated branching structure, and investigators have not reached unanimous agreement about which part to study and whether one part reflects the whole network. Thus some investigators have studied the uterine artery near its origin (Schulman *et al.*, 1986), some the subplacental vasculature (Trudinger, Giles and Cook, 1985) and some have tried to devise overall measures (Bewley and Bower, 1992). Also, the physiological variability and changes in response to stresses and disease have been less extensively documented in the uteroplacental circulation than in the fetoplacental circulation. Uteroplacental flow velocity waveforms (FVW) are thought not to be influenced from day to day, nor by time, meals, smoking or external vibratory acoustic stimulation, but to be affected by maternal heart rate and exercise. Nevertheless, the instability of the circulation makes accurate and reproducible measurements in screening for and diagnosis of pregnancy-induced hypertensive disorders and fetal growth retardation difficult. This variability has led to much wider coefficient of variation measurements for uteroplacental FVWs than for fetal FVWs, ranging from 6–15% (Bewley and Bower, 1992).

The uteroplacental circulation may be identified with a duplex sector scanner and a vaginal probe. The uterine arteries may also be examined abdominally, with identification of the distinctive uterine artery waveform. Alternatively, the arcuate arteries may be examined in a placental or non-placental site. However, abdominal observations of the radial or arcuate arteries represent one vessel in a very complex circulation, so that reproducible identification of an arcuate artery is difficult (Low, 1991). Reference values of uteroplacental FVWs have been reported by a number of investigators, and were recently reviewed by Low (1991). Indices of uteroplacental blood flow velocity decrease in early pregnancy until 20–26 weeks gestation and then remain stable to term. The high end-diastolic blood flow velocity and low ratios during the last half of pregnancy reflect the low peripheral resistance of the uteroplacental vascular bed.

The sampling site must be known. Indices of blood flow velocity tend to be lower in the arcuate artery than in the uterine artery. Indices are lower in placental than in non-placental sites. These differences are particularly striking in the second trimester, when differences of up to 50% may occur between observations from non-placental and placental sites in the arcuate and uterine arteries (Low, 1991).

When continuous wave (CW) equipment is used, the probe is placed 2–3 cm medial to the anterior superior iliac spine. Subsequently, the transducer is pointed toward the paracervical area through the lower abdomen early in pregnancy and toward the lateral part of the uterus later in pregnancy. FVW patterns are used to identify the proper signal. There is an ongoing discussion concerning the use of continuous wave (CW) versus pulsed Doppler ultrasound for the study of the uteroplacental circulation. Although pulsed waved ultrasonography with a range gate may demonstrate the exact depth of insonation, it does not necessarily visualize the vessels accurately, and so presently there is no convincing reason to advocate its use for the study of the uteroplacental circulation. In the third trimester, narrow branching vessels can be identified with real-time ultrasound in the lateral uterine wall, which, in most instances, represent the arcuate arteries. The sample gate is then placed over such a pulsating vessel and FVWs are obtained. However, in the second trimester, the arcuate arteries are difficult to visualize without color Doppler flow equipment. In this setting, pulsed Doppler has no clear advantage as compared to CW equipment. CW has the advantages of cost, maneuverability of the probe and smaller machine size. In the study of the uteroplacental circulation CW and pulsed wave ultrasonography have shown consistent results (Meahalek *et al.*, 1988). In screening for uteroplacental insufficiency, CW ultrasonography has to be preferred (Bewley and Bower, 1992). In using CW for the studying the uteroplacental vascular bed, it is impossible to determine which vessel produces the signal. Therefore, the signals are best described as coming from a uteroplacental vessel.

FVWs of the uterine arteries can also be obtained by transvaginal sonography. The vaginal probe is inserted in the lateral fornix, and a segment of the main branch of the ascending uterine artery is located. This can usually be achieved by identifying the internal cervical os and then directing the beam laterally to the parametrial area.

With the use of color flow Doppler ultrasound, branches of vessels can be followed all over the uterus and under the placenta. It has the potential eventually to measure velocity, volume and pressure gradients. Color flow has improved accuracy when compared with pulsed wave ultrasound (Arduini *et al.*, 1990).

Several sources of error are inherent in the methodology used to quantify mean velocity and volume flow. Obstetric Doppler velocimetry studies have favored the simpler qualitative analysis of waveforms changes using indices. The indices most commonly used are:

Systolic/diastolic (SD) ratio: S/D;
Resistance index (RI): (S–D)/S;
Pulsatility index (PI): (S–D)/mean;
where S = peak systolic flow velocity; D= maximum end diastolic flow.

The indices are simple to calculate, especially the S/D ratio and the RI. All three indices are very highly correlated. The RI and the S/D ratio are related mathematically as follows: $S/D = 1/(1 – RI)$. The PI, unlike the S/D ratio and the RI, involves the whole waveform and not just the maximum and minimum points. A value for the PI can be derived in the absence of end-diastolic frequencies. Because the resistance index (RI) is normally distributed in normal pregnancy, in contrast to the S/D ratio, it is preferable to use the RI for the study of the uteroplacental circulation. The pulsatility index (PI) has not generally been used in the study of the uteroplacental circulation because there are huge variations and errors in its measurement (Ruissen, van Vugt and de Haan, 1988). None of the major studies in the literature have used PI so far and there is no pressing reason why they should (Bewley and Bower, 1992).

There is no standard method of reporting uteroplacental FVWs. Pearce and McParland (1991) have suggested that both sides of the uterus should be examined and the FVWs reported as follows:

1. **Uniform low resistance**: FVWs from both sides of the uterus have a RI less than 0.58;
2. **Uniform high resistance**: FVWs from both sides of the uterus have a RI more than 0.58;
3. **Mixed resistance pattern**: one waveform (almost invariably that from the placental side) is of low resistance (RI < 0.58) while the waveform from the other side is of high resistance.

There is more information in the waveform shape than just a FVW index. In particular, the presence or absence of a notch is very important in this respect (Arsitodou *et al.*, 1990). The early diastolic notch of uteroplacental FVWs has been reported in normal pregnancy until approximately 26 weeks gestation. However, on the placental side of the uterus it has been reported to be rarely found after 20 weeks gestation.

Presently, the studies reported in the literature concerning the clinical value of Doppler ultrasound evaluation of the uteroplacental circulation, have resulted in widely varying results. These differences may be related to wide differences in technique, different definitions of pregnancy-induced hypertensive disorders, fetal growth retardation, fetal distress and adverse perinatal outcome. However, the major reason for the different conclusions concerning the value of Doppler FVWs of the uteroplacental vessels is probably the fact that investigators used different selection processes in dividing populations with a normal or abnormal uteroplacental Doppler flow pattern (Bewley and Bower, 1992). Abnormality was sometimes based on the worst FVW (Campbell *et al.*, 1986; Arduini *et al.*, 1987), an average (Schulman *et al.*, 1986), the four-site averaged resistance index (AVRI; Bewley, Cooper and Campbell, 1991) or even the best FVW (Hanretty, Whittle and Rubin, 1988). Another major influence is the site of insonation, i.e. which vessel in the uteroplacental system is being studied, and placental site. Trophoblastic invasion may be incomplete in the peripheral zones of the placental bed, and unaltered decidual segments of spiral arteries can be found in the margin of the placenta. Doppler flow recordings from vessels in the periphery of the placental bed may consequently show a high RI throughout normal pregnancy (Fairlie, 1991).

## (a) Velocimetry in established hypertensive disease of pregnancy

The clinical use of Doppler ultrasound examination of the uteroplacental circulation as an additional surveillance method for identifying the high risk fetus in established preeclampsia is still controversial. In 1983, Campbell *et al.* studied 31 patients whose pregnancies were complicated by hypertension and/or fetal growth retardation. In the hypertensive group with abnormal FVWs there was a higher incidence of proteinuric hypertension.

Hypertensive patients with abnormal FVWs (RI > 0.58) on average delivered 3 weeks earlier, and the average birthweight was 2.05 kg instead of the 2.94 kg found in hypertensive women with normal FVWs. The incidence of perinatal asphyxia was also much higher in hypertensive patients with an abnormal uteroplacental FVW. Trudinger, Giles and Cook (1985) and Fleischer *et al.* (1986) confirmed the increased uteroplacental FVW resistance indices in cases of pregnancy-induced hypertensive disorders. Fleischer *et al.* (1986) demonstrated similar indices with abdominal pulsed Doppler, abdominal continuous wave and vaginal pulsed Doppler probes, and found that uteroplacental FVW analysis may predict neonatal birthweight in established pregnancy-induced hypertensive disorders.

Uterine artery Doppler velocimetry is useful in the differential diagnosis of hypertensive disorders in pregnancy (Fairlie, 1991). Fleischer *et al.* (1986), using a CW system, demonstrated that an S/D ratio of more than 2.6 or the presence of an early diastolic notch in the uterine artery FVW after 26 weeks gestation correlated significantly with the clinical diagnosis of (superimposed) preeclampsia, but not with chronic hypertension alone.

In contrast, Hanretty, Whittle and Rubin (1988) found no overall difference in uteroplacental waveforms between normotensive and pregnant women with established pregnancy-induced hypertensive disorders. These negative findings are probably caused by the method of FVW collection. FVWs were not collected from a defined site, and the method of FVW collection was designed to find the lowest resistance indices. A recent study by Trudinger and Cook (1990) examined a highly selected population of severe preeclampsia with persistent diastolic blood pressures above 110 mmHg and significant proteinuria (> 1 g/24 h). In this study, abnormalities of uteroplacental artery FVW did not correlate with perinatal outcome. However, when the FVWs were abnormal, the umbilical artery

S/D ratios were found to be abnormal as well. In this study 64% of 37 women with severe preeclampsia had uterine artery S/D ratios within normal limits. In our experience all patients with severe preeclampsia have significantly elevated resistance indices (worst FVW), and a majority have distinct notches. Pregnant women with chronic hypertension without superimposed pregnancy-induced hypertensive disease have consistently normal FVWs. In addition, we found no significant difference between RI indices obtained with CW or pulsed-Doppler equipment.

Ducey *et al.* (1987) proposed a system of classification of hypertensive disorders of pregnancy based on uteroplacental and umbilical FVWs. Hypertensive patients with abnormal waveforms in both the uterine and the umbilical arteries have the worst prognoses. Such patients usually have an early onset of disease and increased severity of symptoms. This is in contrast to those hypertensive patients who have normal uterine and umbilical waveforms; these have an outcome similar to that of the normotensive population. Perinatal outcome is best indicated by the combined use of uteroplacental and umbilical FVWs than by any other clinical means, but umbilical artery velocimetry is a better predictor of perinatal outcome than velocimetry of the uteroplacental circulation. (Ducey *et al.*, 1987; Trudinger and Cook, 1990). Slater *et al.* (1992) classified hypertensive disorders of pregnancy on uteroplacental FVWs. These authors defined preeclampsia as hypertension plus an RI of more than 0.58, and pregnancy-induced hypertensive disease as hypertension plus an RI of less than 0.58. Although this is a completely new approach to classifying hypertensive disorders of pregnancy that has still to be validated in further prospective studies, the concept is good, because it emphasizes the significant clinical difference between near-term non-proteinuric hypertension (pregnancy-induced hypertensive disease) and the real disease preeclampsia (Broughton Pipkin, 1985; de Jong, Dekker and Sibai, 1991).

Kofinas *et al.* (1988, 1989) showed that patients with unilateral placentas have a 2.8-fold greater incidence of preeclampsia than women with central placentas. Among all patients unilateral placental position was more likely to be associated with abnormal uteroplacental FVWs than central placental location. Patients with marked differences in Doppler FVW patterns between the right and left uterine artery have an increased risk of fetal growth retardation, preeclampsia and delivery before 37 weeks gestation (Kofinas *et al.*, 1988, 1989; Schulman *et al.*, 1987). In patients with unilateral placentas the placental uterine artery is a better predictor of poor pregnancy outcome than the non-placental artery or the mean of the two arteries (Kofinas *et al.*, 1992).

Several investigators evaluated the uteroplacental hemodynamic effects of antihypertensive drugs in preeclampsia with Doppler ultrasound. These initial studies appear to yield clinically useful data, but further prospective studies are needed to assess the value of Doppler ultrasound in evaluating uteroplacental hemodynamic effects of antihypertensive drugs (Janbu and Nesheim, 1989; Moretti *et al.*, 1990; Torres *et al.*, 1990; Fairlie, 1991). In summary, the association of pregnancy-induced hypertensive disorders and/or adverse perinatal outcome with abnormal uteroplacental FVWs has not been consistently observed. Presently, the clinical value of velocimetry of the uteroplacental circulation in patients with established hypertensive disorders is confined to the combination of this method and umbilical Doppler velocimetry in predicting adverse perinatal outcome, and perhaps in the near future the assessment of hemodynamic effects of antihypertensive drugs and plasma volume expansion in the treatment of preeclampsia (Karsdorp *et al.*, 1992). In addition, uteroplacental Doppler velocimetry may assist in the differential diagnosis of hypertensive disorders of pregnancy.

## (b) Velocimetry in the early detection of pregnancy-induced hypertensive disorders

In 1986, Campbell *et al.* were the first to report on the use of uteroplacental Doppler velocimetry as a screening test in early pregnancy for hypertension, fetal growth retardation and fetal asphyxia. This first yielded extremely promising results. However, the excellent predictive value found in this study was caused by a complication rate of 25% in the study group. Arduini *et al.* (1987) examined uteroplacental FVWs in 60 pregnancies at risk for hypertension. For pregnancy-induced hypertensive disorders they found a positive predictive value of 70%, a negative predictive value of 80%, a sensitivity of 64% and specificity of 64% and 84%. The predictive values are very high, as this is a high-risk population (prevalence 37%). Steel *et al.* (Steel, Pearce and Chamberlain, 1988, Steel *et al.*, 1990) examined 1198 nulliparous women for early detection of pregnancy-induced hypertensive disorders. A CW ultrasound study was made at 18–20 weeks and repeated at 24 weeks gestation if the result was abnormal. An unspecified number of FVWs on either side of the uterus was obtained and if any had an RI of more than 0.58 the test was considered abnormal. In the pilot study (Steel, Pearce and Chamberlain, 1988) 37% of women were found to have abnormal FVWs at 18–20 weeks, but this had fallen to 11% by 24 weeks gestation. Hypertension was significantly more frequent among women with persistently abnormal FVWs (25%) than in women with normal FVWs, and also correlated with severity of disease and the prevalence of proteinuria (10% *versus* 0.8%). More importantly, the test had a sensitivity of nearly 100% for the early detection of severe preeclampsia associated with fetal growth retardation. Bewley, Cooper and Campbell (1991) studied the resistance indices of the uteroplacental circulation; the four-site averaged resistance index (AVRI) was used in stead of the original cut-off of worst RI > 0.58. Although the risk for an individual woman with a high AVRI to develop a complication was increased by up to 9.8 times, the sensitivity of the test (AVRI > 95th centile) was only 13%. The results of Steel *et al.*(1990) and the scattered occurrence of 'preeclamptic lesions' in the spiral arteries (Pijnenborg *et al.*, 1991) suggest that it is more logical to look for the worst Doppler-flow patterns. Newnham *et al.* (1990) reported a significant association between uteroplacental S/D ratios at 24 weeks gestation and subsequent fetal hypoxia (sensitivity 24%, specificity 93.9%). However, they could not find a relationship between elevated S/D ratios and subsequent development of pregnancy-induced hypertensive disorders. In addition, Jacobson *et al.* (1990) studied the value of uteroplacental Doppler velocimetry in predicting preeclampsia and/or fetal growth retardation. In this study a low fetal abdominal circumference at 20 or 24 weeks gestation or an increasing plasma uric acid level at 24 weeks was as predictive as an elevated resistance index. These authors concluded that although elevated resistance indices identified about 60% of the women in whom preeclampsia and/or fetal growth retardation subsequently developed, the false-positive rates were unacceptably high and the positive predictive values low.

In conclusion, Doppler-flow studies of the uteroplacental circulation are easy, inexpensive and non-invasive. Doppler-flow studies can be done in early pregnancy and are suitable for therapeutic intervention in an attempt to reduce the incidence of preeclampsia and its complications. The results of Doppler ultrasound examination of the uteroplacental circulation as a screening test for any degree of hypertension are somewhat disappointing. In the early diagnosis of severe preeclampsia and/or severe fetal growth retardation Doppler ultrasound has demonstrated a high sensitivity, but this may be sufficient for clinical purposes because most hypertension in pregnancy probably represents an enhanced physiological adaptation to pregnancy (Broughton Pipkin, 1985).

Abdominal and transvaginal color Doppler ultrasonography have recently allowed the assessment of the uteroplacental circulation from 4–18 weeks gestation (Jurkovic *et al.*, 1991). The results from the first major study from King's College Hospital are very promising (Harrington *et al.*, 1991). A total of 2437 women were screened by means of CW equipment, FVWs were obtained from both sides of the uterus at 20 weeks gestation. An abnormal result was considered as a RI of more than 0.58 from either side of the uterus, or the presence of an early diastolic notch. At 20 weeks, 15% of these 2437 women had an abnormal result. At 24 weeks these women were assessed again using of color flow mapping and pulsed Doppler studies and, if these were abnormal, again at 26 weeks gestation. At 24 weeks, 5.4% of women had abnormal findings, and this figure fell to 4.1% at 26 weeks gestation. The high sensitivity (76%) at 20 weeks was retained at 24 and 26 weeks, while the specificity (from 86% to 97%) and positive predictive value (13% to 44%) improved progressively with gestational age and the introduction of color flow mapping. In this study the presence of a dichrotic notch in the FVW was a better predictor than just an abnormal RI.

Transvaginal color Doppler imaging makes it possible to assess the uteroplacental circulation as early as 5 weeks gestation (Jaffe and Warsof, 1991). Transvaginal color flow mapping of the uteroplacental circulation, starting at a very early gestational age, and the recognition of persistence of a dichrotic notch throughout the period from 4–18 weeks, holds great promise for the near future in the prediction of pregnancy-induced hypertensive disorders.

## 7.12 CONCLUSION

An individualized and judicious combination of fetal assessment methods and methods for assessment of the maternal condition can lead the obstetrician in providing optimum management in preeclampsia. The frequency in which these fetal and maternal surveillance

methods should be used depends on the severity of the disease process, gestational age and the results of earlier evaluations. If an increasing rate of deterioration is noted, as determined by laboratory findings, symptoms and clinical signs, the decision to continue the pregnancy is determined day by day. Important clinical signs are blood pressure, urinary output and fluid retention as evidenced by daily weight increase. Laboratory evaluation of the hypertensive pregnant woman complements but does not replace astute, thorough clinical assessment. Individualization based on physician judgment is imperative in every patient. The interval between tests needs to be shortened if there is a change in maternal condition that could result in a reduction in placental perfusion. These changes can either be caused by progression of the preeclamptic disease process, or be iatrogenic, for example the initiation of antihypertensive treatment. The different methods for maternal and fetal surveillance should not be regarded as mutually exclusive investigations for assessing maternal and/or fetal compromise in hypertensive pregnant women; rather they should be integrated in a diagnostic protocol. Optimum obstetric management in pregnancy-induced hypertensive disorders demands meticulous maternal assessment and use of tests of feto-placental function and fetal maturity, and depends on balancing the risks to the mother and fetus from expectant management against the risks of prematurity from immediate delivery.

## REFERENCES

Ackerman, W. E., Porembka, D. T., Juneja, M. M. *et al.* (1990) Use of a pulmonary artery catheter in the management of the severe preeclamptic patient. *Anesthesiol. Rev.*, **17**, 37–40.

Arduini, D., Rizzo, G., Romanini, C. *et al.* (1987) Uteroplacental blood flow velocity waveforms as predictors of pregnancy-induced hypertension. *Eur. J. Obstet. Gynecol. Reprod. Biol.*, **26**, 335–341.

Arduini, D., Rizzo, G., Boccolini, M. R. *et al.* (1990) Functional assessment of uteroplacental and fetal circulations by means of color Doppler ultrasonography. *J. Ultrasound Med.*, **9**, 249–253.

Aristodou, A., van den Hof, M. C., Campbell, S. *et al.* (1990) Uterine artery Doppler in the investigation of pregnancies with raised maternal serum alpha-fetoprotein. *Br. J. Obstet. Gynaecol.*, **97**, 431–435.

Assali, N. S. and Prystowsky, H. (1950) Studies on autonomic blockade. I. Comparison between the effects of tetraethylammonium chloride (TEAC) and high selective spinal anesthesia on blood pressure of normal and toxemic pregnancy. *J. Clin. Invest.*, **29**, 1354–1366.

Assali, N. S. (1977) Blood volume in pre-eclampsia: fantasy and reality. *Am. J. Obstet. Gynecol.*, **129**, 353–359.

Aznar, J., Gilabert, J., Estelles, A. *et al.* (1986) Fibrinolytic activity and protein C in preeclampsia. *Thromb. Haemostasis*, **55**, 314–317.

Ballegeer, V., Mombarts, P., De Clerck, P. J. *et al.* (1987) Fibrinolytic response to venous occlusion and fibrin fragment D-Dimer levels in normal and complicated pregnancy. *Thromb. Haemostasis*, **58**, 1030–1032.

Ballegeer, V., Spitz, B., Kieckens, L. *et al.* (1989) Predictive value of increased plasma levels of fibronectin in gestational hypertension. *Am. J. Obstet. Gynecol.*, **161**, 432–436.

Ballegeer, V. C., Spitz, B., De Baene, L. A. *et al.*, (1992) Platelet activation and vascular damage in gestational hypertension. *Am. J. Obstet. Gynecol.*, **166**, 629–633.

Banner, T., Banner, M. J. (1988) Cardiac output measurement technology, in *Critical Care*, 1st edn, (eds J. M. Civetta, R. W. Taylor and R. R. Kirby), J. B. Lippincott, Philadelphia, PA, p. 361–376.

Barton, J. R., Riely, C. A. and Sibai, B. M. (1992) Baking powder pica mimicking preeclampsia. *Am. J. Obstet. Gynecol.*, **167**, 98–99.

Barton, J. R. and Sibai, B. M. (1991) Cerebral pathology in eclampsia. *Clin. Perinatol.*, **18**, 891–910.

Barton, J. R. and Sibai, B. M. (1992) Acute life-threatening emergencies in preeclampsia–eclampsia. *Clin. Obstet. Gynecol.*, **35**, 402–413.

Bernstein, D. (1986a) A new stroke volume equation for thoracic electrical bioimpedance. Theory and rationale. *Crit. Care Med.*, **14**, 904–909.

Bernstein, D. (1986b) Continuous noninvasive real-time monitoring of stroke volume and cardiac output by thoracic electrical bioimpedance. *Crit. Care Med.*, **14**, 898–901.

Bewley, S. and Bower, S. (1992) The application of continuous wave screening to the uteroplacental circulation, in *Doppler Ultrasound in Perinatal Medicine*, 1st edn, (ed. J. M. Pearce), Oxford University Press, Oxford, p. 112–141.

Bewley, S., Cooper, D. and Campbell, S. (1991) Doppler investigation of uteroplacental blood flow resistance in the second trimester: a screening study for pre-eclampsia and intrauterine growth retardation. *Br. J. Obstet. Gynaecol.*, **88**, 871–879.

Bischof, P. and Klopper, A. (1983) Placental proteins, in *Progress in Obstetrics and Gynaecology 3*, (ed. J. W. W. Studd), Churchill Livingstone, Edinburgh, p. 57–72.

Bletka, M., Hallavaty, V., Trenkova, M. *et al.* (1970) Volume of whole blood and absolute amount of serum proteins in the early stages of late toxemia of pregnancy. *Am. J. Obstet. Gynecol.*, **106**, 10–14.

Boneu, B., Fournie, A., Sie, P. *et al.* (1980) Platelet production time, uricemia, and some hemostasis tests in pre-eclampsia. *Eur. J. Obstet. Gynecol. Reprod. Biol.*, **11**, 85–94.

Bonnar, J., McNicol, G. P. and Douglas, A. S. (1971) Coagulation and fibrinolytic systems in pre-eclampsia and eclampsia. *Br. Med. J.*, **ii**, 12–16.

Bonsnes, R. W. (1956) Concentrations of electrolytes in the serum in normal pregnancy and in toxemia of pregnancy, in *Toxemia of Pregnancy: Report of the First Ross Obstetric Research Conference*, (ed. S. J. Fomon), Ross Laboratories, Columbus OH, p. 27–29.

Borok, Z., Weitz, J., Owen, J. *et al.* (1984) Fibrinogen proteolysis and platelet a-granule release in preeclampsia/eclampsia. *Blood*, **63**, 525–531.

Broughton Pipkin, F. (1985) Hypertension in pregnancy – physiology or pathology? in *The Physiological Development of the Fetus and Newborn*, Academic Press, London, p. 699–709.

Brown, C. E., Purdy, P. and Cunningham, F. G. (1988) Head computed tomographic scans in women with eclampsia. *Am. J. Obstet. Gynecol.*, **159**, 915–920.

Buyon, J. P., Cronstein, B. N., Morris, M. *et al.* (1986) Serum complement values (C3 and C4) to differentiate between systemic lupus activity and pre-eclampsia. *Am. J. Med.*, **81**, 194–200.

Campbell, D. M. and Templeton, A. A. (1980) Is eclampsia preventable?, in *Pregnancy Hypertension*, (eds J. Bonnar, I. MacGillivray and E. M. Symonds), University Park Press, Baltimore, MD, p. 320–340.

Campbell, S., Diaz-Recasens, J. Griffin, D. R. *et al.* (1983) New Doppler technique for assessing uteroplacental blood flow. *Lancet*, **i**, 675–677.

Campbell, S., Pearce, J. M. F., Hackett, G. *et al.* (1986) Qualitative assessment of uteroplacental blood flow; early screening test for high-risk pregnancies. *Obstet. Gynecol.*, **68**, 649–653.

Chard, T. (1982) Placental lactogen: biology and clinical applications, in *Pregnancy Proteins. Biology, Chemistry and Clinical Application*, (eds J. G. Grudzinskas, B. Teisner and M. Seppala), Academic Press, Sydney, p. 101–118.

Chesley, L. C. (1939) The variability of proteinuria in the hypertensive complications of pregnancy. *J. Clin. Invest.*, **18**, 617–620.

Chesley, L. C. (1972) Plasma and red cell volumes during pregnancy. *Am. J. Obstet. Gynecol.*, **112**, 440–450.

Chesley, L. C. (ed. ) (1978) *Hypertensive Disorders in Pregnancy*, Appleton-Century-Crofts, New York.

Chesley, L. C. (1985) Diagnosis of preeclampsia. *Obstet. Gynecol.*, **65**, 423–425.

Chesley, L. C. and Lindheimer, M. D. (1988) Renal hemodynamics and intravascular volume in normal and hypertensive pregnancy, in *Handbook of Hypertension, vol. 10: Hypertension in Pregnancy*, 1st edn, (ed. P. C. Rubin), Elsevier, Amsterdam, p. 38–65.

Chesley L. C. and Williams, L. O. (1945) Renal glomerular and tubular functions in relation to the hyperuricemia of pre-eclampsia and eclampsia. *Am. J. Obstet. Gynecol.*, **50**, 367–375.

Clark, S. L. (1991) The pulmonary artery catheter: insertion technique and complications, in *Critical Care Obstetrics*, 2nd edn, (eds S. L Clark, D. B. Cotton, G. D. V. Hankins and J. P. Phelan), Blackwell Scientific Publications, Boston, MA, p. 62–71.

Clark, C. A. and Harman, E. M. (1988) Hemodynamic monitoring: pulmonary artery catheters, in *Critical Care*, 1st edn, (eds J. M. Civetta, R. W. Taylor and R. R. Kirby), J. B. Lippincott, Philadelphia, PA, p. 293–302.

Clark, S. L., Greenspoon, J. S., Aldahl, D. *et al.* (1986) Severe preeclampsia with persistent oliguria: management of hemodynamic subsets. *Am. J. Obstet. Gynecol.*, **154**, 490–494.

Combes, B. and Adams, R. H. (1972) Disorders of the liver in pregnancy, in *Pathophysiology of Gestation*, 1st edn, (eds N. S. Assali and C. R. Brinkman III), Academic Press, New York, p. 479–522.

Combs, C. A., Wheeler, B. C. and Kitzmiller, J. L. (1991) Urinary protein/creatinine ratio before and during pregnancy in women with diabetes mellitus. *Am. J. Obstet. Gynecol.*, **165**, 920–923.

Consensus Report. (1990) National High Blood Pressure Education Program Working Group report on high blood pressure in pregnancy. *Am. J. Obstet. Gynecol.*, **163**, 1689–1712.

Covi, G., Corsato, M., Paluani, F. *et al.* (1990) Reduced urinary excretion of calcium in pregnancy-induced hypertension: relationship to renal prostaglandin excretion. *Clin. Exper. Hypertens. Pregn.*, **B9**, 151–167.

Crandall, B. F., Robinson, L. and Grau, P. (1991) Risks associated with an elevated maternal serum a-fetoprotein level. *Am. J. Obstet. Gynecol.*, **165**, 581–586.

Crawford, S., Varner, M. W., Digre, K. B. *et al.* (1987) Cranial magnetic resonance imaging in eclampsia. *Obstet. Gynecol.*, **70**, 474–477.

Crosignani, P. G., Trojsi, L., Attanasio, A. E. M. *et al.* (1974) Value of hCG and hCS measurement in clinical practice. *Obstet. Gynecol.*, **44**, 673–681.

Cunningham, F. G., Lowe, T., Guss, S. *et al.* (1985) Erythrocyte morphology in women with severe preeclampsia: preliminary observations with scanning electron microscopy. *Am. J. Obstet. Gynecol.*, **153**, 358–363.

Curzen, P., Lloyd and U. E., Thomas, D. J. (1980) Some epidemiological aspects of dysmaturity. *Biol. Res. Pregn. Perinat.*, **1**, 72–78.

Davey, D. (1985) Hypertensive disorders of pregnancy, in *Progress in Obstetrics and Gynaecology 5*, (ed. J. W. W. Studd), Churchill Livingstone, Edinburgh, p. 89–107.

Dawes, M. G. and Grudzinskas J. G. (1991) Repeated measurement of maternal weight during pregnancy. Is this a useful practice ? *Br. J. Obstet. Gynaecol.*, **98**, 189–194.

de Boer, K., Lecander, I., ten Cate, J. W. *et al.* (1988) Placental-type plasminogen activator inhibitor in preeclampsia. *Am. J. Obstet. Gynecol.*, **158**, 518–522.

de Boer, K., Buller, H. R., ten Cate, J. W. *et al.*, (1991) Coagulation studies in the syndrome of haemolysis, elevated liver enzymes and low platelets. *Br. J. Obstet. Gynaecol.*, **98**, 42–47.

de Jong, C. L. D., Dekker, G. A. and Sibai, B. M. (1991) The renin–angiotensin system in preeclampsia; a review. *Clin. Perinatol.*, **18**, 683–711.

Dekker, G. A. (1989) Prediction and prevention of pregnancy-induced hypertensive disorders: a clinical and pathophysiologic study. Academic Thesis, Erasmus University Rotterdam.

Dekker, G. A., Makovitz, J. W. and Wallenburg, H. C. S. (1990) Comparison of prediction of pregnancy-induced hypertensive disease by angiotensin II sensitivity and supine pressor test. *Br. J. Obstet. Gynaecol.*, **97**, 817–821.

Dekker, G. A. and Sibai, B. M. (1991) Early detection of preeclampsia. *Am. J. Obstet. Gynecol.*, **165**, 160–172.

Dekker, G. A. and van Geijn, H. P (1992) Hypertensive disease in pregnancy. *Curr. Opinion Obstet. Gynecol.*, **4**, 10–27.

den Ouden, M., Cohen-Overbeek, T. E. and Wladimiroff, J. W. (1990) Uterine and fetal umbilical artery flow velocity waveforms in normal first trimester pregnancies. *Br. J. Obstet. Gynaecol.*, **97**, 716–719.

de Swiet, M. and Talbert, D. (1986) The measurement of cardiac output by electrical impedance plethysmography in pregnancy. Are the assumptions valid? *Br. J. Obstet. Gynaecol.*, **93**, 721–726.

de Vries, J. I. P., Vellenga, E. and Aarnoudse, J. G. (1983) Plasma beta-thromboglobulin in normal pregnancy and pregnancy-induced hypertension. *Eur. J. Obstet. Gynecol. Reprod. Biol.*, **14**, 209–216.

Dieckmann, W. J. (1952) *The Toxemias of Pregnancy*, 2nd edn, C. V. Mosby, St Louis, MO, p. 240–249.

Digre, K. B., Varner, M. W. and Schiffman, J. S. (1990) Neuroophthalmologic effects of intravenous magnesium sulfate. *Am. J. Obstet. Gynecol.*, **163**, 1848–1852.

Donaldson, J. O. (1989) *Neurology of Pregnancy*, 2nd edn, W. B. Saunders, London.

Douglas, J. T., Shah, M., Lowe, G. D. O. *et al.* (1982) Plasma fibrinopeptide A and beta-thromboglobulin in pre-eclampsia and pregnancy hypertension. *Thromb. Haemostasis*, **47**, 54–55.

Ducey, J., Schulman, H., Farmakides, G. *et al.* (1987) A classification of hypertension in pregnancy based on Doppler velocimetry. *Am. J. Obstet. Gynecol.*, **157**, 680–685.

Duenhoelter, J. H., Whalley, P. J. and MacDonald, P. C. (1976) An analysis of the utility of plasma immunoreactive estrogen measurements in determining delivery time of gravidas with a fetus considered at high risk. *Am. J. Obstet. Gynecol.*, **125**, 889–898.

Easterling, T. R. (1992) The maternal hemodynamics of preeclampsia. *Clin. Obstet. Gynecol.*, **35**, 375–386.

Easterling, T. R. and Benedetti, T. J. (1991a) Principles of invasive hemodynamic monitoring in pregnancy, in *Critical Care Obstetrics*, 2nd edn, (eds S. L Clark, D. B. Cotton, G. D. V. Hankins and J. P. Phelan), Blackwell Scientific Publications, Boston, MA, p. 72–85.

Easterling, T. R. and Benedetti, T. J. (1991b) Principles of noninvasive hemodynamic monitoring in pregnancy, in *Critical Care Obstetrics*, 2nd edn, (eds S. L Clark, D. B. Cotton, G. D. V. Hankins and J. P. Phelan), Blackwell Scientific Publications, Boston, MA, p. 86–101.

Easterling, T. R., Watts, D. H., Schmucker, B. C. *et al.* (1987) Measurement of cardiac output during pregnancy: validation of Doppler technique and clinical observations in preeclampsia. *Obstet. Gynecol.*, **69**, 845–850.

Easterling, T., Benedetti, T., Carlson, K. *et al.* (1989) Measurement of cardiac output in pregnancy: impedance vs. thermodilution techniques. *Br. J. Obstet. Gynaecol.*, **96**, 67–69.

Easterling, T. R., Benedetti, T. J., Schmucker, B. C. *et al.* (1990) Maternal hemodynamics in normal and preeclamptic pregnancies: a longitudinal study. *Obstet. Gynecol.*, **76**, 1061–1069.

Eden, T. W. (1922) Eclampsia: a commentary on the reports presented to the British Congress of Obstetrics and Gynaecology. *J. Obstet. Gynaecol. Br. Emp.*, **29**, 386–401.

Eden, R. D., Wahbeh, C. J., Williams, A. Y. *et al.* (1984) Serial nephelometric urine IgG measurement and the management of pregnancy-induced hypertension. *Am. J. Obstet. Gynecol.*, **148**, 1080–1088.

Entman, S. S. and Richardson, D. (1983) Clinical applications of the altered iron kinetics of toxemia of pregnancy. *Am. J. Obstet. Gynecol.*, **146**, 568–574.

Entman, S. S., Moore, R. M., Richardson, L. D. *et al.* (1982a) Elevated serum iron in toxemia of pregnancy. *Am. J. Obstet. Gynecol.*, **143**, 398–404.

Entman, S. S., Richardson, L. D., Killam, A. P. (1982b) Elevated serum ferritin in the altered ferrokinetics of toxemia of pregnancy. *Am. J. Obstet. Gynecol.*, **144**, 418–422.

Entman, S. S., Kambam, J. R., Bradley, C. A. *et al.* (1987) Increased levels of carboxyhemoglobin and serum iron as an indicator of increased red cell turnover in preeclampsia. *Am. J. Obstet. Gynecol.*, **156**, 1169–1173.

Estelles, A., Gilabert, J., Espana, F. *et al.* (1987) Fibrinolysis in pre-eclampsia. *Fibrinolysis,* **1,** 209–214.

Estelles, A., Gilabert, J., Espana, F. *et al.* (1991) Fibrinolytic parameters in normotensive pregnancy with intrauterine fetal growth retardation and in severe preeclampsia. *Am. J. Obstet. Gynecol.,* **165,** 138–142.

Fairlie, F. M. (1991) Doppler flow velocimetry in hypertension in pregnancy. *Clin. Perinatol.,* **18,** 749–778.

Fay, R. A., Hughes, A. O. and Farron, N. T. (1983) Platelets in pregnancy; hyperdestruction in pregnancy. *Obstet. Gynecol.,* **61,** 238–240.

Firkin, B. G. (1984) *The Platelet and its Disorders,* MTP Press, Lancaster.

Fleischer, A., Schulman, H., Farmakides, G. *et al.* (1986) Uterine artery Doppler velocimetry in pregnant women with hypertension. *Am. J. Obstet. Gynecol.,* **154,** 806–813.

Forbes, C. D. and Greer, I. A. (1992) Physiology of haemostasis and the effect of pregnancy, in *Haemostasis and Thrombosis in Obstetrics and Gynaecology,* 1st edn, (eds I. A. Greer, A. G. G. Turpie and C. D. Forbes), Chapman & Hall, London, p. 1–25.

Frenkel, Y., Barkai, G. and Mashiach, S. *et al.* (1991) Hypocalciuria of preeclampsia is independent of parathyroid level. *Obstet. Gynecol.,* **77,** 689–691.

Friedman, E. A. and Neff, R. K. (1977) *Pregnancy Hypertension. A Systematic Evaluation of Clinical Diagnostic Criteria,* PSG Publishing, Littleton, MA.

Galbraith, R. M. (1992) Liver disease: general considerations, in *Principles and Practice of Medical Therapy in Pregnancy,* 2nd edn, (ed. N. Gleicher), Appleton & Lange, Norwalk, CT, p. 957–959.

Gallery, E. D. M., Hunyor, S. N. and Gyory, A. Z. (1979) Plasma volume contraction: A significant factor in both pregnancy-associated hypertension (pre-eclampsia) and chronic hypertension in pregnancy. *Q. J. Med.,* **48,** 593–602.

Gant, N. F., Daley, G. L., Chand, S. *et al.* (1973) A study of angiotensin II pressor response throughout primigravid pregnancy. *J. Clin. Invest.,* **52,** 2682–2689.

Garn, S. M., Ridella, A. S., Petzold, A. S. *et al.* (1981) Maternal hematologic levels and pregnancy outcomes. *Semin. Perinatol.,* **5,** 155–162.

Gibson, B., Hunter, D., Neame, P. B. *et al.* (1982) Thrombocytopenia in preeclampsia and eclampsia. *Semin. Thromb. Hemostasis,* **8,** 234–247.

Gilabert, J., Estelles, A., Ridocci, F. *et al.* (1990) Clinical and haemostatic parameters in the HELLP syndrome: relevance of plasminogen activator inhibitors. *Gynecol. Obstet. Invest.,* **30,** 81–86.

Giles, C. (1982) Intravascular coagulation in gestational hypertension and pre-eclampsia: the value of hematologic screening tests. *Clin. Lab. Haematol.,* **4,** 351–358.

Giles, C. and Inglis, T. C. M. (1981) Thrombocytopenia and macrothrombocytosis in gestational hypertension. *Br. J. Obstet. Gynaecol.,* **88,** 1115–1119.

Gonik, B., Cotton, D., Spillman, T. *et al.* (1985) Peripartum colloid osmotic pressure changes: effects of controlled fluid management. *Am. J. Obstet. Gynecol.,* **151,** 812–815.

Greene, J. W. and Touchstone, J. C. (1963) Urinary estriol as an index of placental function. *Am. J. Obstet. Gynecol.,* **85,** 1–15.

Grudzinskas, J. G. and Chard, T. (1991) Protein and hormone products of the human placenta, in *Scientific Foundations of Obstetrics and Gynaecology,* 4th edn, (eds E. Philipp, M. Setchell and J. Ginsberg), Butterworth Heinemann, Oxford, p. 298–304.

Grudzinskas, J. G. and Sinosich, M. J. (1982) Pregnancy specific β1 glycoprotein in normal and abnormal late pregnancy, in *Pregnancy Proteins. Biology, Chemistry and Clinical Application,* (eds J. G. Grudzinskas, B. Teisner and M. Seppala), Academic Press, Sydney, p. 251–259.

Gupta, P. P. and Srivastava, R. K. (1987) Radial immunodiffusion estimation of maternal serum alpha feto-protein in normal pregnancy and pregnancy-induced hypertension. *Indian J. Physiol. Pharm.,* **19,** 273–284.

Hallum, A. V. (1936) Eye changes in hypertensive toxemia of pregnancy, a study of 300 cases. *J. A. M. A.,* **106,** 1649–1651.

Hankins, G. D. V., Wendel, G. D., Cunningham, F. G. *et al.* (1984) Longitudinal evaluation of hemodynamic changes in eclampsia. *Am. J. Obstet. Gynecol.,* **150,** 506–512.

Hanretty, K. P., Whittle, M. J. and Rubin, P. C. (1988) Doppler uteroplacental waveforms in pregnancy-induced hypertension. A reappraisal. *Lancet,* **i,** 850–855.

Harrington, K. F., Campbell, S., Bewley, S. *et al.* (1991) Doppler velocimetry studies of the uterine artery in the early prediction of pre-eclampsia and intra-uterine growth retardation. *Eur. J. Obstet. Gynecol. Reprod. Biol.,* **42S,** 14–20.

Haukland, H. H., Florholmen, J., Oian, P. *et al.* (1987) The effect of severe pre-eclampsia on the pancreas: changes in the serum cationic trypsinogen and pancreatic amylase. *Br. J. Obstet. Gynaecol.*, **94**, 765–767.

Hays, P. M., Cruikshank, D. P. and Dunn, L. J. (1985) Plasma volume determinations in normal and preeclamptic pregnancies. *Am. J. Obstet. Gynecol.*, **151**, 958–966.

Hazoff, R. G., Kahale, S., Zugaib, M. *et al.* (1987) Correlations between ophthalmoscopy and hypertensive pregnant states: Diagnosis and prognostic values. *Arq. Bras. Oftalmol.*, **50**, 264–267.

Heilmann, L., Siekmann, U., Schmid-Schonbein, H. *et al.* (1981) Hemoconcentration and pre-eclampsia. *Arch. Gynecol.*, **23**, 7–21.

Hellgren, M., Egberg, N. and Eklund, J. (1984) Blood coagulation and fibrinolytic factors and their inhibitors in critically ill patients. *Intens. Care Med.*, **10**, 23–28.

Hill, J. A., Devoe, L. D. and Bryans, C. I. (1986) Frequency of asymptomatic bacteriuria in preeclampsia. *Obstet. Gynecol.*, **67**, 529–531.

Hirsch, J. (1987) Laboratory diagnosis of thrombosis, in *Hemostasis and Thrombosis. Basic Principles and Clinical Practice*, 2nd edn, (eds R. W. Colman, J. Hirsch, V. J. Marder and E. W. Salzman), J. B. Lippincott, Philadelphia, PA, p. 1165–1183.

Honger, PE (1968) Albumin metabolism in preeclampsia. *Scand. J. Clin. Lab. Invest.*, **22**, 177–184.

Howell, R. J. S., Perry, L. A., Choglay, N. S. *et al.* (1985) Placental protein 12 (PP12): a new test for the prediction of the small-for-gestational-age infant. *Br. J. Obstet. Gynaecol.*, **92**, 1141–1144.

Howie, P. W., Prentice, C. R. M. and McNicol, G. P. (1971) Coagulation, fibrinolysis and platelet function in pre-eclampsia, essential hypertension and placental insufficiency. *J. Obstet. Gynaecol. Br. Commonw.*, **78**, 992–1003.

Huikeshoven, F. J. M. and Zuijderhoudt, F. M. J. (1990) Hypocalciuria in hypertensive disorders in pregnancy and how to measure it. *Eur. J. Obstet. Gynecol. Reprod. Biol.*, **36**, 81–85.

Huisman, A. and Aarnoudse, J. G. (1986) Increased second trimester hemoglobin concentration in pregnancies later complicated by hypertension and growth retardation. *Acta Obstet. Gynecol. Scand.*, **65**, 605–608.

Hutchesson, A. C. J., MacIntosh, M. C., Duncan, S. L. B. *et al.* (1990) Hypocalciuria and hypertension in pregnancy: a prospective study. *Clin. Exper. Hypertens. Pregn.*, **B9**, 115–134.

Iino, K., Sjoberg, J. and Seppala, M. (1986) Elevated circulating levels of a decidual protein, placental protein 12, in preeclampsia. *Obstet. Gynecol.*, **68**, 58–60.

Inglis, T. C. M., Stuart, J., George, A. J. *et al.* (1982) Haemostatic and rheological changes in normal pregnancy and pre-eclampsia. *Br. J. Obstet. Haemat.*, **56**, 461–465.

Irgens-Moller, L., Hemmingsen, L. and Holm, J. (1986) Diagnostic value of microalbuminuria in pre-eclampsia. *Clin. Chim. Acta*, **157**, 295–298.

Jackson, D. P. (1987) Management of thrombocytopenia, in *Hemostasis and Thrombosis. Basic Principles and Clinical Practice*, 2nd edn, (eds R. W. Colman, J. Hirsch, V. J. Marder and E. W. Salzman), J. B. Lippincott, Philadelphia, PA, p. 530–536.

Jacobson, S. L., Imhof, R., Manning, N. *et al.* (1990) The value of Doppler assessment of the uteroplacental circulation in predicting preeclampsia or intrauterine growth retardation. *Am. J. Obstet. Gynecol.*, **162**, 110–114.

Jaffe, R. and Warsof, S. L. (1991) Transvaginal color Doppler imaging in the assessment of uteroplacental blood flow in the normal first-trimester pregnancy. *Am. J. Obstet. Gynecol.*, **164**, 781–785.

Janbu, T. and Nesheim, B. I. (1989) The effects of dihydralazine on blood velocities in branches of the uterine artery in pregnancy induced hypertension. *Acta Obstet. Gynecol. Scand.*, **68**, 395–400.

Jones, D. D., Bahijri, S., Roberts, E. L. *et al.* (1982) Activity of serum cytidine deaminase during pregnancy. *Br. J. Obstet. Gynaecol.*, **89**, 314–317.

Jorgensen, M., Philips, M., Thorsen, S. *et al.* (1987) Plasminogen activator inhibitor-1 is the primary inhibitor of tissue-type plasminogen activator in pregnancy plasma. *Thromb. Haemostasis*, **58**, 872–878.

Jost, H. (1948) Electroencephalographic records in relation to blood pressure changes in eclampsia. *Am. J. Med. Sci.*, **216**, 57–63.

Jurkovic, D., Jauniaux, E., Kurjak, A. *et al.* (1991) Transvaginal color Doppler assessment of the uteroplacental circulation in early pregnancy. *Obstet. Gynecol.*, **77**, 365–369.

Kalur, J. S., Martin, J. N., Kirchner, K. A. *et al.* (1991) Postpartum preeclampsia-induced shock and death: a report of three cases. *Am. J. Obstet. Gynecol.*, **165**, 1362–1368.

Karsdorp, V. H. M., van Vugt, J. M. G., Dekker, G. A. *et al.* (1992) Reappearance of end-diastolic velocities in umbilical artery following maternal volume expansion: a preliminary study. *Obstet. Gynecol.*

Keller, P. J. (1976) Human chorionic gonadotrophin. *Contr. Gynecol. Obstet.*, **2**, 92–113.

Khong, Y. T. and Pearce, J. M. F. (1987) Development and investigation of the placenta and its blood supply, in *The Human Placenta*, (ed J. P. Lavery), Aspen, Rockville, MD, p. 25–46.

Kincaid-Smith, P. (1985) Pregnancy-related renal disease, in *The Kidney: Physiology and Pathophysiology*, 1st edn, (eds D. W. Seldin and G. Giebish), Raven Press, New York, p. 2043–2058.

Klopper, A. (1982) Biological and clinical aspects of PAPP-A, in *Pregnancy Proteins. Biology, Chemistry and Clinical Application*, (eds J. G. Grudzinskas, B. Teisner and M. Seppala), Academic Press, Sydney, p. 333–344.

Kofinas, A. D., Penry, M., Greiss, F. C. *et al.* (1988) The effect of placental localisation on uterine artery flow velocity waveforms. *Am. J. Obstet. Gynecol.*, **159**, 1504–1508.

Kofinas, A. D., Penry, M., Swain, M. *et al.* (1989) Effect of placental laterality on uterine artery resistance and development of preeclampsia and intrauterine growth retardation. *Am. J. Obstet. Gynecol.*, **161**, 1536–1539.

Kofinas, A. D., Penry, M., Simon, N. V. *et al.* (1992) Interrelationship and clinical significance of increased resistance in the uterine arteries in patients with hypertension or preeclampsia or both. *Am. J. Obstet. Gynecol.*, **166**, 601–606.

Koller, O. (1982) The clinical significance of hemodilution during pregnancy. *Obstet. Gynecol. Surv.*, **37**, 649–655.

Kolstad, P. (1961) The practical value of electroencephalography in pre-eclampsia. *Acta Obstet. Gynecol. Scand.*, **40**, 127–138.

Kruithof, E. K. O., Tran-Thang, C., Gudinchet, A. *et al.* (1987) Fibrinolysis in pregnancy: a study of plasminogen activator inhibitors. *Blood*, **69**, 460–466.

Kubicek, W. G., Karegis, J. N., Patterson, R. P. *et al.* (1966) Development and evaluation of an impedance cardiac output system. *Aerospace Med.*, **37**, 1208–1216.

Kunzig, H. J., Geiger, W. (1976) Estrogens. *Contr. Gynecol. Obstet.*, **2**, 2–74.

Latham, P. S. (1992) Liver diseases, in *Principles and Practice of Medical Therapy in Pregnancy*, 2nd edn, (ed. N. Gleicher), Appleton & Lange, Norwalk, CT, p. 960–969.

Leduc, L., Lederer, E., Lee, W. *et al.* (1991) Urinary sediment changes in severe preeclampsia. *Obstet. Gynecol.*, **77**, 186–189.

Lee, W., Gonik, B. and Cotton, D. B. (1987) Urinary diagnostic indices in preeclampsia-associated oliguria: correlation with invasive hemodynamic monitoring. *Am. J. Obstet. Gynecol.*, **156**, 100–103.

Lee, W. and Pivarnik, P. (1992) Hemodynamic Studies During Pregnancy. *J. Maternal–Fetal Med.*, **1**, 75–77.

Lee, W., Rokey, R. and Cotton, D. B. (1988) Noninvasive maternal stroke volume and cardiac output determinations by pulsed Doppler echocardiography. *Am. J. Obstet. Gynecol.*, **158**, 505–510.

Lee, J. N., Salem, H. T., Huang, S. C. *et al.* (1981) Placental protein 5 in severe pre-eclampsia and eclampsia. *Int. J. Gynecol. Obstet.*, **19**, 65–67.

Letchworth, A. T. (1976) Human placental lactogen. *Contr. Gynecol. Obstet.*, **2**, 114–142.

Letsky, E. A. (1989) Coagulation defects, in *Medical Disorders in Obstetric Practice*, 2nd edn, (ed. M. de Swiet), Blackwell Scientific, Oxford, p. 104–165.

Lever, J. C. W. (1843) Cases of puerperal convulsions, with remarks. *Guy's Hosp. Rep.* (2nd series), **1**, 495–517.

Lockwood, C. J. and Peters, J. H. (1990) Increased plasma levels of ED1+ cellular fibronectin precede the clinical signs of preeclampsia. *Am. J. Obstet. Gynecol.*, **162**, 358–362.

Lopez-Espinoza, I., Dhar, H., Humphreys, S. *et al.* (1986) Urinary albumin excretion in pregnancy. *Br. J. Obstet. Gynaecol.*, **93**, 176–181.

Low, J. A. (1991) The current status of maternal and fetal blood flow velocimetry. *Am. J. Obstet. Gynecol.*, **164**, 1049–1063.

Lowe, G. D. O. (1992) Blood rheology in pregnancy – physiology and pathology, in *Haemostasis and Thrombosis in Obstetrics and Gynaecology*, 1st edn, (eds I. A. Greer, A. G. G. Turpie and C. D. Forbes), Chapman & Hall, London, p. 27–44.

Ludlam, C. A. (1979) Evidence for the platelet specificity of β-thromboglobulin and studies on its plasma concentration in healthy individuals. *Br. J. Haematol.*, **41**, 271–278.

Mabie, M. C. and Sibai, B. M. (1990) Transient diabetes insipidus in a patient with preeclampsia and HELLP syndrome, in *Clinical Decisions in Obstetrics and Gynecology*, (ed. R. C Cefalo), Aspen, Rockville, MD, p. 136–138.

MacGillivray, I. and Campbell, D. M. (1980) The relevance of hypertension and oedema in pregnancy. *Clin. Exper. Hypertens. Pregn.*, **2**, 897–914.

MacGillivray, I. (1983) *Pre-eclampsia. The Hypertensive Disease of Pregnancy*, W. B. Saunders, London.

Maki, M. (1983) Coagulation, fibrinolysis, platelet and kinin forming systems during toxemia of pregnancy. *Biol. Res. Pregn. Perinat.*, **4**, 152–154.

Martin, J. N. and Cowan, B. D. (1990) Biochemical assessment and prediction of gestational well-being. *Obstet. Gynecol. Clin. North Am.*, **17**, 81–93.

Martin, J. N. and Stedman, C. M. (1991) Imitators of Preeclampsia and HELLP syndrome. *Obstet. Gynecol. Clin. North Am.*, **18**, 181–198.

Martin, J. N., Blake, P. G., Lowry, S. L. *et al.* (1990) Pregnancy complicated by preeclampsia-eclampsia with the syndrome of hemolysis, elevated liver enzymes, and low platelet count: how rapid is postpartum recovery? *Obstet. Gynecol.*, **76**, 737–741.

Martin, J. N., Blake, P. G., Perry, K. G. *et al.* (1991) The natural history of HELLP syndrome: Patterns of disease progression and regression. *Am. J. Obstet. Gynecol.*, **164**, 1500–1513.

Masaki, D. I., Greenspoon, J. S. and Ouzounian, J. G. (1989) Measurement of cardiac output in pregnancy by thoracic electrical bioimpedance and thermodilution. A preliminary report. *Am. J. Obstet. Gynecol.*, **161**, 680–684.

Mau, G. (1977) Hemoglobin changes during pregnancy and growth disturbances in the neonate. *J. Perinat. Med.*, **5**, 172–177.

Mehalek, K. E., Berkowitz, G. S., Chitkara, U. *et al.* (1988) Comparison of continuous-wave and pulsed Doppler S/D ratios of umbilical and uterine arteries. *Obstet. Gynecol.*, **72**, 603–606.

Meng Lu, Z., Goldenberg, R. L., Cliver, S. P. *et al.* (1991) The relationship between maternal hematocrit and pregnancy outcome. *Obstet. Gynecol.*, **77**, 190–194.

Milunsky, A., Jick, S. S., Bruell, C. L. *et al.* (1989) Predictive values, relative risks, and overall benefits of high and low maternal serum α-fetoprotein screening in singleton pregnancies: new epidemiologic data. *Am. J. Obstet. Gynecol.*, **161**, 291–297.

Moise, K. J. and Cotton, D. B. (1986) The use of colloid osmotic pressure in pregnancy. *Clin. Perinatol.*, **13**, 827–842.

Moise, K. J. and Cotton, D. B. (1991) Colloid osmotic pressure and pregnancy, in *Critical Care Obstetrics*, 2nd edn, (eds S. L Clark, D. B. Cotton, G. D. V. Hankins and J. P. Phelan), Blackwell Scientific Publications, Boston, MA, p. 35–61.

Moller, B. and Lindmark, G. (1986) Eclampsia in Sweden, 1976–1980. *Acta Obstet. Gynecol. Scand.*, **65**, 307–314.

Moretti, M. M., Fairlie, F. M., Akl, S. *et al.* (1990) The effect of nifedipine therapy on fetal and placental Doppler waveforms in preeclampsia remote from term. *Am. J. Obstet. Gynecol.*, **163**, 1844–1848.

Murphy, J. E., Preuss, H. G. and Henry, J. B. (1984) Evaluation of renal function and water, electrolyte, and acid-base balance, in *Clinical Diagnosis and Management by Laboratory Methods*, 17th edn, (ed. J. B. Henry), W. B. Saunders, London, p. 118–132.

Murphy, J. F., Newcombe, R. G., O'Riordan, J. O. *et al.* (1986) Relation of haemoglobin levels in first and second trimesters to outcome of pregnancy. *Lancet*, **i**, 992–994.

Naeye, R. L. and Friedman, E. A. (1979) Causes of perinatal death associated with gestational hypertension and proteinuria. *Am. J. Obstet. Gynecol.*, **133**, 8–10.

Nakamura, T., Ito, M., Yoshimura, T. *et al.* (1992) Usefulness of the urinary microalbumin/creatinine ratio in predicting pregnancy-induced hypertension. *Int. J. Gynecol. Obstet.*, **37**, 99–103.

Newman, R. L. (1957) Serum electrolytes in pregnancy, parturition, and puerperium. *Obstet. Gynecol.*, **10**, 51–55.

Newnham, J. P., Patterson, L. L., James, I. R. *et al.* (1990) An evaluation of the efficacy of Doppler flow velocity waveform analysis as a screening test in pregnancy. *Am. J. Obstet. Gynecol.*, **162**, 403–410.

Nordenvall, M. and Sandstedt, B. (1990) Placental lesions and maternal hemoglobin levels. A comparative investigation. *Acta Obstet. Gynecol. Scand.*, **69**, 127–133.

Obiekwe, B. C., Sturdee, D., Cockrill, B. L *et al.* (1984) Human placental lactogen in pre-eclampsia. *Br. J. Obstet. Gynaecol.*, **91**, 1077–1080.

Oian, P., Maltau, J. M., Noddeland, H. *et al.* (1985) Oedema-preventing mechanisms in subcutaneous tissue of normal pregnant women. *Br. J. Obstet. Gynaecol.*, **92**, 113–119.

Oian, P., Maltau, J. M., Noddeland, H. and Fadnes, H. O. (1986) Transcapillary fluid balance in pre-eclampsia. *Br. J. Obstet. Gynaecol.*, **93**, 235–239.

Pearce, J. M. and MacParland, P. (1991) Uteroplacental circulation. *Contemp. Rev. Obstet. Gynaecol.*, **3**, 6–12.

Penaz, J. (1973) Photo-electric measurement of blood pressure, volume and flow in the finger. *Digest 10th. Int. Conf. Med. Biol. Eng. (Dresden)*, 104.

Perry, K. G. and Martin, J. N. (1992) Abnormal hemostasis and coagulopathy in preeclampsia and eclampsia. *Clin. Obstet. Gynecol.*, **35**, 338–350.

Philips, O. P., Simpson, J. L., Morgan, C. D. *et al.* (1992) Unexplained elevated maternal serum α-fetoprotein is not predictive of adverse perinatal outcome in an indigent urban population. *Am. J. Obstet. Gynecol.*, **166**, 978–982.

Pickering, T. G. and Blank, S. G. (1990) Blood pressure measurement and ambulatory blood pressure monitoring; evaluation of available equipment, in *Hypertension: Pathophysiology, Diagnosis, and Management*, 1st edn, (eds J. H. Laragh and B. M. Brenner), Raven Press, New York, p. 1429–1441.

Pijnenborg, R., Anthony, J., Davey, D. A. *et al.* (1991) Placental bed spiral arteries in the hypertensive disorders of pregnancy. *Br. J. Obstet. Gynaecol.*, **98**, 648–655.

Pollak, V. E. and Nettles, J. B. (1960) The kidney in toxemia of pregnancy: a clinical and pathologic study based on renal biopsies. *Medicine*, **39**, 469–526.

Porapakkham, S. (1979) An epidemiologic study of eclampsia. *Obstet. Gynecol.*, **54**, 26–30.

Pritchard, J. A., Cunningham, F. G. and Mason, R. A. (1976) Coagulation changes in eclampsia: their frequencies and pathogenesis. *Am. J. Obstet. Gynecol.*, **124**, 855–864.

Ramanathan, J., Sibai, B. M., Vu, T. *et al.* (1989) Correlation between bleeding times and platelet counts in women with preeclampsia undergoing cesarean section. Anesthesiology, **71**, 188–191.

Ramsay, M. (1979) Noninvasive automatic determination of mean arterial pressure. *Med. Biol. Eng. Comp.*, **17**, 11–18.

Redman, C. W. G. (1989a) Hypertension in pregnancy, in *Medical Disorders in Obstetric Practice*, 2nd edn, (ed. M. de Swiet), Blackwell Scientific, Oxford, p. 249–305.

Redman, C. W. G. (1989b) Hypertension in pregnancy, in *Obstetrics*, 1st edn, (eds A. Turnbull and G. Chamberlain), Churchill Livingstone, Edinburgh, p. 515–541.

Redman, C. W. G. (1991) Current topic; pre-eclampsia and the placenta. *Placenta*, **12**, 301–308.

Redman, C. W. G., Beilin, L. J. and Bonnar, J. (1976) Renal function in pre-eclampsia. *J. Clin. Pathol.*, **10**, S91–S94.

Redman, C. W. G., Bonnar, J. and Beilin, L. (1978) Early platelet consumption in pre-eclampsia. *Br. Med. J.*, **i**, 467–469.

Redman, C. W. G., Beilin, L. J., Bonnar, J. *et al.* (1976) Plasma urate measurements in predicting fetal death in hypertensive pregnancy. *Lancet*, **i**, 1370–1373.

Redman, C. W. G., Williams, G. F., Jones, D. D. *et al.* (1977) Plasma urate and serum deoxycytidylate deaminase measurements for the early diagnosis of pre-eclampsia. *Br. J. Obstet. Gynaecol.*, **84**, 904–908.

Riely, C. A., Latham, P. S., Romero, R. *et al.* (1987) Acute fatty liver of pregnancy: a reassessment based on observations in 9 patients. *Ann. Intern. Med.*, **106**, 703–706.

Robson, S. C., Dunlop, W., Moore, M. *et al.* (1987) Combined Doppler and echocardiographic measurement of cardiac output: theory and application in pregnancy. *Br. J. Obstet. Gynaecol.*, **94**, 1014–1027.

Rodriguez, M. H., Masaki, D. I., Mestman, J. *et al.* (1988) Calcium/creatinine ratio and microalbuminuria in the prediction of preeclampsia. *Am. J. Obstet. Gynecol.*, **159**, 1452–145.

Roelofsen, J. M. T., Berkel, G. M., Uttendorfsky, O. T. *et al.* (1988) Urinary excretion rates of calcium and magnesium in normal and complicated pregnancies. *Eur. J. Obstet. Gynecol. Reprod. Biol.*, **27**, 227–236.

Ruissen, C. J., van Vugt, J. M. G. and de Haan, J. (1988) Variability of PI calculations. *Eur. J. Obstet. Gynecol. Reprod. Biol.*, **27**, 213–220.

Sagen, N., Koller, O. and Haram, K. (1982) Haemoconcentration in severe pre-eclampsia. *Br. J. Obstet. Gynaecol.*, **89**, 802–805.

Sagen, N., Nilsen, S. T., Kim, H. C. *et al.* (1984) The predictive value of total estriol, HPL and Hb on perinatal outcome in severe pre-eclampsia. *Acta Obstet. Gynecol. Scand.*, **63**, 603–608.

Said, M. E., Campbell, D. M., Azzam, M. E. *et al.* (1984) Beta-human chorionic gonadotrophin levels before and after the development of pre-eclampsia. *Br. J. Obstet. Gynaecol.*, **91**, 772–775.

Salem, H. T., Seppala, M. and Chard, T. (1981) The effect of thrombin on placental protein 5 (PP5): is PP5 the naturally occurring antithrombin III of the human placenta. *Placenta*, **2**, 205–208.

Samuels, P., Main, E. K., Mennuti, M. T. *et al.* (1987) The origin of increased serum iron in pregnancy-induced hypertension. *Am. J. Obstet. Gynecol.*, **157**, 721–725.

Sanchez-Ramos, L., Sandroni, S., Andres, F. J. and Kaunitz, A. M. (1991) Calcium excretion in preeclampsia. *Obstet. Gynecol.*, **77**, 510–513.

Schmorl, G. (1901) Zur pathologischen Anatomie der Eklampsie. Verhandl. Dtsch. Gesellsch. Gynaekol., **9**, 303–313.

Schulman, H., Fleischer, A., Farmakides, G. *et al.* (1986) Development of uterine artery compliance in pregnancy as detected by Doppler ultrasound. *Am. J. Obstet. Gynecol.*, **155**, 1031–1036.

Schulman, H., Ducey, J., Farmakides, G. *et al.* (1987) Uterine artery Doppler velocimetry: the significance of divergent systolic–diastolic ratios. *Am. J. Obstet. Gynecol.*, **157**, 1539–1542.

Segal, K. R., Burastero, S., Chun, A. *et al.* (1991) Estimation of extracellular and total body water by multiple-frequency bioelectrical-impedance measurement. *Am. J. Clin. Nutr.*, **54**, 26–29.

Shaffer, E. D. (1987) The liver and pregnancy: update. *Curr. Prob. Obstet. Gynecol. Fertil.*, **10**, 445–501.

Sheppard, B. L. and Bonnard, J. (1976) The ultrastructure of the arterial supply of the human placenta in pregnancy complicated by fetal grwotgh retardation. *Br. J. Obstet. Gynaecol.*, **83**, 948–959.

Sibai, B. M. (1988a) Preeclampsia–eclampsia. Maternal and perinatal outcome. *Contemp. Obstet. Gynecol.*, **32**, 109–118.

Sibai, B. M. (1988b) Pitfalls in diagnosis and management of preeclampsia. *Am. J. Obstet. Gynecol.*, **159**, 1–5.

Sibai, B. M. (1990a) Preeclampsia–eclampsia. *Curr. Prob. Obstet. Gynecol. Fertil.*, **13**, 3–45.

Sibai, B. M. (1990b) Eclampsia: VI. Maternal–perinatal outcome in 254 consecutive cases. *Am. J. Obstet. Gynecol.*, **163**, 1049–1055.

Sibai, B. M. (1990c) The HELLP syndrome (hemolysis, elevated liver enzymes, and low platelets): much ado about nothing? *Am. J. Obstet. Gynecol.*, **162**, 311–316.

Sibai, B. M., Anderson, G. D. and McCubbin, J. H. (1982) Eclampsia. II. Clinical significance of laboratory findings. *Obstet. Gynecol.*, **59**, 153–157.

Sibai, B. M., Fairlie, F. M. (1992) Eclampsia, in *Principles and Practice of Medical Therapy in Pregnancy*, 2nd edn, (ed. N. Gleicher), Appleton & Lange, Norwalk, CT, p. 880–888.

Sibai, B. M., Villar, M. A. and Mabie, B. C. (1990) Acute renal failure in hypertensive disorders of pregnancy: pregnancy outcome and remote prognosis in thirty-one consecutive cases. *Am. J. Obstet. Gynecol.*, **162**, 777–783.

Sibai, B. M., Anderson, G. D., Spinnato, J. A. *et al.* (1983) Plasma volume findings in patients with mild pregnancy induced hypertension. *Am. J. Obstet. Gynecol.*, **147**, 16–19.

Sibai, B. M., Spinnato, J. A., Watson, D. L. *et al.* (1984) Effect of magnesium sulfate on electroencephalographic findings in preeclampsia–eclampsia. *Obstet. Gynecol.*, **64**, 261–266.

Sibai, B. M., Abdella, T. N., Spinnato J. A. *et al.* (1986) Eclampsia V. The incidence of nonpreventable eclampsia. *Am. J. Obstet. Gynecol.*, **154**, 581–586.

Sibai, B. M., Maibie, B. C., Harvey, C. J. *et al.* (1987) Pulmonary edema in severe preeclampsia–eclampsia: analysis of thirty-seven consecutive cases. *Am. J. Obstet. Gynecol.*, **156**, 1174–1179.

Sill, P. R., Lind, T. and Walker, W. (1985) Platelet values during normal pregnancy. *Br. J. Obstet. Gynaecol.*, **92**, 480–483.

Simanowitz, M. D., MacGregor, W. G. and Hobbs, J. R. (1973) Proteinuria in pre-eclampsia. *J. Obstet. Gynaecol. Br. Commonw.*, 80, 103–108.

Sipes, S. L. and Weiner, C. P. (1992) Coagulation disorders in pregnancy, in *Medicine of the Fetus and Mother*, 1st edn, (eds E. A. Reece, J. C. Hobbins, M. J. Mahoney and R. H. Petrie), J. B. Lippincott, Philadelphia, PA, p. 1111–1138.

Slater, D., Pearce, J. M. F., Wilson, K. *et al.* (1992) Vasoactive substance in pregnancy: a study based on a Doppler waveform classification of hypertension.

Socol, M. L., Weiner, C. P., Louis, G. *et al.* (1985) Platelet activation in pre-eclampsia. *Am. J. Obstet. Gynecol.*, 151, 494–497.

Soffronoff, E. C., Kaufmann, B. M. and Connaughton, J. F. (1977) Intravascular volume determinations and fetal outcome in hypertensive diseases of pregnancy. *Am. J. Obstet. Gynecol.*, **127**, 4–9.

Spellacy, W. N., Teoh, E. S., Buhi, W. C. *et al.* (1971) Value of human chorionic somatomammotropin in managing high-risk pregnancies. *Am. J. Obstet. Gynecol.*, **109**, 588–598.

Stabile, I., Grudzinskas, J. G. and Chard, T. (1988) Clinical applications of pregnancy protein estimations with particular reference to pregnancy-associated plasma protein A (PAPP-A). *Obstet. Gynecol. Surv.*, **43**, 73–82.

Stahnke, E. (1922) Uber das Verhalten der Bluttplattchen bei Eklampsie. *Zentralbl. Gynäkol.*, **46**, 391.

Steel, S. A., Pearce, J. M. and Chamberlain, G. V. (1988) Doppler ultrasound of the uteroplacental circulation as a screening test for severe preeclampsia with intrauterine growth retardation. *Eur. J. Obstet. Gynecol. Reprod. Biol.*, **28**, 279–287.

Steel, S. A., Pearce, J. M., McParland, P. *et al.* (1990) Early Doppler ultrasound screening in prediction of hypertensive disorders of pregnancy. *Lancet*, **335**, 1548–1551.

Stubbs, T. M., Lazarchick, J., Dorsten van, P., *et al.* (1986) Evidence of accelerated platelet production and consumption in nonthrombocytopenic preeclampsia. *Am. J. Obstet. Gynecol.*, **155**, 263–265.

Studd, J. W. W. (1971) Immunoglobulins in normal pregnancy, pre-eclampsia, and pregnancy complicated by the nephrotic syndrome. *J. Obstet. Gynaecol, Br. Commonwealth*, **78**, 786–790.

Symmers, W. St C. (1952) Thrombotic microangiopathic haemolytic anemia (thrombotic microangiopathy). *Br. Med. J.*, **ii**, 897–908.

Tatum, H. J. and Mule, J. G. (1956) Puerperal vasomotor collapse in patients with toxemia of pregnancy – a new concept of the etiology and a rational plan of treatment. *Am. J. Obstet. Gynecol.*, **71**, 492–501.

Taufield, P. A., Alex, K. L., Resnick, L. M. *et al.* (1987) Hypocalciuria in preeclampsia. *N. Engl. J. Med.*, **316**, 715–718.

Taylor, R. N., Crombleholme, W. R., Friedman, S. A. *et al.* (1991) High plasma cellular fibronectin levels correlate with biochemical and clinical features of preeclampsia but cannot be attributed to hypertension alone. *Am. J. Obstet. Gynecol.*, **165**, 895–901.

Teph, E. S. and Sivasamboo, R. (1968) Immunological chorionic gonadotrophin titres in severe toxaemia of pregnancy. *J. Obstet. Gynaecol. Br. Commonw.*, **75**, 724–727.

Terao, T., Maki, M., Ikenoue, T *et al.* (1991) The relationship between clinical signs and hypercoagulable state in toxemia of pregnancy. *Gynecol. Obstet. Invest.*, **31**, 74–85.

Than, G. N., Csaba, I. F., Szabo, D. G. *et al.* (1984) Serum levels of placenta-specific tissue protein 12 (PP-12) in pregnancies complicated by preeclampsia, diabetes or twins. *Arch. Gynecol.*, **236**, 41–45.

Thomas, R. L. and Blakemore, K. J. (1990) Evaluation of elevations in maternal serum alpha-fetoprotein: a review. *Obstet. Gynecol. Surv.*, **45**, 269–283.

Thomson, A. M., Hytten, R. E. and Billewicz, W. Z. (1967) The epidemiology of oedema during pregnancy. *J. Obstet. Gynaecol. Br. Commonw.*, **74**, 1–10.

Thong, K. J., Howie, A. F., Smith, A. F. *et al.* (1991a) Micro-albuminuria in random daytime specimens in pregnancy-induced hypertension. *J. Obstet. Gynecol.*, **11**, 324–327.

Thong, K. J., Howie, A. F., Smith, A. F. *et al.* (1991b) Distribution of calcium/creatinine ratio in pregnancy induced hypertension. *Clin. Exper. Hypertens. Pregn.*, **B10**, 345–351.

Thornton, J. G., Hughes, R., Davies, J. A *et al.* (1986) Letter to the editor. *Lancet*, **i**, 328–329.

Toop, K. and Klopper, A. (1981) Concentrations of pregnancy-associated plasma protein A (PAPP-A) in patients with preeclamptic toxaemia. *Placenta*, **3S**, 167–173.

Torres, I., Pons, P. J., Fite-Exojo, L. *et al.* (1990) Umbilical and uterine artery blood flow velocities after antihypertensive treatment. *Echocardiography*, **7**, 603–605.

Trofatter, K. F., Howell, M. L., Greenberg, C. S. *et al.* (1989) Use of the fibrin D-dimer in screening for coagulation abnormalities in preeclampsia. *Obstet. Gynecol.*, **73**, 435–440.

Trudinger, B. J. (1976) Platelets and intrauterine growth retardation in pre-eclampsia. *Br. J. Obstet. Gynaecol.*, **83**, 284–286.

Trudinger, B. J. and Cook, C. M. (1990) Doppler umbilical and uterine flow waveforms in severe pregnancy hypertension. *Br. J. Obstet. Gynaecol.*, **97**, 142–148.

Trudinger, B. J., Giles, W. B. and Cook, C. M. (1985) Uteroplacental blood flow velocity-time waveforms in normal and complicated pregnancy. *Br. J. Obstet. Gynaecol.*, **92**, 39–45.

Tygart, S. G., McRoyan, D. K., Spinnato, J. A. *et al.* (1986) Longitudinal study of platelet indices during normal pregnancy. *Am. J. Obstet. Gynecol.*, **154**, 883–887.

Uttendorfsky, O. T., Veersema, D., Mooij, P. N. M. *et al.* (1988) Protein/creatinine ratio in the assessment of proteinuria during pregnancy. *Eur. J. Obstet. Gynecol. Reprod. Biol.*, **27**, 221–226.

van Dam, P. A., Renier, M., Baekelandt, M. *et al.* (1989) Disseminated intravascular coagulation and the syndrome of hemolysis, elevated liver enzymes, and low platelets in severe preeclampsia. *Obstet. Gynecol.*, **73**, 97–102.

Wallenburg, H. C. S (1987) Changes in the coagulation system and platelets in pregnancy-induced hypertension and preeclampsia, in *Hypertension in Pregnancy. Proceedings of the Sixteenth Study Group of the Royal College of Obstetricians and Gynaecologists*, (eds F. Sharp and E. M. Symonds), Perinatology Press, Ithaca, NY, p. 227–248.

Wallenburg, H. C. S. (1988) Hemodynamics in hypertensive pregnancy, in *Handbook of Hypertension, vol. 10: Hypertension in Pregnancy*, 1st edn, (ed. P. C. Rubin), Elsevier, Amsterdam, p. 66–101.

Wallmo, L., Karlsson, K. and Teger-Nilsson, A. C. (1984) Fibrinopeptide and intravascular coagulation in normotensive and hypertensive pregnancy and parturition. *Acta Obstet. Gynecol. Scand.*, **63**, 637–640.

Walker, J. J., Cameron, A. D., Steingrimur, B. *et al.* (1989) Can platelet volume predict progressive hypertensive disease in pregnancy? *Am. J. Obstet. Gynecol.*, **161**, 676–679.

Watson, W. J. and Seeds, J. W. (1990) Acute fatty liver of pregnancy. *Obstet. Gynecol. Surv.*, **45**, 585–593.

Weber, H., Heller, S. and Seulen, P. (1980) Plazentahormone und EPH-Gestose. *Geburtsh. Frauheilk.*, **40**, 339–343.

Weinstein, L. (1982) Syndrome of hemolysis, elevated liver enzymes, and low platelet count: a severe consequence of hypertension in pregnancy. *Am. J. Obstet. Gynecol.*, **142**, 159–167.

West, J. E, Busch-Vishniac, I. J., Harsfield, G. A. and Pickering T. G. (1983) Foil electret transducer for blood pressure monitoring. *J. Acoust. Soc. Am.*, **74**, 680–686.

Westergaard, J. G., Teisner, B., Hau, J. *et al.* (1984) Placental proteins in complicated pregnancies. II. Pregnancy-related hypertension. *Br. J. Obstet. Gynaecol.*, **91**, 1224–1229.

Whigham, K. A. E., Howie, P. W., Drummond, A. H. *et al.* (1978) Abnormal platelet function in pre-eclampsia. *Br. J. Obstet. Gynaecol.*, **85**, 28–32.

White, G. C. II, Marder, V. J., Colman, R. W. *et al.* (1987) Approach to the Bleeding Patient, in *Hemostasis and Thrombosis. Basic Principles and Clinical Practice*, 2nd edn, (eds R. W. Colman, J. Hirsch, V. J. Marder and E. W. Salzman), J. B. Lippincott, Philadelphia, PA, p. 1048–1060.

Wichman, K., Ryden, G. and Wichman, M. (1984) The influence of different positions and Korotkoff sounds on the blood pressure measurements in pregnancy. *Acta Obstet. Gynecol. Scand.*, **118**, 25–28.

Wilde, J. T., Kitchen, S., Kinsey, S. *et al.* (1989) Plasma D-dimer levels and their relationship to serum fibrinogen/fibrin degradation products in hypercoagulable states. *Br. J. Haematol.*, **71**, 65–70.

Will, A. D., Lewis, K. L., Hinshaw, D. B. *et al.* (1987) Cerebral vasoconstriction in toxemia. *Neurology*, **37**, 1555–1557.

Williams, J. L. (1921) Increased amount of uric acid in the blood in the toxemias of pregnancy. *J. A. M. A.*, **76**, 1297–1299.

Williams, G. F. and Jones, D. D (1975) Deoxycytidylate deaminase in pregnancy. *Br. Med. J.*, **11**, 10–12.

Williams, G. F. and Jones, D. D (1982) Serum deoxycytidylate deaminase as an index of high-risk pregnancy. *Br. J. Obstet. Gynaecol.*, **89**, 309–313.

Wiman, B., Csemiczky, G., Marsk, L. *et al.* (1984) The fast inhibitor of tissue-type plasminogen activator in plasma during pregnancy. *Thromb. Haemostasis*, **52**, 124–126.

Wood, S. M. (1977) Assessment of renal functions in hypertensive pregnancies. *Clin. Obstet. Gynecol.*, **4**, 747–758.

Zangmeister, W. (1903) Untersuchungen über die Blutbeschaffenheit unde die Harnsekretion bei Eclampsie. *Zentralbl. Gynaekol.*, **50**, 385–389.

Zeeman, G. G. and Dekker, G. A. (1992) Pathogenesis of preeclampsia: a hypothesis. *Clin. Obstet. Gynecol.*, **35**, 317–337.

Zimmerman, H. J. (1984) Function and integrity of the liver, in *Clinical Diagnosis and Management by Laboratory Methods*, 17th edn, (ed. J. B. Henry), W. B. Saunders, London, p. 217–250.

Zimmerman, H. J. and Henry, J. B. (1984) Clinical enzymology, in *Clinical Diagnosis and Management by Laboratory Methods*, 17th edn, (ed. J. B. Henry), W. B. Saunders, London, p. 251–282.

Zinaman, M., Rubin, J. and Lindheimer, M. D. (1985) Serial plasma oncotic pressure levels and echoencephalography during and after delivery in severe pre-eclampsia. *Lancet*, **i**, 1245–1247.

Zuspan, F. P. (1990) Abnormal placentation in hypertensive disorders of pregnancy, in *Hypertension: Pathophysiology, Diagnosis, and Management*, 1st edn, (eds J. H. Laragh and B. M. Brenner), Raven Press, New York, p. 1779–1788.

Zuspan, F. P. and Rayburn, W. F. (1991) Blood pressure self-monitoring during pregnancy: practical considerations. *Am. J. Obstet. Gynecol.*, **164**, 2–6.

*Fiona M. Fairlie*

## 8.1 INTRODUCTION

Hypertension complicates 10–15% of pregnancies in the UK and in the USA. The complications of hypertension in pregnancy are a major cause of maternal and perinatal mortality and morbidity worldwide. Despite much study over many years, an effective strategy for the prevention or amelioration of hypertensive complications has yet to be determined.

Maternal hypertension is rarely an isolated finding. It is usually one sign of a clinical syndrome which may have adverse effects on maternal and/or fetal health. The fetus is often forgotten in the concern for the mother's wellbeing. As shown in Chapters 4 and 7, the disease in the mother can be widespread and affect multiple organs. In the fetus the problem is simpler because the effect is directly related to a reduction in placental function leading to problems of fetal growth and wellbeing. This chapter considers the influence of hypertensive disorders on the fetus and the role of antepartum monitoring tests to detect fetal compromise.

## 8.2 PERINATAL COMPLICATIONS ASSOCIATED WITH HYPERTENSION IN PREGNANCY

It is not possible to accurately predict perinatal outcome for an individual pregnancy. Perinatal mortality and morbidity are rarely the result of a single insult. Chronic antepartum hypoxia may be compounded by acute intrapartum hypoxia and preterm delivery. The difficulty of assessing fetal and perinatal risks in hypertensive pregnancies has been increased by the many methods used to classify these disorders. However there is no doubt that the risk of fetal compromise, perinatal death and long-term disability is higher for hypertensive pregnancies compared with uncomplicated pregnancies. In Scotland in 1985 there were 47 perinatal deaths associated with pregnancy-induced hypertension. Of these, 31 babies were stillborn (Scottish Stillbirth and Neonatal Death Report, 1985). It would appear obvious that, to improve the outcome for the fetus in this condition, an improved protocol for the assessment and timing of the delivery is required. Prematurity and intrauterine growth retardation are the major causes of perinatal mortality and morbidity in hypertensive pregnancies. Regardless of its underlying etiology, sustained hypertension has an adverse effect on fetal growth, but its relative risk differs from one disease entity to another (Lin *et al.*, 1982). Although an accurate estimation of relative risks is not possible there are some general guidelines. First, hypertension alone carries a lower risk of fetal growth retardation than hypertension and proteinuria. In a study by Ounsted, Moar and Scott (1985) hypertension accompanied by proteinuria was associated with a relative risk of a small-for-gestational infant of 14.6 times that of a normotensive pregnancy (95% confidence limits 5.8–36.5).

*Hypertension in Pregnancy*
Edited by J.J. Walker and N.F. Gant. Published by Chapman & Hall, 1997 ISBN 0 412 30910 6

Chronic hypertension alone was associated with a relative risk of 2.7 (95% confidence limits 1.8–4.0). Second, the earlier the disease presents clinically, the greater is the risk and severity of fetal growth retardation (Sibai *et al.*, 1984).

Premature delivery is a major cause of perinatal mortality and morbidity in hypertensive pregnancies (Martin and Tupper, 1975; Odendaal *et al.*, 1987). It may be necessitated by a deterioration in the maternal and/or fetal condition. For the surviving infant of a pregnancy complicated by hypertension there may be long-term problems. The studies of Lilienfeld, Pasamanick and Kawi were the first to emphasize the importance of pregnancy complications and preterm delivery in the etiology of neurodevelopmental disability. They found a higher incidence of 'toxemia' in pregnancies that resulted in children with cerebral palsy or mental deficiency (Lilienfeld and Pasamanick, 1955), epilepsy (Lilienfeld and Pasamanick, 1954), behavioral disorders (Pasamanick, Rogers and Lilienfeld, 1956) and reading disabilities (Kawi and Pasamanick, 1958). Friedman and Neff (1977) using data collected from the collaborative study of cerebral palsy in the USA showed that the risk of stillbirth increased when diastolic pressures (Korotkoff 5) were 95 mmHg or greater and proteinuria 2 pluses or greater. The British Births Survey (Chamberlain *et al.*, 1978) demonstrated a rise in perinatal mortality and neonatal neurological complications when the diastolic blood pressure was either above 100 mmHg or above 90 mmHg with significant proteinuria. More recently, Taylor *et al.* (1985), in a case-control study, found severe preeclampsia was significantly more common in children with mental retardation (20%) global delay (17.3%) and motor delay (14%) compared with controls (5.3%). In this study severe preeclampsia was defined as a diastolic blood pressure of more than 110 mmHg or blood pressure of 90–120 mmHg with proteinuria more than 1+ on Dipstix testing or more than 300 mg in a 24-hour urine specimen.

Over the last 30 years there has been a gradual improvement in the survival of very low birthweight infants. Most follow-up studies have shown that very low birthweight infants are disadvantaged compared with reference populations. In a recent UK study in which 6-year-old very low birthweight infants (< 1.25 kg) were compared with their age- and sex-matched classmates, the very low birthweight infants performed significantly less well over a range of intelligence quotient, motor and behavioral tests. In multiple regression model, the most significant association of poor motor and intelligence quotient was with very low birthweight and less so with socioeconomic factors (Marlow, Roberts and Cooke, 1989). The effect of severe preeclampsia on the development of very low birthweight infants was studied in a prospective case control study of 35 pairs of infants of comparable length of gestation (Szymonowicz and Yu, 1987). At 2 years of age the children born to severely preeclamptic mothers were still smaller and had a significantly lower mental developmental index, and significantly more of these children had one or more impairments compared with the control group.

In summary, hypertension in pregnancy is associated with an increased risk of fetal or neonatal death, intrauterine growth retardation, abruptio placentae, preterm delivery and long-term physical and/or neurological developmental delay. In order to design a protocol to reduce this morbidity, an understanding of the causes of the fetal compromise is required.

## 8.3 MECHANISMS OF FETAL COMPROMISE IN HYPERTENSIVE PREGNANCIES

The impact of maternal hypertension on fetal wellbeing depends on:

1. gestational age when maternal and/or fetal signs and symptoms first appear;
2. the presence or absence of impaired placental function;

3. whether or not therapies are instituted that may directly or indirectly alter fetal physiology.

In clinical practice maternal hypertension in pregnancy has little or no impact of perinatal outcome if it presents after 30 weeks and a placental vascular abnormality is minimal or absent. In contrast, midtrimester severe preeclampsia is associated with a high perinatal mortality and morbidity and placental vascular abnormalities are usually widespread and severe.

In normal pregnancy the trophoblast disrupts the walls of the spiral arteries destroying muscle and elastic coats and replacing them with fibrinoid tissue (Brosens, Robertson and Dixon, 1967). This process occurs in two waves, the first at the time of implantation and limited to the decidual parts of the spiral arteries. The second invasion occurs between 14 and 22 weeks gestation and invades as far as the radial arteries. Trophoblastic invasion converts muscular spiral arteries into wide, flaccid uteroplacental arteries. The lack of a muscular coat renders these vessels insensitive to circulating vasopressor substances.

The pathophysiological mechanisms responsible for the signs and symptoms of preeclampsia have yet to be elucidated. Endothelial damage secondary to placental ischemia is thought to play a critical role. Vascular endothelium is a complex and active organ. It acts as a semipermeable barrier between the bloodstream and extravascular space, it modulates vascular tone and prevents intravascular coagulation. The placenta from a pregnancy complicated by preeclampsia shows failure of the second wave of trophoblastic invasion. In addition, there is histological evidence of vascular endothelial damage and spiral artery occlusion by aggregates of fibrin, platelet and lipid-filled macrophages. These secondary changes are termed 'acute atherosis' (Robertson, Brosens and Dixon, 1967). Light microscopy has sug-

gested that preeclampsia is associated with a reduction in the normal frequency and distribution of small muscular arteries in the tertiary stem villi. Thus, preeclampsia is associated with widespread endothelial cell damage and histological abnormalities of the uteroplacental and fetoplacental circulations. Fetal wellbeing and perinatal outcome depends on the severity of these changes.

Antihypertensive therapy is administered to stabilize and lower maternal blood pressure. In the presence of already impaired placental perfusion a rapid and/or profound reduction in maternal blood pressure may adversely affect fetal perfusion and precipitate acute fetal hypoxia. In the presence of fetal compromise, the use of antihypertensive therapy must be made with great care.

## 8.4 ANTEPARTUM TESTS OF FETAL CONDITION

The purposes of fetal monitoring are:

1. to establish fetal normality and exclude/detect fetal compromise;
2. to detect as early as possible a deterioration in fetal health and wellbeing;
3. to prevent fetal death and physical and neurological damage.

Fetal monitoring tests are employed to assess the intrauterine health of a specific fetus. This information should enable the obstetrician to determine whether or not the pregnancy should be prolonged or if delivery is indicated and to assess the most appropriate mode of delivery from the fetal point of view.

The increased risk of perinatal mortality and morbidity in hypertensive pregnancies has been discussed. Fetal wellbeing cannot be evaluated by measuring parameters of maternal wellbeing. The fetus must be assessed as an individual. Until the moment of birth, the fetus depends on placenta for growth and development. Tests of fetal wellbeing reflect the function of the fetoplacental unit rather than the fetus alone. Although the risk of fetal hypoxia/asphyxia depends on the etiology and pathophysiology of the maternal hypertension, a uniform approach should be adopted to assessing fetal wellbeing.

The following text critically describes the fetal monitoring tests that are commonly used in Glasgow Royal Maternity Hospital (GRMH) and the Jessop Hospital in Sheffield to assess fetal wellbeing. They are used to a greater or lesser extent in many other units in the UK and the USA.

### 8.4.1 REAL-TIME ULTRASOUND

Real-time ultrasound is essential to the evaluation of fetal wellbeing in a hypertensive pregnancy. We use ultrasound to:

1. Confirm fetal viability
2. Assess fetal growth
3. Assess amniotic fluid volume
4. Study fetal activity (see 'Biophysical profile').

The interpretation of many fetal monitoring tests depends on accurate pregnancy dating. All our patients are scanned at their first visit to confirm viability and gestational age. Decisions concerning fetal wellbeing and delivery require accurate assessment of both fetal state and fetal maturity.

The initial assessment of any hypertensive pregnancy in the unit includes an ultrasound examination to determine fetal viability, growth and amniotic fluid volume. The frequency of subsequent ultrasound examinations depends on gestational age, perceived severity of fetal compromise and stability of the maternal and fetal condition.

### (a) Fetal growth

Intrauterine growth retardation, a consequence of chronic fetal hypoxia, is a well-recognized complication of hypertensive pregnancies. In some cases fetal growth retardation may the first sign of preeclampsia. If pregnancy gestation is accurately known (cer-

tain last menstrual period confirmed by ultrasound fetal measurements before 24 weeks gestation) it is possible to ascertain from a single ultrasound examination whether the fetus is small for gestational age (SGA). In the absence of accurate dating, serial ultrasound measurements are necessary to establish the rate of fetal growth.

It is not possible to predict fetal growth velocity and fetal growth retardation is a gradual process (Seeds, 1984). For these reasons serial ultrasound examinations are performed on all our hypertensive patients at intervals of 10–14 days. There are many publications describing different fetal measurement parameters to detect growth abnormalities. Highly complex formulae have been devised to incorporate the different parameters proposed. In clinical practice the most sensitive ultrasound measurements to detect the SGA fetus are head circumference and abdominal circumference (Chudleigh and Pearce, 1992).

Hypertension in pregnancy may be associated with asymmetric fetal growth retardation, i.e. appropriately grown head with a wasted body or a symmetric fetal growth retardation, i.e. head size and trunk size show a similar degree of growth lag. The term 'intrauterine growth retardation' implies that a pathological process has occurred to restrict fetal growth. 'Small for gestational age' indicates that a fetus or neonate is below a defined reference range of size or weight for gestational age. Intrauterine growth retardation and SGA are not synonymous terms. Not all SGA fetuses suffer from intrauterine growth retardation and not all growth-retarded fetuses are SGA. Ultrasound assessment of fetal growth is thus only one aspect of fetal monitoring in a hypertensive pregnancy and the trend in growth is more significant than the estimated size of the fetus.

### (b) Amniotic fluid volume

It is widely accepted that there is an association between reduced amniotic fluid volume, fetal growth retardation and increased risk of adverse perinatal outcome (Chamberlain *et al.*, 1984; Rutherford *et al.*, 1987). Various non-invasive methods have been described of estimating amniotic fluid volume. Subjective assessment shows a good correlation between extremes of amniotic fluid volume and fetal outcome. However the reliability and reproducibility of this technique depend heavily on operator experience. Semiquantitative assessment has been proposed using either vertical measurement of the single maximal amniotic fluid pocket (Manning, Platt and Sipos, 1980) or the four-quadrant summation of maximal amniotic fluid depth, i.e. the amniotic fluid index (Phelen *et al.*, 1987). Moore and Cayle (1990) published nomograms for amniotic fluid index (AFI) and maximal vertical pocket (MVP) derived from 791 uncomplicated pregnancies. Croom *et al.* (1992) compared semiquantitative methods with actual volume measured by dye-dilution. AFI appeared to be slightly better than MVP for reflecting amniotic fluid volume. However the difference was not sufficient to conclude that one method is unquestionably superior. All non-invasive methods of assessing amniotic fluid volume show maximum errors at extremes of volume, i.e. oligohydramnios and polyhydramnios, and it is important to remember this limitation in clinical practice and to repeat abnormal results before a clinical decision is made, especially if other parameters are satisfactory.

There is little data on the optimum frequency of amniotic fluid volume assessment. Amniotic fluid volume is a chronic marker of fetal wellbeing and frequent testing may not necessarily improve testing sensitivity. Lagrew *et al.* (1992), in a study of high-risk pregnancies at less than 41 weeks gestation (26% were complicated by hypertension and/or fetal growth retardation), found that an amniotic fluid index of more than 8 cm was associated with a low risk of developing oligohydramnios (defined as an AFI of less than 5 cm). A weekly AFI was suggested for

this group. For patients with an AFI between 5 cm and 8 cm, i.e. low–normal, twice-weekly testing was recommended.

In our practice we use both AFI and a subjective assessment of amniotic fluid volume. If the AFV is reduced subjectively and/or AFI is less than 8 cm and other fetal monitoring tests are satisfactory, we repeat the assessment twice weekly. A subjective assessment of oligohydramnios and/or AFI less than 5 cm is an indication for admission for intensive monitoring or delivery if the fetus is mature.

### 8.4.2 FETAL HEART RATE PATTERN

The cardiotocograph (CTG) or non-stress test (NST) relates changes in the fetal heart rate to fetal movement. It has become the most commonly used primary test for antepartum fetal wellbeing in the Western world. The frequent occurrence of fetal heart rate accelerations during a testing period of 10–30 min is generally regarded as a sign of fetal health (Devoe, Castillo and Sherline, 1985).

Keegan and Paul (1980) defined a reactive NST by the following criteria:

1. at least four fetal movements in 20 minutes with two accelerations of the fetal heart rate of at least 5 beats per minute;
2. baseline heart rate within the range of 120–160 beats per minute;
3. long-term variability amplitude of at least six beats per minute.

These criteria are used in our clinical practice to define a reactive NST. If they are not met within 40 min the NST is considered non-reactive. The NST reflects fetal wellbeing at the time of testing. It is not a method of identifying intrauterine growth retardation but it may indicate acute on chronic hypoxia in a growth-retarded fetus. A reactive NST is associated with a low risk of fetal hypoxia. A non-reactive NST, if truly positive, carries a significant risk of adverse perinatal outcome (Devoe *et al.*, 1985). Unfortunately the rate of false positive tests results ranges from 50–80%

depending on the criteria used. Many of the problems come from inconsistent assessment of the fetal heart tracings.

Isolated decelerations of fetal heart in association either with fetal movement or spontaneous contractions are not uncommon in the antepartum period and are usually benign. However, if decelerations are repeated and are associated with absence of accelerations and loss of baseline variability there is an increased incidence of operative delivery for fetal distress, acidosis at delivery and perinatal mortality (Brioschi *et al.*, 1985).

Hypertensive complications often present at less than 37 weeks gestation. Gestational age has an important influence on the interpretation of the NST. The immature fetus has a higher baseline, lower baseline variability, fewer accelerations and the presence of transient decelerations compared with the term fetus. Castillo *et al.* (1989) considered the effects of gestational age on the NST and concluded that before 32 weeks gestation the testing time should be extended to 60 min and the minimum amplitude required of accelerations reduced to 10.

The optimum frequency of non-stress testing is unknown. Test frequency will be influenced by the obstetrician's perception of fetal risk in a particular pregnancy, gestational age and recent NST results. Table 8.1 shows how we use the NST in our assessment of fetal condition in hypertensive pregnancies.

The NST is always used in combination with other fetal monitoring tests. Because of the high false-positive rate, a non-reactive NST is usually an indication for a repeat test later that day unless other fetal monitoring tests are also non-reassuring and delivery is expedited.

Abruptio placentae is an important cause of fetal intrauterine death in patients with severe, proteinuric hypertension (Odendall *et al.*, 1987; Sibai *et al.*, 1985). As a result of their experience of severe proteinuric hypertension before 34 weeks gestation, Odendall *et al.* (1988) concluded that frequent non-stress testing (daily or more frequently when a suspi-

cious pattern was seen) could be useful in detecting fetal distress before abruptio placentae became clinically evident.

It is our practice to carry out weekly NSTs in the outpatient managed group in the Day Unit (Chapter 9), twice weekly for those in hospital and daily or even twice daily in those to be thought to be high risk, especially if there is an abnormality seen or the umbilical Doppler wave form is abnormal.

### 8.4.3 THE BIOPHYSICAL PROFILE

The first report on the use of multiple biophysical variables to predict fetal/neonatal outcome was published by Manning, Platt and Sipos (1980). The aim of this approach was to reduce the false positive and negative results of individual monitoring tests by combining several test results. Each test result was given a score and the total was known as the fetal biophysical profile score. The biophysical profile (BPP) is now widely recognized as a useful method of antepartum fetal assessment. It is a combination of acute (NST, fetal breathing movements and fetal body movements) and chronic (fetal tone and amniotic fluid volume) markers. On the basis of human and animal studies it has been suggested that acute fetal hypoxia will result in a decrease in fetal heart reactivity and fetal breathing movements. A more prolonged hypoxic insult will be associated with loss of fetal body movements and eventually loss of fetal tone (Vintzileos and Tsapanos, 1992).

Fetal activity is subject to a natural periodicity. A low BPP score may be due to fetal sleep, maternal administration of drugs or fetal hypoxia and acidosis. If there is any doubt about the cause of a low score it is advisable to repeat the test after 4–6 hours. It has been suggested that the components of the BPP do not all carry the same significance with respect to fetal wellbeing and relatively high predictive accuracy is only achieved when all variables are abnormal (Manning *et al.*, 1990; Devoe *et al.*, 1992).

**Table 8.1**  The Glasgow Royal Maternity Hospital protocol for fetal monitoring in hypertensive pregnancies

**Initial assessment (all hypertensive pregnancies)**
Real-time ultrasound for:  Fetal viability
Fetal growth parameters
Amniotic fluid volume
Non-stress test
On the basis of these initial test results, pregnancy gestation and the presence or absence of proteinuria the risk of adverse perinatal outcome is assessed. Subsequent intensity of fetal monitoring is based on this risk assessment.

The risk of adverse perinatal outcome is considered to be low if:
● Pregnancy gestation ≥34 weeks
● Hypertension without proteinuria
● Ultrasound suggests adequate fetal growth and normal amniotic fluid volume

Manage as an outpatient with weekly daycare assessment:
1. NST (repeat weekly)
2. Ultrasound assessment of amniotic fluid volume (repeat weekly)
3. Ultrasound assessment of fetal growth (repeat every 2 weeks)

The risk of adverse perinatal outcome is considered to be moderate if:
● Pregnancy gestation < 34 weeks
● Hypertension is associated with proteinuria (> 0.3 g in 24 h)
● Ultrasound suggests adequate fetal growth and normal amniotic fluid volume
● Umbilical artery Doppler FVW indices are within normal range

Manage as an outpatient with twice weekly daycare assessment
1. NST (twice weekly)
2. Ultrasound assessment of amniotic fluid volume (repeat weekly)
3. Ultrasound assessment of fetal growth (repeat every 2 weeks)
4. Umbilical artery Doppler studies (repeat weekly)

The risk of adverse perinatal outcome is considered to be high if:
● Pregnancy gestation < 34 weeks
● Hypertension is associated with proteinuria (> 0.3 g in 24 h)
● Ultrasound suggests inadequate fetal growth (either suspected SGA fetus or a downward trend in fetal growth parameters) and/or ultrasound shows reduced amniotic fluid volume
● Umbilical artery Doppler FVW indices are above the normal range

These patients are admitted for intensive fetal and maternal monitoring. If the NST is non-reactive a BPP is performed daily.

There is little data on the application of BPP specifically in hypertensive pregnancies. Vintzileos *et al.* (1987) reported their experience of the BPP over an 8-year period. They outlined a protocol for fetal evaluation which begins with a NST and subsequent pregnancy management is based on the individual components of the BPP rather than the total score. The BPP requires expertise in real-time ultrasound and NST monitoring. Furthermore it is time-consuming. For these reasons most centers (including our own) do not use the BPP as a primary monitoring test for all hypertensive pregnancies. We reserve the BPP for fetuses judged to be at high risk of intrauterine hypoxia with a non-reactive NST (Table 8.1). We use the scoring system of Manning, Platt and Sipos, 1980 with a modification to amniotic fluid volume as follows: score = 2 if AFI ≥ 5 cm and score = 0 if AFI < 5 cm.

### 8.4.4 DOPPLER ULTRASOUND

Doppler ultrasound is a non-invasive method of measuring changes in blood flow velocity. It application to pregnancy was first described in 1977 by Fitzgerald and Drumm. Doppler equipment, signal acquisition and analysis have been well described (Fairlie, 1991; McParland and Pearce, 1992). In Glasgow and Sheffield we have extensive experience of both continuous wave (CW) Doppler and pulsed wave (PW) Doppler with color flow mapping. In the clinical management of hypertensive pregnancies, we use either CW or PW recordings of the umbilical artery flow velocity waveform (FVW) with analysis of the pulsatility index (PI) and the resistance index (RI). We have not found Doppler studies of the uteroplacental circulation or fetal vessels to offer a clear advantage over the umbilical artery with respect to pregnancy management although we study these vessels for research purposes.

In a sheep model Morrow *et al.* (1989) showed that progressive embolization of the fetal placental vascular bed was associated with a gradual reduction in the end-diastolic component of the umbilical artery Doppler FVW. In human fetuses, loss of end-diastolic frequencies in the umbilical artery FVW is associated with an increased risk of fetal growth retardation, antepartum and intrapartum fetal distress and perinatal death (Trudinger *et al.*, 1985; Berkowitz *et al.*, 1988; Divon *et al.*, 1989). It would appear from clinical and experimental observations that an abnormal umbilical artery Doppler FVW pattern reflects increased fetoplacental vascular resistance. Some fetuses with abnormal umbilical artery FVWs are hypoxic and acidemic (Nicolaides *et al.*, 1988). However fetal hypoxia or acidemia are not responsible for the waveform abnormalities (Copel *et al.*, 1991; Morrow *et al.*, 1990). Suggested mechanisms for increased fetoplacental vascular resistance are obliteration of tertiary stem

arterioles or a failure of their development. However, conclusive evidence to prove either mechanism is still lacking.

Our experience of the role of umbilical artery Doppler FVWs in the management of hypertensive problems in pregnancy has been reported (Fairlie, 1991; Fairlie *et al.*, 1991) and is in agreement with other workers in this field. To summarize:

1. The normal umbilical artery FVW shows a progressive increase in end-diastolic frequencies with advancing gestational age. In pregnancies complicated by hypertension, there is an association between adverse perinatal outcome and an abnormal umbilical artery Doppler FVW (i.e. reduced end-diastolic frequencies), reflected by a PI or RI value above the normal range.
2. The risk of adverse outcome increases as end-diastolic frequencies decrease. Absent end-diastolic frequencies at a gestation of less than 30 weeks is particularly associated with increased perinatal mortality and morbidity.
3. Umbilical artery Doppler is a chronic marker of fetal wellbeing. Return of end-diastolic frequencies has been observed by several authors and this finding is associated with improved pregnancy outcome compared with pregnancies showing persistently absent end-diastolic frequencies (Bell *et al.*, 1992).
4. Umbilical artery Doppler studies must be interpreted in conjunction with other fetal monitoring tests. Delivery should not be based on the umbilical artery Doppler FVW alone. However, umbilical artery Doppler in combination with the NST can provide useful information about fetal wellbeing particularly at gestations less than 30 weeks (Fairlie, 1991).

## 8.5 GLASGOW ROYAL MATERNITY HOSPITAL FETAL MONITORING PROTOCOLS FOR HYPERTENSIVE PREGNANCIES

The ideal antepartum fetal monitoring test should be rapid, non-invasive, repeatable and applicable at all gestations. It should provide unequivocal results with a high sensitivity and specificity for the prediction or early detection of fetal hypoxia. Such a test has yet to be determined.

Fetal wellbeing is an ill-defined term. It implies absence of fetal compromise. The effectiveness of a fetal monitoring test is usually judged by its sensitivity and specificity in predicting adverse perinatal outcome. However, the most clinically appropriate definition of adverse perinatal outcome is controversial. Table 8.2 indicates some of the outcome parameters in common use.

Death is an unequivocal perinatal outcome but in the Western world it is too infrequent to be a clinically useful definition. Thus, although antepartum fetal monitoring tests are widely used, their benefit in terms of reducing perinatal mortality and morbidity is difficult to prove.

In clinical practice obstetricians employ a combination of fetal monitoring tests to assess fetal wellbeing. Their aim is to answer the following questions.

1. What is the state of fetal wellbeing at the time of testing?
2. What is the optimum time of delivery?
3. What is the optimum mode of delivery?

Fetal monitoring tests assess different aspects of fetal physiology. In the absence of 'the ideal test', it is anticipated that a combination of tests provides a more accurate assessment of fetal wellbeing than a single test. The relationship between a monitoring test result and the health of a specific fetus at a specific time can only be inferred on the basis of a previous experience of the test result and its associated perinatal outcome. The fetal monitoring tests in current use predict fetal health more reliably than fetal compromise, i.e. a normal test result usually indicates absence of fetal compromise while an abnormal result has a significant false-positive rate. In our experience (and that of others, e.g. Devoe *et al.*, 1990) multiple tests assessing different parameters are particularly helpful when one test gives an abnormal or equivocal result and when the fetus is immature. Finally, fetal monitoring cannot predict sudden events such as preterm delivery or abruptio placentae.

The protocol outlined in Table 8.1 has been devised as the result of clinical experience in the management of more than 5000 pregnancies complicated by hypertension. Initially all fetuses of hypertensive pregnancies are assessed by ultrasound and NST. On the basis of these test results and the pregnancy characteristics, the risk of adverse perinatal outcome is assessed.

Gestational age is crucial in interpreting fetal monitoring tests. Advancing gestation influences the umbilical artery Doppler waveform pattern, the amniotic fluid volume the fetal activity and the fetal heart rate pattern. The earliest gestation at which testing is commenced depends on the estimated pregnancy risk and the test being considered. In our unit, the earliest gestation at which NST and BPP monitoring are commenced is 26 weeks. The NST and BPP may change acutely and such changes may prompt the obstetrician to deliver the patient. In our unit, we would not consider delivery in the fetal interest before 26 weeks. Serial umbilical artery Doppler and fetal growth assessment may be commenced as early as 20 weeks, since these are chronic markers of fetal wellbeing.

The frequency of testing fetal wellbeing in hypertensive pregnancies depends on gestational age, stability of clinical condition,

---

**Table 8.2** Parameters commonly used to define adverse perinatal outcome

- Fetal distress in labor'
- Perinatal death
- Apgar score below 6 at 1 min, below 8 at 5 min
- Cord blood acid–base at delivery
- Admission to special care baby unit
- Duration of stay in special care baby unit
- Neurological and physical development

degree of fetal compromise and test result. Guidelines for test frequency are given in Table 8.1.

Many of our patients are managed as out-patients through our daycare assessment unit. However intensive, inpatient fetal monitoring is required for a small proportion of cases. The fetal indications for admission are shown in Table 8.3.

### 8.5.1 THE DECISION TO DELIVER

Table 8.4 lists fetal indications for delivery.

It may appear that the criteria are clear and unequivocal. In practice this is often not the case – particularly for the preterm fetus. The decision to deliver for fetal reasons should be reached after balancing the risks to the fetus of remaining *in utero* against the risks to the neonate of being delivered prematurely. As gestational age advances delivery becomes a safer option. There is no precise method of measuring individual risks. An assessment is made based on ultrasound estimated fetal weight, estimated gestational age and current survival rates in the intensive care baby unit.

In certain cases *in utero* transfer will be appropriate. The concept of *in utero* transfer is well established in North America and is becoming more accepted in the UK. With respect to perinatal outcome, *in utero* transfer to a tertiary center with intensive pediatric care facilities is preferable to the transfer of a premature neonate.

---

**Table 8.3** Fetal indications for hospital admission for the purpose of intensive monitoring

- Ultrasonic evidence of static or declining fetal growth profile
- Oligohydramnios (amniotic fluid index < 5 cm)
- Non-reactive non-stress test
- Biophysical profile score of 6 or less

---

**Table 8.4** Fetal indications for delivery

- Fetal maturity
- Non-reactive NST with decelerations
- Biophysical profile score of 4 or less on two occasions 4 h apart

---

### 8.5.2 PREDELIVERY STEROIDS

Recent meta-analysis (Crowley, Chalmers and Keirse, 1990) has shown that, for pregnancies of less than 34 weeks gestation, maternal administration of steroids antepartum is effective in reducing the incidence of neonatal hyaline membrane disease. As described in Chapter 14 it is our practice to administer two doses of 12 mg betamethasone 12 h apart 48 h before delivering a hypertensive patient of less than 34 weeks gestation.

### 8.5.3 ANTIHYPERTENSIVE THERAPY AND FETAL MONITORING TESTS

Antihypertensive therapy is the mainstay of the management protocol in the Glasgow Royal Maternity Hospital (Chapter 14). An acute fall in maternal blood pressure may adversely alter fetal wellbeing but, once maternal blood is stabilized, antihypertensive therapy does not influence the interpretation of fetal monitoring tests. It is important to realize that, even though the blood pressure is controlled, the fetus remains at risk and requires continued close monitoring.

### 8.5.4 MODE OF DELIVERY

We aim for vaginal delivery if gestational age exceeds 34 weeks and there is no antepartum evidence of acute fetal compromise. Montan and Ingemarsson (1989) demonstrated an increased risk of ominous intrapartum fetal heart patterns in hypertensive pregnancies compared with normotensive pregnancies (20.5% *versus* 7.6%). The etiology of the hypertension did not influence the frequency of ominous patterns and the highest frequency was found in growth-retarded fetuses. We advocate continuous intrapartum electronic fetal heart rate monitoring for all hypertensive pregnancies and a low threshold for fetal blood sampling in the event of abnormal patterns.

In our experience the risk of failed induction of labor and/or intrapartum fetal heart rate abnormalities increases significantly as gestational age decreases below 34 weeks. It is our practice to deliver by cesarean section if gestational age is less than 34 weeks, there are antepartum fetal heart rate abnormalities or a biophysical profile score is less than 4/10.

### 8.5.5 PREPARATION OF PARENTS

Severe preeclampsia at less than 28 weeks gestation presents the main challenge to hypertensive pregnancy management in the Western world. If the maternal and fetal wellbeing are stable there is a prospect of prolonging pregnancy. In the presence of deteriorating fetal condition and a stable maternal condition, parents and obstetrician must choose between preterm delivery, with the risks of neonatal death and long-term disability, and non-intervention, with the risk of intrauterine death. In this situation it is particularly important that parents are prepared for all eventualities and spend time visiting the intensive care baby unit discussing options with the pediatricians and obstetricians before a final decision is reached.

### 8.5.6 POSTDELIVERY FOLLOW-UP

Once they have managed the initial postpartum maternal complications, obstetricians often find it difficult to maintain contact with patients who have been delivered prematurely. These patients often leave hospital without a baby. Either they have suffered a stillbirth or they spend many weeks attending the intensive care baby unit. Continued support from their obstetrician during this time is impor-

tant. It is our practice to review our prematurely delivered mothers at our daycare unit 7–10 days after discharge. This provides an opportunity to assess maternal wellbeing, offer emotional support and adjust drug therapy if necessary. Further appointments are made according to the needs of the patient. All women who have suffered a perinatal loss are seen by their obstetrician 4–6 weeks postdelivery and at varying intervals thereafter according to their needs.

### 8.6 SUMMARY

The effect of hypertension in pregnancy on the fetus cannot be judged on the basis of maternal wellbeing. It is thus crucial to apply a comprehensive and clinically useful testing system to assess fetal wellbeing in every hypertensive pregnancy. Multiple parameter testing is recommended using real-time ultrasound, fetal heart rate monitoring and Doppler ultrasound. The significance of the test results must be interpreted in the light of pregnancy gestation and the recent trend in test results.

### REFERENCES

Bell, J. G., Ludomirsky, A., Bottalico, J. *et al.* (1992) The effect of improvement of umbilical artery absent end-diastolic velocity on perinatal outcome. *Am. J. Obstet. Gynecol.*, **167**, 1015–1020.

Berkowitz, G. S., Mehalek, K. E., Chitkara, U. *et al.* (1988) Doppler umbilical velocimetry in the prediction of adverse outcome in pregnancies at risk of intrauterine growth retardation. *Obstet. Gynecol.*, **71**, 742–746.

Brioschi, P. A., Extermann, P., Terracina, D. *et al.* (1985) Antepartum nonstress fetal heart rate monitoring: systematic analysis of baseline patterns and decelerations as an adjunct to reactivity in the prediction of fetal risks. *Am. J. Obstet. Gynecol.*, **153**, 633–639.

Brosens, I., Robertson, W. B. and Dixon, H. G. (1967) The physiological response of the vessels of the placental bed to normal pregnancy. *J. Pathol. Bacteriol.*, **93**, 569–573.

Castillo, R. A., Devoe, L. D., Arthgur, M. *et al.* (1989) The preterm nonstress test: effects of gestational age and length of study. *Am. J. Obstet. Gynecol.*, **160**, 172–175.

Chamberlain, G., Phillip, E., Howlett, B. *et al.* (1978) *British Births 1970, 2: Obstetric Care*, Heinemann, London.

Chamberlain, P. F., Manning, F. A., Morrison, I. *et al.* (1984) The relationship of marginal and decreased amniotic fluid volume to perinatal outcome. *Am. J. Obstet. Gynecol.*, **150**, 245–249.

Chudleigh, P. and Pearce, J. M. (1992) *Obstetric Ultrasound: How, Why and When*, Churchill Livingstone, Edinburgh.

Copel, J. A., Woudstra, B. R., Wentworth, R. *et al.* (1991) Hypoxia cannot be detected by the umbilical S/D ratio in fetal lambs. *J. Maternal–Fetal Invest.*, **1**, 219–221.

Croom, C. S., Banias, B. B., Ramos-Santos, E. *et al.* (1992) Do semiquantitative amniotic fluid indexes reflect actual volume? *Am. J. Obstet. Gynecol.*, **167**, 995–999.

Crowley, P., Chalmers I. and Keirse, M. J. (1990) The effects of corticosteroid administration before preterm delivery: an overview of the evidence from controlled trials. *Br. J. Obstet. Gynaecol.*, **97**, 11–25.

Devoe, L. D., Castillo, R. A. and Sherline, D. M. (1985) The nonstress test as a diagnostic test: a critical reappraisal. *Am. J. Obstet. Gynecol.*, **152**, 1047–1052.

Devoe, L. D., McKenzie, J., Searle, N. S. *et al.* (1985) Clinical sequelae of the extended nonstress test. *Am. J. Obstet. Gynecol.*, **151**,1074–1078.

Devoe, L. D., Gardner, P., Dear, C. *et al.* (1990) The diagnostic values of concurrent nonstress testing, amniotic fluid measurement, and Doppler velocimetry in screening a general high-risk population. *Am. J. Obstet. Gynecol.*, **163**, 1040–1048.

Devoe, L. D., Youssef, A. A., Gardner, P. *et al.* (1992) Refining the biophysical profile with a risk-related evaluation of test performance. *Am. J. Obstet. Gynecol.*, **167**, 346–352.

Divon, M. Y., Girz, B. A., Lieblich, R. *et al.* (1989) Clinical management of the fetus with markedly diminished umbilical artery end-diastolic flow. *Am. J. Obstet. Gynecol.*, **161**, 1523–1527.

Fairlie, F. M. (1991) Doppler flow velocimetry in hypertension in pregnancy. *Clin. Perinatol.*, **18**, 749–778.

Fairlie, F. M., Moretti, M., Walker, J. J. *et al.* (1991) Determinants of perinatal outcome in pregnancy-induced hypertension with absence of umbilical artery end-diastolic frequencies. *Am. J. Obstet. Gynecol.*, **164**, 1084–1089.

Fitzgerald, D. E. and Drumm J. E. (1977) Noninvasive measurement of human fetal circulation using ultrasound: a new method. *Br. Med. J.*, **ii**, 1450–1452.

Friedman, E. A. and Neff, R. K. (1977) *Pregnancy Hypertension: A Systematic Evaluation of Clinical Diagnostic Criteria*, PSG Publishing, Littleton, MA.

Kawi, A. and Pasamanick, B. (1958) The association of factors of pregnancy with the development of reading disorders in childhood. *J. A. M. A.*, **166**, 1420–1423.

Keegan, K. A. and Paul, R. H. (1980) Antepartum fetal heart rate testing IV. The nonstress test as a primary approach. *Am. J. Obstet. Gynecol.*, **136**, 75–80.

Lagrew, D. C., Pircon, R. A., Nageotte, M. *et al.* (1992) How frequently should the amniotic fluid index be repeated? *Am. J. Obstet. Gynecol.*, **169**, 1129–1133.

Lilienfeld, A. and Pasamanick, B. (1954) Association of maternal and fetal factors with the development of epilepsy: 1. Abnormalities in the prenatal and perinatal periods. *J. A. M. A.*, **155**, 719–724.

Lilienfeld, A. and Pasamanick, B. (1955) The association of prenatal and perinatal factors with the development of cerebral palsy and epilepsy. *Am. J. Obstet. Gynecol.*, **70**, 93–101.

Lin, C. C., Lindheimer, M. D., River, P. *et al.* (1982) Fetal outcome in hypertensive disorders of pregnancy. *Am. J. Obstet. Gynecol.*, **142**, 255–260.

McParland, P. and Pearce, J. M. (1992) Signal acquisition and reporting results, in *Doppler Ultrasound in Perinatal Medicine*, (ed. J. M. Pearce), Oxford University Press, Oxford, p. 63–81.

Manning, F. A., Platt, L. D. and Sipos, L. (1980) Antepartum fetal evaluation: development of a fetal biophysical profile. *Am. J. Obstet. Gynecol.*, **136**, 787–795.

Manning, F. A., Morrison, I., Harman, C. R. *et al.* (1990) The abnormal fetal biophysical profile score. V. Predictive accuracy according to score composition. *Am. J. Obstet. Gynecol.*, **162**, 918–927.

Marlow, N., Roberts, B. L. and Cooke, R. W. I. (1989) Motor skills in extremely low birthweight children at the age of 6 years. *Arch. Dis. Child.*, **64**, 839–847.

Martin, T. N. and Tupper, W. R. C. (1975) The management of severe toxaemia in patients less than 36 weeks gestation. *Obstet. Gynecol.*, **54**, 602–605.

Montan, S. and Ingemarsson, I. (1989) Intrapartum fetal heart rate patterns in pregnancies complicated by hypertension. *Am. J. Obstet. Gynecol.*, **160**, 283–288.

Moore, T. R. and Cayle, J. E. (1990) The amniotic fluid index in normal human pregnancy. *Am. J. Obstet. Gynecol.*, **162**, 1168–1172.

Morrow, R. J., Adamson, S. L., Bull, S. B. *et al.* (1989) The effect of placental embolization on the umbilical artery waveform in sheep. *Am. J. Obstet. Gynecol.*, **161**, 1055–1060.

Morrow, R. J., Adamson, S. L., Bull, S. B. *et al.* (1990) Hypoxic acidaemia, hyperviscosity and maternal hypertension do not affect the umbilical artery velocity waveform in fetal sheep. *Am. J. Obstet. Gynecol.*, **163**, 1313–1320.

Nicolaides, K. H., Bilardo, C. M., Soothill, P. W. *et al.* (1988) Absence of end diastolic frequencies in the umbilical artery: a sign of fetal hypoxia and acidosis. *Br. Med. J.*, **297**, 1026–1027.

Odendall, H. J., Pattinson, R. C., DuToit, R. *et al.* (1987) Fetal and neonatal outcome in patients with severe preeclampsia before 34 weeks. *S. Afr. Med. J.*, **71**, 555–558.

Odendall, H. J., Pattinson, R. C., DuToit, R. *et al.* (1988) Frequent fetal heart rate monitoring for early detection of abruptio placentae in severe proteinuric hypertension. *S. Afr. Med. J.*, **74**, 19–21.

Ounsted, M., Moar, V. A. and Scott, A. (1985) Risk factors associated with small-for-dates and large-for-dates infants. *Br. J. Obstet. Gynaecol.*, **92**, 226–232.

Pasamanick, B. Rogers, M. E. and Lilienfeld, A. M. (1956) Pregnancy experience and the development of childhood behaviour disorder. *Am. J. Psychiat.*, **112**, 613–317.

Phelan, J. P., Ahn, M. O., Smith, C. V. *et al.* (1987) Amniotic fluid index measurements. *J. Reprod. Med.*, **32**, 601–604.

Robertson, W. B. Brosens, I. and Dixon, H. G. (1967) The pathological response of the vessels of the placental bed to hypertensive pregnancy *J. Pathol. Bacteriol.*, **93**, 581–592.

Rutherford, S. E., Phelan, J. P., Smith, C. V. *et al.* (1987) The four quadrant assessment of amniotic fluid volume. *Obstet. Gynecol.*, **70**, 353–356.

Scottish Stillbirth and Neonatal Death Report (1985) Scottish stillbirth and neonatal death report, Information Services Division, Scottish Health Services Common Services Agency, Edinburgh.

Seeds, J. W. (1984) Impaired fetal growth: ultrasonic evaluation and clinical management. *Obstet. Gynecol.*, **64**, 577–581.

Sibai, B. M., Spinnato, J. A., Watson, D. L. *et al.* (1984) Pregnancy outcome in 303 cases with severe preeclampsia. *Obstet. Gynecol.*, **64**, 319–325.

Sibai, B. M., Taslimi, M., Abdella T. N. *et al.* (1985) Maternal and perinatal outcome of conservative management of severe preeclampsia in the midtrimester. *Am. J. Obstet. Gynecol.*, **152**, 32–37.

Szymonowicz, W. and Yu, V. Y. H. (1987) Severe pre-eclampsia and infants of very low birthweight. *Arch. Dis. Child.*, **62**, 712–616.

Taylor, D. J., Howie, P. W., Davidson, J. *et al.* (1985) Do pregnancy complications contribute to neurodevelopmental disability? *Lancet*, **i**, 713–716.

Trudinger, B. J., Giles, W. B., Cook, C. M. *et al.* (1985) Fetal umbilical artery flow velocity waveforms and placental resistance: clinical significance. *Br. J. Obstet. Gynaecol.*, **92**, 23–30.

Vintzileos, A. M. and Tsapanos, V. (1992) Biophysical assessment of the fetus. *Ultrasound Obstet. Gynecol.*, **2**, 133–143.

Vintzileos, A. M., Campbell, W. A., Nochimson, D. J. *et al.* (1987) The use and misuse of the fetal biophysical profile. *Am. J. Obstet. Gynecol.*, **156**, 527–533.

# THE MANAGEMENT OF MILD/MODERATE HYPERTENSION IN PREGNANCY – THE USE OF ANTENATAL DAYCARE ASSESSMENT

*James J. Walker*

## 9.1 INTRODUCTION

Hypertension is a common problem, occurring in around 12–15% of all pregnancies (Cunningham and Lindheimer, 1992). It remains one of the major causes of maternal death (Redman, 1988; Turnbull *et al.*, 1989). Because of this perceived risk, obstetricians often admit a patient found to be hypertensive to hospital for closer observation (Chamberlain *et al.*, 1978a; Hall, Chang and MacGillivray, 1980). The result of this approach is that pregnancy hypertension is responsible for around 25% of antenatal admissions (Hall, Chang and MacGillivray, 1980). However, it is obvious that the majority of hypertensive pregnant patients have a satisfactory outcome. This would imply that there is an overdiagnosis of the problem with poor predictive value of antenatal screening and assessment of actual risk.

There are various reasons for this. Blood pressure is a biological measurement and is inherently variable (Redman, Beilin and Bonnar, 1977). Studies carried out with ambulatory blood pressure measurement have demonstrated marked variation on a minute to minute basis (Halligan *et al.*, 1991). Even if the assessments are thought to be accurate, blood pressure measurement is part of a continuum and the definition of hypertension is a relatively arbitrary level (Redman and Jefferies, 1988). It is not the hypertension itself that matters but the risks that any given blood pressure level brings. The risk for the mother would appear to increase after the diastolic blood pressure has reached 110 mmHg (Goldby and Beilin, 1972), whereas an increased risk to the baby has been shown to correlate with a diastolic blood pressure above 95 mmHg (Chamberlain *et al.*, 1970). To allow some leeway in the diagnosis, a diastolic blood pressure measurement of over 90 mmHg at phase 4 (muffling) is generally taken as the level when hypertension in pregnancy is diagnosed and the potential risk is increased for the mother and baby. This does not take into account the normal changes of blood pressure levels or the underlying cause of hypertension.

Blood pressure falls in pregnancy to a low at around 18 weeks (MacGillivray, Rose and Rowe, 1969). It then rises again to reach levels approaching the normal non-pregnant level by term. This implies that a diastolic blood pressure of 95 mmHg is more abnormal at 30

*Hypertension in Pregnancy*
Edited by J.J. Walker and N.F. Gant. Published by Chapman & Hall, 1997 ISBN 0 412 30910 6

weeks than at 39 weeks and the concomitant risks may also be different. The perinatal mortality is far higher in women who were hypertensive below 30 weeks compared with those at term.

Raised blood pressure in pregnancy can be due to various underlying causes, not all of which increase the risk to the mother or baby. Preeclampsia is now generally accepted as a specific syndrome consisting of hypertension occurring in the later half of a primigravid pregnancy with the presence of proteinuria (Barron, 1992). This occurs in around 3–5% of pregnancies. The risk to the mother and baby is highest in this situation as the condition is more likely to be progressive. It is important in the assessment of each woman that she is investigated for evidence of potential progression of the disease, which will highlight those hypertensive pregnancies at increased risk (Walker, 1987)

Preeclampsia is a multisystem disease (Friedman, Taylor and Roberts, 1991). The problem would appear to originate in the placental bed, where there is a failure of adequate trophoblastic invasion. The cause of this is probably an abnormal immunological interaction between the mother and baby. These changes lead to a relative failure of trophoblastic invasion and diminished maternal blood flow to the placenta and can result in placental ischemia. A 'Factor X' is then released that causes the systemic changes noted. This is associated with an increase in free radical activity. This, plus increased cytokine activity, leads to a generalized membrane disorder, particularly the vascular endothelium. Vascular hypertension is one manifestation of these changes. Other membranes are also affected leading to increased platelet activity (Redman, Bonnar and Beilin, 1978; Walker *et al.*, 1989), liver damage (Lubbe, 1984), renal damage (Redman, Beilin and Wilkinson, 1976) and vascular permeability (Goldby and Beilin, 1972). Preeclampsia may have a genetic basis (Arngrimsson *et al.*, 1990, 1993), relating to abnormalities on the

angiotensinogen gene. This may relate to the susceptibility of developing hypertension and accentuates the importance of family history in the prediction of this disease.

Therefore, the condition of hypertension can present in multiple ways with differing effects in each individual patient. There are various investigations that can give information concerning the degree of systemic effect and the probability of progression. This requires that each patient be approached in an individualistic way without preexisting ideas of diagnosis or risk.

## 9.2 RISKS TO THE MOTHER

Hypertension in pregnancy remains a major cause of maternal mortality throughout the world (Duley, 1992). It remains a problem in the UK (Turnbull *et al.*, 1989). There is an increase in maternal morbidity associated with hypertension. Eclampsia is seen as the classic non-fatal complication of preeclampsia but this is now rare in the UK, with a current incidence of around 3/10 000 deliveries. The average obstetrician may not see an eclamptic patient on their on-call day in any 5-year period. However, admission to hospital was still common in the 1970s because of the fear of complications occurring. This management dates from the 1950s (Hamlin, 1952) and led to approximately 25% of all antenatal admissions being due to hypertension. Overdiagnosis of the hypertensive risk was common and over 50% of patients admitted were found to be normotensive on admission. Despite this policy, maternal and perinatal mortality from hypertension in pregnancy did not change over a 30-year period (Turnbull, 1987). This routine admission of patients with hypertension has been challenged (Mathews, Patel and Sengupta, 1971) as there appears to be no evidence to show that bed rest is of benefit (Crowther and Chalmers, 1989; Mathews, 1977). Admission rates have reduced in recent years with the increased use of antihypertensive drugs and the development of daycare units (Hutton *et al.*, 1992).

## 9.3 RISKS TO THE FETUS

Hypertension in pregnancy is a major cause of fetal mortality (Chamberlain *et al.*, 1978b; Connon, 1992). There is also increased morbidity relating to intrauterine growth retardation and long-term neurological damage from the complications of iatrogenic prematurity. In the absence of placental insufficiency, there appears to be little adverse effect of hypertension in pregnancy to the fetus.

## 9.4 THE DILEMMA

Hypertension is an accepted serious complication of pregnancy that can affect all body systems but it is realized that most women with the diagnosis have no increased morbidity or morality. This produces a management dilemma. There is a need to closely assess and monitor the at-risk pregnancies but admission may not be necessary. Each patient should have their risk assessed individually. Blood pressure is very variable and the problem is often overdiagnosed. Other factors should be taken into account. The presence of proteinuria and abnormalities of platelets and uric acid appear to increase the risk. Early-onset disease would appear to more serious (Moore and Redman, 1983) than later-onset disease, with a poorer outcome for mother and baby (Sibai, 1991). Therefore, gestation of onset would also appear to be an important parameter. All this implies that the management of hypertension in pregnancy should not be based on blood pressure alone. All aspects must be taken into account.

## 9.5 A STEPWISE MANAGEMENT OF HYPERTENSION IN PREGNANCY

The basis of the management of hypertension in pregnancy is comprehensive antenatal care. Monitoring of the blood pressure is probably the most important investigation in the second and third trimester. Any change in the antenatal care system should not underestimate this. However, it must be remembered that this is a screening test and does not diagnose hypertension. It is an important method of selecting the at-risk groups. Other, more sensitive methods of prediction of preeclampsia have been proposed (Dekker, 1991) but none has been found to be accurate or clinically useful. Angiotensin infusions have been used successfully but are invasive, time-consuming and potentially dangerous (Dekker, Makovitz and Wallenburg, 1990; Gant *et al.*, 1973). If prediction were possible, close monitoring and prevention of disease development of progression might be possible (Walker, 1987; Dekker and Sibai, 1993). The encouraging studies into the family history and genetics of preeclampsia may help in this area in the future (Arngrimsson *et al.*, 1990, 1993)

Apart from elevated antenatal blood pressure, there are other accepted 'at risk' groups who should be offered closer monitoring. They are those with preexisting hypertension, a past history of preeclampsia in a previous pregnancy and those with a family history of preeclampsia or cardiovascular disease.

Those patients who are thought to be at increased risk, along with those who are discovered to have mild/moderate hypertension during pregnancy, are all suitable for referral for daycare assessment (Walker, 1987)

## 9.6 WHAT IS DAYCARE?

Daycase care is becoming increasingly popular in all aspects of medicine, particularly in surgery (Bartoli *et al.*, 1992). It has been found to reduce costs and increase the efficiency of use of resources (Burn, 1992). There is also a danger that the drive for efficiency can move inappropriate procedures to outpatient facilities. Daycare developments should aim to at least maintain the level of care provided but reduce the need for admission to hospital, which is not only expensive but also inconvenient to the patient.

The system works well when there is a specific protocol for daycare management of a particular problem (Broadbent *et al.*, 1992). Therefore, in principle, daycare obstetrics would appear to be an attractive option for care of the 'at-risk' hypertensive pregnant patient. Standardized protocols can be produced, targeted care and investigations can be provided and women, often with other small children, can be kept as outpatients.

## 9.7 THE PROBLEMS OF SETTING UP AND RUNNING A DAYCARE SYSTEM

Daycare must be part of a comprehensive antenatal care system (Redman, 1982). It is the 'middle ground' between normal antenatal care and admission to hospital. There has to be free access to the system from all providers of antenatal care without judgment or penalty. The system must be flexible to allow patients to be moved from inpatient to daycare and back again if the risk is thought to have changed. The daycare unit must have decision-making powers and not be a simple test area. If the measurement of the blood pressure is seen as similar to cervical screening, the daycare unit should be seen as the colposcopy clinic. It should be able to assess, manage and treat.

Therefore, the factors that are paramount to the safe development and running of the unit are the decision of who and why to refer for daycare, the development of the daycare protocols and rules of assessment of the patient when results are available. These factors influence the benefit that the system will give the hospital.

## 9.8 WHO SHOULD ATTEND

In the Glasgow Royal Maternity Hospital (GRMH), the aim of the developing Daycare Unit was to monitor all patients thought to be at risk of a hypertensive problem during or immediately after pregnancy. No firm guidelines for patient selection were issued, as each obstetrician has different criteria of risk. It was felt that if the unit was too judgmental on the referral criteria, some professionals might be reluctant to refer. However, general guidelines about risk factors were given but there was no criticism of those who did not want to use the system. The consultant obstetrician was free either to refer the patient to daycare or admit her to hospital as he saw fit. The main reason for referral to the Daycare Unit at GRMH was a diagnosis of hypertension in patients attending the antenatal clinic. An important role for the Daycare Unit has been as a referral unit from outlying clinics, particularly those run by GPs and midwives. It has allowed the use of these clinics to be increased with the knowledge that, if there is any concern, easy referral for a second opinion is available.

## 9.9 THE DEVELOPMENT OF THE DAYCARE UNIT

The main role of the Daycare Unit is to provide a diagnostic and assessment service for those thought to be at risk. it is not a simple test center. It must have easy access for the patient, simple referral methods for the clinician and trained staff to receive the patients, carry out the investigations and make a management assessment based on the results. This is the critical factor. No benefit from daycare will be achieved unless there is a management component. A decision is required as to whether the patient requires admission or not. This should be done on site in the unit by those experienced in doing so. This requires senior trained staff to supervise the service and be available daily for advice.

### 9.9.1 THE METHOD OF REFERRAL

When there is a decision to refer to daycare, the unit is phoned and an appointment made. The patient can be seen either on the same day or on a day suitable to the patient and the unit. Generally, the attendance will be within the next 4 days. The referring professional is free to attend the Unit on the day of referral to be involved in any management decision if he or she desires, although this is not necessary.

### 9.9.2 FACILITIES

In GRMH, the unit initially used the day area of one of the antenatal wards and then gradually took over larger areas when space was released by the reduction of admissions. It is presently housed in a ward area adjacent to the ultrasound department. It comprises three separate rooms: a sitting area where patients stay most of the time; a center room for the nursing station, computer center and two cubicles for counseling; and a third area, which is used for monitoring, with four beds, each with a cardiotocograph monitor. There is also a dedicated continuous wave Doppler ultrasound machine available.

The unit has been open for five days a week from 8 a.m. until 5 p.m. since August 1981. It now opens on a Saturday morning as well as most public holidays. Initially, the antenatal ward staff ran the unit. From 1983 a dedicated midwifery sister was allocated and the present staff comprises two midwifery sisters, a staff midwife and a student midwife. This level of nursing staff had become necessary because of the increasing use of daycare for other areas of

high-risk antenatal monitoring. It now houses the clinics for women with twins, diabetes, small-for-dates and recurrent miscarriage. It was also appreciated that if student midwives were not allocated to the unit they would not be exposed to many patients requiring antenatal monitoring, as the admission rates dropped.

### 9.9.3 UNIT PROTOCOLS

Another purpose of the unit was to centralize and standardize the monitoring of the hypertensive patient. It was felt that it was important to have a comprehensive monitoring program for these at-risk patients. Also, by standardizing the monitoring protocols, it has been possible to assess the value of the various tests available.

As blood pressure was known to vary, it was decided to use five blood pressure readings taken over 3 hours and average the results. As progressive preeclampsia is characterized by a fall in platelet count, a rise in uric acid and the presence of proteinuria, these investigations are used as the mainstay of maternal assessment and are available at 12 noon on the day of attendance to allow an accurate risk assessment (Table 9.1).

Full estimation of urea and electrolytes and liver function tests are also carried out but these results are not available on the day of attendance. The patient attends between 9.00 and 9.30 in the morning. Venesection is performed

**Table 9.1**   The monitoring tests carried out at the daycare unit; the results should be available on the day of attendance to allow for an accurate risk assessment

| *Maternal* | *Fetal* |
| --- | --- |
| Five blood pressure readings over 3 hours | Cardiotocograph |
| Abdominal palpation | Fetal weight estimation |
| Serum uric acid | Liquor volume estimation |
| Serum urea | Umbilical Doppler |
| Hemoglobin | Biophysical profile |
| Platelet count | |
| Urinalysis for protein | |

and a blood sample is taken. The laboratory results are telephoned or faxed directly to the unit when available. No investigation should be looked at in isolation, as correlation is not absolute. The patient assessments are based on the results of all these tests taken together.

Fetal assessment is based on seperate targeted investigations. After 28 weeks gestation, a cardiotocograph is carried out on all patients for 40 minutes. A normal cardiotocograph was taken as one with four accelerations within the 40-minute period, beat-to-beat variation of at least 20 bpm and the absence of decelerations. This is the mainstay investigation of fetal wellbeing.

An ultrasound examination for fetal weight estimation, liquor volume assessment using the amniotic fluid index and Doppler ultrasound of the umbilical artery are used to assess intrauterine environment in pregnancies that are thought to be at particular risk, either because of past history or after initial assessment. A full biophysical profile has added value but is time-consuming and, if the fetus is thought to be at that high a risk, the patient should be admitted to hospital for closer monitoring.

### 9.9.4 PATIENT ASSESSMENT

All results are available by 12 noon on the day of attendance. The patient is then interviewed and further management is discussed. Although the referring consultant is able to assess the patient if he wishes, most of the assessments are carried out by the medical staff who are, at least, specially trained registrars.

Patients are classified as being of normal/low risk, mild/moderate risk or high risk of blood pressure problems using the four main parameters: blood pressure (average of five readings), platelet count, uric acid and urinalysis (Table 9.2).

The results of the assessment of fetal wellbeing are used as a seperate consideration regarding further management. If there is evidence of poor growth or diminished liquor

volume, further monitoring is arranged. If there is any sign of fetal compromise, the patient is admitted for further investigation and the need for delivery is assessed.

If thought to be normal or low-risk, the patient is referred back to the referring antenatal clinic. This return appointment must be within 10 days of their Daycare appointment unless she is less than 20 weeks gestation, when an appointment within a month is arranged. If the patient's blood pressure is found to be elevated in the future, she can be referred back to the Daycare Unit at any time. If moderate risk, the patient is brought back for a return visit at the Daycare Unit, either the same or the following week to assess any progress of the disease. If the risk is thought to be high, because of persistent blood pressure elevation above 100 mmHg diastolic, low platelets, high uric acid or evidence of fetal compromise, the patient is admitted to hospital on either the same or the next day, when further observation and management would be carried out.

If the patient is reassessed at Daycare, all investigations are repeated, along with the ultrasound estimations of fetal wellbeing, and the same criteria are used for management decisions. Obviously, a clearer picture of progression can be seen with serial values. If there is evidence of disease progression because of rising uric acid or falling platelets, the patients will be followed closely in Daycare or admitted, depending on the risk assessment.

If the patient is near term, induction can be arranged from Daycare without need to refer back to the patient's consultant. This allows consistency of care provision and streamlining of patient care without repetition of attendance and conflicting advice.

### 9.9.5 ADMISSION TO HOSPITAL

It is important to realize that daycare is only a component in the overall management of hypertensive patients in pregnancy. After

**Table 9.2** The risk categories used at daycare for the assessment of patients. To be low-risk, all the parameters must be met. If any of the parameters in the moderate- or high-risk category are met, the patient is classified into that group. Therefore, the patient is classified into the highest-risk category that any of the parameters met. Those at low risk are referred back to the antenatal clinic, moderate-risk patients are referred back to daycare and high-risk patients are admitted to hospital

**Low risk (if all of the following are found)**
- Average diastolic blood pressure < 90 mmHg
- Uric acid < 350 mmol/l
- Platelet count ≥ 200 × 10⁹
- Absence of proteinuria
- Reactive cardiotocograph
- Absence of signs IUGR and normal liquor volume

**Moderate risk (if any of the following are found)**
- Average diastolic blood pressure ≥ 90 but < 100 mmHg
- Uric acid ≥ 350 but < 450 mmol/l
- Platelet count < 200 but ≥ 100 × 10⁹
- Proteinuria < ++ or < 1.5 g/24 h
- Reactive cardiotocograph
- Signs of IUGR but adequate liquor volume

**High risk (if any of the following are found)**
- Average diastolic blood pressure ≥ 100 mmHg
- Uric acid ≥ 450 mmol/l
- Platelet count < 100 × 10⁹
- Proteinuria ≥ ++ or ≥ 1.5 g/24 h
- Non-reactive cardiotocograph
- Signs of IUGR and reduced liquor volume

admission, further monitoring is required along similar protocols. If the patient is treated with antihypertensive drugs, the blood pressure may settle enough to allow discharge from hospital, when further monitoring can be provided in the antenatal daycare unit as an outpatient with continuing medication (Walker, 1991).

At all times, the system allows flexibility to overrule the protocol and bring the patient back to daycare or to admit them to hospital if there is any doubt about the safety of the mother or the fetus. A patient may have several admissions/discharges over the length of her pregnancy. The aim is keep her out of hospital as much as possible as long as it is thought to be safe.

Another important role of daycare is the postnatal follow-up of patients who have not settled to normal after delivery. They can be allowed home on therapy for close (often daily) monitoring. Many will be attending the hospital to visit their baby in the special care unit anyway. This means that there is no need to wait for the patient's blood pressure to return to normal before discharge from hospital. She can be allowed home, often still on antihypertensive therapy, and her management can be continued by the same team that managed her in the hospital. If the blood pressure does not settle by 6 weeks, further investigations should be instigated, with referral to other professionals for help. The most likely cause is underlying renal disease.

## 9.10 ASSESSMENT OF THE EFFECT OF DAYCARE

In an attempt to assess the effects of daycare, all patients who attended the Daycare Unit in Glasgow Royal Maternity Hospital between the years 1981 and 1989 were followed up until delivery and the outcome was noted. Hospital admissions, the number of inpatient days and the final diagnoses were obtained from the hospital records department and from the Information Services Department of the Scottish Home and Health Department. Antenatal inpatient nights were counted for every April and averaged as confirmation of the reduction of antenatal bed occupancy. Statistical comparisons of the changes seen were carried out using Fisher's exact test.

### 9.10.1 NUMBER OF REFERRALS

Daycare began with referrals from only two consultant units in August 1981. Only 25 patients were seen before the end of the first year. As the success of daycare became recognized, more of the consultants utilized the service and by 1984 all the doctors (eight) in GRMH referred patients to daycare. The number of attendances remained steady following this and by the end of 1989 a total of 3156 patients had attended in the 10-year period. Over the last 6 years of the decade around 12% of the total number of deliveries were referred to the Unit because of a perceived risk of hypertension. Most (59%) of the referrals were primigravidae but 41% were parous women, who would potentially benefit most from non-admission. The most significant change has been the reduction in the number of inpatient days due to hypertension. In the years 1980–81 there were over 2200 inpatient days as compared to under 750 for 1988–89. This is a highly significant reduction of 70% ($p < 0.0001$).

The average antenatal bed occupancy for all reasons during April for the year 1981 was 57 per night and this had fallen to 20 per night in 1989 ($p < 0.0001$). Obviously, this is not purely due to a reduction in admissions of hypertensive patients and it reflects the increasing use of daycare for all high-risk monitoring.

### 9.10.2 REASONS FOR REFERRAL

By far the most common reason for referral was a diagnosis of pregnancy-induced hypertension at the antenatal clinic (2773 referrals). The rest were mostly related to essential hypertension or renal disease (221 referrals) and a further 142 who were seen because of past history of hypertension in pregnancy and who were normotensive at the time of referral. A number of patients were referred because of isolated proteinuria or some other sign of potential development of preeclampsia. Most of them were found not to have a problem.

### 9.10.3 GESTATION AT REFERRAL

The average gestation at referral was $33 \pm 6$ weeks and most patients (1925) were between 32 and 40 weeks. However, 568 presented before 28 and 190 after 40 weeks. Therefore, the bulk of the patients present near term and can be monitored closely until labor occurs or induction is planned. This allows a reduction in planned induction unless there are signs of increased risk. There is no need to routinely induce hypertensive patients at around term. The value of daycare to the earlier group is to assess the likelihood of progression and the need for admission and/or treatment with antihypertensive drugs.

### 9.10.4 REFERRAL BLOOD PRESSURE

Since the main reason for referral is pregnancy hypertension, it is not surprising that most referral diastolic blood pressures (DBP) were between 90 and 100 mmHg diastolic (68%), but 9% of the patients were normotensive at the time of referral. Since many obstetricians feel that admission is mandatory when the (DBP) is at or above 100 mmHg, it is interesting to note that 23% of the referrals were in this category and 5% had a DBP above 110 mmHg. The average DBP found at daycare was 10 mmHg lower than the referral DBP, and the majority of the patients had an average DBP of below 90 mmHg and were considered to be normal. Of the patients with referral DBP of over 90 mmHg only 25% came under the same category at daycare assessment. This demonstrates the relative over-diagnosis of hypertension at the outpatient clinic and confirms the value of reassessment of the risk at an Antenatal Day Unit. Obviously not all these women would have been admitted but many would, even if only for 24 hours.

## 9.10.5 ATTENDANCES

The Daycare Unit was primarily a Daycare Assessment Unit. The majority (62%) of the patients were seen only once. However, the average number of visits was $2.1 \pm 0.7$ and 461 patients had more than three visits. If the patients are seen as high-risk because of the results of the monitoring tests or past history, it is normal to follow them on a weekly basis to assess disease progression and continued fetal wellbeing. No patient is seen more than three times in one week. If the patient is thought to require more frequent attendances than this, she is admitted to hospital.

## 9.10.6 DAYCARE DIAGNOSIS

At the first Daycare attendance, patients were grouped into three risk categories: normal, low-risk or high-risk. Most of the patients were assessed as normal or low-risk. Overall, 68% were referred back to the antenatal clinic for continuing care after either their first or subsequent visit. Only 4% required immediate admission to hospital. A number of the patients were referred back to Daycare at a later date. In total, 16% of the patients eventu-

ally required admission to hospital but this was delayed in around 75% of cases. If low risk was diagnosed, only 6% of the women were later admitted to hospital because of hypertension. If moderate risk was diagnosed, the risk of admission was 29%. Therefore, of the patients with moderate risk at the time of daycare assessment, a significant number developed worsening hypertension, highlighting the need for continuing vigilance at the antenatal clinic or further Daycare attendances. No patient who was assessed as high-risk reduced their risk assessment at a later date.

## 9.10.7 MATERNAL OUTCOME

There are those who claim that, even if the blood pressure settles after initial diagnosis, the women are still at risk. Because of this concern that severe hypertension may occur, all patients are advised about worsening clinical signs, particularly headache, visual disturbances and abdominal pain. In fact, of all those managed as outpatients, only three patients developed severe hypertension with symptoms prior to their next appointment, one of whom had failed to return for her scheduled follow-up appointment. Apart from these three patients, all the rest did well and there were no cases of maternal death or eclampsia in the outpatient group.

## 9.10.8 FETAL OUTCOME

The overall perinatal mortality was 3.5/1000, about 35% of the average for the hospital over this period. The outcome was worse in patients admitted compared to those managed as outpatients, because of the selection of severity. There were three perinatal deaths in the outpatient group. One patient was seen on a Friday and thought to be of moderate risk, but returned after the weekend with an intrauterine death. Another perinatal death was due to a placental abruption (one of the two abruptions in the overall group) and the third was due to a congenital heart defect. The overall perinatal mortality rate was 1.1/1000 for the 2650 patients managed totally as outpatients.

### 9.11 HAS DAYCARE ACHIEVED ITS AIM?

If others are to copy the daycare system, it is important to assess whether it has achieved its aims. It does appear to be a safe method of caring for and assessing the hypertensive patient.

Daycare would appear to have achieved its primary aim of providing inpatient facilities on an outpatient basis. It has allowed the standardization of protocols for the management of hypertension in the hospital. It has reduced the number of antenatal admissions to hospital and the number of beds occupied. These findings have been confirmed by a randomized trial carried out in St James's Hospital in Leeds (Tuffnell *et al.*, 1992) and other audits of centers that have set up day units. The Leeds study randomized women to either admission or day unit care. The results demonstrated that the majority of the women did not require admission and could be managed through the day unit, reducing admissions. This study was far too small to demonstrate absolute safety with any confidence.

### 9.12 COMPARISON WITH OTHER HOSPITALS

Comparison with other hospitals appear to demonstrate benefits to the patients (Twaddle and Harper, 1992) and to hospital costs (Rosenburg and Twaddle, 1990). A comparison with four other large maternity hospitals in Central Scotland, which did not have daycare units is shown in Table 9.3.

These hospitals were chosen as being those nearest the Glasgow Royal Maternity Hospital and delivering around the same number of patients. The figures are for 1986 and 1987 and are taken from the Information Services Department of the Scottish Home and Health

Department. There is wide variation between the hospitals but the Glasgow Royal Maternity Hospital had fewer admissions and inpatient days per 1000 deliveries than any of the other hospitals. The size of the difference ranged from 41% to over 60%.

In the USA, admission for mild preeclampsia is common. Three studies carried out in Dallas and Memphis, in a total of 945 patients, appear to show benefit from hospital admission, but the results are similar in the gestation of referral and perinatal outcome to those seen in the GRMH with the use of the Antenatal Day Unit. In the USA, the patients were induced with favorable cervix at 36 weeks. Practice in Glasgow has demonstrated that, with daycare, routine induction is not necessary and the patients can be monitored through up to and past term in the Antenatal Day Unit. Previous studies have demonstrated that ambulatory care in mild/moderate hypertension does not increase perinatal or maternal morbidity (Crowther and Chalmers, 1989; Mathews, 1977). Therefore, it would appear that, with proper protocols and control, outpatient ambulatory care of the mildly/moderately hypertensive pregnant women is not only feasible but safe.

### 9.13 DISADVANTAGES

The main disadvantage of daycare is the perceived loss of control of patient care from the referring doctor to a central management unit. This requires a change of practice for many consultants. This change, with the trend for all normals to be seen by midwives or general practitioners, has led to a potential reduction in the role of the average consultant in antenatal care. This is resisted by many. The patients like the Antenatal Daycare Unit, with the reassurance it gives, and do not appear to object to the loss of contact with 'their' consultant. The patients can remain under their consultant's care and still benefit from the daycare facilities.

**Table 9.3** A comparison of number of admissions and inpatient days spent due to hypertension in pregnancy in Glasgow Royal Maternity Hospital and four other large maternity hospitals in Scotland without daycare units (totals for the years 1986–87)

| Hospital | No. of deliveries | Admissions | Admissions/ 1000 deliveries | No. of inpatient days | Inpatient days/ 1000 deliveries |
|---|---|---|---|---|---|
| A | 9077 | 478 | 53 | 1353 | 149 |
| B | 8641 | 446 | 52 | 2628 | 304 |
| D | 7200 | 349 | 48 | 1283 | 178 |
| GRMH | 8609 | 256 | 30 | 804 | 93 |

The reduction in bed requirement may be seen as an excuse to reduce numbers of attendant staff. This must be resisted, as the same number of patients are being looked after. However, daycare can facilitate a reduction in 'out of hours working' and the targeting of expensive, rationed resources to areas of need.

### 9.14 ALTERNATIVES TO DAYCARE

There are other, well-established alternatives to daycare management, leading many to believe that it is not necessary to develop the service in their hospitals. One alternative is home monitoring using community midwives. The GRMH unit has been compared favorably with this system as practiced in Aberdeen (Twaddle and Harper, 1992). General practitioners can also assess the patient as an outpatient, by getting the patient to see him or her in the surgery or at her home. The main advantage of daycare is the access to laboratory tests, methods of fetal assessment and the ability to make decisions on the day of testing. The concept has been developed and tested successfully in other units (Soothill *et al.*, 1991).

Blood pressure can be assessed at home with various electronic equipment, some able to transmit the results to the hospital (Dawson, Middlemiss and Vanner, 1989; Dawson *et al.*, 1989) This can also be done with home fetal monitoring using the cardiotocograph (James *et al.*, 1988) but this lacks personal contact and is more suited to patients requiring serial screening because of a bad past history, where reassurance is the main aim. It would be sensible, at least in the short term, to use existing facilities in obstetric hospitals before investing in the equipment required for home monitoring.

### 9.15 OTHER USE OF DAYCARE FACILITIES

One of the major benefits of the development of the Daycare Unit has been the expansion of its use into other areas of maternal/fetal surveillance (Soothill *et al.*, 1991). The patient groups that can benefit include those suspected as having intrauterine growth retardation (IUGR) and lack of fetal movements, but other specialized clinics can also be developed within the facilities where space and staff are available.

### 9.16 CONCLUSIONS

As a common disorder, hypertension has been a burden on the health service's resources in terms of manpower and hospital accommodation . The high prevalence of the condition, with its potential harmful effects for the mother and baby, makes it a difficult management problem for the obstetrician.

Pregnancy hypertension is thought to be unpredictable and most obstetricians would admit the hypertensive patient for closer monitoring of both mother and baby. This 'play-safe approach' can cause much inconvenience to the patient and her family. Mild to moderate disease carries little risk unless there is progression to the more severe form. Therefore, the majority of the patients can be managed safely at home if there is access to adequate fetal and maternal monitoring. The idea of outpatient management is not new, and Mathews (1977) showed that, in the absence of proteinuria, non-admission to hospital had no detrimental effect on the hypertensive patient. Inpatient management may vary between different hospitals but the cornerstone is to admit the patient to allow serial monitoring of blood pressure. Strict bedrest has been suggested as having therapeutic value but this has never been substantiated. As some patients will progress to more severe forms of the disease, it is important that there is early recognition of any signs of progression (Walker, 1987)

Daycare was envisaged as a system of reducing admissions to the hospital by providing a third option of antenatal care for the 'at-risk' patient. The aim was to provide inpatient monitoring facilities on an outpatient basis. This would allow an increased access to monitoring for all the hypertensive patients.

Other forms of monitoring have become available that allow closer monitoring of the fetus to be carried out on an outpatient basis. Home cardiotocography, district midwives measuring blood pressure at home and home blood pressure monitoring using battery sphygmomanometers have all been advocated. None of these methods use the adjunctive biochemical and hematological investigations normally available in the hospital setting. Studies have shown the predictive value of platelet count and uric acid estimation for the assessment of ongoing risk. The protocol that was developed encompassed all the facilities used for inpatient management and made them available for outpatients.

Daycare has developed rapidly because of the management flexibility it offers and the increasing faith in it that has developed among consultants in the hospital. This is

reflected by the steadily increasing number of referrals. A greater percentage of hypertensive patients are now fully monitored. There has been a fall in hypertensive admissions by nearly 70%. This has allowed a targeting of inpatient care to those requiring intensive monitoring and treatment. There is no evidence that the mothers or babies have suffered from non-admissions after introduction of the daycare system.

The advantage of daycare is that more than two-thirds of the patients were diagnosed as normal and were returned back to the routine antenatal system after the first visit. Follow-up of the patients shows that there is a chance that the patient may develop worsening hypertension. In those with increased risk of this, daycare also allows continuous close monitoring as an outpatient.

Initially, all the patients were assessed by a single trained doctor but, more recently, other members of staff have been trained in antenatal day unit management. It is important to provide relatively senior medical cover for daycare to make sure that there is adequate surveillance of the patients and that management decisions are maintained. This is important not only for patient safety but for the confidence of the consultants in the hospital. This confidence has been successfully built up, after some initial resistance, as the benefits of daycare were appreciated by both doctor and patient.

Daycare units are now well established in Scotland, over 75% of hospitals now having a designated daycare area, and many hospitals in England and other parts of Europe are following this example. The use of these areas varies widely. In Glasgow Royal Maternity Hospital and St James's University Hospital, Leeds, all forms of intensive monitoring are now offered to outpatients. This has helped to further reduce the inpatient load. The units also provide facilities for other specialist clinics such as diabetic, twin, epileptic, recurrent miscarriage, prepregnancy and prenatal diagnosis.

Three problems remain before daycare can be recommended as the main method of management of the 'at-risk' antenatal patient.

### 9.16.1 IS IT SAFE?

This was not a controlled trial. Daycare evolved out of a desire to improve the monitoring and diagnosis of hypertensive patients. Many obstetricians were wary of allowing patients home with a DBP above 90 mmHg. A controlled trial has been carried out in Leeds but it is too small to show evidence of safety. Since in the Glasgow experience there were only 11 perinatal deaths in 3156 patients, it would be difficult to show that admission to hospital is any safer for the mother or baby or that daycare is more dangerous.

### 9.16.2 IS IT COST-EFFECTIVE?

With a nearly 70% reduction in inpatient days, one would predict considerable saving on running costs. This, however, is difficult to prove. The hospital still needs most of the midwifery staff, as it delivers the same number of patients. The most significant saving would be on capital cost when designing a new maternity hospital with a purpose-built daycare facility or for a larger number of deliveries to be managed through the existing facilities. The cost comparison study carried out between the Glasgow Royal Maternity Hospital and Aberdeen Maternity Hospital, which uses domiciliary midwifes to check the patient's blood pressure at home, suggested that Glasgow is cheaper on a patient cost basis for the majority of the patients referred. There is a suggestion that a daycare unit might increase the overall hospital workload, despite reducing admission days, because of the daily load of patients requiring monitoring.

### 9.16.3 ARE ALL THESE TESTS NECESSARY?

The Daycare Unit was set up to provide blanket monitoring to make sure that the system did not miss any potential problems. It became obvious that many of the patients could have been diagnosed as low-risk without many of the adjunctive tests. The problem is that it was not possible to know which patients fell into this category before the Daycare appointment. It may be that many patients could be managed with a reduced battery of tests.

The overall conclusion for the experience in Glasgow and now in other parts of the UK and Europe is that daycare works and should be part of the available management protocol for all hypertensive patients.

### REFERENCES

Arngrimsson, R., Bjornsson, S., Geirsson, R. T. *et al.* (1990) Genetic and familial predisposition to eclampsia and preeclampsia in a defined population. *Br. J. Obstet. Gynaecol.*, **97**, 762–769.

Arngrimsson, R., Purandare, S., Connor, M. *et al.* (1993) Angiotensinogen – a candidate gene involved in preeclampsia. *Nat. Genet.*, **4**, 114–115.

Barron, W. M. (1992) The syndrome of preeclampsia. *Gastroenterol. Clin. North. Am.*, **21**, 851–872.

Bartoli, C., Zurrida, S., Clemente, C. and Cascinelli, N. (1992) Outpatient surgical treatment of cutaneous melanoma. *Melanoma Res.*, **1**, 385–390.

Broadbent, J. A., Hill, N. C., Molnar, B. G. *et al.* (1992) Randomized placebo controlled trial to assess the role of intracervical lignocaine in outpatient hysteroscopy. *Br. J. Obstet. Gynaecol.*, **99**, 777–779.

Burn, J. M. (1992) Costs of day case surgery. *Br. Med. J.*, **304**, 11–18.

Chamberlain, G. V. P., Lewis, P. J., De Swiet, M. and Bulpitt, C. J. (1978) How obstetricians manage hypertension in pregnancy. *Br. Med. J.*, **1**, 626–630.

Chamberlain, G. V. P., Phillip, E., Howlett, B. and Masters, K. (1978) *British Births 1970, 2: Obstetric Care*, Heinemann, London, 80–84.

Connon, A. F. (1992) An assessment of key aetiological factors associated with preterm birth and perinatal mortality. *Aust. NZ J. Ohstet. Gynaecol.*, **32**, 200–203.

Crowther, C. A. and Chalmers, I. (1989) Bed rest and hospitalisation during pregnancy, in *Effective Care in Pregnancy and Childbirth*, vol. 1, (eds I. Chalmers, M. Enkin and M. J. N. C. Keirse), Oxford University Press, Oxford, p. 624–632.

Cunningham, F. G. and Lindheimer, M. D. (1992) Hypertension in pregnancy. *N. Engl. J. Med.*, **326**, 927–932.

Dawson, A. J., Middlemiss, C. and Vanner, T. F. (1989a) Miniature electronic blood pressure monitor compared with a blind-reading mercury sphygmomanometer in pregnancy. *Eur. J. Obstet. Gynecol. Reprod. Biol.*, **33**, 147–153.

Dawson, A. J., Middlemiss, C., Gough, N. A. J. and Jones, M. E. (1989b) A randomised study of a domiciliary antenatal care scheme: the effect on hospital admissions. *Br. J. Obstet. Gynaecol.*, **96**, 1319–1322.

Dekker, G. A. (1991) Prediction of pregnancy-induced hypertensive disease. *Eur. J. Obstet. Gynecol. Reprod. Biol.*, **42** (Suppl), S36–S44.

Dekker, G. A., Makovitz, J. W. and Wallenburg, H. C. (1990) Prediction of pregnancy-induced hypertensive disorders by angiotensin II sensitivity and supine pressor test. *Br. J. Obstet. Gynaecol.*, **97**, 817–821.

Dekker, G. A. and Sibai, B. M. (1993) Low-dose aspirin in the prevention of preeclampsia and fetal growth retardation: rationale, mechanisms and clinical trials. *Am. J. Obstet. Gynecol.*, **168**, 214–227.

Duley, L. (1992) Maternal mortality associated with hypertensive disorders of pregnancy in Africa, Asia, Latin America and the Caribbean. *Br. J. Obstet. Gynaecol.*, **99**, 547–553.

Friedman, S. A., Taylor, R. N. and Roberts, J. M. (1991) Pathophysiology of preeclampsia. *Clin. Perinatol.*, **18**, 661–682.

Gant, N., Daley, G. l., Chand, S. *et al.* (1973) A study of angiotensin II pressor response throughout primigravid pregnancy. *J. Clin. Invest.*, **52**, 2682–2686.

Goldby, F. S. and Beilin, L. J. (1972) Relationship between arterial pressure and the permeability of arterioles to carbon particles in acute hypertension. *Cardiovasc. Res.*, **6**, 384–388.

Hall, M., Chang, P. K. and MacGillivray, I. (1980) Is routine antenatal care worthwhile? *Lancet*, **ii**, 78–80.

Halligan, A., O'Brien, E., O'Malley, K. *et al.* (1991) Clinical application of ambulatory blood pressure measurement in pregnancy. *J. Hypertens.*, **9** (Suppl), S75–S77.

Hamlin, R. H. J. (1952) The prevention of eclampsia and pre-eclampsia. *Lancet*, **i**, 64–68.

Hutton, J. D., James, D. K., Stirrat, G. M. *et al.* (1992) Management of severe pre-eclampsia and eclampsia by UK consultants. *Br. J. Obstet. Gynaecol.*, **99**, 554–556.

James, D., Paralta, B., Porter, S. *et al.* (1988) Fetal heart rate monitoring by telephone II. Clinical experience in four centres with a commercially produced system. *Br. J. Obstet. Gynaecol.*, **95**, 1024–1029.

Lubbe, W. F. (1984) Hypertension in pregnancy. Pathophysiology and management. *Drugs*, **28**, 170–188.

MacGillivray, I., Rose, G. and Rowe, B. (1969) Blood pressure survey in pregnancy. *Clin. Sci.*, **37**, 395–399.

Mathews, D. D. (1977) A randomised controlled trial of bed rest and sedation of normal activity and non-sedation in the management of non-albuminuric hypertension in pregnancy. *Br. J. Obstet. Gynaecol.*, **84**, 108–112.

Mathews, D. D., Patel, I. E. and Sengupta, S.M. (1971) Outpatient management of toxaemia. *J. Obstet. Gynaecol.*, Br Cwlth, **78**, 610–614.

Moore, M. P. and Redman, C. W. G. (1983) Case control study of severe pre-eclampsia of early onset. *Br. Med. J.*, **ii**, 580–584.

Redman, C. W. G. (1982) Screening for preeclampsia, in *Effectiveness and Satisfaction in Antenatal Care*, (eds M. Enkin and I. Chalmers), Spastics International Medical Publications, Heinemann Medical, London, p. 69–80.

Redman, C. W. G. (1988) Eclampsia still kills. *Br. Med. J.*, **296**, 1209–1210.

Redman, C. W. G., Beilin, L. J. and Bonnar, J. (1977) Variability of blood pressure in normal and abnormal pregnancy, in *Hypertension in Pregnancy*, (eds M. D. Lindheimer, A. l. Katz and F. P. Zuspan), John Wiley, New York, p. 53–57

Redman, C. W. G., Beilin, L. J. B. and Wilkinson, B. H. (1976) Plasma urate measurements in predicting fetal death in hypertensive pregnancy. *Lancet*, **i**, 1370–1374.

Redman, C. W. G., Bonnar, J. and Beilin, L. J. (1978) Early platelet consumption in pre-eclampsia. *Br. Med. J.*, **i**, 146–150.

Redman, C. W. G. and Jefferies, M. (1988) Revised definition of pre-eclampsia. *Lancet*, **i**, 809–812.

Rosenberg, K. and Twaddle, S. (1990) Screening and surveillance of pregnancy hypertension – an economic approach to the use of daycare, in *Baillières Clinical Obstetrics And Gynaecology, vol. 4: Antenatal Care*, (ed. M. Hall), Baillière Tindall, London, p. 89–107.

Sibai, B. M. (1991) Management of pre-eclampsia remote from term. *Eur. J. Obstet. Gynecol. Reprod. Biol.*, **42**(Suppl), S96–S101.

Soothill, P. W., Ajayi, R., Campbell, S. *et al.* (1991) Effect of a fetal surveillance unit on admission of antenatal patients to hospital. *Br. Med. J.*, **303**, 269–271.

Tuffnell, D. J., Lilford, R. J., Buchan, P. C. *et al.* (1992) Randomised controlled trial of day care for hypertension in pregnancy. *Lancet*, **339**, 224–227.

Turnbull, A. C. (1987) Maternal mortality and present trends, in *Hypertension in Pregnancy. Proceedings of the Sixteenth Study Group of the Royal College of Obstetricians and Gynaecologists*, (eds F. Sharp and E. M. Symonds), Perinatology Press, Ithaca, NY, p. 135–144.

Turnbull, A., Tindall, V. R., Beard, R. W. *et al.* (1989) *Report on Confidential Enquiries Into Maternal Deaths in England and Wales 1982–1984*, DHSS, London, vol. 34, p. 1–166.

Twaddle, S. and Harper, V. (1992) An economic evaluation of daycare in the management of hypertension in pregnancy. *Br. J. Obstet. Gynaecol.*, **99**, 459–463.

Walker, J. J. (1991) Hypertensive drugs in pregnancy. Antihypertension therapy in pregnancy, preeclampsia and eclampsia. *Clin. Perinatol.*, **18**, 845–873.

Walker, J. J., Cameron, A. D., Bjornsson, S. *et al.* (1989) Can platelet volume predict progressive hypertensive disease in pregnancy? *Am. J. Obstet. Gynecol.*, **161**, 676–679.

Walker, J. J. (1987) The case for early recognition and intervention in pregnancy induced hypertension, in *Hypertension in Pregnancy. Proceedings of the Sixteenth Study Group of the Royal College of Obstetricians and Gynaecologists*, (eds F. Sharp and E. M. Symonds), Perinatology Press, Ithaca, NY, p. 289 99.

# MANAGEMENT OF MILD PREGNANCY HYPERTENSION: THE DALLAS EXPERIENCE

*Lawrence Nathan and Larry C. Gilstrap*

## 10.1 INTRODUCTION

Hypertension complicates approximately 15% of all pregnancies and remains an important cause of both maternal and neonatal morbidity and mortality. Although the exact etiology of pregnancy-induced hypertension remains a mystery, improvements in both prenatal and neonatal care have contributed to drastically reduced maternal and perinatal mortality rates.

Many terms have been used to classify the hypertensive disorders of pregnancy but the most commonly used classification is the one detailed in the 1990 report of the Working Group on High Blood Pressure in Pregnancy. The four categories of hypertension associated with pregnancy are preeclampsia and eclampsia, chronic hypertension, preeclampsia superimposed on chronic hypertension and transient hypertension. This chapter will focus on the management of mild hypertension remote from term that develops as a consequence of pregnancy and regresses postpartum, i.e. pregnancy-induced hypertension. The ideas and techniques described are those practiced in Parkland Memorial Hospital, Dallas. They are also widely followed throughout the rest of the United States.

## 10.2 DEFINITION

Pregnancy-induced hypertension is divided into three categories:

1. hypertension alone;
2. preeclampsia;
3. eclampsia.

Pregnancy-induced hypertension may be divided into mild or severe disease (Cunningham *et al.*, 1993). This differentiation is significant in guiding the care of gravidas throughout gestation. Mild and severe disease can be distinguished by careful consideration of symptoms, signs and laboratory findings (Table 10.1).

### 10.2.1 PREECLAMPSIA

The classic triad of preeclampsia includes hypertension, proteinuria and generalized edema. Blood pressure criteria include an increase of 30 mmHg systolic or 15 mmHg diastolic over baseline on at least two occasions 6 hours apart, or a blood pressure of 140/90 mmHg or greater after 20 weeks gestation. Proteinuria is defined as 300 mg or more of urinary protein in a 1-hour collection or 100 mg/dl or more in at least two random urine specimens collected 6 or more hours apart.

*Hypertension in Pregnancy*
Edited by J.J. Walker and N.F. Gant. Published by Chapman & Hall, 1997 ISBN 0 412 30910 6

**Table 10.1**  Pregnancy-induced hypertension: indications of severity (Source: Cunningham *et al.*, *Williams Obstetrics* 19th edn, Published by Appleton & Lange, 1993.)

| Abnormality | Mild | Severe |
|---|---|---|
| Diastolic blood pressure | < 100 mmHg | 100 mmHg or higher |
| Proteinuria | Trace to 1+ | Persistently 2+ or more |
| Headache | Absent | Present |
| Visual disturbances | Absent | Present |
| Upper abdominal pain | Absent | Present |
| Oliguria | Absent | Present |
| Convulsions | Absent | Present (eclampsia) |
| Serum creatinine | Normal | Elevated |
| Thrombocytopenia | Absent | Present |
| Hyperbilirubinemia | Absent | Present |
| Liver enzyme elevation | Minimal | Marked |
| Fetal growth retardation | Absent | Obvious |
| Pulmonary edema | Absent | Present |

## 10.2.2 HYPERTENSION ALONE

This category is defined as the development of an elevated blood pressure during pregnancy or in the first 24 hours postpartum without signs of preeclampsia or chronic hypertension.

## 10.2.3 ECLAMPSIA

Eclampsia is defined as the occurrence of convulsions in women with pregnancy-induced hypertension and no underlying cerebral disease.

## 10.3 MANAGEMENT

### 10.3.1 OBJECTIVES

Delivery is recognized as the only definitive cure for the pathophysiological events of pregnancy-induced hypertension and the ultimate goal of the management plan should be the successful termination of the pregnancy with the least harm to both mother and fetus. There are several key points in such a management plan. Of paramount importance is the stabilization of maternal hemodynamic status and the prevention and/or control of convulsions. Next, it is important to evaluate the effects of the disease on maternal and fetal wellbeing. Finally, it is important to ascertain the optimal time for delivery to provide the fetus with the maximum potential for survival without jeopardizing maternal wellbeing. It cannot be overemphasized that, in the presence of overt signs and symptoms of severe preeclampsia, temporizing and delaying delivery for the sake of the fetus is often fraught with hazards from the maternal standpoint and is rarely, if ever, justified.

### 10.3.2 INITIAL EVALUATION

Within the United States, it is generally accepted that women with mild disease who have a favorable cervix at or near term should undergo induction of labor for delivery (American College of Obstetricians and Gynecologists, 1996; Cunningham and Leveno, 1988; Gant and Worley, 1980). However, in the patient with mild disease remote from term it is often possible to gain significant time *in utero* for the fetus with temporizing or conservative therapy, with little risk to maternal wellbeing.

There is no unanimity of opinion regarding the optimal management of patients with mild pregnancy-induced hypertension prior to 37 weeks (Sibai and Watson, 1985; Chamberlain *et al.*, 1978; Lindberg and Sandstrom, 1981; Trudinger and Rarik, 1982). However, it is generally agreed that when the diagnosis is first suspected patients should be hospitalized for an evaluation of maternal and fetal health (National High Blood Pressure Education Working Group, 1990; Cunningham and Leveno, 1988; Cunningham and Lindheimer, 1992; Chesley, 1978). The initial assessment should include a thorough history and complete physical examination. The exact methodology of blood pressure measurements has recently been reviewed (Cunningham and Lindheimer, 1992) and is beyond the scope of this chapter. Nevertheless, an appropriate size of cuff and a consistent approach are mandatory. Initial laboratory evaluation should include a urinalysis as well as determination of hemoglobin, hematocrit, platelet count, serum creatinine and oxaloacetic transaminase. Fibrinogen and a thrombin clot test should be evaluated as indicated. Gestational age should be established and supported by ultrasound if necessary. Amniotic fluid volume, fetal activity and heart rate should be assessed in the evaluation of fetal health. Following the initial assessment the patient should be hospitalized for a few days for serial observations of symptoms, blood pressure excursions, weight gain, urinary protein excretion and fetal status.

The management of the patient with established mild disease subsequent to a few days of hospitalization is controversial. Dietary manipulation, the value of bed rest, inpatient versus ambulatory care and antihypertensive therapy are components of conservative management that will be reviewed.

## 10.3.3 DIET

Several dietary manipulations have been proposed in the management of pregnancy-induced hypertension. In the early 19th and 20th centuries it was theorized that protein restriction would prevent or improve the outcome of PIH (Chesley, 1978), however, more recently it has been shown that maternal protein intake has no impact on the course of the disease (MacGillivray, 1983). Therefore, withholding protein is not recommended in the treatment of these women. Historically, caloric restriction was also recommended for women with PIH (Chesley, 1978); however, this too has been abandoned. Studies investigating dietary salt intake in pregnancies complicated by hypertension have yielded conflicting results with similarly contrasting conclusions, but there appears to be no conclusive support for salt restriction (Brown, 1990) and undoubtedly the debate will continue.

## 10.3.4 BED REST

Since Hamlin (1952) first popularized bed rest for the management of hypertension in pregnancy, reduction in activity has been advocated by many to arrest progression of the disease. Reasons for the beneficial effect of bed rest are not clear. It was initially thought that bed rest contributed to the restoration of angiotensin refractoriness in women who had become angiotensin-sensitive (Gant and Worley, 1980). However, research in this area failed to detect changes in pressor responsiveness to angiotensin in the face of improving hypertension (Everett *et al.*, 1978). Furthermore, Mathews, Patel and Sengupta (1971) reported a favorable outcome for women managed as outpatients over a 2-year period. This was followed by a randomized controlled trial (Mathews, 1977) comparing bed rest and sedation to normal activity in 135 patients with non-albuminuric hypertension in late pregnancy. No significant differences in the incidence of eclampsia, perinatal mortality and low birthweight were found between the two groups. Despite the lack of data to support its efficacy, bed rest continues to be recommended by many workers, although others recommend ambulatory care (Chapter 9).

### 10.3.5 OUTPATIENT CARE VERSUS HOSPITALIZATION

Gilstrap, Cunningham and Whalley (1978) reported an improved perinatal outcome and reduced maternal morbidity in 545 women with mild pregnancy-induced hypertension remote from term treated with prolonged hospitalization. Similarly, Sibai and co-workers (1987) found that early and prolonged hospitalization for patients with mild hypertension was associated with improved pregnancy outcome. In contrast, Feeney (1984) compared outcomes between women who were hospitalized ($n = 438$) and a group who were evaluated at home two to three times per week by midwives. Infrequent admissions to the hospital for hypertensive disease were noted in those managed as outpatients and the authors concluded that uncomplicated hypertension in pregnancy may be safely managed by community midwives. More recently, two studies have addressed this area of dispute. Tuffnell *et al.* (1992) randomized 54 women with non-proteinuric hypertension after 26 weeks to daycare or traditional hospital management.

Hospitalization, the development of proteinuria and labor inductions were all significantly increased in the control group. Crowther, Bouwmeester and Ashurst (1992) compared outpatient management to hospitalization in a randomized controlled trial in 218 women with non-proteinuric hypertension between 28 and 38 weeks gestation. They found that the hospitalized patients had a decreased risk of developing severe hypertension but found no differences in fetal growth or neonatal morbidity. The authors concluded that outpatient antenatal care provides a safe alternative to hospital admission for patients with mild pregnancy-induced hypertension remote from term.

In view of the conflicting data, further investigations are warranted before outpatient management is uniformly recommended over the traditional in-hospital approach. It would seem reasonable to assume that patient compliance and results may vary among different populations. The experience in the UK is more fully covered in Chapter 9.

### 10.3.6 ANTIHYPERTENSIVES

The role of antihypertensive therapy in the management of severe hypertension is well defined (American College of Obstetricians and Gynecologists, 1996; Cunningham *et al.*, 1993; Walker, 1991; Cunningham and Pritchard, 1984; Lindheimer, 1989); however the value of such drugs in mild pregnancy-induced hypertension is less clear.

Many studies have reported the use of antihypertensive medications to prolong gestation and improve outcome in mild pregnancy-induced hypertension remote from term. However, the results of such studies are difficult, if not impossible, to interpret as heterogeneous populations are frequently studied and appropriate control groups are lacking.

Rubin and associates (1983) compared atenolol (100–200 mg daily) with placebo in a randomized, double-blind trial of 120 women with mild to moderate preeclampsia. They concluded that atenolol reduced the development of proteinuria, decreased hospital admission rate and was associated with lower neonatal morbidity especially respiratory distress syndrome. In 1984, a Swedish group (Wichman, Ryden and Karlberg, 1984) compared metoprolol (100 mg daily) to placebo in 52 women with mild pregnancy-induced hypertension in a randomized fashion. The authors concluded that metoprolol lowers blood pressure in pregnancies complicated by hypertension but fails to prevent the development of preeclampsia and does not impact on perinatal outcome. Sibai *et al.* (1987) randomized 200 primigravidae with mild preeclampsia to treatment with labetalol (600–2400 mg daily) or hospitalization alone. Fewer women were delivered for severe hypertension in the treatment group but there were no differences in progression of proteinuria. Furthermore, labetalol was associated with a greater incidence of fetal growth retardation. Pickles, Symonds and Broughton-Pipkin (1989) compared labetalol (300–600 mg daily) to placebo in a multicenter randomized double-blind trial in 152 women with mild to moderate non-proteinuric pregnancy-induced hypertension and reported no differences in fetal growth but a decrease in preterm delivery and respiratory distress syndrome.

Plouin *et al.* (1990) randomized 155 women with pregnancy-induced hypertension to oxprenolol (150–320 mg daily) or placebo. Participants with diastolic blood pressure above 105 mmHg were given hydralazine (50–100 mg) to control hypertension. A greater number of cesarean sections were performed for severe hypertension in the placebo group but there were no differences in perinatal morbidity or mortality. Finally, Phippard and colleagues (1991) compared clonidine plus hydralazine to placebo in 52 primigravid women with early third-trimester hypertension in a double-blind randomized study. Worsening hypertension developed in eight women in the placebo group compared to one receiving medication. Proteinuria developed only in the placebo group. Moreover, the incidence of neonatal respiratory distress was increased in infants delivered to women who received placebo. They concluded that early control of mild hypertension in pregnancy can prevent progression of disease and preterm delivery.

Unfortunately, pregnancy-induced hypertension and chronic hypertension were not clearly distinguished in many of the studies. In conclusion, we believe that there is no convincing evidence that antihypertensive therapy in mild pregnancy-induced hypertension remote from term will significantly prolong gestation and/or impact favorably on perinatal outcome.

## 10.4 THE DALLAS EXPERIENCE

### 10.4.1 PROTOCOL

In 1955 a standardized treatment regimen was developed to manage women with pregnancy-induced hypertension at Parkland Memorial Hospital (Pritchard, 1980), and since the early 1970s these women have been cared for in a 31-bed high-risk pregnancy unit established to provide long-term care for women with certain pregnancy complications. The clinical management of women with mild pregnancy-induced hypertension remote from term is based on the premise that limited physical activity under close observation in the hospital is a safe and effective means of modifying the hypertensive disease process while awaiting fetal maturity.

Following admission, initial laboratory evaluation includes a complete blood count, platelet count, serum creatinine, 24-hour urine collection for urinary protein and creatinine clearance and aspartate aminotransferase. These laboratory tests are performed weekly or more frequently if indicated. Ultrasound examination is performed to confirm gestational age and serial sonography for fetal growth is performed every 3–4 weeks. Strict bed rest is neither enforced nor encouraged and patients are permitted to ambulate as desired. Each patient is given a general hospital diet with no sodium restriction and food from outside the hospital is allowed. The only medication provided is ferrous fumarate, 200 mg twice daily; diuretics, antihypertensives and sedatives are not administered. The mother is requested to report complaints such as headache, visual disturbance, abdominal pain, decreased fetal movement or vaginal bleeding. Blood pressure is measured four times daily, while maternal weight and urinary protein is determined daily. Uterine and fetal size and amniotic fluid volume are assessed daily, and fetal heart rate tracings are recorded twice weekly. The patients are seen daily by obstetric residents and the hospital course is reviewed with a faculty member and recorded on the high-risk pregnancy unit flow sheet (Figures 10.1, 10.2).

This careful maternal and fetal surveillance is directed towards immediate recognition of any compromise of maternal or fetal health. The gestation is allowed to proceed until spontaneous labor ensues or the cervix becomes favorable for induction of labor at or near term. Prompt delivery is accomplished if any findings of severe pregnancy-induced hypertension are detected.

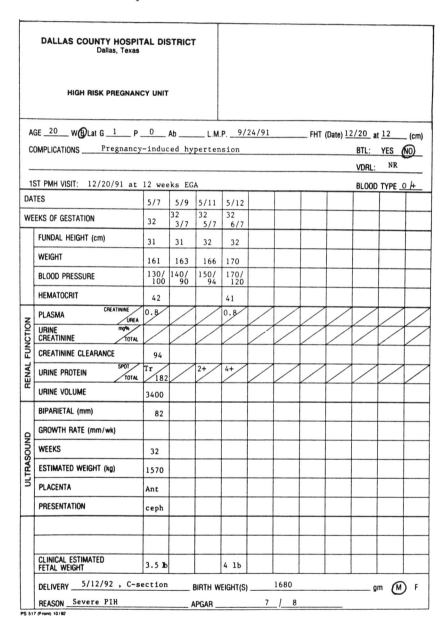

**Figure 10.1**   High Risk Pregnancy Unit flow sheet for patient A. K., who responded well to bed rest (see text).

**DALLAS COUNTY HOSPITAL DISTRICT**
Dallas, Texas

**HIGH RISK PREGNANCY UNIT**

AGE __17__ (W)B Lat G __1__ P __0__ Ab __0__ L.M.P. __9/14/91__    FHT (Date) _____ at _____ (cm)

COMPLICATIONS __Pregnancy-induced hypertension__    BTL: YES (NO)

VDRL: NR

1ST PMH VISIT: 11/25/91 at 10 weeks EGA    BLOOD TYPE _A +_

| DATES | | 5/2 | 5/9 | 5/16 | 5/26 | 6/2 | 6/10 | | | | |
|---|---|---|---|---|---|---|---|---|---|---|---|
| WEEKS OF GESTATION | | 32 | 33 | 34 | 36 | 37 | 38 | | | | |
| | FUNDAL HEIGHT (cm) | 31 | 32 | 33 | 34 | 35 | 37 | | | | |
| | WEIGHT | 153 | 154 | 158 | 161 | 164 | 168 | | | | |
| | BLOOD PRESSURE | 130/90 | 120/80 | 120/74 | 120/80 | 120/80 | 130/88 | | | | |
| | HEMATOCRIT | 35.3 | 36.4 | | 34.5 | 35.4 | | | | | |
| RENAL FUNCTION | PLASMA CREATININE/UREA | 0.6 | | | | 0.7 | 0.7 | | | | |
| | URINE CREATININE mg% /TOTAL | | | | | | | | | | |
| | CREATININE CLEARANCE | 106 | | | | | | | | | |
| | URINE PROTEIN SPOT /TOTAL | Tr / 99 | Tr | Tr | Nrg | Tr | Tr | | | | |
| | URINE VOLUME | 1640 | | | | | | | | | |
| ULTRASOUND | BIPARIETAL (mm) | 80 | | | 85 | | | | | | |
| | GROWTH RATE (mm/wk) | | | | 1.7 | | | | | | |
| | WEEKS | 32 | | | 34 | | | | | | |
| | ESTIMATED WEIGHT (kg) | 1716 | | | 2255 | | | | | | |
| | PLACENTA | post | | | post | | | | | | |
| | PRESENTATION | ceph | | | ceph | | | | | | |
| | | | | | | | | | | | |
| | CLINICAL ESTIMATED FETAL WEIGHT | 3 lb | 4 lb | | 5 lb | | 6 lb | | | | |

DELIVERY __6/10/92__    BIRTH WEIGHT(S) __2805__ gm (M) F

REASON __PIH at term__    APGAR __9__ / __9__

PS 517 (9 mm) 10/92

**Figure 10.2**  High Risk Pregnancy Unit flow sheet for patient L. N., with a poor response of hypertension to hospitalization.

## 10.4.2 DATA

Results of this management regimen were first reported in 1976 (Hauth, Cunningham & Whalley, 1976) and updated in 1978 (Gilstrap, Cunningham and Whalley, 1978). Hauth, Cunningham and Whalley (1976) reported on the initial 372 primigravidae who were managed on the unit from October 1971 through April 1975. In the update by Gilstrap, Cunningham and Whalley (1978), 576 nulliparous women with pregnancy-induced hypertension were admitted and 545 remained on the high-risk unit until delivery. As detailed in Table 10.2, 441 (81%) had a good response and became normotensive within 5 days, 70 (13%) had a moderate response and continued to have intermittent hypertension which was not severe enough to mandate delivery, and 34 (13%) women had a poor response characterized by either worsening or persistence of significant hypertension.

As illustrated in Table 10.3, prolongation of pregnancy was possible in a significant number of patients, and over 80% delivered after 37 weeks gestation.

A total of 71% of the women were delivered vaginally and approximately half of those delivered by cesarean section followed a failed induction for hypertension. The perinatal outcome for those infants of the women who remained hospitalized was 9/1000 compared to 129/1000 for those who left against medical advice. Of the infants, 418 (77%) weighed more than 2500 g at birth and the incidence of growth retardation compared favorably with the general obstetrical population delivered at Parkland Hospital during the same period. Through 1992, more than 3000

nulliparous women with mild pregnancy-induced hypertension have been cared for on the high-risk unit with similar results. The following cases illustrate the hospital courses of two women who were recently managed on the unit.

**Case 1.** A. K., whose hospital course is depicted in Figure 10.1, was a 17-year-old white primigravida admitted at 32 weeks gestation with mild pregnancy-induced hypertension. She remained mildly hypertensive for 6 weeks and was induced at 38 weeks when her cervix was favorable. She delivered a 2805 g male infant with Apgars 9/9 without incident.

**Case 2.** L. N., whose hospital course is summarized in Figure 10.2, was a 20-year-old black primigravida at 32 weeks gestation admitted to the high-risk unit after being observed in labor and delivery for hypertension. Over the course of her hospital stay her blood pressure worsened, and she was induced at 32–33 weeks for severe pregnancy-induced hypertension. Despite an adequate trial of pitocin she was delivered by cesarean section for failure to progress of a male infant weighing 1680 g with Apgars 7/8.

### 10.4.3 FINANCIAL CONSIDERATIONS

In the current environment of escalating health care costs the financial impact of this

**Table 10.2** Blood pressure response of 545 nulliparae with pregnancy-induced hypertension on the High Risk Pregnancy Unit (Source: modified with permission from Gilstrap, Cunningham and Whalley, 1978. Management of pregnancy-induced hypertension in the nulliporous patient remote from term. *Semin. Perinatol.*, **2**, 73–81.)

| Response | n | % |
|---|---|---|
| Good response (normotensive after admission) | 441 | 81 |
| Recurrent hypertension prior to labor | 183 | 42 |
| Recurrent hypertension in labor | 199 | 45 |
| Remained normotensive | 59 | 13 |
| Moderate response (improved but intermittent hypertension) | 70 | 13 |
| Poor response (persistent hypertension) | 34 | 6 |

**Table 10.3** Gestational age at times of admission and to delivery in 545 women with pregnancy-induced hypertension admitted to the High Risk Pregnancy Unit (Source: modified with permission from Gilstrap, Cunningham and Whalley, 1978)

| Gestational age (weeks) | Admission (%) | Delivery (%) |
|---|---|---|
| Less than 30 | 25 (4.8) | 1 (0.2) |
| 30–32 | 86 (15.8) | 11 (2.0) |
| 33–36 | 261 (47.9) | 59 (10.8) |
| 37 or greater | 172 (31.5) | 474 (87.0) |
| Totals | 545 | 545 |

management must be considered. Prolonged hospitalization creates a financial burden for the patient, her family, the insurance carrier or the society that provides this care. The cost for maternal hospitalization on the high-risk unit at Parkland Memorial Hospital is approximately $300 per day, which is actually much less than the cost of protracted care of the preterm infant in the Neonatal Intensive Care Unit, which can average $1800 per day. Hospitalization, therefore, would appear to be cost-effective and financially prudent in order to maximize fetal maturity.

## 10.5 SUMMARY

The goal in the management of patients with pregnancy-induced hypertension is delivery of infants who will thrive physically and mentally without compromising maternal health. Many therapeutic approaches have been recommended; however, none except delivery are curative. In the interests of maternal health, delivery is essential when severe preeclampsia or eclampsia are diagnosed regardless of gestational age. On the other hand, the patient with mild pregnancy-induced hypertension remote from term may be managed conservatively with effort directed to prolonging the gestation to maximize perinatal outcome. The regimen used at Parkland Memorial Hospital has proved to be safe and effective and thus warrants continuation of inpatient care for the gravida until well-controlled studies yield comparably safe and efficacious outcomes.

## REFERENCES

American College of Obstetricians and Gynecologists (1996) *Technical Bulletin Hypertension in Pregnancy* no. **2**, 91, American College of Obstetricians and Gynecologists, Washington, DC

Brown, M. A. (1990) Editorial review: non-pharmacological management of pregnancy-induced hypertension. *J. Hypertens.*, **8**, 295–301.

Chamberlain ,G. V. P., Lewis, P. J., deSweit, M. *et al.* (1978) How obstetricians manage hypertension in pregnancy. *Br. Med. J.*, **i**, 626.

Chesley, L. C. (ed. ) (1978) *Hypertensive Disorders in Pregnancy*, Appleton-Century-Crofts, New York.

Crowther, C. A., Bouwmeester, A. M. and Ashurst, H. M. (1992) Does admission to hospital for bed rest prevent disease progression or improve fetal outcome in pregnancy complicated by non-proteinuric hypertension? *Br. J. Obstet. Gynaecol.*, **99**, 13–17.

Cunningham, F. G. and Leveno, K. J. (1988) Management of pregnancy-induced hypertension, in *Handbook of Hypertension*, vol. 10: *Hypertension in Pregnancy*, 1st edn, (ed. P. C. Rubin), Elsevier, New York, p. 290–319.

Cunningham, F. G. and Lindheimer, M. D. (1992) Hypertension in pregnancy. *N. Engl. J. Med.*, **326**, 927–32.

Cunningham, F. G., MacDonald, P. C., Gant, N. F. *et al.* (1993) *Williams Obstetrics*, 19th edn, Appleton & Lange, Norwalk, CT, p. 797.

Cunningham, F. G. and Pritchard, J. A. (1984) How should hypertension during pregnancy be managed? *Med. Clin. North. Am.*, **68**(2), 505–26.

Everett, R. B., Cox, K., Gant, N. F. *et al.* (1978) Vascular reactivity to angiotensin-II (A-II) in human pregnancy: the effect of hospitalization and modified bedrest in women with pregnancy-induced hypertension (PIH). *Proc. Soc. Gynecol. Invest.*, **March**, Abstract 113.

Feeney, J. G. (1984) Hypertension in pregnancy managed at home by community midwives. *Br. Med. J.*, **288**, 1046–47.

Gant, N. F. Jr. and Worley, R. J. (1980) *Hypertension in Pregnancy: Concepts and Management*, Appleton-Century-Crofts, New York, p. 108.

Gilstrap, L. C. III, Cunningham, F. G. and Whalley, P. J. (1978) Management of pregnancy-induced hypertension in the nulliparous patient remote from term. *Semin. Perinatol.*, **2**(1), 73–81.

Hamlin, R. H. J. (1952) The prevention of eclampsia and preeclampsia. *Lancet*, **i**, 64–68.

Hauth, J. C., Cunningham, F. G. and Whalley, P. J. (1976) Management of pregnancy-induced hypertension in the nullipara. *Obstet. Gynecol.*, **48**(3), 253–259.

Lindberg, B. S. and Sandstrom, B. (1981) How Swedish obstetricians manage hypertension in pregnancy: a questionnaire study. *Acta Obstet. Gynecol. Scand.*, **60**, 327.

Lindheimer, M. D. (1989) Diagnosis and management of hypertension complicating pregnancy. *Am. J. Kidney Dis.*, **13**(6, Supp. 1), 17–27.

MacGillivray, I. (1983) *Preeclampsia: The Hypertensive Disease of Pregnancy*. W. B. Saunders, London.

Mathews, D. D. (1977) A randomized controlled trial of bed rest and sedation of normal activity and non-sedation in the management of non-albuminuric hypertension in late pregnancy. *Br. J. Obstet. Gynaecol.*, **84**, 108–114.

Mathews, D. D., Patel, I. R. and Sengupta, S. M. (1971) Out-patient management of toxaemia. *J. Obstet. Gynaecol. Br. Commonw.*, **78**, 610–619.

National High Blood Pressure Education Working Group (1990) Report on high blood pressure during pregnancy. *Am. J. Obstet. Gynecol.*, **163**, 1689–1712.

Phippard, A. F., Fischer, W. E., Horvath, J. S. *et al.* (1991) Early blood pressure control improves pregnancy outcome in primigravid women with mild hypertension. *Med. J. Aust.*, **154**, 378–382.

Pickles, C. J., Symonds, E. M. and Broughton Pipkin, F. (1989) The fetal outcome in a randomized double-blind controlled trial of labetolol versus placebo in pregnancy-induced hypertension. *Br. J. Obstet. Gynaecol.*, **96**, 38–43.

Plouin, P-F., Breart, G., Llado, J. *et al.* (1990) A randomized comparison of early with conservative use of antihypertensive drugs in the management of pregnancy-induced hypertesion. *Br. J. Obstet. Gynaecol.*, **97**, 134–141.

Pritchard, J. A. (1980) Management of preeclampsia and eclampsia. *Kidney Int.*, **18**, 259–266.

Rubin, P. C., Clark, D. M., Sumner, D. J. *et al.* (1983) Placebo-controlled trial of atenolol in treatment of pregnancy-associated hypertension. *Lancet*, **i**, 431–434.

Sibai, B. M., Watson, D. L. (1985) How American obstetricians manage hypertension during pregnancy (abstract). Annual Meeting of American College of Obstetricians and Gynecologists, Washington, DC.

Sibai, B. M., Gonzalez, A. R., Mabie, W. C. and Moretti, M. (1987) A comparison of labetolol plus hospitalization versus hospitalization alone in the management of preeclampsia remote from term. *Obstet. Gynecol.*, **70**(3), 323–327.

Trudinger, B. J. and Rarik, I. (1982) Attitudes to the management of hypertension in pregnancy: a survey of Australian fellows. *Aust. NZ J. Obstet. Gynaecol.*, **22**, 191.

Tuffnell, D. J., Lilford, R. J., Buchan, P. C. *et al.* (1992) Randomised controlled trial of day care for hypertension in pregnancy. *Lancet*, **339**, 224–228.

Walker, J. J. (1991) Hypertensive drugs in pregnancy: antihypertension therapy in pregnancy, preeclampsia and eclampsia. *Clin. Perinatol.*, **18**(4), 845–873.

Wichman, K., Ryden, G. and Karlberg, B. E. (1984) A placebo controlled trial of metroprolol in the treatment of hypertension in pregnancy. *Scand. J. Clin. Lab. Invest.*, **44**, 90–95.

# THE MANAGEMENT OF KNOWN ESSENTIAL HYPERTENSION IN PREGNANCY

*Eileen Gallery*

## 11.1 INTRODUCTION

The expected incidence of chronic hypertension in pregnancy is 5–10%, higher values being found with increasing age. The majority of these women will have essential hypertension, although this diagnosis can only be reached after exclusion of causes of secondary hypertension. The final diagnosis is often retrospective, as most of the investigations are best performed after the effects of pregnancy on the anatomy and physiology of the renal tract have resolved.

## 11.2 DEFINITION OF HYPERTENSION IN PREGNANCY

There is controversy about the level of blood pressure that should be called abnormal in pregnancy, as the normal range is reset downwards in the first trimester by 10–15 mmHg, predominantly as a result of vasodilatation, with a slow rise towards non-pregnant levels during the second half of gestation. Concerns that the conventional borderline value of 140/90 mmHg may be too high led to the adoption of an alternative definition of a rise from the first trimester value of ≥ 25/15 mmHg by the American Committee on Maternal Welfare. For ease of use in practice, and as a

guide in therapy, the Australasian Society for the Study of Hypertension in Pregnancy has recommended maintenance of a value of 140/90 mmHg as the arbitrary dividing line between normal and abnormal.

## 11.3 MEASUREMENT OF BLOOD PRESSURE IN PREGNANCY

There is current controversy about the relative merits of measuring Korotkoff phase IV or V as the diastolic endpoint, neither of which is exactly correlated with intra-arterially measured pressure. In our institution, phase IV is routinely used, as the majority of published reports describing risks, outcomes and the effects of treatment have correlated their findings with phase IV. Of much greater practical importance than which Korotkoff phase to record are other variables in making the measurement of blood pressure. Factors of importance include the following:

1. **Position of the patient**. If the patient is lying on her left side, the blood pressure measured in her right arm will be 8–10 mmHg lower than that measured when she is sitting, predominantly because of the hydrostatic effect of the cuff being 8–10 cm higher than the heart. If she lies on her

*Hypertension in Pregnancy*
Edited by J.J. Walker and N.F. Gant. Published by Chapman & Hall, 1997 ISBN 0 412 30910 6

back in late pregnancy, the measured blood pressure may be very low because of the supine hypotensive syndrome, due to reduced venous return of blood to the heart.

2. **Position of the arm**. If the patient sits with her arm by her side, the antecubital fossa may be 8–10 cm lower than the heart, resulting in a spurious increase in the blood pressure of 8-10 mmHg.

3. **Relaxation of the arm**. If the arm is not supported, the static exercise involved in holding it still may result in a spurious increase in the measured blood pressure of several millimeters of mercury.

4. **Correct cuff size and cuff applied correctly**. If the cuff is too small, the measured blood pressure will be spuriously elevated, if too large, falsely low values will be obtained. Again, the differences are often of the order of 8–10 mmHg, and can be as much as 20 mmHg. In general, for women with an arm circumference of 35 cm or above, a large cuff should be used (with a bladder 15 × 33 cm).

5. **Errors in measuring technique**. A mercury sphygmomanometer should be used, the mercury read at eye level, the column lowered slowly with enough time to observe a change over a 2 mm space, and the recording made to the nearest 2 mm (rather than reading to the nearest 5 or even 10 mmHg).

More than 30% of women with underlying chronic hypertension will experience an exaggerated fall in their blood pressure, reaching levels within the normal range by the end of the first trimester. In these women, it is often possible to reduce or stop antihypertensive treatment for a variable period of time.

## 11.4 CLASSIFICATION OF CHRONIC HYPERTENSION IN PREGNANCY

A clear understanding of the potential causes of hypertension simplifies the management plan considerably. One of the most widely used and practical classification systems is listed in Table 11.1, and will form the basis for this relatively brief management review.

## 11.5 DIAGNOSTIC APPROACH TO HYPERTENSION IN PREGNANCY

The most appropriate time to plan the management of a woman with any of these disorders is prior to the index pregnancy. Although essential hypertension is a common disorder in our society, the accuracy of the diagnosis clearly depends on the completeness of investigations searching for an underlying cause. In addition to a careful history and thorough physical examination at the first consultation, it is our usual practice to perform formal testing of renal function (both glomerular and medullary, with careful examination of the centrifuged urinary sediment), and a renal imaging procedure (usually intravenous pyelogram) in all pre-menopausal hypertensive women. A decision about the necessity for more sophisticated or invasive investigations

---

**Table 11.1**   Causes of chronic hypertension in pregnancy

1. **Essential ('primary')**

2. **Secondary**
   (a) *Renal disease*
       Glomerulonephritis (idiopathic or secondary)
       Tubulo-interstitial (inherited, infective, toxic, metabolic )

   (b) *Vascular disease*
       Vasculitis
       Coarctation of the aorta

   (c) *Endocrine disease*
       Adrenal (cortical or medullary)
       Thyroid
       Pancreatic
       Ovarian

   (d) *Drug-induced*

depends on the clinical situation and the results of these basic tests.

### 11.5.1 EXAMPLES

#### (a) In addition to hypertension, the patient has central obesity and hirsutism, with irregular menstruation

In this case, the direction of focus would be towards the polycystic ovary syndrome, hyperadrenocorticism or perhaps one of the forms of congenital adrenal hyperplasia. Further investigations to elucidate the situation might include a glucose tolerance test, 24-hour free urinary cortisol, 17-hydroxyprogesterone and androgens, plasma cortisol and dexamethasone suppression testing.

#### (b) There is a history of episodic palpitations and unstable hypertension

It will be essential to exclude pheochromocytoma as a diagnosis. This is readily achieved by measurement of 24-hour urinary catecholamine excretion; usually it is sufficient to measure adrenalin, noradrenalin and dopamine. (All 24-hour urine collections should have creatinine measurements to assess the completeness of the collection.)

#### (c) The patient has been taking oral contraceptives for 5 years

The combined oral contraceptive pill can cause hypertension in susceptible women, and its cessation may result in a slow return of the blood pressure to normal, without a need for further treatment.

#### (d) Physical examination reveals an upper abdominal vascular bruit, radiating to one side

Consideration must be given to the possibility of renal artery stenosis, which in the young woman is likely to be due to fibromuscular hyperplasia. As this may be a bilateral condition, it is not excluded by a normal intravenous pyelogram, or by ultrasound or isotope flow studies. The definitive investigation is bilateral renal angiography.

#### (e) The blood pressure is elevated in the right arm but normal on the left side

This suggests an occlusive vascular problem (e.g. coarctation) in the aortic arch proximal to the origin of the left arm vessels. Confirmation will require angiographic evidence of the narrowing.

#### (f) Among the initial results is a serum potassium of 3.2 mmol/l, in a woman who is not taking diuretics

This would prompt consideration of primary hyperaldosteronism; this could be addressed in the first instance by measurement of plasma renin activity, plasma aldosterone and 24-hour urinary aldosterone, sodium, potassium and creatinine. (Although renin and aldosterone levels rise in pregnancy, there are normal values available for different stages of pregnancy.)

#### (g) Initial investigations reveal protein, red blood cells and casts in the urine

These findings are indicative of glomerular disease and would prompt referral of the patient for possible renal biopsy and further investigation of secondary causes such as systemic lupus erythematosus.

### 11.6 RISKS OF CHRONIC HYPERTENSION TO MOTHER AND FETUS

After making a definitive diagnosis, any correctable causes of hypertension can be addressed prior to embarking on a pregnancy, and associated disorders can be given specific treatment as indicated. Appropriate advice about the potential interaction of the underlying disease and pregnancy can be given.

If there is no evidence of end-organ damage and the tests outlined above are normal, then a presumptive diagnosis of essential hypertension may be made and no specific contraindication to pregnancy is seen. The major risks of this disorder to mother and fetus are:

1. the development of 'superimposed pre-eclampsia' (i.e. the appearance of proteinuria, usually with worsening of the hypertension);
2. acceleration of hypertension with resultant end-organ damage (in particular bleeding secondary to a generalized coagulopathy, cerebral hemorrhage, cardiac, renal or hepatic failure);
3. uteroplacental insufficiency, leading to intrauterine growth retardation and/or fetal death.

The magnitude of these risks is variable within the hypertensive population. In two early series reported by Chesley and Annitto (1947) and Browne and Dodds (1942), there was a high incidence of proteinuria developing in women with pre-existing chronic essential hypertension (32% and 17% respectively), but in neither case was this risk apparently related to the initial severity of the hypertension, above a threshold level of the order of 130–140/85–95 mmHg.

In contrast, the risk of accelerated hypertension seemed to be closely related to the level of blood pressure at first presentation, a finding confirmed by many subsequent authors. The reduction in this risk by control of moderate degrees of hypertension (initial BP 140/90 mmHg) is impressive, as shown by Redman, Beilin and Bonnar (1977), who described acute exacerbations of hypertension to levels in excess of 170/110 mmHg in 21% of untreated, compared with 9% of treated hypertensive pregnant women.

A highly significant relationship between the severity of untreated chronic essential hypertension and fetal death was first described by Chesley and Annitto (1947) and Browne and Dodds (1942), and has been confirmed by many subsequent authors. Silverstone *et al.* (1980) described a midtrimester abortion rate of 2.4%, compared to 0.7% for the total antenatal population of one British center. Page and Christianson, in California (1976), found a direct correlation between the level of maternal blood pressure in the second trimester and subsequent fetal death and intrauterine growth retardation.

## 11.7 EFFECTS OF TREATMENT IN HYPERTENSIVE PREGNANCY

Several studies of groups of pregnant women with chronic hypertension of various etiologies have shown a reduction in the crude perinatal mortality rate in response to antihypertensive treatment. Leather *et al.* (1968) studied 47 women presenting prior to 20 weeks amenorrhea, whom they randomized to control ($n = 24$) or treatment ($n = 23$) groups. There were five fetal losses in the former (two midtrimester spontaneous abortions), none in the latter group. In a later study (Redman, Beilin and Bonnar, 1977), dealing with less severe hypertension in women presenting before 28 weeks gestation, patients were randomized to control ($n = 107$) or treatment ($n = 101$) groups, and again a reduction was found in the incidence of spontaneous midtrimester abortion (3% *versus* 0). In this overall study, which also included 34 subjects recruited after 28 weeks gestation, there was a higher incidence of late perinatal deaths in the control group (4% *versus* 0.8%).

There is general agreement that control of hypertension throughout pregnancy is associated with a reduction in the occurrence of accelerated hypertension, but some disagreement exists about the effect of treatment in reducing the rate of 'superimposed pre-eclampsia' as defined above. However, as this complication was described in up to 60% of women in the early reports cited and is now encountered much less frequently, it is likely that therapeutic practices have had an impact. A recent review of several studies of the natural course of chronic hypertension in pregnancy and the impact of therapy (Gallery *et al.*, 1991) showed a general reduction in:

1. the incidence of accelerated hypertension;
2. the incidence of significant proteinuria;
3. the crude perinatal mortality rate in response to antihypertensive therapy with a variety of agents.

## 11.8 PRINCIPLES OF MANAGEMENT OF THE HYPERTENSIVE PREGNANT WOMAN

### 11.8.1 INITIAL EVALUATION

As outlined above, the ideal time to assess a woman with chronic hypertension is prior to a planned pregnancy, when the diagnosis can be established with some certainty and any corrective treatment can be applied, or control of blood pressure achieved with an agent suitable for use in pregnancy.

Often patients are not seen until pregnancy has already occurred and hypertension is noted. Here again, history and physical examination will give much valuable information and will help rule out many causes of secondary hypertension. There are published normal values for renal function in pregnancy, so tests performed should be compared with these. Radiological procedures can usually be postponed until after the index pregnancy, but if renal imaging is needed, either an ultrasound or a limited series intravenous pyelogram can be performed.

### 11.8.2 ASSESSMENT OF MATERNAL WELLBEING

After baseline clinical and laboratory evaluation, the patient should be closely observed throughout her pregnancy and into the early postpartum period. This may involve alternate visits to the obstetrician and a physician experienced in the care of pregnant women, or more frequent visits to a high-risk antenatal center. Clinical assessment of maternal wellbeing, in addition to measurement of blood pressure, should include inspection of the optic fundi for evidence of arteriolar vasospasm, an early sign of the superimposition of the vasospasm of preeclampsia. If a positive dipstick urine protein test is found at any time, it should be confirmed by 24-hour urine measurement (Kuo *et al.*, 1992). If there is any clinical suspicion of worsening maternal condition, estimation of renal function (in particular serum uric acid and creatinine concentrations), hepatic function (serum albumin and transaminases), volume status (hematocrit or plasma volume measurement) and coagulation status (platelet count) should be performed. In all well hypertensive pregnant women seen in our institution, these minimum investigations are repeated at 28–30 and at 34–36 weeks gestation. A summary of the protocol followed for patient supervision is shown in Table 11.2.

### 11.8.3 ASSESSMENT OF FETAL WELLBEING

Early uterine ultrasound examination is of great value for accurate dating of the duration of pregnancy, and serial ultrasound is a useful adjunct to clinical assessment of fetal growth. From 30 weeks amenorrhea onwards, it is the usual practice in our institution to perform weekly unstressed fetal heart rate monitoring in all high-risk pregnancies (Table 11.2). The place and value of Doppler umbilical vessel flow studies in management is less clear. It is most likely that they are of benefit in early detection of patients at high risk of fetal problems related to placental insufficiency, who can then be followed closely, both clinically and by serial cardiotocography.

### 11.8.4 THERAPEUTIC MANEUVERS

The principal aims of treatment of hypertension in pregnancy are to prevent maternal

**Table 11.2**  Management guide for chronic hypertension in pregnancy (+ indicates the frequency of performance of the indicated procedure)

| Event | Weeks gestation | | | | | | | |
|---|---|---|---|---|---|---|---|---|
| | *0–12* | *13–16* | *17–20* | *21–24* | *25–28* | *29–32* | *33–36* | *37–40* |
| Examination | + | + | + | + | + | ++ | ++++ | ++++ |
| BP | + | + | + | + | + | ++ | ++++ | ++++ |
| Uterine size | + | + | + | + | + | ++ | ++++ | ++++ |
| Urinalysis | + | + | + | + | + | ++ | ++++ | ++++ |
| FBC | | + | | | + | | + | + |
| S creatinine | | + | | | + | | + | + |
| S uric acid | | + | | | + | | + | + |
| U catecholamines | | + | | | | | | |
| Uterine ultrasound | + | | | + | | + | | |
| Cardiotocography | | | | | | ++ | ++++ | ++++ |

complications and achieve a satisfactory pregnancy outcome – a mature healthy neonate.

## (a) Delivery

Delivery of the baby will not cure the chronically hypertensive woman, but often results in much easier control, and resolution of complications. It also allows a wider range of therapeutic and investigation options. The general principle is that, if continued pregnancy is of significant risk to the mother's life, it should be terminated, whether this be at 14 or at 40 weeks amenorrhea. If pregnancy can be continued with no danger to the mother, and the fetus has a potential gain, then it may be allowed to progress for as long as the situation remains manageable. If, at any time, it is judged that there is more risk to the fetus in the uterus than in the Nursery, then delivery should be expedited for fetal indications.

## (b) Rest

Although the place of rest has never been the subject of a formal trial in women with chronic hypertension, it has become an integral part of the management. It is not necessary, or even desirable, to confine the patient to bed throughout her pregnancy, but a reduction in her overall work load, perhaps stopping work outside the home if it is physically or mentally stressful, is often of great value in resetting the blood pressure downwards. There is no need for admission to hospital in the antenatal period, unless the blood pressure is unstable or a specific indication appears (e.g. intrauterine fetal growth retardation, threatened premature labor, antepartum hemorrhage, etc.). It is our usual practice to admit patients to hospital if commencement of antihypertensive therapy is contemplated for the first time after 26 weeks gestation. This gives the opportunity to observe the patient closely and detect any other problems, and to assess the therapeutic response to rest under supervision.

## (c) Diet

Clearly, all pregnant women, including those with chronic hypertension, should eat a well-balanced diet that is not deficient in any essential nutrients. However, no convincing association has been described between the development or aggravation of hypertension and any particular dietary manipulation. In particular, although sodium restriction has benefits for a proportion of non-pregnant hypertensive patients, there is nothing to be gained by prescribing a low sodium diet for the hypertensive pregnant woman. Salt restriction may, in fact, be hazardous in this group of patients who already have inappropriate intravascular volume contraction (Gallery, Hunyor and Gyory, 1980).

### (d) Antihypertensive therapy

Many women with known essential hypertension experience a significant fall in blood pressure in early pregnancy and therefore do not require consideration of treatment until the third trimester. Some women who required antihypertensives for control of hypertension prior to pregnancy are able to reduce the dose and occasionally stop treatment entirely for a variable period of time in the first and second trimesters. As outlined above, it is our usual practice to treat women whose blood pressure is persistently in excess of 140/90 mmHg despite non-pharmacological measures, at any stage of pregnancy. The aim of treatment, once started, is to lower the sitting phase IV diastolic BP to < 80 mmHg. Specific therapeutic regimens employed depend on the severity of the hypertension and the stage of pregnancy.

If there is mild hypertension in the last 4 weeks of gestation, bed rest at home or in hospital, followed by delivery, may be the only treatment needed. The earlier in pregnancy the patient presents with hypertension, and the more severe the hypertension is, the more likely she is to require antihypertensive medication. If the diastolic BP is 90–109

mmHg, oral therapy is usually sufficient. However, if the diastolic BP is $\geq$ 110 mmHg, initial parenteral treatment may be needed to achieve rapid control, followed by oral maintenance therapy. The guide employed at the Royal North Shore Hospital to assist in decisions about urgency and mode of antihypertensive therapy is shown briefly in Table 11.3.

The antihypertensive drugs most commonly used in pregnancy (Redman, Beilin and Bonnar, 1977; Rubin *et al.*, 1983; Gallery, Ross and Gyory, 1985; Weitz *et al.*, 1987; Plouin *et al.*, 1988; Phippard *et al.*, 1991), and their common dosage regimens, are listed in Table 11.4. Angiotensin converting enzyme inhibitors are best avoided at all stages of pregnancy, because of a high reported rate of fetal loss in experimental animals, while the newer calcium channel blockers should be avoided in early pregnancy, because of lack of information about their potential teratogenicity.

### (e) Other treatment

The pregnant woman with chronic hypertension may have underlying renal disease, or other cause for her hypertension. If so, treatment for these problems should be addressed separately. She will have the same risks of iron or folate deficiency, and these should be managed as for any pregnant woman. Because she has an increased risk of developing 'superimposed preeclampsia', constant vigilance should be kept for symptoms or signs of this syndrome. If labor is to be induced or a cesarean section performed, con-

**Table 11.3** Guide to urgency and mode of antihypertensive therapy

| Sitting diastolic BP (mmHg) | Duration (h) | Mode of treatment |
| --- | --- | --- |
| 90–95 | 24 | Oral |
| 96–100 | 12 | Oral |
| 101–105 | 8 | Oral |
| 106–110 | 4 | Parenteral |
| > 110 | 1 | Parenteral |

**Table 11.4** Antihypertensive agents most commonly used in pregnancy

| Acute parenteral therapy | | Oral maintenance therapy | |
|---|---|---|---|
| Drug | Dose range | Drug | Daily dose range |
| Hydralazine | IM or IV, 5–20 mg | Methyl DOPA | 250–2500 mg |
| Diazoxide | IV, 50–300 mg | Oxprenolol | 80–320 mg |
| Nifedipine | Sublingual, 5–10 mg | Labetalol | 100–400 mg |
| | | Metoprolol | 100–400 mg |
| | | Hydralazine | 25–200 mg |
| | | Clonidine | 150–600 µg |
| | | Verapamil | 40–320 mg |

sideration should be given to epidural anesthetic, provided that she does not have a significant disturbance of her coagulation mechanisms. In addition to excellent analgesia, this offers an opportunity for smooth BP control. Since many hypertensive pregnant women are relatively volume-depleted (and therefore at risk of acute hypotension in the presence of sympathetic blockade of the lower limbs), preloading with intravenous fluid may be desirable in preparation for the epidural insertion.

## 11.9 SUMMARY

I have attempted, in this relatively brief review, to outline the possible causes of secondary hypertension that are most commonly encountered in the pregnant woman with chronic hypertension, and a logical diagnostic approach to these. The remainder of the discussion has involved the risks to both mother and baby of hypertension *per se*, and the principles of management. Although there are undoubted risks involved for any woman with chronic hypertension contemplating pregnancy, these are usually manageable. Provided that her prepregnancy renal function is reasonable and her hypertension well controlled, the woman with chronic hypertension has a good chance of a relatively uncomplicated antenatal course, and a successful pregnancy outcome.

## REFERENCES

Browne, F. J. and Dodds, G. H. (1942) Pregnancy in the patient with chronic hypertension. *J. Obstet. Gynaecol. Br. Emp.*, **49**, 12.

Chesley, L. C. and Annitto, J. E. (1947) Pregnancy in the patient with hypertensive disease. *Am. J. Obstet. Gynecol.*, **53**, 372.

Gallery, E. D. M., Hunyor, S. N. and Gyory, A. Z. (1980) Plasma volume contraction: a significant factor in both pregnancy-associated hypertension (pre-eclampsia) and chronic hypertension in pregnancy. *Q. J. Med.*, **48**, 553.

Gallery, E. D. M., Ross, M. and Gyory, A. Z. (1985) Antihypertensive treatment in pregnancy: analysis of different responses to oxprenolol and methyl dopa. *Br. Med. J.*, **291**, 563.

Gallery, E. D. M., Boyce, E. S., Saunders, D. M. and Gyory, A. Z. (1991) Chronic hypertension in pregnancy, in *Hypertension in Pregnancy*, (eds E. V. Cosmi and G. C. Di Renzo), Monduzzi Editore, Bologna, p. 67–79.

Kuo, V., Gallery, E. D. M., Koumantakis, G. and Ross, M. (1992) Proteinuria and its assessment in normal and hypertensive human pregnancy. *Am. J. Obstet. Gynecol.*, **167**, 723–728.

Leather, H. M., Humphrey, D. M., Baker, P. and Chadd, M. A. (1968) A controlled trial of hypotensive agents in hypertension in pregnancy. *Lancet*, **ii**, 488.

Page, E. W. and Christianson, R. (1976) The inpact of mean arterial blood pressure in the middle trimester upon the outcome of pregnancy. *Am. J. Obstet. Gynecol.*, **125**, 740.

Phippard, A. F., Fischer, W. E., Horvath, J. S. *et al.* (1991) Early blood pressure control improves pregnancy outcome in primigravid women with mild hypertension. *Med. J. Aust.*, **154**, 378.

Plouin, P. F., Breart, G., Maillard, F. *et al.* (1988) Comparison of antihypertensive efficacy and perinatal safety of labetalol and methyldopa in the treatment of hypertension in pregnancy: a randomized controlled trial. *Br. J. Obstet. Gynaecol.*, **95**, 868.

Redman, C. W. G., Beilin, L. J. and Bonnar, J. (1977) Treatment of hypertension in pregnancy with methyldopa: blood pressure control and side effects. *Br. J. Obstet. Gynaecol.*, **84**, 419.

Rubin, P. C., Butters, L., Clark, D. M. *et al.* (1983) Placebo-controlled trial of atenolol in treatment of pregnancy-associated hypertension. *Lancet*, **i**, 431.

Silverstone, A., Trudinger, B. J., Lewis, P. J. and Bulpitt, C. J. (1980) Maternal hypertension and intrauterine fetal death in mid-pregnancy. *Br. J. Obstet. Gynaecol.*, **87**, 457.

Weitz, C., Khouzami, V., Maxwell, K. and Johnson, J. W. C. (1987) Treatment of hypertension in pregnancy with methyldopa: a randomised double blind study. *Int. J. Gynecol. Obstet.*, **25**, 35.

# PREGNANCY IN THE PATIENT WITH RENAL DISEASE

*John Davison and Christine Baylis*

## 12.1 INTRODUCTION

Alterations in a woman's appearance are obvious as pregnancy advances. Less obvious, but just as significant, are the alterations in the mother's internal environment, whereby her homeostatic mechanisms are overridden and reset in the interests of the pregnancy. The changes in the renal tract are particularly important aspects of this adaptation and a pregnant woman cannot be judged by the ordinary standards of renal function for a non-pregnant individual. Accurate information has been slow to accrue from clinical practice and animal models have therefore been carefully developed in order to rigorously examine the mechanisms controlling the altered renal function of normal pregnancy as well as the long-term renal consequences of pregnancy in health and disease.

This review of current knowledge, including data derived from animal models, provides an insight into the factors controlling the striking gestational renal alterations, which is a prerequisite for the detection, understanding and management of renal problems in pregnancy.

## 12.2 NORMAL PREGNANCY

### 12.2.1 STRUCTURAL CHANGES IN THE URINARY TRACT

The kidneys of normal pregnant women enlarge because both vascular volume and interstitial space increase (Cietak and Newton, 1985a). Evidence from intravenous excretory urography performed immediately after delivery reveals that renal size is consistently greater than that predicted by standard height–weight nomograms and repeat investigation 6 months later indicates a decrease in renal length of approximately 1 cm (Bailey and Rolleston, 1971). Ultrasound studies suggest that renal parenchymal volumes increase during pregnancy with a 70% increment by the beginning of the third trimester and reductions commencing during the first weeks postpartum (Cietak and Newton, 1985a, b).

The most striking anatomical change in the urinary tract is dilatation of the calyces, renal pelvis and ureter (Croce *et al*, 1994) (Figure 12.1). These changes, invariably more prominent on the right side, can be seen as early as the first trimester, are present in 90% of

*Hypertension in Pregnancy*
Edited by J.J. Walker and N.F. Gant. Published by Chapman & Hall, 1997 ISBN 0 412 30910 6

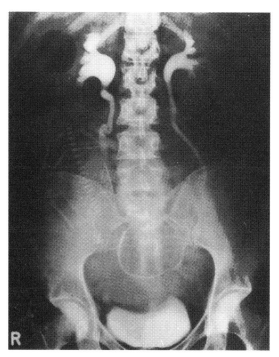

**Figure 12.1** Intravenous excretory urogram showing ureteral dilation of pregnancy. The right ureter is abruptly cut off at the pelvic brim where it crosses the iliac artery (the so-called 'iliac sign') (Dure-Smith, 1970).

women by the third trimester and resolve completely and spontaneously postpartum (Cietak and Newton, 1985b; Brown, 1990).

### 12.2.2 RENAL HEMODYNAMIC CHANGES

#### (a) Time course and magnitude of renal hemodynamic changes

Inulin clearance is used experimentally to measure glomerular filtration rate (GFR), which increases by about 50% during pregnancy (Figure 12.2), reaching the maximum at the end of the first trimester and maintained at this augmented level until at least the 36th gestational week (Davison and Dunlop, 1980; Davison and Hytten, 1974).

Since GFR increases less than renal plasma flow during early pregnancy, the ratio of GFR to RPF, i.e. the filtration fraction, falls. Late

pregnancy is associated with an increase in filtration fraction to values similar to the non-pregnant norm (Dunlop, 1976). Endogenous 24-hour creatinine clearance is a convenient, non-invasive method that measures GFR when inulin infusion studies are impracticable. Studies performed at weekly intervals after conception have shown that 24-hour creatinine clearance increases by 25% 4 weeks after the last menstrual period and by 45% at 9 weeks (Davison and Noble, 1981) (Figure 12.3). During the 3rd trimester a consistent and significant decrease to non-pregnant values occurs preceding delivery (Davison, Dunlop and Ezimokhai, 1980); and daily investigations have suggested a small increase during the first few days of the puerperium (Davison and Dunlop, 1984).

### 12.3 RENAL HEMODYNAMIC CHANGES IN PREGNANT ANIMALS

Pregnancy-induced increases in GFR have been reported in a number of animal species including the rat (Conrad, 1987), which is a particularly good animal model for study of both renal and systemic hemodynamic changes in pregnancy, discussed below.

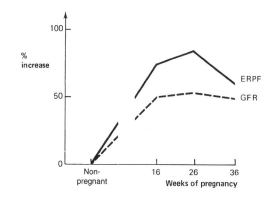

**Figure 12.2** Relative changes in renal hemodynamics during normal human pregnancy (calculated from data by Davison, 1985; Davison and Hytten, 1975; Dunlop, 1976; Davison, Dunlop and Ezimokhai, 1980).

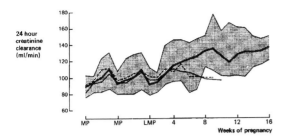

**Figure 12.3**  Changes in 24-hour creatinine clearance measured weekly before conception and through to uncomplicated spontaneous abortion in two women. Solid line represents the mean and stippled area the range for nine women with successful obstetric outcome. MP = menstrual period; LMP = last menstrual period. (Source: reproduced with permission from Davison and Noble, 1981).

### 12.3.1 TIME COURSE AND MAGNITUDE OF RENAL HEMODYNAMIC CHANGES

Gestation in the rat lasts 22 days. As shown in Figure 12.4a, GFR rises early in the conscious rat and has increased maximally by midterm, to 30–40% above the virgin value.

The elevated GFR is maintained throughout the pregnancy, although close to term a return towards the non-pregnant value is evident (Conrad, 1987). To gain insight into the intrarenal mechanisms that control glomerular ultrafiltration, the micropuncture technique can be employed; however, this requires major surgery under general anesthesia.

When plasma volume is carefully controlled, a rise in GFR is detected in this preparation that is maximal by midterm pregnancy and has begun to decline close to term (day 20) (Figure 12.4b); thus the pregnant, volume-maintained rat prepared for micropuncture is a good model for study of renal hemodynamic changes in pregnancy (Baylis, 1987a).

### 12.3.2 DETERMINANTS OF GLOMERULAR HEMODYNAMICS IN PREGNANCY IN THE RAT

Glomerular filtration rate is the product of the single nephron glomerular filtration rate (SNGFR) and the number of filtering

glomeruli. There is no change in glomerular number in pregnancy and thus the increased GFR is due to increases in SNGFR. Glomerular micropuncture allows calculation of SNGFR and all of its determinants; i.e.:
1. glomerular plasma flow ($Q_A$), which varies directly with SNGFR;
2. the hydrostatic pressure gradient ($\Delta P$) across the wall of the glomerulus, i.e. the difference between glomerular blood pressure and the hydrostatic pressure of Bowman's space fluid, which varies directly with SNGFR;

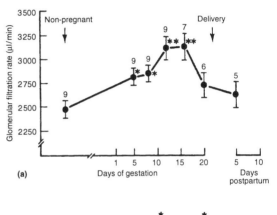

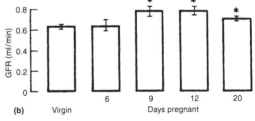

**Figure 12.4**  **(a)** Magnitude and time course of the gestational change in GFR (for both kidneys) measured in the conscious, chronically catheterized Long-Evans rat by Conrad (1984). **(b)** GFR (left kidney measured in the anesthetized, euvolemic Munich-Wistar rat before and during pregnancy. In both **(a)** and **(b)** data are shown as mean ± s.e. A significant difference from the virgin value is denoted by * $p < 0.05$ and ** ($p < 0.0001$). Composite drawn from Baylis (1987a) Glomerular Filtration and Volume Regulation in Gravid Animal Models, Baillières Clin. Obstet. Gynecol., 1(4), 789-813 with permission.)

3. the oncotic pressure of the plasma arriving at the glomerulus (due to the plasma proteins) ($P_A$), which varies inversely with SNGFR;

4. the glomerular capillary ultrafiltration coefficient, $K_f$, the product of the intrinsic glomerular wall water permeability and glomerular filtration surface area (Baylis, 1986). $K_f$ varies directly with SNGFR up to a threshold value above which further increases have no further effect.

The pressures and flows at the glomerulus that determine SNGFR are controlled by the preglomerular and postglomerular (efferent) resistance vessels. By variations in tone in the preglomerular ($R_A$) and efferent resistances ($R_E$), it is possible to control glomerular blood pressure ($P_{GC}$) independently of systemic blood pressure (BP). Figure 12.5 shows the possible combinations of resistance changes at the glomerulus and the predicted effect on SNGFR and its determinants, assuming no change in systemic BP.

The first four examples are all consistent with a net renal vasodilation. If preglomerular resistance decreases and efferent resistance stays constant, a greater percentage of sys-

temic pressure is transmitted through to the glomerulus, so glomerular blood pressure increases and glomerular plasma flow also rises, thereby increasing SNGFR. If both preglomerular resistance and efferent resistance decrease, and those decreases are proportional, then no change will occur in glomerular blood pressure, but glomerular plasma flow will increase and SNGFR will increase. If preglomerular resistance decreases and efferent resistance increases, a large increase will occur in glomerular blood pressure; glomerular plasma flow will probably increase, but may not change if the increase in efferent resistance is sufficiently marked; however the net effect will be an increase in SNGFR. Finally, if preglomerular resistance is constant and efferent resistance decreases, glomerular blood pressure will decrease, glomerular plasma flow will increase a little and SNGFR will either decrease or remain unchanged. Thus, the control of glomerular blood pressure, glomerular plasma flow and SNGFR by the segmental arteriolar resistances is complex and cannot be predicted from whole kidney renal vascular resistance measurements.

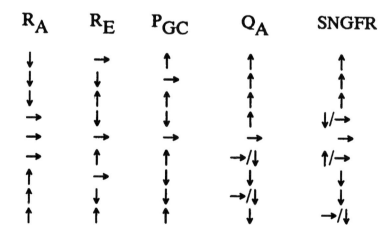

**Figure 12.5**  How changes in preglomerular ($R_A$) and efferent arteriolar ($R_E$) resistances control glomerular capillary blood pressure, $P_{GC}$, glomerular plasma flow, $Q_A$ and SNGR, assuming no change in arterial BP. (Redrawn with permission from Baylis and Reckelhoff, 1991, Renal Hemodynamics in Normal and Hypertensive Pregnancy Lessons; from Micro-puncture. *Am. J. Kidney Diseases*, **17(2)**, 98-104.)

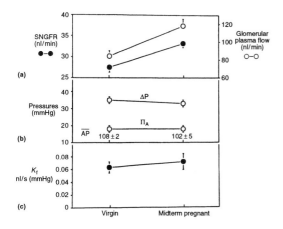

**Figure 12.6** Determinants of glomerular filtration in the virgin and midterm pregnant Munich-Wistar rat studied under anesthetized, volume-restored conditions. In **(a)**, single-nephron GFR (SNGFR) is given by the solid circles and glomerular plasma flow by open circles; **(b)** summarizes the mean ultrafiltration pressures; the transglomerular hydrostatic pressure differences ($\Delta P$) and the preglomerular (systemic) oncotic pressures ($\pi_A$) are given by open circles; **(c)** gives the mean, minimum value of the glomerular capillary ultrafiltration coefficient, K $_f$. Data given as mean ± s.e., by Baylis (1982). Redrawn with permission from Baylis and Reckelhoff, 1991, Renal Hemodynamics in Normal and Hypertensive Pregnancy: Lessons from Micropuncture. *Am. J. Kidney Diseases,* **17**(2), 98-104.)

Micropuncture studies performed in the euvolemic pregnant Munich–Wistar rat demonstrated approximately 30% increases in superficial cortical SNGFR by midterm (Figure 12.6).

The increase in SNGFR (solid symbols, Figure 12.6(a)) is the result exclusively of a proportional increase in glomerular plasma flow rate (open symbols, Figure 12.6(a)). As shown in Figure 12.6(b), the oncotic pressure of systemic blood (at the beginning of the glomerulus, $\pi_A$) is unchanged. Also, the glomerular blood pressure and Bowman's space fluid pressure change little; thus the glomerular hydrostatic pressure gradient $\Delta P$ (Figure 12.6(b)) is also unchanged and cannot be contributing to the gestational rise in

SNGFR. Mean arterial blood pressure (AP) is unaltered at midterm. As shown in Figure 12.6(c), the glomerular capillary ultrafiltration coefficient, $K_f$, does not change markedly with pregnancy and does not contribute to the gestational rise in SNGFR.

Micropuncture studies have now been carried out early (day 6); at midterm (days 9 and 12) and late (days 19–20) in the euvolemic Munich–Wistar rat (Baylis, 1979/80, 1980, 1982, 1987b). One significant finding is that no sustained rise occurs in glomerular capillary blood pressure at any time during the gestation period, despite the renal vasodilation of pregnancy, because of close proportionality in the declines in preglomerular and efferent arteriolar resistances. Clinicians are concerned at the possibility that prolonged periods of renal vasodilation may damage the glomerulus as a result of chronic increase in glomerular blood pressure, secondary to reductions in preglomerular tone (Brenner, Meyer and Hostetter, 1982; Meyer *et al.*, 1987). As discussed above, pregnancy is a state in which the kidneys are chronically vasodilated, although pregnancy is a physiological condition which proceeds without loss of nephron number or underlying disease. Also, there is no sustained increase in glomerular blood pressure during a single gestation period. Multiple, closely spaced pregnancies in normal rats produced no elevation in glomerular blood pressure despite prolonged renal vasodilation (Baylis and Rennke, 1985). Also, there was no evidence of either proteinuria or morphological damage in repetitively pregnant or age-matched virgin rats despite their advancing age. Thus, pregnancy *per se* does not lead to any acceleration in the non-specific age-dependent deterioration seen in renal function in rats whose kidneys were previously normal.

In pregnant women the evidence so far, albeit limited, also argues against the possibility that glomerular injury is produced by normal pregnancy (Davison, 1988). Furthermore, the consensus is that there is no irreversible deterioration in renal function during normal pregnancy or as a result of successive pregnancies, whether assessed by 24-hour creatinine clearance, by inulin clearance or by total protein excretion. Women studied in consecutive pregnancies show similar GFR increments in the later compared with the first pregnancy and it is known that women do not show any tendency for GFR to decline during the reproductive years; overall they show less age-dependent decline than men (Brown *et al.*, 1986).

In summary, therefore, the gestational rise in GFR in the rat is entirely due to renal vasodilation, with consequent increases in renal plasma flow. The reductions in vascular tone in both preglomerular and efferent arteriolar resistances are in proportion, with the result that glomerular blood pressure is constant throughout the entire gestation period. The rise in GFR in the pregnant woman is also most probably the result of a selective rise in RPF. The small fall in filtration fraction, seen throughout most of the gestational period in the normal woman, is probably due to the development of filtration pressure **dis**equilibrium (Baylis, 1987a 1994) because of the large increase in RPF. At filtration pressure disequilibrium further increases in RPF produce disproportionately smaller increases in GFR (for reasons discussed elsewhere; Baylis, 1986); thus filtration fraction falls without any change in the other determinants of GFR. Based on whole kidney human data (Sturgiss *et al,* 1994) and the animal studies reviewed above, it is most unlikely that $\Delta P$ increases significantly during pregnancy in the normal woman (Roberts *et al,* 1996). The available evidence indicates that the chronic renal vasodilation of pregnancy has no long-term damaging effects on the maternal kidney.

## 12.4 FUNCTIONAL CHARACTERISTICS OF THE RENAL VASCULATURE IN PREGNANCY

### 12.4.1 RENAL AUTOREGULATION DURING PREGNANCY

The ability of the kidney to maintain blood flow and GFR over a range of blood pressure

(i.e. to autoregulate) has been extensively investigated in non-gravid animals and variations in preglomerular arteriolar tone are the main mechanisms of autoregulatory maintenance of RPF (Navar, 1978). However, reciprocal alterations in pre- and postglomerular resistance also maintain glomerular blood pressure at near-constant levels over a wide range of systemic blood pressures (Robertson *et al.*, 1972). Arterial blood pressure falls during a normal pregnancy and, since normal blood pressure is quite close to the lower level at which renal autoregulation occurs, autoregulatory failure might present a potential problem in pregnancy. The chronic renal vasodilation of pregnancy might also compromise the autoregulatory vasodilatory requirements of the kidney.

Renal autoregulatory behavior was investigated in pregnant rats, and at midterm, when renal blood flow and GFR were elevated, the autoregulatory ability of the kidney was similar in pregnant and virgin rats (Reckelhoff, Yokota and Baylis, 1992). Similar findings have also been reported in the pregnant rabbit (Woods, Mizelle and Hall, 1987); therefore the gestational renal vasodilation does not alter the intrinsic renal autoregulatory ability. Studies in late-pregnant rats where a gestational fall in blood pressure has occurred have also indicated unimpaired autoregulation of renal blood flow together with a downward resetting in the 'threshold' for renal autoregulation of blood flow. This may represent a protective mechanism whereby late-pregnant animals are protected from periods of renal hypoperfusion (Reckelhoff, Yokota and Baylis, 1992).

### 12.4.2 RESPONSIVITY OF THE RENAL VASCULATURE IN PREGNANCY; RENAL VASODILATORY CAPACITY

In normal non-pregnant humans and experimental animals, a meal high in protein or an amino acid infusion elicit substantial increases in GFR due to a selective renal vasodilation and increased RPF (Bosch *et al.*, 1983; Castellino, Coda and Defronzo, 1986; Hostetter, 1984; Meyer *et al.*, 1983). The normal midterm pregnant rat, which exhibits the maximal gestational renal vasodilation, responds to an acute amino acid infusion with further substantial rises in both GFR and SNGFR due solely to further increases in plasma flow (Baylis, 1988). To date, observations in normal women have been conflicting, since one group observed a substantial rise in endogenous creatinine clearance following a meat meal in third-trimester women (Brendolan *et al.*, 1985) whereas others have suggested that inulin and PAH clearances rise marginally, if at all, following a meat meal in normal gravidas (Barron, Bailin and Lindheimer, 1989). In response to intravenous amino acids, however, normal pregnant women show a marked renal vasodilatory response (Sturgiss, Wilkinson and Davison, 1992). Thus, the kidneys of gravid rats and women possess significant reserve vasodilatory capacity despite the chronic renal vasodilation of pregnancy.

### 12.4.3 RESPONSES TO VASOACTIVE HORMONES

Increased *urinary prostaglandin $E_2$* and *prostacyclin* levels have been reported in normal pregnant women and rats and these elevations in prostaglandins are probably involved in the vascular refractoriness to administered vasopressor agents that develops in normal pregnancy (Conrad and Colpoys, 1986; Pedersen *et al.*, 1983; Ferris, 1988). However, studies in animals provide no support for a role of prostaglandins as mediators of the gestational rise in GFR (Baylis, 1987b; Conrad and Colpoys, 1986; Venuto and Donker, 1982).

The *renin–angiotensin II (AII) system* is substantially modified and has been extensively studied during pregnancy. The changes include increases in plasma renin activity and plasma AII with a decreased responsivity to the vasopressor action of administered AII (Gant *et al.*, 1973, 1987; Broughton and Pipkin, 1988; Paller, 1984; Bay and Ferris, 1979; Brown, Broughton Pipkin and Symonds, 1988). Whether this loss of sensitivity to the vasoconstrictor actions of AII extends to the renal resistance vessels and the glomerulus is not clear. *In vitro* studies in pregnant rabbits and rats suggest downregulation of glomerular AII receptors (Brown and Venuto., 1986; Barbour, Stonier and Aber, 1990); however, recent indirect, functional evidence suggests that the glomeruli of midterm pregnant rats do not develop a reduced responsivity to AII, since the glomerulotoxic effects of gentamicin (mediated by AII) are not blunted by pregnancy (Baylis, 1989a). Recent *in vitro* studies also report no difference in AII receptors in rabbit renal preglomerular vessels from pregnant and virgin animals (Brown and Venuto, 1988). A mild blunting of the renal vasoconstrictor response to administered AII has been reported in conscious pregnant rabbits (Brown and Venuto, 1991), although studies in the late-pregnant conscious rat show normal renal vascular responsiveness to administered AII despite loss of pressor responsivity (Masilamani and Baylis, 1992). However, since renal hemodynamics are not dependent on AII in the normal unstressed animal (Baylis and Collins, 1986; Baylis *et al.*, 1992a), loss of renal responsivity to endogenous AII cannot be the mechanism of the renal vasodilation of pregnancy. Furthermore, studies in rats have indicated that AII-mediated renal vasoconstriction is unlikely to cause the close-to-term fall in GFR and renal plasma flow (Baylis and Collins, 1986).

Vascular sensitivity to other vasoconstrictors is also influenced during pregnancy and some workers report reduced peripheral responsivity to administered noradrenaline and arginine vasopressin (Conrad and Colpoys, 1986; Paller, 1984; Gant *et al.*, 1987). These systems have not been extensively studied with regard to control of renal hemodynamics in pregnancy; however, acute $\alpha_1$-adrenoceptor blockade has similar depressor and renal vasoconstrictor effects on virgin, midterm and late-pregnant, conscious rats (Baylis, 1991) and acute blockade of the vascular AVP ($V_1$) receptor is without BP or renal hemodynamic effect in conscious virgin, mid- and late-pregnant rats (Baylis, 1993). Dopamine is a unique catecholamine, which produces a selective renal vasodilation, and it has been suggested as the gestational renal vasodilatory agent since elevated urinary dopamine excretion has been reported during pregnancy (Gregoire *et al.*, 1990; Perkins *et al.*, 1981). At present, there is no evidence for a causal relationship between dopamine and the gestational renal vasodilation, in fact, preliminary studies in the rat show similar renal hemodynamic responses to acute inhibition of the DA1 (renal vascular) dopamine receptor in virgin and pregnant animals (Reckelhoff and Baylis, unpublished data).

*Atrial natriuretic peptides* have been studied by a number of workers in both human and animal pregnancy. In the rat, plasma ANP and responsiveness to ANP are essentially unchanged during gestation (Kristensen *et al.*, 1986; Nadel *et al.*, 1988), whereas normal women show moderate increases in plasma ANP during the second and third trimester, although there is substantial variability in the data (Fournier *et al.*, 1991; Gregoire *et al.*, 1990; Steegers *et al.*, 1991). The increased plasma ANP in late pregnancy is unlikely to reflect a physiological response to volume expansion because:

1. atrial size does not change during normal pregnancy (Steegers *et al.*, 1991);
2. plasma ANP levels remain elevated long after delivery (Gregoire *et al.*, 1990) when plasma volume has normalized;
3. even greater increases are seen in preeclamptic pregnancies, which exhibit volume contraction (Fournier *et al.*, 1991; Lowe *et al.*, 1991).

The stimulus and physiological significance of the gestational rise in plasma ANP is currently unknown. In studies on male rats, pharmacological doses of ANP raise GFR but via a complex mechanism that includes increased tone in the efferent arteriole and elevation in glomerular blood pressure (Dunn *et al.*, 1986). Since normal pregnancy is associated with dilation of both preglomerular and efferent arteriolar resistances with no change in glomerular blood pressure, ANP is unlikely to be involved in the renal hemodynamic alterations of pregnancy.

*The vasodilatory nitric oxide (NO) system,* which acts via a second messenger, cGMP (cyclic guanosine monophospate), is now known to exert a major impact on the regulation of renal function and blood pressure (Moncada *et al.*, 1991). Toxically produced NO controls, peripheral resistance and blood pressure, both by direct vasodilatory actions and by blunting the responsiveness to vasoconstrictor factors (Conrad and Whittemore, 1992).

Several investigations have examined whether enhanced production and/or sensitivity to NO occurs in normal pregnancy. Plasma and urinary cGMP levels increase during pregnancy in rats, and urinary cGMP increases in pseudopregnant rats (Conrad and Vernier, 1989), which probably reflects increased tissue production of cGMP since metabolic clearance is not affected. NO is unstable *in vivo* with rapid oxidation to $NO_2$ and $NO_3$ ($N_x$) and the $NO_x$ content of body fluids provides an index of NO production, after correcting for dietary $NO_x$ intake, In the pregnant rat 24 h urinary $NO_x$ excretion increases along with the plasma $NO_x$, both of which correlate perfectly with cGMP increases and cannot be accounted for by increased dietary $NO_x$ intake (Conrad *et al.*, 1993).

NO production in pregnant rats is resistant to NO synthesis inhibition, suggesting enhanced basal production, and *in vitro* studies in guinea pigs suggest enhancement of agonist-stimulated NO in pregnancy (Weiner *et al.*, 1991). *In vitro* and *in vivo* studies suggest that NO is responsible for the pregnancy-associated refractoriners to administered vasoconstrictors (Molkar and Hertelendy,

1992; Weiner *et al.*, 1992). Pregnancy also increases mRNA for constitutive NO synthase (cNOS) in a variety of locations, with oestrogen likely to be a primary stimulus (Wiener *et al.*, 1994). There is relative arginine deficiency in pregnant rats since orotic acid excretion increases progressively during pregnancy (Milner and Visek, 1978). There is controversy about the extent to which increased NO is involved in the normal reduction in blood pressure in pregnancy but on balance NO does have a role in the systemic cardiovascular responses to normal pregnancy (Umaus *et al.*, 1990); St-Louis and Sicotte, 1992; Morris *et al.*, 1996; Baylis *et al.*, 1996).

Specifically, increased NO production may play a role in the renal vasodilation of pregnancy. It is indeed an important physiological renal vasodilator (Raij and Baylis, 1995) and recent work in the conscious, pregnant rat suggests that the renal vasodilator is due to the increased NO production (Danielson and Conrad, 1995). It is important to note that chronic NO blockade in pregnancy suppresses the normal peripheral and renal vasodilation, with reductions in GFR, enhanced protein excretion as well as increased maternal and fetal morbidity and mortality, in a pattern reminiscent of pre-eclampsia (Baylis, 1994).

The recently discovered peptide hormone *endothelin* (Yanagisawa *et al.*, 1988) provides the counterregulatory vasoconstrictor influence for EDRF, although a physiological role for endothelin has not yet been described. Plasma endothelin levels are either unchanged (Ihara *et al.*, 1991) or reduced in normotensive pregnancy (Schiff *et al.*, 1992; Florijn *et al.*, 1991). There is unanimity, however, that plasma endothelin levels rise in preeclampsia but not in pregnant essential hypertensives (Florijn *et al.*, 1991; Ihara *et al.*, 1991; Nova *et al.*, 1991; Schiff *et al.*, 1992; Taylor *et al.*, 1990) and a primary pathogenic role for endothelin in preeclampsia has therefore been suggested. Of interest, *in vivo* studies in pregnant rats suggest that unlike AII and other vasoconstrictors, the pressor responsiveness to administered endothelin is not blunted in normal pregnancy and that subpressor doses of endothelin greatly potentiate the pressor response to other vasoconstrictors, particularly in the pregnant rat (Molnar and Hertelendy, 1990). One preliminary *in vitro* study suggests that the renal vasculature from normal late-pregnant rats, either makes less or is less responsive to endogenous endothelin (Griggs and McLaughlin, 1990) but no *in vivo* studies have yet investigated the possibility that diminished endothelin activity is involved in the gestational renal vasodilation and/or late fall in BP; this is unlikely, since urinary endothelin excretion increases during normal human pregnancy (Begigni *et al.*, 1991).

## 12.5 VOLUME HOMEOSTASIS IN PREGNANCY

In normal pregnancy the average weight gain is 12.5 kg. Much of this increase consists of fluid, since total body water increases by 6–8 liters, of which 4–6 liters is extracellular. There are also increases in plasma volume (maximum during the second trimester and approaching 50% above non-pregnant values) and in fluid accumulations within the fetal and maternal interstitial spaces, which are greatest in late pregnancy (Gallery and Brown, 1994). During normal pregnancy, there is a gradual cumulative retention of about 900 mmol of sodium, distributed between the products of conception and maternal extracellular space. These changes in maternal intravascular and interstitial spaces produce the so-called 'physiological hypervolemia'. However, the volume receptors seem to sense these large gains as normal and when diuretics or salt restriction limit volume expansion the maternal response is similar to that observed in salt-depleted non-pregnant women (Lindheimer and Katz, 1985).

Plasma volume expansion will cause renal vasodilation with resultant increases in RPF and GFR in non-gravid rats, providing the volume expansion is of sufficient magnitude.

A cumulative volume expansion occurs during pregnancy in both women and rats such, that close to term, plasma volume is enormously expanded (Chesley, 1978; Lindheimer and Katz, 1985; Baylis, 1994). There is, however, a dissociation between the plasma volume increase and the elevation in RPF and GFR in pregnancy since the renal hemodynamic alterations are maximal quite early, before any substantial rise in plasma volume; thus the plasma volume expansion of pregnancy is not the primary determinant of the gestational rise in GFR (see Baylis and Davison, 1990 for expanded discussion).

## 12.6 CLINICAL RELEVANCE OF RENAL ALTERATIONS

### 12.6.1 URINE COLLECTION

Dilatation of the urinary tract may lead to collection errors in tests based on timed urine volume, e.g. 24-hour creatinine clearance and/or protein excretion. Such errors may be minimized if the pregnant woman is sufficiently hydrated to give a high urine flow and/or if she is positioned in a lateral recumbency for an hour before and at the end of the collection (Dure-Smith, 1970). These precautions standardize the procedure and minimize dead space errors.

### 12.6.2 INTERPRETATION OF RADIOGRAPHS

Acceptable norms of kidney size should be increased by 1 cm if estimated during pregnancy or immediately after delivery (Bailey and Rolleston, 1971). Dilatation of the ureters may persist until the 16th postpartum week and elective intravenous excretory urography during this period should be deferred (Rasmussen and Nielsen, 1988). Ureteric dilation is permanent in up to 11% of parous women with no history of urinary tract infection (Fried *et al*, 1982) and whether this is a harmless sequel of normal pregnancy or represents the residuum of missed infection is not certain.

### 12.6.3 INTERPRETATION OF ULTRASOUND FINDINGS

Even in the face of massive ureteral and renal pelvic dilatation as well as slight reduction in cortical width in pregnancy, provided the patient is without symptoms and there is no evidence of renal impairment it is in order to allow the pregnancy to progress without intervention (Brown, 1990). It is known, however, that renal pelvicalyceal dilatation in pyelonephritis in pregnancy is significantly increased compared to normal pregnancy but as there is no consistent decrement in renal dilatation after treatment this suggests that the dilatation may antedate the infection (Twickler *et al.*, 1991). Acute renal failure due to obstruction by the gravid uterus is a rare complication and, as well as ultrasound changes, there are biochemical alterations and anuria that invariably resolve immediately following amniotomy (Brandes and Fritsche, 1991), or if delivery is not appropriate then ultrasound-guided percutaneous nephrostomy is safe and reliable (Van Sonnenberg *et al.*, 1992).

### 12.6.4 PLASMA CREATININE AND UREA

Plasma creatinine decreases from a non-pregnant value of 70 $\mu$mol/l to 65, 50 and 50 mmol/l, respectively in successive trimesters; plasma urea levels fall from non-pregnancy values of 4 mmol/l to pregnancy values of 3.5, 3 and 3 mmol/l respectively (Kuhlback and Widholm, 1966). Familiarity with the changes is vital, because values considered normal in non-pregnant women may signify decreased renal function in pregnancy. As a rough guide, values of plasma creatinine of 75 $\mu$mol/l and urea of 4.5 mmol/l should alert the clinician to assess renal function further. It should be remembered, however, that caution is necessary when serially assessing renal function on the basis of plasma creatinine levels alone, especially in the presence of renal disease. Even when up to 50% of renal function has been lost, it is still possible to have a plasma creatinine level of less than 130 μmol/l.

## 12.6.5 CREATININE CLEARANCE

Although the reciprocal or logarithm of plasma (or serum) creatinine is often used to estimate GFR (in relation to age, height and weight) (Trollfors, Alestig and Jagenburg, 1987), this approach has recently been questioned (Dunlop and Davison, 1987; Levey, Perrone and Madias, 1988) and in any case should not be used in pregnancy, because body weight or size does not reflect kidney size. Ideally, evaluation of renal function in pregnancy should be based on the clearance rather than the plasma concentration of creatinine. To overcome such problems as 'washout' from changes in urine flow and to avoid difficulties caused by diurnal variations, 24-hour urine samples should be used for clearances. Many methods of determining creatinine concentration in plasma also measure non-creatinine chromogens, leading to overestimates that must be taken into account when calculating creatinine clearances. In addition, recent intake of cooked meat can acutely increase plasma creatinine levels (because cooking converts preformed creatine into creatinine) and awareness of this governs the timing of blood sampling during a clearance period (Jacobsen *et al.*, 1980).

## 12.6.6 PROTEINURIA

Urine flow normally varies over a wide range from moment to moment so that the protein concentration of a random specimen can give only a semiquantitative appraisal of the degree of proteinuria. Although this estimate recorded on a scale of 'pluses' (or as an approximate concentration) is valuable, a more accurate quantitation is needed.

Proteinuria should not be considered abnormal until it exceeds 500 mg in 24 h. Albumin excretion averages 12 mg in 24 h, with 29 mg in 24 h as the upper limit of normal in pregnancy (Higby *et al.*, 1994).

Currently there is debate about the independent effect of normal pregnancy on long-term renal function, using microalbuminuria to detect any damage (Davison, 1985). As discussed in detail elsewhere in this chapter, the consensus is that pregnancy does not damage the kidney; and in any case, better markers are needed than albumin excretion alone.

## 12.6.7 VOLUME HOMEOSTASIS AND DIURETICS

In view of the mechanisms involved in the control of renal sodium reabsorption and the many hemodynamic and humoral alterations that occur during pregnancy (Baylis and Davison, 1990), it is remarkable that problems related to sodium and water homeostasis do not constantly beset pregnant women. Admittedly, many pregnant women have asymptomatic edema at some time during pregnancy but, in the absence of preeclampsia, infants born to women with edema of the hands and face actually weigh more at birth than do infants of non-edematous women (Hytten and Thomson, 1976).

It remains to be established whether the increment in maternal extracellular fluid volume is required for optimal utero-placental perfusion. Of interest, in preeclampsia intravascular volume is decreased (Gallery and Brown, 1994) with compromised placental perfusion and function and the administration of a thiazide or frusemide further can reduce placental function.

Diuretics are sometimes given during pregnancy to prevent and to treat preeclampsia. Carefully controlled studies (Collins, Yusuf and Peto, 1985) have not confirmed the claim that prophylaxis with thiazides reduces the incidence of preeclampsia. Many diuretics effect the renal handling of uric acid and with few exceptions cause hyperuricemia, which can obviously be confusing (Kahn, 1988). Furthermore, diuretics are not without risk, causing maternal pancreatitis, severe hypokalemia, neonatal electrolyte imbalance, cardiac arrhythmias and thrombocytopenia (Collins, Yusuf and Peto, 1985).

## 12.7 CHRONIC RENAL DISEASE IN PREGNANCY

While there are dissenting opinions (Lindheimer and Katz, 1994; Lancet editorial, 1975, 1989; Packham *et al.*, 1989; Jungers *et al.*, 1995, 1996) the majority view is that provided non-pregnant renal function is only mildly compromised and hypertension is absent or minimal, then obstetric outcome is usually successful and there is little or no adverse effect on long-term renal prognosis, except in a few specific disease entities (see below).

## 12.8 CLINICAL IMPLICATIONS OF RENAL DYSFUNCTION IN PREGNANCY

An individual may lose approximately 50% of function and yet maintain a plasma creatinine level of less than 130 mmol/l (Figure 12.7).

If renal function is more severely compromised, however, then small further decreases in glomerular filtration rate (GFR) cause plasma creatinine to increase markedly (Levey, Perrone and Madias, 1988). Nevertheless, a patient who has severe impairment in 75% of her nephrons may have lost only 50% of function and may have a deceptively normal plasma creatinine level. Thus, evaluation of renal function should be based on the clearance of creatinine rather than on its plasma concentration.

### 12.8.1 PATHOPHYSIOLOGY OF RENAL INSUFFICIENCY

In patients with renal disease, pathological conditions may be both chemically and clinically silent. Most individuals remain symptom-free until their GFR falls to less than 25%

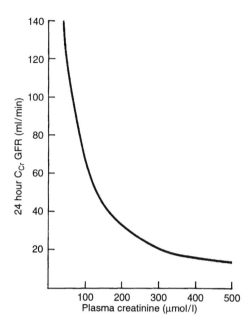

**Figure 12.7** Relationship between GFR (ml/min), determined by clearance of creatinine (24-h $C_{Cr}$), and plasma creatinine concentration ($\mu$mol/l) assuming a constant 24-h creatinine excretion of about 11.5 mmol. (Source: Davison, unpublished observations.)

of its original level, and many plasma constituents are frequently normal until a late stage of the disease. As renal function declines, the ability to conceive and to sustain a viable pregnancy decreases (Surian *et al.*, 1984; Kincaid-Smith and Fairley, 1987; Abe, 1991a; Imbasciati and Ponticelli, 1991). Degrees of functional impairment that do not cause symptoms or appear to disrupt homeostasis in non-pregnant individuals can jeopardize pregnancy.

### 12.8.2 PREPREGNANCY COUNSELING

Normal pregnancy is rare when renal function decreases to such a degree that non-pregnant plasma creatinine and urea levels exceed 275 $\mu$mol/l and 10 mmol/l respectively. These increments above normal non-pregnant levels are moderate but they represent considerable loss of function. The basic question for a woman with renal disease must be 'Is pregnancy advisable?' If it is, then the sooner she starts to have her family the better since in many cases renal function will continue to decline with time. Women are not always counseled prior to pregnancy and may therefore present as a '*fait accompli*', with suspected or known renal disease and then the question must be 'Does pregnancy continue?'

### 12.8.3 RENAL IMPAIRMENT AND THE IMPACT OF PREGNANCY

Obstetric and remote renal prognoses differ in women with different degrees of renal insufficiency and the impact of pregnancy is best considered by categories of functional renal status prior to conception (Tables 12.1, 12.2).

### 12.8.4 PRESERVED/MILDLY IMPAIRED RENAL FUNCTION

Women with normal or mildly decreased prepregnancy renal function (plasma creatinine < 125 μmol/l), usually have a successful obstetric outcome and pregnancy does not adversely affect the course of their disease (Jungers, Houilliet and Forget, 1987; Lindheimer and Katz, 1994). Although true for most patients, some authors suggest that this statement should be tempered somewhat in lupus nephropathy, membranoproliferative glomerulonephritis, focal glomerular sclerosis and perhaps IgA and reflux nephropathies, which appear to be more sensitive to intercurrent pregnancy (Abe, 1991a; Hayslett, 1991; Nicklin, 1991).

Most women with mild underlying renal disease show increments in GFR during pregnancy although the magnitude is less than seen in normal pregnant women (Figure 12.8) (Katz *et al.*, 1980).

Increased proteinuria is common, occurring in 50% of pregnancies (although rarely in women with chronic pyelonephritis) and it can be massive (often exceeding 3 g in 24 h) leading to nephrotic edema. The prevalence of hypertension, renal functional abnormalities and proteinuria, as well as their severity, are considerably lower between pregnancies and during long-term follow-up. When renal failure does supervene, it usually reflects the inexorable course of a particular renal disease.

**Table 12.1** Pre-pregnancy classification of renal functional status

| *Renal status* | *Plasma creatinine (μmol/l)* |
|---|---|
| Preserved/mildly impaired renal function | ≤ 125 |
| Moderate renal insufficiency (± hypertension) | ≤ 125 |
| Severe renal insufficiency (usually with hypertension) | ≤ 250 |

**Table 12.2** Pregnancy implications for women with chronic renal disease. Estimates based on 2350 women/3404 pregnancies (1973–1996) that attained at least 28 weeks gestation. Figures in brackets refer to implications when complication(s) developed prior to 28 weeks gestation. Collagen diseases are not included. (Source: data from Davison, Katz and Lindheimer, 1985; Lindheimer and Katz, 1987; Davison and Lindheimer, 1989; Jungers *et al.*, 1995, 1996; Jones and Hayslett, 1996; Davison and Baylis, unpublished.)

| *Renal status* | *Problems in pregnancy (%)* | *Successful obstetric outcome (%)* | *Problems in long term (%)* |
|---|---|---|---|
| Mild | 26 | 96 (85) | > 3 (9) |
| Moderate | 47 | 89 (59) | 25 (71) |
| Severe | 86 | 46 (8) | 53 (92) |

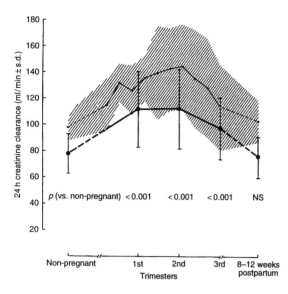

**Figure 12.8** Serial 24-h creatinine clearances (mean ± s.d.) before, during and after pregnancy in 26 women with mild chronic renal disease (solid line). Data from ten healthy subjects (mean ± s.d. shown by hatched area. (Source: reproduced with permission from Katz et al., 1980.)

### 12.8.5 MODERATE RENAL INSUFFICIENCY

Prognosis is more guarded when renal function is moderately impaired before pregnancy (plasma creatinine 125–250 μmol/l) (Cunningham *et al.*, 1990; Hou, 1994). It is difficult to draw firm conclusions about pregnancy in these women, chiefly because the number of cases reported is still relatively small. Suffice it to say that the major worries are serious renal deterioration (particularly early in pregnancy), uncontrolled hypertension (Tables 12.3, 12.4), variable obstetric outcome and accelerated

postdelivery decline in renal function (Surian *et al.*, 1984; Abe, 1991b; Sibai, 1991; Jungers *et al*, 1995 & 1996).

### 12.8.6 SEVERE RENAL INSUFFICIENCY

Most women in this category (plasma creatinine < 250 μmol/l) are amenorrheic and/or anovulatory (Lim, 1987). The likelihood of conception, let alone having a normal pregnancy and delivery, is low but it is not, as some have been misled to believe, impossible (Cunningham *et al.*, 1990; Jones and Hayslett, 1996). The risk of severe maternal complications is much greater than the probability of a successful obstetric outcome (Epstein, 1996). Realistically, these patients should not take additional health risks; therefore pregnancy should be vigorously discouraged. The aim should be to preserve what little renal function remains in these patients and/or to achieve renal rehabilitation via a dialysis and transplant program, after which the question of pregnancy can be reconsidered, if appropriate (Davison, Katz and Lindheimer, 1986).

### 12.9 ANTENATAL STRATEGY AND DECISION-MAKING

Patients with renal disease who become pregnant should be seen at 2-week intervals until 32 weeks gestation, after which assessment should be weekly. Routine serial antenatal observations should be supplemented with:
1. assessment of renal function by 24-hour creatinine clearance and protein excretion;
2. careful monitoring of blood pressure for early detection of hypertension and then assessment of its severity;

**Table 12.3** Effect of blood pressure on pregnancy complications in 86 women/123 pregnancies with chronic renal disease (Source: data from Surian *et al.*, 1984)

|  | Intrauterine growth retardation (%) | Preterm delivery (%) | Renal deterioration (%) |
|---|---|---|---|
| Normotension | 2.3 | 11.4 | 3.0 |
| Hypertension | 15.6 | 20.0 | 15.0 |

**Table 12.4** Effect of blood pressure and/or renal deterioration on fetal mortality (%) in 122 women/240 pregnancies with chronic renal disease (Source: data from Jungers *et al.*, 1986)

| | Hypertension | Renal deterioration | Both |
|---|---|---|---|
| Absent throughout pregnancy | 18 | 12 | 10 |
| Present at some time during pregnancy | 34 | 27 | 40 |
| Present from 1st trimester and controlled | 20 | — | — |
| Present from 1st trimester and uncontrolled | 100 | — | — |
| Present only during 3rd trimester | 12 | | |

3. early detection of preeclampsia;
4. biophysical assessment of fetal size, development and wellbeing;
5. early detection of covert bacteriuria or confirmation of urinary tract infection (reviewed by Cox *et al.*, 1991; Imbasciati and Ponticelli, 1991; Lowe and Rubin, 1992; Sibai, 1996).

The crux of management is the balance between maternal prognosis and fetal prognosis – the effect of pregnancy on a particular disease and the effect of that disease on pregnancy. The various problems specifically associated with particular kidney diseases are summarized in Table 12.5 while the following guidelines apply to all clinical situations, as described in the accompanying case histories.

### 12.9.1 RENAL FUNCTION

If renal function deteriorates significantly at any stage of pregnancy, then reversible causes, such as urinary tract infection, subtle dehydration or electrolyte imbalance (occasionally precipitated by diuretic therapy), should be sought. Near term, as in normal pregnancy, a 15–20% decrement in function, which affects blood creatinine minimally, is permissible. Failure to detect a reversible cause of a significant decrement is grounds to end the pregnancy by elective delivery. When proteinuria occurs and persists, but blood pressure is normal and renal function is preserved, pregnancy can be allowed to continue.

### CASE HISTORY 1

A 28-year-old Gravida 2 (Para 1 + 0) had mesangial IgA nephropathy (Berger's nephritis or focal proliferative glomerulonephritis) diagnosed by biopsy 4 years earlier. The course of her pregnancy is summarized in Figure 12.9.

She had stable renal function (minimal dysfunction – plasma creatinine < 125 μmol/l), was normotensive prepregnancy and was booked at 10 weeks gestation, with no problems in early pregnancy and all routine screen-

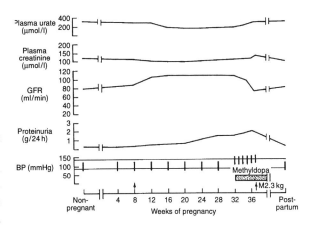

**Figure 12.9** Summary of Case History 1. Blood pressure (BP) denoted by vertical solid line; upper value = systolic, lower value = diastolic pressure. The solid, continuous horizontal lines denote systolic BP = 140 mmHg and diastolic BP = 90 mmHg. BP data are represented in this format in Figures 12.9–12.12. For further details, see text.

**Table 12.5** Pregnancy and specific renal diseases, from Jungers et al, 1986, 1987, 1995, 1996; Cunningham *et al,* 1987; Lindheimer and Katz, 1987, 1994; Packham *et al,* 1988; Magmon and Fejgin, 1989; Baylis and Wilson, 1989; Hill *et al,* 1990; Abe 1991a; Davison and Lindheimer, 1991; Easterling *et al,* 1991; Fields *et al,* 1991; Hayslett, 1991; Heyborne *et al,* 1991; Imbasciati and Ponticelli, 1991; Murty *et al,* 1991; Petri et al, 1991; Lindheimer and Katz, 1994; Jungers *et al,* 1995, 1996; Jones and Hayslett, 1996.

| Renal disease | Effects |
| --- | --- |
| Chronic glomerulonephritis | Usually no adverse effect in the absence of hypertension. One view is that glomerulonephritis is adversely affected by the coagulation changes of pregnancy. Urinary tract infections may occur more frequently. |
| IgA nephropathy | Risks of uncontrolled and/or sudden escalating hypertension and worsening of renal function. |
| Pyelonephritis | Bacteriuria in pregnancy can lead to exacerbation. Multiple organ system derangements may ensue, including adult RDS. |
| Reflex nephropathy | Risks of sudden escalating hypertension and worsening of renal function. |
| Urolithiasis | Infections can be more frequent, but ureteral dilatation and stasis do not seem to affect natural history. |
| Polycystic disease | Functional impairment and hypertension usually minimal in childbearing years. |
| Diabetic nephropathy | Usually no adverse effect on the renal lesion, but there is increased frequency of infection, edema and/or preeclampsia. |
| Systemic lupus erythematosus | Controversial; prognosis most favorable if disease in remission > 6 months prior to conception. Steroid dosage should be increased postpartum. |
| Periarteritis nodosa | Fetal prognosis is dismal and maternal death often occurs. |
| Scleroderma (SS) | If onset during pregnancy then can be rapid overall deterioration. Reactivation of quiescent scleroderma may occur postpartum. |
| Previous urinary tract surgery | Might be associated with other malformations of the urogenital tract. Urinary tract infection common during pregnancy. Renal function may undergo reversible decrease. No significant obstructive problem but cesarean section often needed for abnormal presentation and/or to avoid disruption of the continence mechanism if artificial sphincter present. |
| After nephrectomy, solitary kidney and pelvic kidney | Might be associated with other malformations of urogenital tract. Pregnancy well tolerated. Dystocia rarely occurs with a pelvic kidney. |

**Table 12.5 continued**

| Renal disease | Effects |
|---|---|
| Wegener's granulomatosis | Limited information. Proteinuria (hypertension) is common from early in pregnancy. Immunosuppressives are safe but cytotoxic drugs are best avoided. |
| Renal artery stenosis | May present as chronic hypertension or as recurrent isolated preeclampsia. If diagnosed then transluminal angioplasty can be undertaken in pregnancy if appropriate. |

ing negative. She had a satisfactory maternal adaptation to pregnancy for the first 24 weeks as evidenced by a decrement in plasma creatinine and increment in GFR. Significant proteinuria ($< 500$ mg/24 h) appeared at 24 weeks with otherwise stable renal function and blood pressure. By 32 weeks gestation there had been further increments in proteinuria, GFR had decreased and blood pressure attained levels above 160/110. Changes in plasma urate were unremarkable. Methyldopa was commenced and increased up to 750 mg q.d.s. but even then BP did not stabilize satisfactorily. Because of further deterioration in renal function (with increasing proteinuria) and inadequate control of blood pressure, labor was induced at 36 weeks gestation. A vaginal delivery of a live male child weighing 2.3 kg was achieved. By 10 weeks postpartum she was normotensive and renal function was within normal limits, without proteinuria.

There is usually a favorable obstetric and maternal outcome in any woman with chronic renal disease entering pregnancy in the mild renal dysfunction category and without hypertension. IgA nephropathy can behave unpredictably and in particular escalating hypertension can be a problem. This woman had significant proteinuria by mid-pregnancy and as early as 32 weeks gestation, renal function had started to decline in advance of the usual 15% decrement seen after 36 weeks in normal pregnancy.

Concomitantly hypertension was increasing and in retrospect attempts to control it with methyldopa were unsatisfactory; perhaps other antihypertensive agents should have been used and/or earlier intervention undertaken.

### 12.9.2 BLOOD PRESSURE

Most of the specific risks of hypertension in pregnancy appear to be mediated through superimposed preeclampsia (Sibai, 1996). There is confusion about the true incidence of superimposed preeclampsia in women with preexisting renal disease because the diagnosis cannot be made with certainty on clinical grounds alone, since hypertension and proteinuria may be manifestations of the underlying renal disease. Treatment of mild hypertension (diastolic blood pressure $< 95$ mmHg in the second trimester or less than 100 mmHg in the third) is not necessary during normal pregnancy, but many would treat women with underlying renal disease more aggressively, believing that this preserves function. Most patients can be taught to take their own blood pressure, thereby making monitoring more effective, but there are debates (nearing settlement) regarding the determination of diastolic pressure — Korotkoff's phase IV versus phase V (Johenning and Barron, 1992; Halligan *et al.*, 1993).

## CASE HISTORY 2

A 20-year-old Gravida 3 (Para 0 + 2) with chronic pyelonephritis (infectious interstitial nephritis), stable renal function (minimal dysfunction – plasma creatinine 125 μmol/l) was normotensive pre-pregnancy. She had suffered frequent urinary tract infections in childhood and at 15 years old radiological and ultrasound assessment followed by renal biopsy had established the diagnosis of chronic pyelonephritis.

As summarized in Figure 12.10, during early pregnancy there was a moderate GFR augmentation response with corresponding decrements in plasma creatinine and plasma urea.

Regular urine cultures were negative and she did not have any symptoms or signs of urinary tract infection. At 24 weeks gestation, significant proteinuria appeared and substantial decrements in GFR were evident over the next 4 weeks or so. Urine cultures were negative. At 28 weeks gestation she was pyrexial and had bilateral loin tenderness. From the overall clinical assessment she was diagnosed as having an acute urinary tract infection (acute UTI) and intravenous antibiotics were commenced. She mentioned that she had not felt fetal movements for 24 h and fetal car-

diotocography revealed poor beat-to-beat variation and prolonged late decelerations. Delivery was expedited by lower segment cesarean section (LSCS) with delivery of a live female child weighing 720 g. By 24 h postdelivery there were further increments in maternal temperature, she become breathless and renal function further deteriorated. On clinical, radiological and biochemical grounds a diagnosis of adult respiratory distress syndrome (adult RDS) was made. Thereafter she spent 2 weeks on assisted ventilation in an intensive therapy unit (ITU). She ultimately made a complete recovery. By 10 weeks postpartum she was normotensive, renal function was within normal limits and urine cultures were negative.

Occasionally the course of pregnancy in women with chronic pyelonephritis can be unpredictable even when urine cultures are negative. In this case the proteinuria may have been related to covert pyelonephritis and by the time this was clinically evident and treatment was commenced other systems had become involved. Respiratory involvement is now well recognized, often with the development of adult RDS. Early diagnosis is the key to successful treatment. It might be argued that any woman with her history should have been given prophylactic antibiotics regardless of negative urine cultures.

## CASE HISTORY 3

A 24-year-old Gravida 2 (Para 0 + 1) had membranous nephropathy, diagnosed by biopsy 5 years earlier during investigation of hypertension. She had stable renal function (minimal dysfunction – plasma creatinine 125 μmol/l) and hypertension significant enough to warrant treatment with a beta blocker (atenolol 100 mg daily) for 3 years prepregnancy. In pregnancy atenolol was maintained. As shown in Figure 12.11, during the first trimester there was a moderate GFR augmentation response.

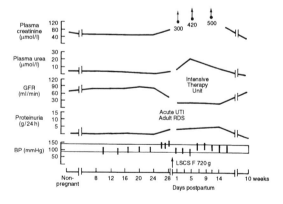

**Figure 12.10** Summary of Case History 2. For details see text.

From 25 weeks gestation onwards there were several changes in antihypertensive treatment (each marked * in Figure 12.11) because of escalating blood pressure. Initially the dose of atenolol was increased, then methyldopa was added with subsequent increments. Blood pressure was adequately controlled until 32 weeks, when a further increment prompted cessation of methyldopa and addition of a calcium channel blocker to the beta blocker. GFR had declined over this time and proteinuria increased. Within 3 days of the fourth change in antihypertensive therapy an intrauterine death occurred. Labor was induced and a vaginal delivery of a stillborn (SB) male weighing 1220 g was achieved. By 10 weeks postpartum she was normotensive (on atenolol ≈ 100 mg daily) and renal function was normal.

Attempts were made to control blood pressure to 'buy time' for fetal maturation. In retrospect this was a mistake because a physical sign (blood pressure) was merely being controlled without any knowledge and/or modification of the underlying pathology. Furthermore, cardiotocography was falsely reassuring that the fetal condition remained satisfactory and by inference that placental perfusion was not being affected. Better control of the blood pressure failed to halt the decline in GFR or increments in proteinuria. This multiple drug approach was not satisfactory and it should have been a warning that the situation was deteriorating and that delivery was needed, at least in the interests of the fetus.

### 12.9.3 FETAL SURVEILLANCE AND TIMING OF DELIVERY

Serial assessment of fetal wellbeing is essential because renal disease can be associated with intrauterine growth retardation and, when complications do arise, the judicious moment for intervention is influenced by fetal status. Current technology should minimize intrauterine fetal death as well as neonatal morbidity and mortality. Regardless of ges-

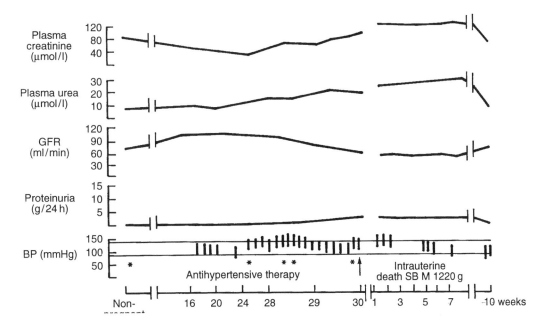

**Figure 12.11**   Summary of Case History 3. For details see text.

tational age, most babies weighing 1500 g or more survive better in a special care nursery than in a hostile intrauterine environment. Deliberate preterm delivery may be necessary if there are signs of impending intrauterine fetal death, if renal function deteriorates substantially, if uncontrollable hypertension supervenes or if eclampsia occurs.

Antenatal fetal heart rate monitoring is the most widely accepted diagnostic test for assessing fetal wellbeing. Non-stress antenatal cardiotocography (CTG) is the most commonly used and needs to be done frequently to identify the changing fetal heart rate pattern associated with hypoxia. Dynamic ultrasound imaging has now advanced from merely assessing fetal age (fetal biometry) to examination of placental architecture and fetal biophysical profile scoring. Doppler ultrasound also allows cardiovascular assessments, particularly in the umbilical vessels, the fetal aorta and cerebral circulation, as well as the maternal uterine and arcuate arteries.

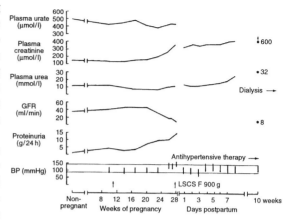

**Figure 12.12** Summary of Case History 4. For details see text.

## CASE HISTORY 4

A 22-year-old Gravida 1 had minimal change glomerulonephritis, diagnosed on biopsy 3 years earlier during investigation of 'pill hypertension'. She had stable renal function (moderate dysfunction – plasma creatinine 125–250 μmol/l) and minimal hypertension when the 'pill' was stopped. Antihypertensive therapy was not considered necessary. In early pregnancy the GFR augmentation response was poor (Figure 12.12).

Antihypertensive therapy was commenced by her family doctor for reasons unknown at 11 weeks gestation and then stopped at 14 weeks gestation. The antenatal course was uneventful until 20 weeks gestation when GFR decreased and proteinuria increased significantly. By 27 weeks gestation BP was 180/110 and antihypertensive therapy (labetalol) was commenced. At this time plasma creatinine was 320 mmol/l and urea 11

mmol/l with proteinuria of 15 g in 24 h. Plasma urate levels were consistently 'high' without specific trends. Fetal cardiotocography revealed fetal compromise. An emergency lower segment cesarean section (LSCS) was undertaken with delivery of a live female child weighing 900 g. The antihypertensive therapy was continued postoperatively, with a sustained fall in BP which did not initially respond to withdrawal of the labetalol. By the fourth postoperative day BP had stabilized at 140/90 without any treatment. Over the next 10 weeks there were progressive increases in plasma creatinine and urea and peritoneal dialysis was instituted.

Although this primigravida had chronic renal disease, was the clinical deterioration and eventual renal failure due to interaction between the renal lesion and pregnancy or did she have (superimposed) preeclampsia? There was marked renal deterioration and proteinuria, which preceded the escalating hypertension. Proteinuria with chronic renal disease in pregnancy is commonplace and in the absence of other biochemical and clinical stigmata can usually be ignored provided the patient does not develop significant nephrotic syndrome. The 'late' appearance of the hypertension in the face of renal deterioration was deceptive and attempts to control the blood pressure might be considered overzealous such that fetal compromise ensured. In the immediate postoperative phase there was a prolonged period of significant hypotension with BP slow to normalize within 24 h of stopping the labetalol. She developed significant renal failure persisting at 10 weeks postpartum such that dialysis had been commenced.

### 12.9.4 ROLE OF RENAL BIOPSY IN PREGNANCY

In pregnancy experience with renal biopsy is sparse mainly because clinical circumstances rarely justify the risks. Biopsy is therefore usually deferred until after delivery (Lindheimer, Spargo and Katz, 1975). Reports of excessive bleeding and other complications in pregnant women have led some to consider pregnancy a relative contraindication to renal biopsy (Schewitz, Friedman and Pollak, 1965), although others have not observed any increased morbidity (Lindheimer *et al.*, 1981). When renal biopsy is undertaken in the immediate postdelivery phase in women with well-controlled blood pressure and normal coagulation indices, the morbidity is certainly similar to that reported in non-pregnant patients.

A recent report on 111 biopsies in pregnant women, all preterm, confirms and extends the impression that risks of the procedure resemble those in the non-pregnant population (Packham and Fairley, 1987). In fact, the incidence of transient gross hematuria, 0.9% (all patients undergoing biopsy have microscopic hematuria unless the kidney has been missed!), was considerably lower than in non-pregnant patients, where it is 3–5%. Such excellent statistics no doubt reflect the experience and technical skills of the unit and statistics have also been improved by refinement of the prebiopsy evaluation.

It is still important, however, to have specific indications for renal biopsy in pregnancy.

Packham and Fairley (1987) suggest that closed (percutaneous) needle biopsy should be undertaken quite often, because they believe that certain glomerular disorders are adversely influenced by pregnancy and that specific therapy, such as antiplatelet agents, might be beneficial. The consensus, however, goes against such broad indications and reiterates that renal biopsy should be performed infrequently during pregnancy (Lindheimer and Davison, 1987). Indeed, even in the nonpregnant individual the reasons for renal biopsy are not clearly defined and experts categorize indications as 'most useful', 'possibly useful' and/or 'of little or no use'.

The few widely agreed indications for antepartum biopsy are as follows.

1. Sudden deterioration of renal function prior to 30–32 weeks gestation with no obvious cause. Certain forms of rapidly progressive glomerulonephritis may respond to aggressive treatment with steroid 'pulses', chemotherapy and perhaps plasma exchange, when diagnosed early.
2. Symptomatic nephrotic syndrome prior to 30–32 weeks gestation. While some might consider a therapeutic trial of steroids in such cases, it is best to determine beforehand whether the lesion is likely to respond to steroids, because pregnancy is itself a hypercoagulable state prone to worsening by such treatment. On the other hand, proteinuria alone with well-preserved renal function in a non-eclamptic pregnant woman without gross edema and/or hypoalbuminemia suggests the need for close monitoring but biopsy can be deferred until the puerperium.
3. Presentation characterized by 'active urinary sediment', proteinuria and border line renal function in a woman who has not been evaluated in the past. This is a controversial area and it could be argued that diagnosis of a collagen disorder such as scleroderma or periarteritis would be grounds for terminating the pregnancy, or that classifying the type of lesion in a

woman with lupus would determine the type and intensity of therapy.

## 12.10 LONG-TERM EFFECTS OF PREGNANCY IN RENAL DISEASE

### 12.10.1 CLINICAL OBSERVATIONS

As discussed earlier, pregnancy does not cause any deterioration or otherwise affect the rate of progression of the disease beyond what might be expected in the non-pregnant state, provided prepregnancy kidney dysfunction was minimal and hypertension absent during pregnancy. However, an important factor in remote prognosis could be that gestational renal vasodilation might potentiate sclerosis in residual glomeruli in kidneys of women with renal disease. The situation may be worse in a single diseased kidney where more sclerosis has occurred within fewer glomeruli. Theoretically, further progressive loss of renal function could ensue in pregnancy. Although the limited evidence in women with ablation-induced renal disease argues against hemodynamic-induced damage in pregnancy (Davison, 1988) there is little doubt that in some women with moderate dysfunction there is accelerated and irreversible declines in renal function in pregnancy or immediately afterwards (Jones and Hayslett, 1996).

### 12.10.2 STUDIES IN ANIMALS

Recent studies have investigated the long-term effect of superimposition of multiple pregnancies on a state of chronic underlying renal vasodilation induced by uninephrectomy plus high-dietary-protein feeding (Baylis and Wilson, 1989). The SNGFR and GFR were somewhat lower in repetitively pregnant compared to virgin rats but, interestingly, the functional renal vasodilatory response to intravenous amino acid was intact in repetitively pregnant rats whereas renal reserve was absent in the virgins. Neither morphological evidence of damage nor proteinuria were worse in repetitively pregnant *versus* virgin rats. Glomerular blood pressures are elevated by long-term uninephrectomy plus high-dietary-protein feeding but are not worsened by pregnancy (Deng and Baylis, 1995), which may explain the lack of exacerbation of the underlying glomerular impairment due to multiple pregnancies.

The spontaneously hypertensive rat (SHR) develops glomerular injury with advancing age although the evolution of injury is much slower in females than in males (Feld *et al.*, 1977; Feld, Brentjens and Van Liew, 1981). Multiple pregnancies have no long-term effect on glomerular function, structure or protein excretion in 1-year-old SHRs nor is the already high glomerular blood pressure elevated further by repetitive pregnancies (Baylis, 1989b). It had been anticipated that in the presence of severe systemic hypertension (as occurs in the SHR) superimposed pregnancy would expose the kidney to additional increases in glomerular blood pressure and injury; however, the normal gestational renal vasodilation was not seen in the midterm pregnant SHR (Baylis, 1989b). This finding was quite unexpected since, as discussed elsewhere in this chapter, pregnancy is almost always associated with increases in GFR and RPF providing renal function is not already seriously impaired. This lack of a renal vasodilatory response in the pregnant SHR despite peripheral vasodilation (BP falls markedly in pregnancy) (Aoi *et al.*, 1976; Takeda, 1964) may reflect a protective mechanism, guarding the maternal kidney.

Studies on a new model of systemic hypertension with renal disease produced by chronic NO blockade revealed that both the renal and peripheral vasodilation were absent and proteinuria developed close to term (Baylis and Engels, 1992). In contrast to other hypertensions, chronic NO blockade in pregnancy results in high blood pressures close to term, suppression of the normal midterm GFR increment and renal plasma flow, suppression of the cumulative plasma volume expansion and the development of protinuria (see Baylis, 1994). Pregnancy outcome is also impaired with increased maternal and fetal morbidity and mortality. The pattern seen resembles the changes in human pre-eclampsia.

The glomerular hemodynamic consequences of experimentally induced, immune-mediated glomerulonephritis have been studied by a number of workers in the male rat. With specific antibodies it has been possible to create lesions of varying severity that can be characterized with regard to glomerular function, using micropuncture techniques (Wilson and Blantz, 1985). In recent studies in the rat, the effect of superimposition of midterm pregnancy was studied on the glomerular functional alterations produced in a model of antiglomerular basement membrane – glomerulonephritis (Baylis, Reese and Wilson, 1989). This lesion was associated with significant proteinuria, high glomerular capillary blood pressure, low $K_f$ and mild impairment in function such that SNGFR and GFR were maintained at near normal values. Despite the underlying glomerulonephritis, a moderate gestational renal vasodilation occurred at midterm with increases in RPF; however, pregnancy did not worsen the increase in glomerular blood pressure due to the glomerulonephritis (Baylis, Reese and Wilson, 1989). There was no evidence of any exacerbation of the glomerular disease by pregnancy in the short term with this lesion, since proteinuria and glomerular morphology were similar in virgin and pregnant rats.

The Fx1A antibody produces Heymann nephritis, which provides a model of membranous glomerulonephritis (Wilson and Blantz, 1985), the most common cause of nephrotic syndrome in adults (Couser and Abrass, 1988). In virgin female rats, passive Heymann nephritis leads to sustained and heavy proteinuria (< 0.5 g/day/250 g rat) with mild impairment in glomerular function and high glomerular blood pressure (Baylis *et al.*, 1992b). Superimposition of late pregnancy does not worsen the proteinuria but substantially lowers SNGFR and GFR and normalizes glomerular blood pressure, predominantly as a result of increased preglomerular tone. Since pregnancy is not associated with increased glomerular pressure in either of these immune-mediated models of renal disease, there is no hemodynamic basis to anticipate a long-term exacerbation of the renal disease by pregnancy (Baylis *et al*, 1995).

Adriamycin-induced nephropathy involves progressive glomerular disease and slowly evolving hypertension – which is accelerated by the superimposition of pregnancy with worsening hypertension, increasing protinuria and suppression of the normal gestational renal hemodynamic response (Podjarny *et al.*, 1992). The changes are probably irreversible one they have taken place (Pomeranz *et al.*, 1995). This is, however, partially alleviated with L-arginine supplementation during pregnancy suggesting that a generalised endothelial dysfunction is involved (Podjarny *et al.*, 1993).

Future studies are necessary to investigate both short- and long-term effects of pregnancy in various models of primary glomerular disease, specifically with the aim of generating animal models in which pregnancy exacerbates underlying renal disease.

## 12.11 LONG-TERM HEMODIALYSIS

### 12.11.1 CLINICAL IMPLICATIONS OF HEMODIALYSIS IN PREGNANCY

Despite reduced libido and relative infertility, women on hemodialysis can conceive and must therefore use contraception if they wish to avoid pregnancy. Although conception is not common (an incidence of 1 in 200 patients has been quoted), its true frequency is unknown, because most pregnancies in dialyzed women probably end in early spontaneous abortion (Hou, 1994). Furthermore, there is a high therapeutic abortion rate in this group of patients, suggesting that those who become pregnant do so inadvertently, probably because they are unaware that pregnancy is possible.

Some women do achieve delivery of a viable infant but most authorities do not advise attempts at pregnancy, or its continuation if present, when the woman has severe renal insufficiency. Clinicians are reluctant to publish unsuccessful cases as well as those that end in disaster, so that the true incidence of successful pregnancies is probably less than suggested in published reports (Brem *et al.*, 1988; Cohen *et al.*, 1988; Gaucherand *et al.*, 1988; Nageotte and Grundy, 1988; Barri *et al.*, 1991; Elliott *et al.*, 1991; Souqiyyeh *et al.*, 1992). These women are prone to volume overload, severe exacerbations of their hypertension and/or superimposed preeclampsia and polyhydramnios (Redrow *et al.*, 1988; Dominguez *et al.*, 1991). They also have high fetal wastage at all stages of pregnancy. Pregnancy poses excessive risks for the mother, and even when therapeutic terminations are excluded the live birth outcome at best is 19% (Davison, 1991). However, as the debate continues more and more women are choosing to take the chance. Multidisciplinary cooperation is essential.

### 12.11.2 ANTENATAL STRATEGY AND DECISION-MAKING

Women frequently present for care in advanced pregnancy because pregnancy was not suspected. Irregular menstruation is common in dialysis patients and missed periods are usually ignored (Lim, 1994) but, with the introduction of recombinant human erythropoietin (rHuEpo) in the treatment of anemia, normal periods often return, probably due to correction of hyperprolactinemia and/or improved general health (Schaefer, Kokot and Werntze, 1989).

Urine pregnancy tests are unreliable (even if there is any urine available) and sonar is needed to confirm and to date the pregnancy. For a successful outcome, scrupulous attention must be paid to increased hours of dialysis, fluid balance, blood pressure control and provision of good nutrition (Redrow *et al.*, 1988; Yasin and Bey Doun, 1988; Durant, 1989).

### 12.11.3 DIALYSIS POLICY

Some patients show increments in GFR despite the fact that the actual level of renal function is too poor to sustain life without hemodialysis. The planning of dialysis strategy has several aims:

1. to maintain plasma urea below 20 mmol/l; some would argue below 15 mmol/l, as intrauterine death is more likely if levels are much in excess of 20 mmol/l; success has occasionally been achieved despite levels of 25 mmol/l for many weeks;
2. to avoid hypotension during dialysis, which could be damaging to the fetus; in late pregnancy the gravid uterus and the supine posture may aggravate this by decreasing venous return;
3. to ensure rigid control of blood pressure;
4. to avoid rapid fluctuations in intravascular volume, by limiting interdialysis weight gain to about 1 kg until late pregnancy;
5. to scrutinize carefully for preterm labor, as dialysis and uterine contractions are associated;
6. to watch calcium levels closely to avoid hypercalcemia. Pregnant women with end-stage renal disease usually require a 50% increase in hours and frequency of dialysis, a policy that renders dietary management and control of weight gain much easier (Amoah and Arab, 1991).

### 12.11.4 ANEMIA

Dialysis patients are usually anemic, which is invariably aggravated further in pregnancy as part of the effect of plasma volume expansion, if indeed this occurs in these women. Blood transfusion may be needed, especially before delivery. Caution is necessary because transfusion may exacerbate hypertension and impair the ability to control circulatory overload, even with extra dialysis. Fluctuations in blood volume can be minimized if packed red cells are transfused during dialysis.

Treatment of anemia with low-dose rHuEpo has been used in pregnancy without ill effect (Barri *et al.*, 1991; McGregor *et al.*, 1991). The theoretical risks of hypertension and thrombotic complications have not so far been encountered. No adverse effects have been noted on neonates and normal hematological indices and erythropoietin concentration for gestational age suggest that rHuEpo does not have a significant transplacental effect.

Unnecessary blood sampling should be avoided in the face of anemia and lack of venepuncture sites. The protocol for tests usually performed in a one's own unit should be followed strictly, with no more blood removed per venepuncture than is absolutely necessary.

### 12.11.5 HYPERTENSION

A normal blood pressure prepregnancy state is reassuring. Some patients have abnormal lipid profiles and possibly accelerated atherogenesis so it is difficult to predict the cardiovascular capacity to tolerate pregnancy. Diabetic women on dialysis who have become pregnant are those in whom cardiovascular problems are most evident. As a generalization, blood pressure tends to be labile and hypertension is common, although it may be possible to help control it by dialysis.

### 12.11.6 NUTRITION

Despite more frequent dialysis, an uncontrolled dietary intake should be discouraged. A daily oral intake of 70 g protein, 1500 mg calcium, 50 mmol potassium and 80 mmol sodium is advised, with supplements of dialyzable vitamins. Vitamin D supplements can be difficult to judge in patients who have had parathy-

roidectomy. All this poses risks for fetal nutrition, plus the fact that the exact impact of the uraemic environment is difficult to assess.

### 12.11.7 FETAL SURVEILLANCE AND TIMING OF DELIVERY

What has been said regarding chronic renal disease applies here. Preterm labor is generally the rule and may commence during hemodialysis. Cesarean section should be necessary only for purely obstetric reasons. It could be argued, however, that elective cesarean section in all cases would minimize potential problems during labor.

### 12.12 LONG-TERM PERITONEAL DIALYSIS (PD)

Since 1976 chronic ambulatory peritoneal dialysis (CAPD) and chronic cycling peritoneal dialysis (CCPD) have been used more frequently in the management of patients with cell forms of renal insufficiency. Several features of PD make it an attractive approach for the management of renal failure in pregnancy.

1. Theoretically it should maintain a more stable environment for the fetus in terms of fluid and electrolyte concentrations.
2. Episodes of abrupt hypotension are avoided – a frequent occurrence during hemodialysis, which can cause fetal distress.
3. Better maternal nutrition is achieved by allowing an unrestricted diet.
4. Continuous extracellular fluid volume control is allowed for and blood pressure control is consequently augmented.
5. The lack of systemic heparin use is useful but whether the incidence of placental abruption and other bleeding proteins are reduced is as yet unknown.
6. In patients with diabetes mellitus blood sugar control via intraperitoneal insulin can be useful.
7. Theoretically it should allow the safe use of intraperitoneal magnesium, facilitating the prevention and treatment of premature labor and possibly treating preeclampsia.

Women can be managed with this approach and successful pregnancies have been reported (Kioko *et al.*, 1983; Hou, 1987; Redrow *et al.*, 1988; Elliott *et al.*, 1991). Although anticoagulation and some of the fluid balance and volume problems of hemodialysis are avoided in these women, they nevertheless face the same problems as hemodialysis patients – hypertension, anemia, placental abruption, premature labor and sudden intrauterine death. Furthermore, it should be remembered that peritonitis can be a severe complication of PD and when superimposed on a pregnancy can present a confusing diagnostic picture as well as a whole series of management dilemmas (Bennett-Jones, Aber and Barker, 1989).

In women with borderline renal failure it has been suggested that dialysis be instituted prophylactically during pregnancy to increase the chances of successful outcome (Redrow *et al.*, 1988; Jakobi *et al.*, 1992). Furthermore, it has been argued that if dialysis is to be used in pregnancy then CAPD is the method of choice and if a woman is already on hemodialysis then a change in modality should be considered (Redrow *et al.*, 1988).

**12.13 RENAL TRANSPLANTATION**

12.13.1 CLINICAL IMPLICATIONS OF RENAL TRANSPLANTATION AND PREGNANCY

After transplantation renal, endocrine and sexual functions return rapidly. About 1 in 50 women of childbearing age with a functioning transplant becomes pregnant. Of the conceptions, 40% do not go beyond the initial trimester because of spontaneous or therapeutic abortion; however, over 90% of pregnancies that do continue past early pregnancy end successfully (Davison, 1994).

Transplants have been performed with the surgeons unaware that the recipient was in early pregnancy. Obstetric success in such cases does not negate the importance of contraception counseling for all renal failure patients and the exclusion of pregnancy prior to transplantation.

12.13.2 PRECONCEPTION COUNSELING

A woman should be counseled from the time the various treatments for renal failure and the potential for optimal rehabilitation are discussed (Davison and Lindheimer, 1989). Couples who want a child should be encouraged to discuss all the implications, including the harsh realities of maternal survival prospects (Table 12.6).

Team work is essential (Lindheimer and Katz, 1992) and individual centers have their own guidelines (Ehrich *et al.*, 1991; Rizzoni *et al.*, 1992). In most, a wait of 18 months to 2 years post-transplant is advised. By then, the patient will have recovered from the surgery and any sequelae, graft function will have stabilized and immunosuppression will be at maintenance levels (Ahlswede *et al.*, 1993). Also, if function is well maintained at

**Table 12.6** Pregnancy implications for renal allograft recipients. Estimates based on 6740 women/5310 pregnancies that attained at least 28 weeks gestation (1961-1996). Figures in brackets refer to implications when complication(s) developed prior to 28 weeks gestation. (Source: data from Davison, Katz and Lincheimer, 1986; Davison, 1987, 1991 and 1994; Davison and Lindheimer, 1989; Davison and Baylis, unpublished).

| Problems in pregnancy (%) | Successful obstetric outcome (%) | Problems in long term (%) |
|---|---|---|
| 49 | 94 (70) | 12 (25) |

2 years, there is a high probability of allograft survival at 5 years.

### 12.13.3 CLINICAL GUIDELINES

A suitable set of guidelines is given here, but the criteria are only relative:

1. good general health for about 2 years post-transplant;
2. stature compatible with good obstetric outcome;
3. no or minimal proteinuria;
4. no hypertension;
5. no evidence of graft rejection;
6. no pelvicalyceal distention on a recent intravenous urogram;
7. stable renal function with plasma creatinine of 180 μmol/l or less (preferably less than 125 μmol/l);
8. drug therapy reduced to maintenance levels: prednisone (prednisolone), 15 mg per day or less and azathioprine 2 mg/kg body weight per day or less. Safe doses of cyclosporin A have not yet been established because of limited clinical experience (Cockburn, Krupp and Monka, 1989), but currently 5 mg/kg body weight per day or less is being quoted anecdotally.

### 12.13.4 ANTENATAL STRATEGY AND DECISION-MAKING

Management requires serial assessment of renal function, early diagnosis and treatment of rejection, blood pressure control, early diagnosis or prevention of anemia, treatment of any infection and meticulous assessment of fetal wellbeing (Hadi, 1986; Hou, 1989) (Table 12.7).

As well as regular renal assessments liver function tests, plasma protein and calcium and phosphate levels should be checked at 6-weekly intervals (Davison, 1991). Cytomegalovirus and Herpesvirus hominis should be checked during each trimester. Hematinics are needed if the various hematological indices show deficiency.

**Table 12.7** Antenatal problems in renal transplant patients

- Transplant function
- Hypertension/preeclampsia
- Transplant rejection
- Maternal infection
- Premature rupture of membranes
- Preterm labor
- Fetal surveillance/intrauterine growth retardation
- Decisions on timing and method of delivery
- Effects of drugs on fetus and neonate

### 12.13.5 TRANSPLANT FUNCTION

Serial renal function data must supplement routine antenatal assessments. Several points (Davison, 1991; Lindheimer and Katz, 1992) should be remembered.

1. The anatomical changes (Absy *et al.*, 1987) and the sustained increase in GFR characteristic of early pregnancy in normal women is evident in renal transplant recipients (Davison, 1985), even though the transplant is ectopic, denervated, often derived from a male donor, potentially damaged by previous ischemia and immunologically different from both the recipient and her fetus.
2. Immediate graft function after transplantation and the better the prepregnancy GFR, then the greater is the increment in pregnancy.
3. Transient reductions in GFR can occur during the third trimester and do not usually represent a deteriorating situation with permanent impairment.
4. In 15% of patients significant renal functional impairment develops during pregnancy and may persist following delivery. However, as a gradual decline in function is common in non-pregnant patients it is difficult to delineate the specific role of pregnancy. Subclinical chronic rejection with declining renal function may occur as a late result of acute rejection or when immunosuppression has not been adequate.

Interestingly, there is a report in the literature of one renal transplant recipient tolerating five term pregnancies and one spontaneous abortion with no deterioration of renal function (Scott and Branch, 1986).

5. Proteinuria occurs near term in 40% of patients but disappears postpartum and in the absence of hypertension is not significant.

6. Whether or not cyclosporin A is more nephrotoxic in pregnancy compared to the non-pregnant is not known (Bennett, Elzinga and Kelley, 1988). Consequently, advice to switch to standard immunosuppressive regimes in gravidae is based purely on clinical anecdote and evaluations are urgently needed in pregnancy.

## 12.13.6 TRANSPLANT REJECTION

Serious rejection episodes occur in 9% of pregnant women. While this incidence is no greater than that seen in non-pregnant individuals it is unexpected because it has been assumed that the privileged immunological status of pregnancy might benefit the allograft. Rejection often occurs in the puerperium and may be due to a return to a normal immune state (despite immunosuppression) or possibly a rebound effect from the altered gestational immunoresponsiveness.

Chronic rejection may be a problem in all recipients, having a progressive subclinical course. Whether a pregnancy influences the course of subclinical rejection is unknown. No factors consistently predict which patients will develop rejection during pregnancy. There may also be a non-immune contribution to chronic graft failure, as a result of the damaging effect of hyperfiltration through remnant nephrons, perhaps even exacerbated during pregnancy (Feehally *et al.*, 1986). From the clinical viewpoint the following points are important.

1. Rejection is difficult to diagnose.
2. If any of the clinical hallmarks are present – fever, oliguria, deteriorating renal function, renal enlargement and tenderness – then the diagnosis should be considered.
3. Although ultrasound may be helpful, without renal biopsy rejection cannot be distinguished from acute pyelonephritis, recurrent glomerulopathy, possibly severe preeclampsia and even cyclosporin a nephrotoxicity.
4. Renal biopsy is indicated before embarking upon antirejection therapy.

## 12.13.7 IMMUNOSUPPRESSIVE THERAPY

This is usually maintained at prepregnancy levels, but adjustments may be needed if maternal leukocyte or platelet counts decrease. When white blood cell counts are maintained within physiological limits for pregnancy, the neonate usually is born with a normal blood count (Davison, Dellagrammatikas and Parkin, 1985). Azathioprine-induced liver toxicity has been noted occasionally during pregnancy and responds to dose reduction. At present there are few good published reports of pregnancies in patients taking cyclosporin A (Derfler *et al.*, 1988; Flechner *et al.*, 1985; Pickrell, Sawers and Michael, 1988; Haugen *et al.*, 1991). Numerous adverse effects are attributed to this drug in non-pregnant transplant recipients, including renal toxicity, hepatic dysfunction, tremor, convulsions, diabetogenic effects, hemolytic uraemic syndrome and neoplasia (Myers, 1986; Al-Khader *et al.*, 1988; Bennett, Elzinga and Kelley, 1988). In pregnancy some of the maternal adaptations could theoretically be blunted by cyclosporin A (Devarajan *et al.*, 1989), including vascular volume expansion and renal hemodynamic augmentation.

The recently established United States National Transplantation Registry has provided encouraging information, with over 198 patients by 1995, (in 288 pregnancies) on cyclosporin A, of whom over 50% required antihypertensive medication(s) (Armenti *et al.*, 1995 and 1996). Birth weights were reduced, but this could also be related to concomitant renal dysfunction and/or hypertension.

## 12.13.8 HYPERTENSION AND PREECLAMPSIA

Hypertension, particularly before 28 weeks gestation, is associated with adverse perinatal outcome (Sturgiss and Davison, 1991), which may be due to the covert cardiovascular alterations that accompany or are aggravated by chronic hypertension. In the third trimester the appearance of hypertension and its relationship to deteriorating renal function, as well as the possibility of chronic underlying pathology and preeclampsia, pose diagnostic problems. Preeclampsia is actually diagnosed clinically in about 30% of pregnancies.

## 12.13.9 INFECTION

Throughout pregnancy patients should be carefully monitored for all types of infection, bacterial and viral. Prophylactic antibiotics must be given before any surgical procedure, however trivial.

## 12.13.10 DIABETES MELLITUS

The results of renal transplantation have been progressively improving in those women whose renal failure was caused by juvenile-onset diabetes mellitus and, inevitably, pregnancies are now being reported in such women. It is evident that problems occur with at least twice the frequency seen in non-diabetic pregnant renal transplant recipients, which may be due to the presence of generalized cardiovascular pathology (Vimicor *et al.*, 1984; Ogburn *et al.*, 1986; Endler *et al.*, 1987; Barrou *et al.*, 1995).

Interestingly, a few successful pregnancies have been reported after combined kidney–pancreas transplantation (Calne *et al.*, 1988; Tyden *et al.*, 1989). In one woman, however, the pancreatic graft was lost unexpectedly in acute rejection immediately postdelivery, having functioned normally for 3 years prior to the pregnancy.

## 12.13.11 FETAL SURVEILLANCE AND TIMING OF DELIVERY

The strategy enunciated for chronic renal disease is equally applicable to renal transplant recipients. Preterm delivery is common (45–60%) because of intervention for obstetric reasons and the common occurrence of premature labor or premature rupture of membranes. Premature labor is commonly associated with poor renal function, but in some it has been postulated that long-term steroid therapy may weaken connective tissues and contribute to the increased incidence of premature rupture of the membranes.

## 12.13.12 METHOD OF DELIVERY

Vaginal delivery should be the aim and usually there are no obstructive problems and/or mechanical injury to the transplant. Unless there are specific obstetric problems then spontaneous onset of labor can be awaited.

## 12.13.13 MANAGEMENT DURING LABOR

Careful monitoring of fluid balance, cardiovascular status and temperature is mandatory. Aseptic technique is essential for every procedure. Surgical induction of labor (by amniotomy) and episiotomy warrant antibiotic cover. Pain relief can be conducted as for healthy women. Augmentation of steroids should not be overlooked.

## 12.13.14 ROLE OF CESAREAN SECTION

This is necessary for obstetric reasons only. The following may be important in connection with this delivery route.
1. Transplant patients may have pelvic osteodystrophy related to their previous renal failure (and dialysis) or prolonged steroid therapy, particularly before puberty. Patients with pelvic problems must be recognized antenatally and delivered by cesarean section.

2. If there is a question of disproportion or kidney compression then simultaneous intravenous urogram and X-ray pelvimetry may be performed at 36 weeks gestation (Figure 12.13).
3. When a cesarean section is performed a lower segment approach is usually feasible but previous urological surgery and/or pelvic infection may make it difficult.

### 12.13.15 PEDIATRIC MANAGEMENT

Over 50% of liveborns have no neonatal problems (Hadi, 1986; Davison, 1994). Preterm delivery is common (45–60%), small-for-gestational-age infants are delivered in at least 20–30% of pregnancies and occasionally the two problems coexist (Pickerell *et al.*, 1988). Although management is the same as in neonates of other mothers, there are some other specific worries (Table 12.8).

### 12.13.16 BREAST FEEDING

Little is known about the quantities of aza-thioprine and its metabolites in breast milk and whether or not the levels are biologically

| Table 12.8 Neonatal problems in offspring of renal transplant patients |
|---|
| • Preterm delivery/small for gestational age |
| • Respiratory distress syndrome |
| • Depressed hematopoiesis |
| • Lymphoid/thymic hypoplasia |
| • Adrenocortical insufficiency |
| • Septicemia |
| • CMV infection |
| • Hepatitis B surface antigen carrier state |
| • Congenital abnormalities |
| • Immunological problems |
|    – Reduced lymphocyte PHA-reactivity |
|    – Reduced T-lymphocytes |
|    – Reduced immunoglobulin levels |
|    – Chromosome aberrations in leukocytes |

trivial or substantial. Even less is known about cyclosporin A in breast milk, except that levels are usually greater than those in a simultaneously taken blood sample (Flechner *et al.*, 1985; Haugen *et al.*, 1991). Until the many uncertainties are resolved, breast feeding should not be encouraged.

### 12.13.17 LONG-TERM ASSESSMENT

Azathioprine can cause abnormalities in the chromosomes of leukocytes, which may take almost 2 years to disappear spontaneously. In tissues not yet studied, however, these anomalies may not be temporary. The sequelae could be the eventual development of malignancies in affected offspring or abnormalities in the reproductive performance in the next generation (reviewed by Davison and Baylis, 1992; Davison, 1994).

### 12.13.18 MATERNAL FOLLOW-UP AFTER PREGNANCY

The ultimate measure of transplant success is the long-term survival of the woman and the transplant. As it is only 30 years since this procedure became widely employed in the management of end-stage renal failure, there is a paucity of information from sufficiently large

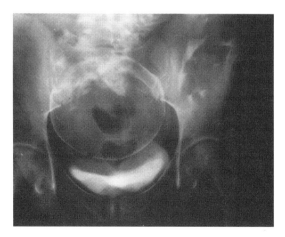

**Figure 12.13** Single-injection intravenous excretory urogram at 37th week of pregnancy in a renal transplant. The left-sided transplant did not interfere with and was not damaged by vaginal delivery.

series from which to draw conclusions. Furthermore, it must be remembered that long-term results for renal transplants relate to a period when many aspects of management would be unacceptable by present-day standards. Average survival figures of large numbers of patients from all over the world indicate that 70–80% of recipients of kidneys from related living donors are alive 5 years after transplantation, and with cadaver kidneys the figure is 40–50% (Morris, 1988; Briggs and Junor, 1992). If renal function is normal 2 years post-transplant, then survival increases to about 80%, which is why women are counseled to wait about 2 years before attempting conception.

Occasionally and sometimes unpredictably pregnancy does cause irreversible declines in renal function but the consensus at present is that pregnancy has no effect on graft function or survival (Whetham *et al.*, 1983; Ehrich *et al.*, 1991; Sturgiss and Davison, 1992).

In isolation, a study from Finland concluded that pregnancy carries a much increased risk of long-term renal deterioration and reduced graft survival and furthermore, that success in one post-transplant pregnancy does not guarantee success in a subsequent one (Salmela *et al.*, 1993). This study was flawed for several reasons and its conclusions have not been endorsed by more recent investigations (First et al., 1995). In addition, there is now evidence that repeated pregnancies do not necessarily adversely affect graft function and/or fetal development provided that graft function was well preserved at the time of conception (Ehrich *et al.*, 1996).

A major concern is that the mother may not survive or remain well enough to rear the child she bears (Kirk, 1991). It has been calculated that 10% of these mothers will be dead within 7 years of pregnancy and 50% dead within 15 years (Crespigny and d'Apice, 1986). Nevertheless, many women will choose parenthood in an effort to renew a normal life and possibly in defiance of the sometimes negative attitudes of medical establishment.

As immunosuppression regimens have been further enhanced an undesired byproduct has been a disproportionately high incidence of neoplasia in these patients. Lest undue concern be aroused by reports of cancers occurring after transplantation it must be emphasized that, although cancer develops in 6% of all transplant recipients, only 1% will die of the disease (Penn, 1990; Briggs and Junor, 1992). Gynecological review is particularly important in this group of women.

## REFERENCES

Abe, S. (1991a) Pregnancy in IgA nephropathy. *Kidney Int.*, **40**, 1098–1102.

Abe, S. (1991b) An overview of pregnancy in women with underlying renal disease. *Am. J. Kidney Dis.*, **17**, 112–115.

Absy, M., Metreweli, C., Matthews, C. and Al-Khader, A. (1987) Changes in transplanted kidney volume measured by ultrasound. *Br. J. Radiol.*, **60**, 525–529.

Ahlswede, K.M., Ahlswede, B.A., Jarrell, B.E., Moritz, M.J., Armeni, V.T. (1993) Effect of transplant to conception interval on outcomes in pregnancies from 266 female renal transplant recipients. *Surg. Forum* **44**, 535-538

Al-Khader, A., Absy, M., Al-Hasani, M. K. *et al.* (1988) Successful pregnancy in renal transplant recipients treated with cyclosporine. *Transplantation*, **45**, 987–988.

Amoah, E. and Arab, H. (1991) Pregnancy in a hemodialysis patient with no residual renal function. *Am. J. Kidney Dis.*, **17**, 585–587.

Aoi, W., Gable, D., Cleary, R. E. *et al.* (1976) The antihypertensive effect of pregnancy in spontaneously hypertensive rats. *Proc. Soc. Exper. Biol. Med.*, **153**, 13–15.

Armenti, V.T., Ahlwede, K.M., Ahlswede, B.A., Moritz, M.J., Jarrell, B.E. (1995) Variables affecting birth weight and graft survival in 197 pregnancies in cyclosporine-treated female kidney transplant recipients *Transpl.* 59, 476-479.

Armenia, V.T., Jarrell, B.E., Radomski, J.S., McGrory, C.H., Gaughan, W.J., Moritz, M.J. (1996) National Transplantation Pregnancy Registry (NTPR): Cyclosporin (CSA) dosing and pregnancy outcome in female renal transplant recipients. *Trans. Proc. In press.*

Bailey, R. R. and Rolleston, G. L. (1971) Kidney length and ureteric dilatation in the puerperium. *J. Obstet. Gynaecol. Br. Commonw.*, **78**, 55–61.

Barbour, C. J., Stonier, C. and Aber, G. M. (1990) Pregnancy-induced changes in glomerular angiotensin II receptors in normotensive and spontaneously hypertensive rats. *Clin. Exper. Hypertens.*, **B9**, 43–56.

Barri, Y. M., Al-Furayh, O., Qunibi, W. Y. and Rahman, F. (1991) Pregnancy in women on regular ÿhemodialysis. *Dialysis Transplantation*, **20**, 652–657.

Barron, W. M., Bailin, J. and Lindheimer, M. D. (1989) Effect of oral protein loading in pregnant and postpartum women: How well does it predict renal reserve? *Clin. Exper. Hypertens.*, **B8**, 208.

Barrou, B., Vidait, A., Bitker, M.O. (1995) Pregnancy after pancreas transplantation: report of a new case. *Transpl. Proc.* **27**, 1751-1759.

Bay, W. H. and Ferris, T. F. (1979) Factors controlling plasma renin and aldosterone during pregnancy. *Hypertension*, **1**, 410–415.

Baylis, C. (1979/1980) Effect of early pregnancy on glomerular filtration rate and plasma volume in the rat. *Renal Physiol.*, **2**, 333–339.

Baylis, C. (1980) The mechanism of the increase in glomerular filtration rate in the 12 day pregnant rat. *J. Physiol.*, **305**, 405–414.

Baylis, C. (1982) Glomerular ultrafiltration in the pseudopregnant rat. *Am. J. Physiol.*, **243**, F300–F305.

Baylis, C. (1986) Glomerular filtration dynamics, in *Advances in Renal Physiology*, (ed. C. J. Lote), Croom Helm, London, p. 33–83.

Baylis, C. (1987a) Glomerular filtration and volume regulation in gravid animal models. *Clin. Obstet. Gynaecol. (Baillière)*, **1**, 789–813.

Baylis, C. (1987b) Renal effects of cyclooxygenase inhibition in the pregnant rat. *Am. J. Physiol.*, **253**, F158–F163.

Baylis, C. (1988) Effect of amino acid infusion as an index of renal vasodilatory capacity in pregnant rats. *Am. J. Physiol.*, **254**, F650–F656.

Baylis, C. (1989a) Gentamicin-induced glomerulotoxicity in the pregnant rat. *Am. J. Kidney Dis.*, **13**, 108–113.

Baylis, C. (1989b) Immediate and long term effects of pregnancy on glomerular function in the SHR. *Am. J. Physiol.*, **257**, F1140–F1145.

Baylis, C. (1991) Effects of acute blockade of ÿα-1 adrenoceptors in virgin, midterm pregnant and late pregnant conscious rats. *Clin. Exper. Hypertens.*, **B10**, 212A.

Baylis, C. (1993) Blood pressure and renal hemodynamic effects of acute blockade of the vascular actions of arginine vasopressin in normal pregnancy in the rat. *Clin. Exper. Hypertens.*, **12**, 93–102.

Baylis, C. (1994) Glomerular filtration and volume regulation in gravid animal models. *Clin. Obstet. Gynaecol (Baillière)* **8**, 235-264

Baylis, C. and Collins, R. C. (1986) Angiotensin II inhibition on blood pressure and renal hemodynamics in pregnant rats. *Am. J. Physiol.*, **250**, F308–F314.

Baylis, C. and Davison, J. (1990) The urinary system, in *Clinical Physiology in Obstetrics*, (eds F. Hytten and G. Chamberlain), Blackwell Scientific, Oxford, p. 245–302.

Baylis, C. and Engels, K. (1992) Adverse interactions between pregnancy and a new model of systemic hypertension produced by chronic blockade of endothelial derived relaxing factor (EDRF) in the rat. *Clin. Exper. Hypertens.*, **11**, 117–129.

Baylis, C., Mitruka, B., Couser, W.G. (1995) Glomerular hemodynamic effects of the late pregnancy in rats with experimental membranous glomerulonephropathy. *J.Am.Soc.Nephrol.* **6**, 1197-1201.

Baylis, C., Mitruka, B. and Deng, A. (1992) Chronic blockade of nitric oxide synthesis in the rat produces systemic hypertension and glomerular damage. *J. Clin. Invest.*, **90**, 278–281.

Baylis, C. and Reckelhoff, J. F. (1991) Renal hemodynamics in normal and hypertensive pregnancy; lessons from micropuncture. *Am. J. Kidney Dis.*, **17**, 98–104.

Baylis, C., Reese, K. and Wilson, C. B. (1989) Glomerular effects of pregnancy in a model of glomerulonephritis in the rat. *Am. J. Kidney Dis.*, **14**, 452–460.

Baylis, C. and Rennke, H. G. (1985) Renal hemodynamics and glomerular morphology in repetitively pregnant, aging rats. *Kidney Int.*, **28**, 140–145.

Baylis, C. and Wilson, C. B. (1989) Sex and the single kidney. *Am. J. Kidney Dis.*, **13**, 290–298.

Baylis, C., Engels, K., Harton, P. and Samsell, L. (1992a) The acute effects of endothelial derived relaxing factor (EDRF) blockade in the normal conscious rat are not due to angiotensin II. *Am. J. Physiol.*, **264**, F74–F78.

Baylis, C., Deng, A., Samsell, L. *et al.* (1992b) Superimposition of pregnancy in the Fx1A model of membranous glomerulonephritis is antihypertensive and lowers glomerular blood pressure. *J. Am. Soc. Nephrol.*, **6**, 1197–1201.

Baylis C., Suto, T., Conrad, K.P., (1996) Importance of nitric oxide in control of systemic and renal hemodynamics during normal pregnancy: studies in the rat and implications for preeclampsia. *Hypert.in Preg.* **15**, 147–169.

Benigni, A., Gaspari, F., Orisio, S. *et al.* (1991) Human placenta expresses endothelin gene and corresponding protein is excreted in urine in increasing amounts during normal pregnancy. *Am. J. Obstet. Gynecol.*, **164**, 844–848.

Bennett, W. M., Elzinga, L. and Kelley, V. (1988) Pathophysiology of cyclosporine nephrotoxicity: role of eicosanoids. *Transplant. Proc.*, **20**, 628–633.

Bennett-Jones, D. N., Aber, G. M. and Barker, K. (1989) Successful pregnancy in a patient with continuous ambulatory peritoneal dialysis. *Nephrol. Dialysis Transplant.*, **4**, 583–585.

Bosch, J. P., Saccaggi, A., Lauer, A. *et al.* (1983) Renal functional reserve in humans: effect of protein intake on glomerular filtration rate. *Am. J. Med.*, **75**, 943–950.

Brandes, J. C. and Fritsche, C. (1991) Obstructive acute renal failure by a gravid uterus: a case report and review. *Am. J. Kidney Dis.*, **18**, 398–401.

Brem, A. S., Singer, D., Anderson, L. *et al.* (1988) Infants of azotemic mothers: a report of three live births. *Am. J. Kidney Dis.*, **12**, 299–303.

Brendolan, A., Bragantini, L., Chiaramonte, S. *et al.* (1985) Renal functional reserve in pregnancy. *Kidney Int.*, **28**, 232A.

Brenner, B. M., Meyer, T. W. and Hostetter, T. H. (1982) Dietary protein intake and the progressive nature of kidney disease: the role of hemodynamically mediated glomerular injury in the pathogenesis of progressive glomerular sclerosis in ageing, renal ablation and intrinsic renal disease. *N. Engl. J. Med.*, **307**, 652–659.

Briggs, J. D. and Junor, B. J. R. (1992) Long term complications and results in the transplant patient, in *Oxford Textbook of Nephrology*, (eds J. S. Cameron, A. M. Davison, J.-P. Grunfeld *et al.*), Oxford University Press, Oxford, p. 1570–1594.

Broughton-Pipkin, F. (1988) The renin–angiotensin system in normal and hypertensive pregnancies, in *Handbook of Hypertension, vol. 10: Hypertension in Pregnancy*, 1st edn, (ed. P. C. Rubin), Elsevier, Amsterdam, p. 118–151.

Brown, M. A. (1990) Urinary tract dilatation in pregnancy. *Am. J. Obstet. Gynecol.*, **164**, 641–643.

Brown, M. A., Broughton-Pipkin, F. and Symonds, E. M. (1988) The effects of intravenous angiotensin II upon blood pressure and sodium and urate excretion in human pregnancy. *J. Hypertens.*, **6**, 457–464.

Brown, G. P. and Venuto, R. C. (1986) Angiotensin II receptor alterations during pregnancy in rabbits. *Am. J. Physiol.*, **251**, E58–E64.

Brown, G. P. and Venuto, R. C. (1988) Angiotensin II receptors in rabbit renal preglomerular vessels. *Am. J. Physiol.*, **255**, E16–E22.

Brown, G. P. and Venuto, R. C. (1991) Renal blood flow response to angiotensin II infusions in conscious pregnant rabbits. *Am. J. Physiol.*, **261**, F51–F59.

Brown, W. W., Davis, B. B., Spray, L. A. *et al.* (1986) Aging and the kidney. *Arch. Intern. Med.*, **146**, 1790–1797.

Calne, R. Y., Brons, E. G. M., Williams, P. F. *et al.* (1988) Successful pregnancy after paratopic segmental pancreas and kidney transplantation. *Br. Med. J.*, **296**, 1709.

Castellino, P., Coda, B. and Defronzo, R. A. (1986) Effect of amino acid infusion on renal hemodynamics in humans. *Am. J. Physiol.*, **251**, F132–F140.

Chesley, L. C. (1978) Blood pressure and circulation, in *Hypertensive Disorders in Pregnancy*, (ed. L. C. Chesley), Appleton-Century-Crofts, New York, p. 119–154.

Cietak, K. A. and Newton, J. R. (1985a) Serial quantitative nephronosonography in pregnancy. *Br. J. Radiol.*, **58**, 405–409.

Cietak, K. A. and Newton, J. R. (1985b) Serial qualitative nephrosonography in pregnancy. *Br. J. Radiol.*, **58**, 399–404.

Cockburn, I., Krupp, P. and Monka, C. (1989) Present experience of Saudimmun in pregnancy. *Transplant. Proc.*, **21**, 3730–3732.

Cohen, D., Frenkel, Y., Maschiach, S. and Eliahou, H. E. (1988) Dialysis during pregnancy in advanced chronic renal failure patients: outcome and progression. *Clin. Nephrol.*, **29**, 144–148.

Collins, R., Yusuf, P. and Peto, R. (1985) Overview of randomised trials of diuretics in pregnancy. *Br. Med. J.*, **290**, 17–23.

Conrad, K. (1987) Possible mechanisms for changes in renal hemodynamics during pregnancy: studies from animal models. *Am. J. Kidney Dis.*, **9**, 253–259.

Conrad, K. P. and Colpoys, M. C. (1986) Evidence against the hypothesis that prostaglandins are the vasodepressor agents of pregnancy. *J. Clin. Invest.*, **77**, 236–245.

Conrad, K.P., Vernier, K.A. (1989) Plasma levels, urinary excretion and metabolic production of cGMP during gestations in rats. *Am. J. Physiol* **257**, R847–R853.

Conrad, K.P. and Whittemore, S.L. (1992) N^G-monomethyl-L-arginine and nitroarginine potentiate pressor responsiveness of vasoconstrictors in conscious rats. *Am. J. Physiol.* **262**, R1137–1144.

Couser, W. G. and Abrass, C. K. (1988) Pathogenesis of membranous nephropathy. *Annu. Rev. Med.*, **29**, 517–530.

Cox, S. M., Shelburne, P., Mason, R. A. *et al.* (1991) Mechanisms of hemolysis and anemia associated with acute antepartum pyelonephritis. *Am. J. Obstet. Gynecol.*, **164**, 587–590.

Crespigny, P. C. D. and D'apice, A. J. F. (1986) Parenthood after renal transplantation. *Aust. NZ J. Med.*, **16**, 245–249.

Croce, J.F., Signorelli, P., Chapparini, I. (1994). Hydro-nephrosis in pregnancy: ultrasongraphic study. *Minerv. Clinical* **46**, 147-153

Cunningham, F. G., Lucas, M. J. and Hankins, G. D. (1987) Pulmonary injury complicating antepartum pyelonephritis. *Am. J. Obstet. Gynecol.*, **156**, 797–807.

Cunningham, F. G., Cox, S. M., Harstad, T. W. *et al.* (1990) Chronic renal disease and pregnancy outcome. *Am. J. Obstet. Gynecol.*, **163**, 453–459.

Danielson, L.A. and Conrad, K.P. (1995) Nitric oxide mediates renal vasodilation and hyperfiltration during pregnancy in chronically instrumented conscious rats. *J.Clin.Invest* **96**, 482–490

Davison, J. M. (1985) The effect of pregnancy on kidney function in renal allograft recipients. *Kidney Int.*, **27**, 74–79.

Davison, J. M. (1988) The effect of pregnancy on long term renal function in women with chronic renal disease and single kidneys. *Clin. Exper. Hypertens.*, **B8**, 226.

Davison, J. M. (1991) Dialysis, transplantation and pregnancy. *Am. J. Kidney Dis.*, **27**, 127–132.

Davison, J. M. (1994) Pregnancy in renal allograft recipients: problems, prognosis and practicalities. *Clin. Obstet. Gynecol. (Baillière)*, **8**, 501–505.

Davison, J. M. and Baylis, C. (1992) Pregnancy in patients with underlying renal disease, in *Oxford Textbook of Nephrology*, (eds J. S. Cameron, A. M. Davison, J.-P. Grunfeld *et al.*), Oxford University Press, Oxford, p. 1936–1956.

Davison, J. M., Dellagrammatikas, H. and Parkin, J. M. (1985) Maternal azathioprine therapy and depressed haemopoiesis in the babies of renal allograft recipients. *Br. J. Obstet. Gynaecol.*, **92**, 233–239.

Davison, J. M. and Dunlop, W. (1980) Renal haemodynamics and tubular function in normal human pregnancy. *Kidney Int.*, **18**, 152–161.

Davison, J. M. and Dunlop, W. (1984) Changes in renal haemodynamics and tubular function induced by normal human pregnancy. *Semin. Nephrol.*, 198–207.

Davison, J. M., Dunlop, W. and Ezimokhai, M. (1980) Twenty-four hour creatinine clearance during the third trimester of normal pregnancy. *Br. J. Obstet. Gynaecol.*, 87, 106–109.

Davison, J. M. and Hytten, F. E. (1974) Glomerular filtration during the after pregnancy. *J. Obstet. Gynaecol. Br. Commonw.*, **81**, 588–595.

Davison, J. M., Katz, A. I. and Lindheimer, M. D. (1986) Pregnancy in women with renal disease and renal transplants. *Proc. EDTA ERA*, **22**, 439A.

Davison, J. M. and Lindheimer, M. D. (1989) Pregnancy and renal transplantation: look before you leap. *Int. J. Artificial Organs*, **12**, 144–146.

Davison, J. M. and Lindheimer, M. D. (1991) Renal disease in pregnancy. *Curr. Obstet. Med.*, **1**, 197–228.

Davison, J. M. and Noble, M. C. B. (1981) Serial changes in 24-hour creatinine clearance during normal menstrual cycles and the first trimester of pregnancy. *Br. J. Obstet. Gynaecol.*, **88**, 10–17.

Deng, A. and Baylis, C. (1995) Glomerular hemodynamic responses to pregnancy in rats with severe reduction of renal mass. *Kid Intl* **4**, 39–44

Derfler, K., Schaller, A., Herold, C. H. *et al.* (1988) Successful outcome of a complicated pregnancy in a renal transplant recipient taking cyclosporine-A. *Clin. Nephrol.*, **29**, 96–102.

Devarajan, P., Kaskel, F. J., Arbeit, L. A. and Moore, L. C. (1989) Cyclosporine nephrotoxicity: blood volume, sodium conservation and renal hemodynamics. *Am. J. Physiol.*, **256**, F71–F78.

Dominguez, N., Cruz, N., Ramos-Barroso, A. and Ramos-Umpierre, E. (1991) Pregnancy in chronic hemodialysis. *Transplant. Proc.*, **23**, 1836–1837.

Dunlop, W. (1976) Investigations into the influence of posture on renal plasma flow and glomerular filtration rate during late pregnancy. *Br. J. Obstet. Gynaecol.*, **83**, 17–23.

Dunlop, W. and Davison, J. M. (1987) Renal haemodynamics and tubular function. *Clin. Obstet. Gynaecol. (Baillière)*, **1**, 769–787.

Dunn, B. R., Ichikawa, I., Pfeffer, J. M. *et al.* (1986) Renal and systemic hemodynamic effects of synthetic atrial natriuretic peptide in the anesthetized rat. *Circ. Res.* **59**, 237–246.

Durant, A. Q. (1989) Treatment guidelines in a pregnant hemodialysis patient. *Dialysis Transplant.*, **18**, 86–90.

Dure-Smith, P. (1970) Pregnancy dilatation of the urinary tract: the iliac sign and its significance. *Radiology*, 96, 545–550.

Easterling, T. R., Brateng, D., Goldman, M. L. *et al.* (1991) Renal vascular hypertension during pregnancy. *Obstet. Gynecol.*, 78, 921–925.

Ehrich, J.H.H., Loirat C, Davison, J.M., Rizzoui, G., Whittkop, B., Selwood, N.H., Mallisk, N.P. (1996) Repeated successful pregnancies after kidney transplantation in 102 women (Report by CDTA Registry) *Nephrol. Dial Transpl.* 11, 1314–1317

Ehrich, J. H. H., Rizzoni, G., Brunner, F. P. *et al.* (1991) Combined report on regular dialysis and transplantation of children in Europe 1989. *Nephrol. Dialysis Transplant.*, 6, 37–47.

Elliott, J. P., O'Keefe, D. F., Schon, D. A. and Cherem, L. B. (1991) Dialysis in pregnancy: a critical review. *Obstet. Gynecol. Surv.*, 46, 319–324.

Endler, M., Derfler, K., Schaller, A. and Nowotny, C. (1987) Schwangerschaft und Geburt nach Nierentransplantation unter Cyclosporin A. Fallbericht und Literatur Übersicht. *Geburtsh. Frauenheilk.*, 47, 660–663.

Epstein Fit (1996) Pregnancy and renal disease. *N Eng J Med* 335, 277–278

Feehally, J., Bennett, S. E., Harris, P. K. G. and Walls, J. (1986) Is chronic renal transplant rejection a non-immunological phenomenon? *Lancet*, ii, 486–488.

Feld, L. G., Brentjens, J. R. and Van Liew, J. B. (1981) Renal injury and proteinuria in female spontaneously hypertensive rats. *Renal Physiol.*, 4, 46–56.

Feld, L. G., Van Liew, J. B., Galaske, R. G. and Boylan, J. W. (1977) Selectivity of renal injury and proteinuria in the spontaneously hypertensive rat. *Kidney Int.*, 12, 332–343.

Ferris, T. F. (1988) Prostanoids in normal and hypertensive pregnancy, in *Handbook of Hypertension, vol. 10: Hypertension in Pregnancy*, 1st edn, (ed. P. C. Rubin), Elsevier, Amsterdam, p. 102–117.

Fields, C. L., Ossorio, M. A., Roy, T. M. and Bunke, C. M. (1991) Wegener's granulomatosis complicated by pregnancy: a case report. *J. Reprod. Med.*, 36, 463–466.

First, M.R., Combs, A., Weiskittel, P., Miodovnik, M. (1995) Lack of effect of pregnancy on renal allograft survival or function. *Transpl.* 59, 472–476.

Flechner, S. M., Katz, A. R., Rogers, A. J. *et al.* (1985) The presence of cyclosporine in body tissues and fluids during pregnancy. *Am. J. Kidney Dis.*, 5, 60–63.

Florijn, K. W., Derkx, F. H. M., Visser, W. *et al.* (1991) Plasma immunoreactive endothelin-1 in pregnant women with and with pre-eclampsia. *J. Cardiovasc. Pharmacol.*, 17, S446–S448.

Fried, A.M., Woodring, J.H., Thompson, D.S. (1982) Hydronephrosis in pregnancy. A prospective sequential study of course of dilation. *J. Ultrasound Med.* 2, 255–259.

Fournier, A., El Esper, G. N., Lalau, J. D. *et al.* (1991) Atrial natriuretic factor in pregnancy and pregnancy-induced hypertension. *Can. J. Physiol. Pharmacol.*, 69, 1601–1608.

Gallery, E. D. M. and Brown, M. (1994) Volume homeostasis in normal and pre-eclampsia: physiology and clinical implications *Clin. Obstet. Gynaecol. (Baillière)*, 8, 287–310.

Gant, N. F., Daley, G. L., Chand, S. *et al.* (1973) A study of angiotensin II pressor response throughout primigravid pregnancy. *J. Clin. Invest.*, 52, 2682–2689.

Gant, N. F., Whalley, P. J., Everett, R. *et al.* (1987) Control of vascular reactivity in pregnancy. *Am. J. Kidney Dis.*, 9, 303–307.

Gaucherand, P., Chalabreysse, J. P., Audra, P. *et al.* (1988) Pregnancy in women undergoing dialysis in chronic renal insufficiency. *J. Gynecol. Obstet. Reprod. Biol.*, 17, 889–895.

Gregoire, I., El Esper, N., Gondry, J. *et al.* (1990) Plasma atrial natriuretic factor and urinary excretion of a ouabain displacing factor and dopamine in normotensive pregnant women before and after delivery. *Am. J. Obstet. Gynecol.*, 162, 71–76.

Griggs, K. C. and McLaughlin, M. K. (1990) Intrinsic tone of isolated rat renal interlobar arteries in pregnancy; role of the endothelium. *J. Am. Soc. Nephrol.*, 1, 664A.

Hadi, H. A. (1986) Pregnancy in renal transplant recipients: a review. *Obstet. Gynecol. Surv.*, 41, 264–271.

Halligan, A., O'Brien, E., O'Malley, K. (1993) 24h ambulatory blood pressure measurement in a prima-gravid population. *J. Hypertension* 11, 869–873.

Haugen, G., Fauchald, P., Sodal, G. *et al.* (1991) Pregnancy outcome in renal allograft recipients: influence of cyclosporin A. *Eur. J. Obstet. Gynaecol. Reprod. Biol.*, 29, 25–29.

Hayslett, J. P. (1991) Maternal and fetal complications in pregnant women with systemic lupus erythematosus. *Am. J. Kidney Dis.*, 17, 123–126.

Heybourne, K. D., Schultz, M. F., Goodlin, R. C. and Durham, J. D. (1991) Renal artery stenosis during pregnancy: a review. *Obstet. Gynecol. Surv.*, 46, 509–514.

Higby, K., Suiter, C.R., Phelps, J.Y., Siler-Khodr, T., Langer, O. (1994) Normal value of urinary albumen and total protein excretion during pregnancy. *Am. J. Obstet Gynaecol* **171**, 984–989

Hill, D. E., Chantigian, P. M. and Kramer, S. A. (1990) Pregnancy after augmentation cystoplasty. *Surg. Gynecol. Obstet.*, **170**, 485–487.

Hostetter, T. H. (1984) Human renal response to a meat meal. *Am. J. Physiol.*, **250**, F613–F618.

Hou, S. (1994) Pregnancy in women on peritoneal and haemodialysis. *Clin. Obstet. Gynaecol. (Baillière)*, **8**, 481–500.

Hou, S. H., Grossman, S. D. and Madias, N. E. (1985) Pregnancy in women with renal disease and moderate renal insufficiency. *Am. J. Med.*, **78**, 185–194.

Hou, S. (1989) Pregnancy in organ transplant recipients. *Med. Clin. North Am.*, **73**, 667–683.

Hytten, F. E. and Thomson, A. M. (1976) Weight gain in pregnancy, in *Hypertension in Pregnancy*, (eds M. D. Lindheimer, A. I. Katz and, F. P. Zuspan), John Wiley, New York.

Ihara, Y., Sagawa, N., Hasegawa, M. *et al.* (1991) Concentrations of endothelin-1 in maternal and umbilical cord blood at various stages of pregnancy. *J. Cardiovasc. Pharmacol.*, **17**, S443–S445.

Imbasciati, E. and Ponticelli, C. (1991) Pregnancy and renal disease: predictors for fetal and maternal outcome. *Am. J. Nephrol.*, **11**, 353–362.

Jacobsen, F. K., Christensen, C. K., Mogensen, C. E. and Heilskow, H. C. S. (1980) Evaluation of kidney function after meals. *Lancet*, **i**, 319.

Jakobi, P., Ohel, G., Szylman, P. *et al.* (1992) Continuous ambulatory peritoneal dialysis as the primary approach in the management of severe renal insufficiency in pregnancy. *Obstet. Gynecol.*, **79**, 808–810.

Johenning, A.R., Baron, W.M (1992) Indirect blood pressure measurement in pregnancy: Korotkoff phase IV versus phase V. *Am. J.Obstet Gynaecol* **167**, 577–580

Jones, D.C., Hayslett, J.P. (1996) Outcome of pregnancy in women with moderate or severe renal insufficiency. *N. Eng. J. Med.* **335**, 226–232.

Jungers, P., Houillier, P. and Forget, D. (1987) Reflux nephropathy and pregnancy. *Clin. Obstet. Gynaecol. (Baillière)*, **1**, 955–969.

Jungers, P., Forget, D., Henry-Amar, M. and Grunfeld, J.-P. (1986) Chronic kidney disease and pregnancy. *Adv. Nephrol.*, **15**, 103–141.

Jungers, P., Houillier, P., Forget, D., Labrunie, M., Skhiri, H., Giatius, I., Descamps-Latscha, B. (1995). Influence of pregnancy on the course of primary glomerulonephritis. *Lancet* **346**, 1122–1124.

Jungers, P., Houillier, P., Chauveau, D., Choukroun, G., Moynot, A., Skhiri, H., Labrunie, M., Descamps-Latscha, B., Grunfeld, J-P (1996) Pregnancy in women with reflux nephrology. *Kid. Intl.*, **50**, 596–599.

Kahn, A. M. (1988) Effect of diuretics on the renal handling of urate. *Sem. Nephrol.*, **8**, 305–314.

Katz, A. I., Davison, J. M., Hayslett, J. P. *et al.* (1980) Pregnancy in women with kidney disease. *Kidney Int.*, **18**, 192–206.

Kincaid-Smith, P. and Fairley, K. F. (1987) Renal disease in pregnancy. Three controversial areas. Mesangial IgA nephropathy, focal glomerulosclerosis (focal and segmental hyalinosis and sclerosis) and reflux nephropathy. *Am. J. Kidney Dis.*, **9**, 328–333.

Kioko, E. M., Shaw, K. M., Clark, A. D. and Warren, D. J. (1983) Successful pregnancy in a diabetic patient treated with continuous ambulatory peritoneal dialysis. *Diabetes Care*, **6**, 298–300.

Kirk, E. P. (1991) Organ transplantation and pregnancy. *Am. J. Obstet. Gynecol.*, **164**, 1629–1634.

Kristensen, C. G., Nakagawa, Y., Coe, F. L. and Lindheimer, M. D. (1986) Effect of atrial natriuretic factor in rat pregnancy. *Am. J. Physiol.*, **250**, R589–R594.

Kuhlback, B. and Widholm, O. (1966) Plasma creatinine in normal pregnancy. *Scand. J. Clin. Lab. Invest.*, **18**, 654–658.

Lancet editorial (1975) Pregnancy and renal disease. *Lancet* **ii**, 801–802.

Lancet editorial (1989) Pregnancy and glomerulonephritis. *Lancet* **ii**, 253–254.

Levey, A. S., Perrone, R. D. and Madias, N. E. (1988) Serum creatinine and renal function. *Annu. Rev. Med.*, **39**, 465–490.

Lim, V. S. (1994) Reproductive endocrinology in uraemia. *Clin. Obstet. Gynaecol. (Baillière)*, **8**, 469–480.

Lindheimer, M. D. and Davison, J. M. (1987) Renal biopsy during pregnancy: 'To b... or not to b...'. *Br. J. Obstet. Gynaecol.*, **94**, 932–934.

Lindheimer, M. D. and Katz, A. I. (1985) Normal and abnormal pregnancy, in *Fluid, Electrolyte and Acid–Base Disorders*, (eds A. I. Arieff and R. DeFronzo), Churchill Livingstone, New York, p. 1041–1080.

Lindheimer, M. D. and Katz, A. I. (1994) Gestation in women with kidney disease: prognosis and management. *Clin. Obstet. Gynaecol. (Baillière)*, **8**, 387–404.

Lindheimer, M. D. and Katz, A. I. (1992) Pregnancy in the renal transplant patient. *Am. J. Kidney Dis.*, **19**, 173–176.

Lindheimer, M. D., Spargo, B. H. and Katz, A. I. (1975) Renal biopsy in pregnancy-induced hypertension. *J. Reprod. Med.*, **15**, 189–194.

Lindheimer, M. D., Fisher, K. A., Spargo, B. H. and Katz, A. I. (1981) Hypertension in pregnancy: a biopsy study with long term follow up. *Cont. Nephrol.*, **25**, 71–77.

Lowe, S. A. and Rubin, P. C. (1992) The pharmacological management of hypertension in pregnancy. *J. Hypertens.*, **10**, 201–207.

Lowe, S. A., Zammit, V. C., Mitar, D. *et al.* (1991) Atrial natriuretic peptide and plasma volume in pregnancy-induced hypertension. *Am. J. Hypertens.*, **4**, 897–903.

McGregor, E., Stewart, G., Junor, B. J. R. and Rodger, R. S. C. (1991) Successful use of recombinant human erythropoietin in pregnancy. *Nephrol. Dialysis Transplant.*, **6**, 292–293.

Magmon, R. and Fejgin, M. (1989) Scleroderma in pregnancy. *Obstet. Gynecol. Surv.*, **44**, 530–534.

Masilamani, S. and Baylis, C. (1992) The renal vasculature does not participate in the peripheral refractoriness to administered angiotensin II in the late pregnancy rat. *J. Am. Soc. Nephrol.*, **3**, 566A.

Meyer, T. M., Ichikawa, I., Zatz, R. and Brenner, B. M. (1983) The renal hemodynamic response to amino acid infusion in the rat. *Trans. Assoc. Am. Phys.*, **96**, 76–83.

Meyer, T. W., Anderson, S., Rennke, H. G. and Brenner, B. M. (1987) Reversing glomerular hypertension stabilizes glomerular injury. *Kidney Int.*, **31**, 752–759.

Molnar, M. and Hertelendy, F. (1990) Pressor responsiveness to endothelin is not attenuated in gravid rats. *Life Sci.*, **47**, 1463–1468.

Milner, J.A., Visek, W.J. (1978) Orotic acidura in the female rat and its relation to dietary regimes. *J. Nutr.* **108**, 1281–1288

Molnar, M. and Hertelendy, F. (1992) N[Ω]-nitro-L-arginine, an inhibitor of nitric oxide synthesis, increases blood pressure in rats and reverses the pregnancy-induced refractoriness to vasopressor agents. *Am. J. Obstet. Gynecol.*, **166**, 1560–1567.

Moncada, S., Palmer, R. M. J. and Higgs, E. A. (1991) Biosynthesis and endogenous roles of nitric oxide. *Pharmacol. Rev.*, **43**, 109–142.

Morris, N.H., Eaton, B.M., Dekker, G. (1996) Nitric oxide, the endothelium, pregnancy and preeclampsia. *Brit. J. Obstet. Gynaecol.*, **103**, 4–15.

Morris, P. J. (1988) Renal transplantation: indications, outcome, complications and results, in (eds R. W. Schrier and C. W. Gottschalk), Little, Brown & Co., Boston, MA, p. 3211–3234.

Murty, G. E., Davison, J. M. and Cameron, D. S. (1991) Wegener's granulomatosis complicating pregnancy: first report of a case with a tracheostomy. *J. Obstet. Gynecol.*, **10**, 399–403.

Myers, B. D. (1986) Cyclosporine nephrotoxicity. *Kidney Int.*, **30**, 964–970.

Nadel, A. S., Ballerman, B. J., Anderson, S. and Brenner, B. M. (1988) Interrelationships among atrial peptides, renin and blood volume in pregnant rats. *Am. J. Physiol.*, **254**, R793–R800.

Nageotte, M. P. and Grundy, H. O. (1988) Pregnancy outcome in women requiring chronic hemodialysis. *Obstet. Gynecol.*, **72**, 456–459.

Navar, L. G. (1978) Renal autoregulation: perspectives from whole kidney and single nephron studies. *Am. J. Physiol.*, **234**, F357–F370.

Nicklin, J. L. (1991) Systemic lupus erythematosus and pregnancy at the Royal Women's Hospital, Brisbane 1979–1989. *Aust. NZ J. Obstet. Gynaecol.*, **31**, 128–133.

Nova, A., Sibai, B. M., Barton, J. R. *et al.* (1991) Maternal plasma level of endothelin is increased in preeclampsia. *Am. J. Obstet. Gynecol.*, **165**, 724–727.

Ogburn, P. L., Kitzmiller, J. L., Hare, J. W. *et al.* (1986) Pregnancy following renal transplantations in Class T diabetes mellitus. *J. A. M. A.*, **255**, 911–915.

Packham, D. and Fairley, K. F. (1987) Renal biopsy: indications and complications in pregnancy. *Br. J. Obstet. Gynaecol.*, **94**, 935–939.

Packham, D. K., Whitworth, J. A., Fairley, K. F. and Kincaid-Smith, P. (1988) Histological features of IgA glomerulonephritis as predictors of pregnancy outcome. *Clin. Nephrol.*, **30**, 22–26.

Packham, D. K., North, R. A., Fairley, K. F. *et al.* (1989) Primary glomerulonephritis and pregnancy. *Q. J. Med.*, **266**, 537–553.

Paller, M. S. (1984) Mechanism of decreased pressor responsiveness to ANG II, NE and vasopressin in pregnant rats. *Am. J. Physiol.*, **247**, H100–H108.

Pedersen, E. B., Christensen, N. J., Christensen, P. *et al.* (1983) Preeclampsia – a state of prostaglandin deficiency? Urinary prostaglandin excretion, the renin–aldosterone system, and circulating catecholamines in preeclampsia. *Hypertension*, **5**, 105–110.

Penn, I. (1990) Cancers complicating organ transplantation. *N. Engl. J. Med.*, **323**, 1767–1768.

Perkins, C. M., Hancock, K. W., Cope, C. F. and Lee, M. R. (1981) Urine free dopamine in normal primigrand pregnancy and women taking oral contraceptives. *Clin. Sci.*, **61**, 423–427.

Petri, M., Howard, D. and Repke, J. (1991) Frequency of lupus flare in pregnancy: the Hopkins Lupus Pregnancy Center experience. *Arthritis Rheumat.*, **34**, 1538–1545.

Pickrell, M. D., Sawers, R. and Michael, J. (1988) Pregnancy after renal transplantation: severe intrauterine growth retardation during treatment with cyclosporin A. *Br. Med. J.*, **296**, 825.

Podjarny, E., Bernheim, J.L., Rathams, M., Pomeranz, A. (1992) Adriamycin nephrology: a model to study the effects of pregnancy on renal disease in rats. *Am. J. Physiol.*, **263**, F711–F715.

Podjarny, E., Pomeranz, A., A., Raham, M., M. Bernheim, J.L. (1993) Effect of L-Arginine treatment in pregnant rats with adriamycin nephropathy. *Hypertension Preg.* **12**, 517–524.

Pomeranz, E., Podjarny, E., Bernheim, J., Ratham, M., Green, J. (1995) Effect of recurrent pregnancies on the evolution of adriamycin nephropathy. *Nephrol. Dial. Transpl.*, **10**, 2049–2052.

Rasmussen, P. E. and Nielsen, F. R. (1988) Hydronephrosis during pregnancy: a literature survey. *Eur. J. Obstet. Gynecol. Reprod. Biol.*, **27**, 249–259.

Raij, L., and Bayli, C. (1995) Nitric oxide and the glomerulus. *Kid. Intl.*, **48**, 20-32.

Reckelhoff, J. F., Yokota, S. and Baylis, C. (1992) Renal autoregulation in mid-term and late pregnant rats. *Am. J. Obstet. Gynecol.*, **166**, 1546–1550.

Redrow, M., Cherem, L., Elliott, J. *et al.* (1988) Dialysis in the management of pregnant patients with renal insufficiency. *Medicine*, **67**, 199–208.

Rizzoni, G., Ehrich, J. H. H., Broyer M. *et al.* (1992) Successful pregnancies in women on renal replacement therapy: report from the EDTA Registry. *Nephrol. Dialysis Transplant.*, **7**, 1–9.

Roberts, M., Lindheimer, M.D., Davison, J.M. (1996) Altered permselectivity to neutral dextrous and heteroporous membrane modelling in human pregnancy. *Am. J. Physiol.*, **270**, F338–F343

Robertson, C. R., Deen, W. M., Troy, J. L. and Brenner, B. M. (1972) Dynamics of glomerular ultrafiltration in the rat. III. Hemodynamics and autoregulation. *Am. J. Physiol.*, **223**, 1191–1200.

Salmella, K.T., Kyllonen, L.E.J., Holmberg-Riska, C (1993) Impaired renal function after pregnancy in renal transplant recipients. *Transpl.*, **56**, 1372–1375.

Schaefer, R. M., Kokot, F. and Wernze, H. (1989) Improved sexual function in hemodialysis patients on recombinant erythropoietin: a possible role for prolactin. *Clin. Nephrol.*, **31**, 1–5.

Schewitz, L. J., Friedman, E. A. and Pollak, V. E. (1965) Bleeding after renal biopsy in pregnancy. *Obstet. Gynecol.*, **26**, 295–304.

Schiff, E., Ben-Baruch, G., Peleg, E. *et al.* (1992) Immunoreactive circulating endothelin-1 in normal and hypertensive pregnancies. *Am. J. Obstet. Gynecol.*, **166**, 624–628.

Scott, J. R. and Branch, D. W. (1986) The effect of repeated pregnancies on renal allograft function. *Transplantation*, **42**, 695–696.

Sibai, B. M. (1991) Diagnosis and management of chronic hypertension in pregnancy. *Obstet. Gynecol.*, **78**, 451–461.

Sibai, B. (1996) Treatment of hypertension in pregnant women. *N. Eng. J. Med.*, **335**, 257–264.

Souqiyyeh, M. Z., Huraib, S. O., Mohd Saleh, A. G. and Aswad, S. (1992) Pregnancy in chronic hemodialysis patients in the Kingdom of Saudi Arabia. *Am. J. Kidney Dis.*, **19**, 235–238.

Spiro, F. I. and Fry, I. K. (1970) Ureteric dilatation in non-pregnant women. *Proc. Roy. Soc. Med.*, **63**, 462–464.

St-Louis, J. and Sicotte, B. (1992) Prostaglandin- or endothelium-mediated vasodilation is not involved in the blunted responses of blood vessels to vasoconstrictors in pregnant rats. *Am. J. Obstet. Gynecol.*, **166**, 684–692.

Steegers, E. A. P., Van Lakwijk, H. P. J. M., Fast, J. H. *et al.* (1991) Atrial natriuretic peptide and atrial size during normal pregnancy. *Br. J. Obstet. Gynaecol.*, **98**, 202–206.

Sturgiss, S. N. and Davison, J. M. (1991) Perinatal outcome in renal allograft recipients: prognostic significance of hypertension and renal function before and during pregnancy. *Obstet. Gynecol.*, **78**, 573–577.

Sturgiss, S. N. and Davison, J. M. (1992) Effect of pregnancy on long-term function of renal allografts. *Am. J. Kidney Dis.*, **19**, 167–172.

Sturgiss, S.N., Davison, J.M. (1995) Effect of pregnancy on the long term function of renal allographs: an update. *Am. J. Kid. Dis.*, **26**, 54–56.

Sturgiss, S.N., Dunlop, W., Danson, J.M. (1994) Renal haemodynamics and lobular function in human pregnancy. *Clin Obstet. Gynaecol (Baillière).*, **8**, 209–234.

Sturgiss, S. N., Wilkinson, R. and Davison, J. M. (1992) Renal haemodynamic reserve (RHR) during normal human pregnancy. *J. Physiol. (Lond.)*, **452**, P317.

Surian, M., Imbasciati, E., Cosci, P. *et al.* (1984) Glomerular disease and pregnancy: a study of 123 pregnancies in patients with primary and secondary glomerular disease. *Nephrology*, **36**, 101–105.

Takeda, T. (1964) Experimental study on the blood pressure of pregnant hypertensive rats. I. Effect of pregnancy on the course of experimentally and spontaneously hypertensive rats. *Jpn. Circ. J.*, **28**, 49–54.

Taylor, R. N., Varma, M., Teng, N. N. H. and Roberts, J. M. (1990) Women with preeclampsia have higher plasma endothelin levels than women with normal pregnancies. *J. Clin. Endocrinol. Metab.*, **71**, 1675–1677.

Trollfors, B., Alestig, K. and Jagenburg, R. (1987) Prediction of glomerular filtration rate from serum creatinine, age, sex and body weight. *Acta Med. Scand.*, **221**, 495–498.

Twickler, D., Little, B. B., Satin, A. J. and Brown, C. E. (1991) Renal pelvicalyceal dilation in antepartum pyelonephritis: ultrasonographic findings. *Am. J. Obstet. Gynecol.*, **165**, 1115–1119.

Tyden, G., Brattstrom, C., Bjorkman, U. *et al.* (1989) Pregnancy after combined pancreas–kidney transplantation. *Diabetes*, **38**(Suppl 1), 43–45.

Umans, J. G., Lindheimer, M. D. and Barron, W. M. (1990) Pressor effect of endothelium derived relaxing factor inhibition in conscious virgin and gravid rats. *Am. J. Physiol.*, **259**, F293–F296.

Van Sonnenberg, E., Casola, G., Talner, L. B. *et al.* (1992) Symptomatic renal obstruction or urosepsis during pregnancy: treatment by sonographically guided percutaneous nephrostomy. *Am. J. Roentgenol.*, **158**, 91–94.

Venuto, R. C. and Donker, A. J. M. (1982) Prostaglandin $E_2$, plasma renin activity and renal function throughout rabbit pregnancy. *J. Lab. Clin. Med.*, **99**, 239–246.

Vinicor, F., Golichowski, A., Filo, R. *et al.* (1984) Pregnancy following renal transplantations in a patient with insulin-dependent diabetes mellitus. *Diabetes Care*, **7**, 280–284.

Weiner, C., Liu, K. Z., Thompson, L. *et al.* (1991) Effect of pregnancy on endothelium and smooth muscle: their role in reduced adrenergic sensitivity. *Am. J. Physiol.*, **261**, H1275–H1283.

Weiner, C.P., Lizasoain, I., Baylis, S.A., Knowles, R.G., Charles, I.G., Moncada, S. (1994) Induction of calcium-dependent nitric oxide syntheses by sex hormones. *Proc. Nat. Acad. USA.*, 91, 5215–5216.

Weiner, C. P., Thompson, L. P., Liu, K. Z. and Herrig, J. E. (1992) Endothelium-derived relaxing factor and indomethacin-sensitive contracting factor alter arterial contractile responses to thromboxane during pregnancy. *Am. J. Obstet. Gynecol.*, **166**, 1171–1181.

Whetham, J. C. G., Cardelle, C. and Harding, M. (1983) Effect of pregnancy on graft function and graft survival in renal cadaver transplant-recipients. *Am. J. Obstet. Gynecol.*, **145**, 193–197.

Wilson, C. B. and Blantz, R. C. (1985) Nephroimmunopathology and pathophysiology. *Am. J. Physiol.*, **248**, F319–F331.

Woods, L. L., Mizelle, H. L. and Hall, J. E. (1987) Autoregulation of renal blood flow and glomerular filtration rate in the pregnant rabbit. *Am. J. Physiol.*, **252**, R69–R72.

Yanagisawa, M., Kurihara, H., Kimura, S. *et al.* (1988) A novel potent vasoconstrictor peptide produced by vascular endothelial cells. *Nature*, **222**, 411–415.

Yasin, S. Y. and Bey Doun, S. N. (1988) Hemodialysis in pregnancy. *Obstet. Gynecol. Surv.*, **43**, 655–668.

# THE USE OF ANTIHYPERTENSIVE DRUGS IN PREGNANCY  13

*James J. Walker*

## 13.1 INTRODUCTION

Eclampsia was recognized by the ancient Greeks and it remains the main presentation of preeclampsia–eclampsia in many parts of the world today. It is not surprising that many treatment regimes are directed at anticonvulsant therapy rather then antihypertensive treatment. This is despite the fact that more mothers die without convulsion than die following convulsion. The aim of this chapter is to discuss the role of antihypertensive therapy in the management of hypertension in pregnancy.

## 13.2 THE USE OF ANTIHYPERTENSIVE DRUGS IN PREGNANCY

Antihypertensive drugs reduce blood pressure. They may have different modes of action but the end results are the same. All antihypertensive drugs have side-effects, some of which may produce further benefits and others harmful results (Pandurski, 1991). Since they are powerful cardiovascular agents, it would be surprising if they did not have some adverse maternal or fetal effect. The obstetrician must balance any potential benefit of antihypertensive therapy against any potential side-effect that might occur. Although there is no consensus about therapy for pregnancy hypertension and the role of antihypertensive drugs (Pandurski, 1991), it

has been felt by many that their use during pregnancy may reduce fetal mortality and the incidence of severe preeclampsia (Walker, 1987; Kincaid Smith, 1994). The recent Cochrane Collaboration of Clinical Trials confirms that use of antihypertensive therapy reduces the incidence of hypertensive crises and improves perinatal mortality rate (Collins and Duley, 1995). It has been accepted for some time that antihypertensive drugs are needed to protect the mother from the dangers of severe hypertension ($\geq 170/110$ mmHg), particularly cerebral hemorrhage. There is, however, still disagreement as to whether treatment of a lower level of hypertension confers any benefit. Some believe that there is little indication for treating mild to moderate hypertension (140–169/90–109 mmHg) (Kyle and Redman, 1992). Delaying the treatment of hypertension of pregnancy to diastolic blood pressure of 100 mmHg is not associated with additional maternal or fetal risk and will reduce the number of patients previously receiving treatment to about half (BottKanner *et al.*, 1992).

Therefore, women with mild hypertension in pregnancy do not require antihypertensive therapy if they are closely observed during pregnancy and delivery, especially if there has been no hypertension before pregnancy and no proteinuria develops (Hjertberg, Belfrage and Hanson, 1992) (also Chapter 9).

*Hypertension in Pregnancy*
Edited by J.J. Walker and N.F. Gant. Published by Chapman & Hall, 1997 ISBN 0 412 30910 6

Patients with severe hypertension early in pregnancy and those with preexisting cardio-vascular and renal disease are at significant risk of maternal and fetal complications and antihypertensive drugs can be life-saving. In contrast, women with mild uncomplicated chronic hypertension will achieve a good perinatal outcome irrespective of the use of antihypertensive medications (Sibai, 1991)

Decisions regarding the need for antihy-pertensive treatment during pregnancy and the selection of a specific antihypertensive agent should be based upon an assessment of the relative risks and benefits for the individ-ual patient. The effects of antihypertensive agents upon the underlying pathophysiologi-cal processes involved in PIH/preeclampsia may help therapeutic decision making (Lowe and Rubin, 1992). A number of agents have a favorable benefit–risk profile for use in this condition; these include centrally acting drugs, beta-blockers and vasodilators. How-ever, angiotensin converting enzyme inhib-itors are contraindicated as there is an unacceptable risk to the fetus (Walker, 1991).

In the USA, hydralazine and methyldopa are the drugs of choice for the acute hyper-tensive crisis and management of chronic hypertension. Parenteral magnesium sulfate remains the preferred therapeutic approach for avoiding or treating the convulsive com-plication, eclampsia (Lindheimer *et al.*, 1993). In the UK, the antihypertensive drugs most commonly used are labetalol (35%), methyl-dopa (23%) and parenteral hydralazine (29%). Diuretics are not used. Anticonvulsants are still prescribed by 85% of consultants to pre-vent seizures and the drugs used are diazepam (41%), phenytoin (30%) and chlormethiazole (24%). Very few consultants in the UK use magnesium sulfate (2%) (Hutton *et al.*, 1992).

Most Swedish obstetricians would not treat a woman in the second trimester with blood pressure 140/95 mmHg with antihypertensive medication (83%) and would monitor her as an outpatient (81%). The corresponding fig-ures according to a similar study published in, 1981 were 33% and 71% respectively. So the use of antihypertensive drugs may be decreasing. However, almost all Swedish obstetricians (95%) would give antihyperten-sive treatment if the blood pressure was 170/110 mmHg or more. Beta-blockers and hydralazine were the most commonly used drugs, and 16% of Swedish obstetricians would use calcium antagonists. Treatment with diuretics, methyldopa or diazepam in pregnancy hypertension was rare (Wide-Swensson, Montal and Ingemarsson, 1994).

Since the benefits of the use of antihyper-tensive agents are now accepted, clinicians caring for pregnancies complicated by hyper-tension require to have a well-formulated management plan and guidelines for the assessment of the need for antihypertensive drugs (Chapter 9). In general, antihypertensive medications should be reserved for those con-sidered as having high-risk hypertension. If the gestation is between 24 and 34 weeks, pro-phylactic steroids can be used in combination with hypertensive therapy to the proven bene-fit of the fetus. After therapy has been com-menced, close monitoring of the maternal and fetal condition is necessary for the rest of the pregnancy. An individualized management plan and a referral to a tertiary care center will improve maternal and perinatal outcome in those women who are remote from term and in those with the HELLP syndrome (Sibai, 1992). Protocol implementation increases the level of care offered to the pregnant hyperten-sive women (Tuffnell *et al.*, 1994).

There are some particular instances where treatment is particularly of benefit. Pregnant women with diabetic nephropathy should have early antihypertensive treatment to reduce progression of diabetic nephropathy (Girndt, 1994), although control may not be possible despite intensive antihypertensive therapy (Biesenbach, Stoger and Zazgornik, 1992).

## 13.3 AVAILABLE DRUGS

Drugs exist that can alter the responses of every known blood pressure control system (Table 13.1). They can be divided into five main groups:

1. centrally acting drugs;
2. drugs that alter cardiac output;
3. drugs that affect the peripheral vascular resistance;
4. angiotensin converting enzyme inhibitors;
5. diuretics.

### 13.3.1 CENTRALLY ACTING DRUGS

The main centrally acting drugs that are commonly used are methyldopa and clonidine. They act by central inhibition of the sympathetic drive (Pandurski, 1991). They are associated with troublesome side-effects, which has led to the move away from these products in the non-pregnant patient (Reid and Elliot, 1984). However, methyldopa is still the most widely used drug for pregnancy hypertension throughout the world. This is partly because of its relative inexpensiveness but also because of its apparent safety (Leather *et al.*, 1968; Redman, Beilin and Wilkinson, 1976). For long-term therapy, methyldopa is the only drug which has been fully assessed and shown to be safe for the neonate and infant (Kyle and Redman, 1992) The effects of methyldopa on fetal heart rate pattern were analyzed by computed cardiotocography.

**Table 13.1** Antihypertensive drugs available for use in pregnancy

|  | *Benefits* | *Side-effects* |
|---|---|---|
| **Centrally acting drugs** | | |
| Methyldopa | Proven | Tiredness/dry mouth |
| | | Not good in the acute situation |
| Clonidine | None | Little experience |
| **Drugs that affect cardiac output** | | |
| Atenolol | Simple | IUGR |
| | | Neonatal hypoglycemia |
| Oxprenolol | Fewer side-effects | Neonatal hypoglycemia |
| | ISA | |
| Metoprolol | Fewer side-effects | Neonatal hypoglycemia |
| Labetalol | α-blockade | Neonatal hypoglycemia |
| | IV and oral use | Tremor |
| **Drugs that affect the peripheral vascular resistance** | | |
| Hydralazine | Proven | Headache/tremor |
| | | IV only of value |
| | | Fetal distress |
| Nifedipine | Oral | Headache |
| | | Tachycardia |
| Nicardipine | Oral | Little experience |
| Nimodipine | Cerebral vasodilator | Little experience |
| **Angiotensin converting enzyme inhibitors** | | |
| Captopril | Contraindicated | Fetal loss |
| Enalapril | Contraindicated | Postpartum only |
| | | Little experience |
| **Diuretics** | | |
| Frusemide | Potent | Postpartum only |

Compared with the pretreatment value, the mean arterial blood pressure decreased significantly. Fetal heart rate characteristics were not significantly changed during drug treatment or bed rest. The various features of the fetal heart rate pattern evaluated by computerized methods were not influenced by treatment with methyldopa (WideSwensson *et al.*, 1993)

### 13.3.2 DRUGS THAT ALTER CARDIAC OUTPUT

The consistent hemodynamic feature of beta-adrenergic blockade is a reduction in the cardiac output (Lund Johansen, 1980). In the non-pregnant hypertensive patient, the cardiac output is often increased and the peripheral resistance is normal. Therefore, beta-blockers are well suited for the treatment of chronic hypertension. As cardiac output is not necessarily increased in pregnancy hypertension, and may be reduced, they may not be the most sensible for use in pregnancy.

Beta-blockers can be subdivided into those that are blockers to both beta-1 and beta-2 receptors, selective beta-1 receptor blockers, those with intrinsic sympathomimetic activity (ISA), different lipid solubility and membrane stabilizing effects. These different properties can alter both the beneficial and harmful effects of these drugs. Adrenoceptor antagonists are now widely used in the treatment of preeclampsia in Europe and Australia (Pandurski, 1991). They are widely accepted as being safe to use although those without intrinsic sympathomimetic activity may increase the chance of intrauterine growth restriction (IUGR) (Dubois *et al.*, 1982; Lardoux *et al.*, 1983). IUGR is one of the main contributory factors in the increased perinatal morbidity and mortality associated with pregnancy-induced hypertension.

Doppler changes have been studied during therapy with atenolol. There was an increase in the fetal aortic PI and the resistance index (RI) of the uterine artery after 7 days. The authors felt that other therapies would be safer than atenolol in hypertensive pregnancies, with less harmful effects on fetal–maternal circulation (Danti *et al.*, 1994). There is also concern that very-low-birthweight ($\leq 1500$ g) infants born to mothers with pregnancy-induced hypertension or preeclampsia, where beta-blockers have been used, are at particular danger of side-effects from these drugs. In one study, it was found that during the first year of life, seven out of 19 infants died when the mothers' antihypertensive regimen included beta-blockers. Four of the deaths occurred within 15 days. There were no deaths in 16 infants whose mothers were treated with other antihypertensive treatment ($p = 0.006$). These results suggest that maternal beta-blocker therapy may have adverse effects on very-low-birthweight infants (Kaaja *et al.*, 1992).

The drugs that have been studied the most are the non-selective blockers pindolol and oxprenolol, the selective blockers atenolol and metoprolol and the combined alpha/beta-blocker labetalol (Pandurski, 1991). Labetalol is a unique adrenoceptor antagonist as it has both alpha-1-adrenoceptor antagonist and non-selective beta-adrenoceptor-antagonist properties. The beta-blocking effect of labetalol is four times less potent than that of propranolol. It appears to produce its hypotensive effects without compromising the maternal cardiovascular system by producing peripheral vasodilatation (Lund Johansen, 1984). This may help to maintain renal and uterine blood flow. The acute administration of labetalol causes a reduction in blood pressure, heart rate and peripheral resistance, but there is no change in the cardiac output in standing and supine positions. In a comparison of the neonatal effects of maternal treatment with labetalol or hydralazine, the median cord pH was lower and the number of infants with a cord pH less than 7.20 was higher in the hydralazine group. However, as with other beta-blockers, blood glucose levels were lower in the labetalol group at 6 hours of age ($p$ 0.05). No clinical signs of adrenergic blockade were found at 24 hours of age (Hjertberg, Faxelius and Lagercrantz, 1993). There is some evidence to suggest that labetalol may diminish the amount of proteinuria in patients who have already developed proteinuric pre-eclampsia. It has been suggested labetalol therapy, despite its vasodilator properties, also may contribute to intra-uterine growth retardation (Cruickshank *et al.*, 1992).

Labetalol therapy does have some other effects, such as a significant reduction in the aggregability of erythrocytes (Tranquilli *et al.*, 1992) and platelets (Greer *et al.*, 1985), which may be beneficial.

### 13.3.3 DRUGS THAT AFFECT THE PERIPHERAL VASCULAR RESISTANCE

These drugs act on the vascular wall to reduce peripheral resistance. The main examples are among the oldest and the newest antihypertensive drugs.

Diazoxide is a benzothiadiazine derivative that is closely related to the thiazide diuretics and is now rarely used. In large doses it is associated with acute fetal distress and intrauterine death (Ayromlooi *et al.*, 1982).

Hydralazine is the oldest antihypertensive drug still in regular clinical use. It acts directly on the vascular wall, requiring an intact endothelium to produce its effect, and acts best with the patient lying flat in bed. The fall in blood pressure results from vasodilation. Used as monotherapy, hydralazine produces side-effects such as tachycardia, flushing, nasal congestion, tremors, headaches, nausea and vomiting (Koch Weser, 1974). A few subjects may be unusually sensitive to hydralazine because of a reduced capacity to metabolize the drug. The use of hydralazine is usually restricted to single or short-term use, as prolonged use leads to both the stimulation of the renin–angiotensin–aldosterone system and a reduction in renal perfusion pressure, causing fluid retention with blunting of the drug's hypotensive effect and an increase in

the chances of cardiac failure. It is more effective in lowering diastolic blood pressure than systolic blood pressure. Acute administration is associated with reduced placental blood flow (Lipshitz, Ahokas and Reynolds,1987) and fetal distress (Vink, Moodley and Philpott, 1980). The effect of a single dose of hydralazine wears off in about 2–3 h. Orally, the effect is minimal but it can be used as an adjunct to beta-blocker therapy (Pandurski, 1991). After intravenous dihydralazine, the mean arterial blood pressure decreased significantly but the Doppler pulsatility index (PI) in the uterine artery increased. These findings would imply an increased resistance in the uteroplacental circulation when the blood pressure is acutely reduced with dihydralazine treatment (Grunewald *et al.*, 1993). In North America, hydralazine is the most commonly used antihypertensive medication, usually in combination with magnesium sulfate (Barron, 1992; Lindheimer, 1993)

Cadralazine, a 6-substituted derivative of 3-hydrazinopyridoxine structurally related to hydralazine, is effective in lowering blood pressure levels in pregnant hypertensive women. No adverse effects from the drug were observed on fetal development or immediate postnatal adaptation to stress during labor, and only mild maternal side-effects were detected such as headache (Voto *et al.*, 1992).

Sodium nitroprusside is an effective intravenous drug for the management of acute hypertension in the non-pregnant patient. It has been used in pregnancy but there is concern about the effects on the placental blood flow and the potential toxic effects. Because it is light-sensitive, it is difficult to give. There are easier and as effective drugs that are preferable.

Calcium channel blockers act primarily by inhibiting extracellular calcium influx into cells through slow calcium channels. They reduce peripheral resistance and their action is proportional to the amount of vasoconstriction (Olivari *et al.*, 1979). They are antagonistic against any form of vasoconstrictor and have a mild tocolytic effect. The drugs most used in primary hypertension are nifedipine, nicardipine and verapamil. They are potent orally and are used alone or in combination with beta-adrenergic blockers (Pandurski, 1991). They can be used in the acute situation or chronically. Animal studies have suggested that placental blood flow is reduced by nicardipine (Parisi, Salinas and Stockmar, 1989a) and there is an increase in fetal hypoxia (Parisi, Salinas and Stockmar, 1989b). Other studies do not support this (Ahokas *et al.*, 1988) and human experience suggests that with therapeutic dosage, calcium channel blockers are safe (Catanzarite, 1992). They may have a direct cerebral vasodilator effect (Belfort *et al.*, 1994). After acute administration of nimodipine, there was a significant reduction in the pulsatility index in the maternal ophthalmic and central retinal arteries and in the fetal middle cerebral artery, suggesting vasodilatation of the cerebral vessels. The umbilical artery systolic/diastolic ratio was also significantly reduced. Maternal blood pressure was controlled without the need for other antihypertensive medication and it was well tolerated, although there was an increase in heart rate. This study suggests that nimodipine is an effective, easily administered antihypertensive agent and may have some advantages.

In another study, no significant differences were found in umbilical and uterine circulation in the patients treated with nifedipine; although there was a short-term significant percentage increase in pulsatility index (PI) in the middle cerebral artery at 60 min ($p < 0.03$), this had returned to normal at 120 min and 48 h. In the group of patients treated with atenolol, no significant percentage changes were noted in the umbilical artery, but there was an increase in the aortic PI ($p < 0.03$) and the resistance index (RI) of the uterine artery ($p < 0.05$) at 7 days. The authors felt that the use of nifedipine could be safer than atenolol in hypertensive pregnancies, with less harm-

ful effects on fetal–maternal circulation (Danti *et al.*, 1994).

Maternal and feto-placental Doppler flow velocity waveforms were studied during acute treatment with nicardipine and chronic antihypertensive therapy with pindolol in patients with pregnancy-induced hypertension. Eight primigravidae were acutely treated with oral nicardipine. Diastolic blood pressure fell at 30, 45 and 60 min after nicardipine. The uteroplacental systolic/diastolic ratio rose significantly at 30 min, but this change was no longer apparent at 60 min. Umbilical artery and maternal brachial artery systolic/diastolic ratios were unchanged. A total of 15 patients with mild preeclampsia were chronically treated with oral pindolol. Diastolic blood pressure fell significantly within 24 h. The uteroplacental systolic/diastolic ratio rose 3 days after pindolol. Brachial artery or umbilical artery systolic/diastolic ratios were unchanged. A control group of 15 patients with untreated mild preeclampsia showed a significant rise in uteroplacental and umbilical artery systolic/diastolic ratios within 7 days of starting recordings. In patients with pregnancy-induced hypertension, acute and chronic blood pressure reduction was associated with no change in umbilical artery or maternal brachial artery Doppler systolic/diastolic ratios and a transient rise in the uteroplacental systolic/diastolic ratio (Walker *et al.*, 1992)

Nifedipine therapy reverts erythrocyte aggregation to normal. Increased erythrocyte aggregation may be due to either changes of the cell membrane occurring during hypertension or a redistribution of the ionic charges on the two surfaces of the membrane. The effect of nifedipine in restoring the ionic charges may be due to this latter event (Tranquilli *et al.*, 1992). The half-life of nifedipine appears to be shorter than in the non-pregnant and the findings indicate that nifedipine may achieve greater antihypertensive efficacy in pregnant women if administered at shorter intervals. Nifedipine can be detected in samples of fetal cord blood and amniotic fluid at concentrations approximately 93% and 53% those of simultaneous maternal vein samples, respectively (Prevost *et al.*, 1992).

Urapidil is an antagonist of postsynaptic alpha-1 receptors, which leads to a diminution of the increased blood pressure by reducing the peripheral vascular resistance. When used postpartum, a declining blood pressure in all treated women without any tachycardia or serious side-effects. Further studies will have to classify the rank of urapidil in the treatment of hypertension in preeclampsia (Wacker *et al.*, 1994)

### 13.3.4 ANGIOTENSIN CONVERTING ENZYME (ACE) INHIBITORS

ACE inhibitors are relatively new, very effective drugs for treatment of hypertension in the non-pregnant patient. They act by inhibiting the action of the angiotensin converting enzyme. This reduces the production of angiotensin II and reduces peripheral vascular resistance (Cody *et al.*, 1978). There is no reflex tachycardia. This action may seem attractive for use in preeclampsia with its abnormalities of angiotensin II. However, the original ACE inhibitor, captopril, has been found to have unacceptable side-effects both in animal experiments and clinical practice (Broughton Pipkin, Turber and Symonds, 1980). Fetal deformity, neonatal renal failure, intrauterine death and a significant reduction in placental blood flow have all been reported. When captopril was given to pregnant sheep and rabbits, there was an appallingly high fetal and neonatal death rate in both species. It was concluded that this treatment should not be used in humans (Broughton Pipkin, Turber and Symonds, 1980).

Enalapril is a newer drug, with fewer side-effects, but adverse reports have begun to appear in the literature. For these reasons the use of ACE inhibitors in pregnancy must be restricted. However, they may be used in the postpartum period when blood pressure control is difficult to achieve. Enalapril is effective in lowering blood pressure in all grades of essential and renovascular hypertension. It is at least as effective as other established and newer ACE inhibitors. This favorable profile of efficacy and tolerability and the substantial weight of clinical experience, explain the increasing acceptance of enalapril as a major antihypertensive treatment in the immediate postpartum period (Todd *et al.*, 1992) .

### 13.3.5 DIURETICS

Diuretics probably act by a mild vasodilator action and by reducing plasma volume by altering sodium balance. The thiazide diuretics are the most commonly used, often in combination with other drugs. Thiazides do not significantly lower the blood pressure in pregnancy and have proved dangerous by inducing of severe hyponatremia and causing acute pancreatitis in the mother and the fetus (Pandurski, 1991). A rise in blood urea and uric acid, neonatal thrombocytopenia, and hyperglycemia and glycosuria in diabetic or prediabetic patients can all be produced by the use of thiazide diuretics. There is some evidence to indicate that they can decrease placental function. However, Sibai (1983) showed that patients with chronic hypertension on diuretics can have the normal blood volume changes of pregnancy. In conclusion, diuretics have a relatively weak action and their use *de nouveau* in pregnancy cannot be recommended. Patients already on diuretic therapy will probably have chronic hypertension mild enough to allow cessation of therapy for the duration of the pregnancy.

The main use of diuretics in preeclampsia should be restricted to the use of frusemide in the postpartum period to help treat fluid overload and pulmonary edema (Chapter 14).

### 13.4 IS TREATMENT OF ANY BENEFIT?

Since these drugs have varying modes of action, beneficial results achieved with one preparation may not be seen with another and failure of action of one antihypertensive drug does not mean that all will fail to work. Side-effects seen with some medications will not be seen with others. Before giving any patient antihypertensive therapy, the obstetrician must assess whether the patient would benefit from the medication and which drug would be best to use. In the non-pregnant patient, the potential benefits are balanced against the potential risks of therapy. With the advent of safer drugs with fewer side-effects, the use of antihypertensive therapy has greatly increased without any clear evidence of benefit to the patients. In pregnancy, the situation is complicated by the presence of the fetus. Although the benefits of therapy may be directed at the mother, the side-effects may be experienced by both the mother and her unborn child. The fear of teratogenicity and other fetal complications has meant that most new drugs are contraindicated for use in pregnancy although there is no evidence of their harm. With the increasing cost of litigation and the relatively low profits from pregnancy use, few companies support or fund antihypertensive studies in pregnancy. This has led to contradictions and other difficulties in this area of research. Labetalol is a drug licensed for use in pregnancy in the UK but it is contraindicated for use in the USA. Both these decisions were based on the same available evidence.

The most recent meta-analysis of antihypertensive trials, published by the Cochrane Collaboration, suggests that these drugs can benefit both the mother and the baby by reducing hypertensive crises and perinatal death (Collins and Duley, 1995). Therefore, judicious use of antihypertensive medication would appear to be beneficial.

### 13.4.1 CHRONIC HYPERTENSION

Most of the studies in hypertension in pregnancy have been conducted on chronic hypertensive patients. Methyldopa was assessed in hypertension occurring in pregnancy as long ago as 1968 (Leather *et al.*, 1968). The most comprehensive study of its use in pregnancy was performed by Redman, Beilin and Wilkinson (1976). They concluded that it was safe and that it appeared to reduce fetal loss from midtrimester abortions. There was no difference in perinatal mortality rate or the incidence of superimposed preeclampsia. The children of the women who took part in this study were followed up for 7 years, and there was no obvious difference between the children from the treatment group and those from the control group, in terms of physical and mental handicap, behavior, vision, hearing and intellectual ability, thus emphasizing the drug's safety but also the lack of measurable benefit. These results have led the authors to state that methyldopa should be the drug of choice in pregnancy as it has been proved to be safe. It should be remembered that the other drugs have not been shown to be unsafe. In this study, maternal side-effects were troublesome enough to cause 15% of the women to be withdrawn. Another study showed that methyldopa was associated with reduced neonatal blood pressure.

In the 1970s increasing studies have been carried out into the use of beta-blockers. Initially, studies with propranolol demonstrated fetal side-effects, but more recent work has shown increasing safety (Pandurski, 1991). Beta-blockers are now well established in the management of chronic hypertension. Metoprolol, oxprenolol, labetalol, sotalol, pindolol and atenolol have all been used in pregnancy, singly or in combination with vasodilators. Although blood pressure control was achieved with all, few studies showed any measurable benefit to the mother or baby.

Oxprenolol has been compared with methyldopa. Both drugs had similar effects on blood pressure control, but one study showed that the oxprenolol group had a better outcome in terms of fetal and placental weight. Labetalol was also compared with methyldopa and was found to be as efficient at lowering blood pressure and reducing the progression to proteinuria. There were fewer side-effects found with the beta-blockers (Walker, 1991).

Different beta-blockers have been compared. Both pindolol and labetalol have been compared with atenolol in pregnancy. All drugs controlled blood pressure but birth-weights were significantly higher in the pindolol and labetalol groups, possibly as a result of increased uteroplacental blood flow (Walker, 1991). Atenolol has been associated with intrauterine growth retardation and fetal heart rate abnormalities (Pandurski, 1991).

Therefore, no great benefit has been shown by the treatment of chronic hypertension in pregnancy. If treatment is desired, no drug appears to be significantly superior, although methyldopa has a high incidence of side-effects and the vasodilator beta-blockers oxprenolol, pindolol and labetalol may allow increased fetal growth compared to the others.

### 13.4.2 PREECLAMPSIA (PET)

In preeclampsia, the mother is at risk of vascular, renal, hepatic and neurological damage, all of which are partly related to the hypertension itself. Therefore, antihypertensive therapy may be of benefit to the mother by reducing these risks. The fetus is at risk from placental damage leading to intrauterine growth retardation and intrauterine death. The placental pathology is not directly related to the hypertension and lowering blood pressure is unlikely to improve placental function, and may be detrimental.

Therefore, the purpose of antihypertensive treatment is to control the blood pressure in order to protect the mother from the effects of hypertensive crisis, especially during labor, and to prolong the pregnancy sufficiently to avoid the complications of prematurity for the fetus without increasing the risk to the mother.

### 13.5 CAN THIS BE ACHIEVED? ARE THERE UNACCEPTABLE SIDE-EFFECTS OF THERAPY?

### 13.5.1 SEVERE HYPERTENSION

There has been no randomized study that has evaluated treatment in severe hypertension, although there is general consensus about starting hypotensive treatment when diastolic blood pressure is above 110 mmHg (Kyle and Redman, 1992; Walker, 1991). This is to protect the mother from cerebrovascular accident, the largest cause of maternal death in hypertensive disease of pregnancy. Many centers manage severe hypertension with prophylactic anticonvulsants. Magnesium sulfate (in the injectable, hydrated form) is the agent used most often for seizure prophylaxis in the preeclamptic patient in the USA. As many as 18% of all patients may be given this therapy, although it has not been evaluated by controlled trial. It is also used widely to control seizures once they develop and its role in established convulsions would appear to be beneficial (Pritchard, 1955). In the USA, diazepam is used to supplement magnesium sulfate if necessary to control seizures, but its use is not routine. If blood pressure is not controlled, IV hydralazine is the therapy preferred (McCombs, 1992). In Germany, magnesium is also the therapy of first choice (Lechner *et al.*, 1993)

Magnesium sulfate is not an antihypertensive agent. In an *in vivo* rat study, magnesium sulfate alone had no significant effect on MAP but attenuated the pressor response to both noradrenalin and angiotensin II (Aisenbrey, Corwin and Catanzarite, 1992). After discontinuation of the magnesium sulfate infusion, the pressor responses returned to normal. Although magnesium sulfate is not an efficient primary antihypertensive agent, it may have effects on blood pressure by attenuating the actions of circulating vasoconstrictors. However, outside the USA, magnesium sulfate is not so widely used, with less than 2% of obstetricians in the UK having any experience with it. Sedation with diazepam and chlormethiazole, or the use of phenytoin, is more common in the UK.

If antihypertensive drugs are to be used, hydralazine is still the most commonly used in acute hypertension, given intravenously by injection or infusion. Satisfactory control of the blood pressure can also be easily achieved with intravenous infusion of labetalol in severe hypertension in pregnancy (Michael, 1979, 1986). There were no maternal hypotensive episodes or side-effects. A slow intravenous injection of 50 mg of labetalol is an effective treatment of severe hypertension. It has been shown to minimize the normal hypertensive effect of intubation at cesarean section (Ramanathan *et al.*, 1988).

Nifedipine has also been proved to be effective in pregnancy and the puerperium (Walters and Redman, 1984; Barton, Hiett and Conover, 1990). In comparison with hydralazine, nifedipine has been found to be as effective in lowering blood pressure and has the advantage of being an oral therapy. One possible serious problem is the possible interaction between calcium channel blockers and magnesium sulfate leading to sudden excessive fall in blood pressure, although this risk may have been overstated.

A prospective randomized study compared the antihypertensive effects of epoprostenol sodium (prostacyclin) with those of dihydralazine in acute hypertensive crises of pregnancy. There were no statistically significant differences in the antihypertensive effects between the two treatment groups. Epoprostenol infusion caused less tachycardia compared with the group treated with dihydralazine ($p = 0.0024$). The place of epoprostenol in pregnancy might be in patients with severe hypertension and tachycardia and in those requiring acute control of severe hypertension on the operating table before general anesthesia (Moodley and Gouws, 1992)

## 13.5.2 MILD TO MODERATE HYPERTENSION

It is less well accepted that treatment should be started with diastolic blood pressure between 90 and 100 mmHg. However, the use of drugs to control blood pressure in pregnancy is gradually increasing, as a result of the greater knowledge about the drugs and their safety in pregnancy.

Despite the initial reservations, adrenoceptor antagonists have now been studied fairly extensively in preeclampsia, and they have been shown to be both safe and effective in controlling blood pressure. They are also relatively free of side-effects, making them acceptable to patients.

The first randomized controlled study of an adrenoceptor antagonist in preeclampsia was performed with atenolol, a selective beta-receptor antagonist (Rubin *et al.*, 1983). This was a study of 120 women. Atenolol effectively controlled blood pressure and reduced the subsequent development of proteinuria, suggesting a possible beneficial effect on the disease process. It is not a surprise, however, if antihypertensive therapy reduces the incidence of proteinuria, as this is probably a result of the reduction in the perfusion pressure to the kidney.

There was no difference in fetal and neonatal complications such as intrauterine growth retardation, neonatal hypoglycemia or hyperbilirubinemia between the two groups. Respiratory distress was seen only in the control group. However, neonatal bradycardia was more common in the atenolol group, although there was no effect on neonatal blood pressure. The children from this study have all been followed up for 1 year and atenolol has not been shown to have any adverse effects on their development. Other studies have confirmed these findings. Some workers recommend the use of a vasodilator like nifedipine as concomitant therapy to overcome the vasoconstriction of preeclampsia. Labetalol, which has built-in vasodilator ability, has also been shown to be effective (Pandurski, 1991).

It would seem from these studies that adrenoceptor antagonists are both safe and effective in the treatment of preeclampsia and may have some beneficial effects on the disease process. Whether any particular adrenoceptor antagonist is more effective than the others is not certain. Labetalol has been shown to be as good as or superior to methyldopa, while both labetalol and pindolol appear to have advantages over atenolol (Pandurski, 1991). In a prospective double-blind randomized placebo controlled study of labetalol in 144 women who developed PIH after 20 weeks gestation, labetalol significantly lowered the blood pressure and reduced the incidence of proteinuria. The placebo-treated group had more patients who developed severe hypertension (> 150/110 mmHg) and a greater requirement for additional antihypertensive therapy prior to labor than the group treated with labetalol. Therefore, the maximum blood pressure prior to labor and the incidence of proteinuria was reduced in women on labetalol therapy. However, since late onset disease did not appear to benefit, the appropriateness of pharmacological therapy for late-onset PIH may be questioned (Pickles, Broughton Pipkin and Symonds, 1992).

Labetalol controls the blood pressure in most women within 24 hours of commencement of therapy. This control is often short-lived, requiring dose escalation after 3–5 days in the majority of cases. Labetalol is well tolerated and no significant maternal toxicity has been noted (Cruickshank *et al.*, 1992b). In various studies, labetalol treated patients had a reduction in hospital inpatient antenatal stay. There is a trend suggesting a possible prolongation of pregnancy for parous patients, a reduction in emergency cesarean sections and an increase in spontaneous vaginal deliveries for labetalol treated women (Cruickshank *et al.*, 1991).

In a double-blind study of pindolol, in 60 women presenting with a diastolic blood pressure of 85–99 mmHg before the 35th week of pregnancy, early treatment of the hypertension was not associated with adverse effects in either mother or newborn.

However, 15 patients receiving placebo required additional treatment, compared with six in the pindolol group ($p = 0.015$). It is thus estimated that 50% of pregnant females with mild–moderate hypertension will eventually require antihypertensive therapy, while the remainder will be able to complete the pregnancy without treatment. (BottKanner *et al.*, 1992)

Hydralazine is frequently used as a 'second-line' drug to augment the effects of adrenoceptor antagonists and methyldopa when satisfactory control is not achieved with a single agent. Erratic metabolism yields unpredictable responses by the oral route and nifedipine has largely superseded hydralazine for this indication.

### 13.5.3 ANTIOXIDANT THERAPY

This evidence that there is an increase in the free radical activity in preeclampsia (Wisdom *et al.*, 1991). This may be due to an oxidant/antioxidant imbalance among the pathogenic factors involved in preeclampsia. A non-randomized controlled trial of vitamin E supplementation showed that vitamin E did not improve fetal outcome in established severe preeclampsia. Furthermore, it does not show favorable effects on maternal hypertension and proteinuria (Stratta *et al.*, 1994)

### 13.6 DISCUSSION

There is no doubt that hypertension in pregnancy is associated with an increased risk to the mother and fetus. However, there appears to be no consensus concerning the best treatment regimes. It appears clear that many of the patients do not require special care but vigilance is probably required to distinguish those that do from those that do not. Hospitalization is not necessary for all. Lowering blood pressure appears to be possible and easy to achieve and its early use may reduce the number of women who develop severe hypertension.

As therapy during pregnancy is directed at the mother, there is concern that the fetus might be subjected to adverse effects without benefit to itself. If antihypertensive therapy prolongs pregnancy, the fetus will indirectly benefit from this and this may counterbalance any harmful effects. Not all therapies would appear to be beneficial and some drugs have greater side-effects than others. Close monitoring is required for any fetus of a hypertensive mother and this need is heightened if she is given antihypertensive therapy. It is difficult to distinguish between side-effects produced by therapy and the problems of the disease itself. All drugs will cross the placenta to a greater or lesser degree. It would be surprising if these drugs produced no side-effects in the neonate.

The ACE inhibitors appear to produce direct complications that are harmful to the fetus and neonate. There would have to be strong reasons for their use in pregnancy. Diuretics have only a weak effect and the potentially harmful changes to placental blood flow would count against their use except in life-threatening pulmonary edema postpartum.

Atenolol is a very effective drug in pregnancy, especially in those with an increased cardiac output, but there are reports of fetal heart rate abnormalities, high levels of cord blood drug concentration and a slow neonatal clearance. One of the main fears concerning antihypertensive drugs is the effect they might have on the placental blood flow. Labetalol has been shown in both animal and human studies to lower blood pressure and maintain placental blood flow. Hydralazine and nicardipine have been shown to reduce placental blood flow but nifedipine does not. It is difficult to know whether these findings are clinically relevant but it would appear advisable to use drugs that have not been shown to have adverse effects.

All the beta-blockers are known to be associated with hypoglycemia, bradycardia and hypotension in some infants. This does not appear to be clinically significant, although awareness of this possibility is important. These problems are also common in babies born of hypertensive mothers not on therapy. It is difficult, therefore, to distinguish the side-effects of drugs from manifestations of the disease process. The following chapters will outline the use of antihypertensive therapy in various management regimes.

## REFERENCES

Ahokas, R. A., Sibai, B. M., Mabie, W. C. and Anderson, G. D. (1988) Nifedipine does not adversely affect uteroplacental blood flow in the hypertensive term-pregnant rat. *Am. J. Obstet. Gynecol.*, 159, 1440–1445.

Aisenbrey, G. A., Corwin, E. and Catanzarite, V. (1992) Effect of magnesium sulfate on the vascular actions of norepinephrine and angiotensin II. *Am. J. Perinatol.*, 9, 477–480.

Ayromlooi, J., Tobias, M., Berg, P. and Leff, R. (1982) The effects of diazoxide upon fetal and maternal hemodynamics and fetal brain function and metabolism. *Pediatr. Pharmacol.*, 2, 293–304.

Barron, W. M. (1992) The syndrome of preeclampsia. *Gastroenterol. Clin. North Am.*, 21, 851–872.

Barton, J. R., Hiett, A. K. and Conover, W. B. (1990) The use of nifedipine during the postpartum period in patients with severe preeclampsia. *Am. J. Obstet. Gynecol.*, 162, 788–792.

Belfort, M. A., Saade, G. R., Moise, K. J. Jr. *et al.* (1994) Nimodipine in the management of preeclampsia: maternal and fetal effects. *Am. J. Obstet. Gynecol.*, 171, 417–424.

Biesenbach, G., Stoger, H. and Zazgornik, J. (1992) Influence of pregnancy on progression of diabetic nephropathy and subsequent requirement of renal replacement therapy in female type I diabetic patients with impaired renal function. *Nephrol. Dialysis Transplant.*, 7, 105–109.

BottKanner, G., Hirsch, M., Friedman, S. *et al.* (1992) Antihypertensive therapy in the management of hypertension in pregnancy: a clinical double-blind study of pindolol. *Clin. Exper. Hypertens. – B: Hypertension in Pregnancy*, 11, 207–220.

Broughton Pipkin, F., Turber, S. R. and Symonds, E. M. (1980) Possible risk with catopril in pregnancy. *Lancet*, i, 1256–1260.

Catanzarite, V. A. (1992) The natural history of thrombocytopenia associated with preeclampsia. *Am. J. Obstet. Gynecol.*, 166, 770–771.

Cody, R. J., Tarazi, R. C., Bravo, E. L. and Fouan, F. M. (1978) Haemodynamics of orally active converting enzyme inhibitor (SQ-14, 225) in hypertensive patients. *Clin. Sci. Mol. Med.*, 55, 453–457.

Collins, R. and Duley, L. (1995) Any antihypertensive therapy for pregnancy hypertension, in *Pregnancy and Childbirth Module* (eds M. W. Enkin, M. J. N. C. Keirse, M. J. Renfrew and J. P. Neilson), Cochrane Database of Systematic Reviews, review no. 04426. Published through Cochrane Updates on Disk, Update Software, Oxford.

Cruickshank, D. J., Robertson, A. A., Campbell, D. M. and MacGillivray, I. (1991) Maternal obstetric outcome measures in a randomised controlled study of labetalol in the treatment of hypertension in pregnancy. *Clin. Exper. Hypertens. – B: Hypertension in Pregnancy*, 10, 333–344.

Cruickshank, D. J., Campbell, D., Robertson, A. A. and MacGillivray, I. (1992a) Intra-uterine growth retardation and maternal labetalol treatment in a random allocation controlled study. *J. Obstet. Gynecol.*, 12, 223–227.

Cruickshank, D. J., Robertson, A. A., Campbell, D. M. and MacGillivray, I. (1992b) Does labetalol influence the development of proteinuria in pregnancy hypertension? A randomised controlled study. *Eur. J. Obstet. Gynecol. Reprod. Biol.*, 45, 47–51.

Danti, L., Valcamonico, A., Soregaroli, M. *et al.* (1994) Fetal and maternal Doppler modifications during therapy with antihypertensive drugs. *J. Maternal–Fetal Invest.*, 4, 19–23.

Dubois, D., Petitcolas, J., Temperville, B. *et al.* (1982) Treatment of hypertension in pregnancy with beta-adrenoceptor antagonists. *Br. J. Clin. Pharmacol.*, 13, 375S–3379.

Girndt, J. (1994) Pregnancy in women with diabetic nephropathy – a clear indication for antihypertensive treatment. (Schwangerschaft bei Frauen mit diabetischer Nephropathie – eine klare Indikation zu einer antihypertensiven Behandlung.) *Zentralbl. Gynäkol.*, 116, 362–364.

Greer, I. A., Walker, J. J., Calder, A. A. and Forbes, C. D. (1985) Inhibition of platelet aggregation in whole blood by adrenoceptor antagonists. *Thromb. Res.*, 40, 631–635.

Grunewald, C., Carlstrom, K., Lunell, N. O. *et al.* (1993) Dihydralazine in preeclampsia: acute effects on atrial natriuretic peptide concentration and feto-maternal hemodynamics. *J. Maternal–Fetal Med.*, 3, 21–24.

Hjertberg, R., Belfrage, P. and Hanson, U. (1992) Conservative treatment of mild and moderate hypertension in pregnancy. *Acta Obstet. Gynecol. Scand.*, 71, 439–446.

Hjertberg, R., Faxelius, G. and Lagercrantz, H. (1993) Neonatal adaptation in hypertensive pregnancy – a study of labetalol vs hydralazine treatment. Journal of Perinatal Medicine 21, 69–75.

Hutton, J. D., James, D. K., Stirrat, G. M. *et al.* (1992) Management of severe pre-eclampsia and eclampsia by UK consultamts. *Br. J. Obstet. Gynaecol.*, 99, 554–556.

Kaaja, R., Hiilesmaa, V., Holma, K. and Jarvenpaa, A. L. (1992) Maternal antihypertensive therapy with beta-blockers associated with poor outcome in very-low birthweight infants. *Int. J. Gynecol. Obstet.*, 38, 195–199.

KincaidSmith, P. (1994) Hypertension in pregnancy. *Blood Pressure*, 3, 18–23.

Koch Weser, J. (1974) Vasodilator drugs in the treatment of hypertension. *Arch. Intern. Med.*, 133, 1017–1020.

Kyle, P. M. and Redman, C. W. G. (1992) Comparative risk–benefit assessment of drugs used in the management of hypertension in pregnancy. *Drug Safety*, 7, 223–234.

Lardoux, H., Gerard, J., Elazquez, G. and Flouvat, B. (1983) Which beta-blocker in pregnancy-induced hypertension? *Lancet*, ii, 1194–1198.

Leather, H. M., Humphries, D. M., Baker, P. and Chadd, M. A. (1968) A control trial of hypotensive agents in hypertension in pregnancy. *Lancet*, ii, 488–492.

Lechner, W. (1993) Calcium antagonists in pregnancy as antihypertensive and tocolytic agents. *Wiener Med. Wochenschr.*, 143, 519–521.

Lindheimer, M. D. (1993) Hypertension in pregnancy. *Hypertension*, 22, 127–137.

Lipshitz, J., Ahokas, R. A. and Reynolds, S. L. (1987) The effect of hydralazine on placental perfusion in the spontaneously hypertensive rat. *Am. J. Obstet. Gynecol.*, 156, 356–359.

Lowe, S. A. and Rubin, P. C. (1992) The pharmacological management of hypertension in pregnancy. *J. Hypertens.*, 10, 201–207.

Lund Johansen, P. (1980) The effect of beta-blocker therapy on chronic hemodynamics. *Prim. Cardiol.*, 1, 20–26.

Lund Johansen, P. (1984) Pharmacology of combined alpha-beta-blockade. *Drugs*, 28, 35–50.

McCombs, J. (1992) Treatment of preeclampsia and eclampsia. *Clin. Pharm.*, 11, 236–245.

Michael, C. A. (1979) Use of labetalol in the treatment of severe hypertension during pregnancy. *Br. J. Clin. Pharmacol.*, **8**, 211–215.

Michael, C. A. (1986) Intravenous labetalol and intravenous diazoxide in severe hypertension complicating pregnancy. *Aust. NZ J. Obstet. Gynaecol.*, **26**, 26–29.

Moodley, J. and Gouws, E. (1992) A comparative study of the use of epoprostenol and dihydralazine in severe hypertension in pregnancy. *Br. J. Obstet. Gynaecol.*, **99**, 727–730.

Olivari, M. T., Bartorelli, C., Polese A. *et al.* (1979) Treatment of hypertension with nifedipine, a calcium antagonistic agent. *Circulation*, **59**, 1056–1058.

Pandurski, F. (1991) [Electrolyte studies of the amniotic fluid]. *Akush Ginekol. Sofiia*, **30**, 5–7.

Parisi, V. M., Salinas, J. and Stockmar, E. J. (1989a) Placental vascular responses to nicardipine in the hypertensive ewe. *Am. J. Obstet. Gynecol.*, **161**, 1039–1043.

Parisi, V. M., Salinas, J. and Stockmar, E. J. (1989b) Fetal vascular responses to maternal nicardipine administration in the hypertensive ewe. *Am. J. Obstet. Gynecol.*, **161**, 1035–1039.

Pickles, C. J., Broughton Pipkin, F. and Symonds, E. M. (1992) A randomised placebo controlled trial of labetalol in the treatment of mild to moderate pregnancy induced hypertension. *Br. J. Obstet. Gynaecol.*, **99**, 964–968.

Prevost, R. R., Akl, S. A., Whybrew, W. D. and Sibai, B. M. (1992) Oral nifedipine pharmacokinetics in pregnancy-induced hypertension. *Pharmacotherapy*, **12**, 174–177.

Pritchard, J. A. (1955) The use of the magnesium ion in the management of eclamptogenic toxemias. *Surg. Gynecol. Obstet.*, 100, 131–135.

Ramanathan, J., Sibai, B. M., Mabie, W. C. *et al.* (1988) The use of labetalol for attenuation of the hypertensive response to endotracheal intubation in preeclampsia. *Am. J. Obstet. Gynecol.*, **159**, 650–654.

Redman, C. W., Beilin, L. J., Bonnar, J. and Ounsted, M. K. (1976) Fetal outcome in a trial of antihypertensive treatment in pregnancy. *Lancet*, **ii**, 754–758.

Reid, J. L. and Elliot, H. L. (1984) Methyldopa, in *Handbook of Hypertension: vol 5: Clinical Pharmacology of Antihypertensive Drugs*, (ed. A. E. Doyle), Elsevier, Amsterdam, p. 92–112.

Rubin, P. C., Clark, D. M., Sumner, D. J. *et al.* L. (1983) Placebo controlled trial of atenolol in treatment of pregnancy associated hypertension. *Lancet*, **i**, 431–435.

Sibai, B. M. (1991) Chronic hypertension in pregnancy. *Clin. Perinatol.*, **18**, 833–844.

Sibai, B. M. (1992) Hypertension in pregnancy. *Obstet. Gynecol. Clin. North Am.*, **19**, 615–632.

Sibai, B. M., Abdella, T. N., Anderson, G. D. and Dilts, P. V. (1983) Plasma volume findings in pregnant women with mild hypertension: therapeutic considerations. *Am. J. Obstet. Gynecol.*, **145**, 539–543.

Stratta, P., Canavese, C., Porcu, M. *et al.* (1994) Vitamin E supplementation in preeclampsia. *Gynecol. Obstet. Invest.*, **37**, 246–249.

Todd, P. A. and Goa, K. L. (1992) Enalapril. A reappraisal of its pharmacology and therapeutic use in hypertension. *Drugs*, **43**, 346–381.

Tranquilli, A. L., Garzetti, G. G., De Tommaso, G. *et al.* (1992) Nifedipine treatment in preeclampsia reverts the increased erythrocyte aggregation to normal. *Am. J. Obstet. Gynecol.*, **167**, 942–945.

Tuffnell, D. J., Currie, I., Bicford Smith, P. *et al.* (1994) A complete audit cycle of the management of severe pre-eclampsia 1990–92. *Contemp. Rev. Obstet. Gynaecol.*, **6**, 36–40.

Vink, G. J., Moodley, J. and Philpott, R. W. (1980) The effect of dihydalazine on the fetus in the treatment of maternal hypertension. *Obstet. Gynecol.*, **55**, 519–523.

Voto, L. S., Lapidus, A. M., Catuzzi, P. *et al.* (1992) Cadralazine for the treatment of preeclampsia: an open, noncomparative, dose-finding pilot study. *Hypertension*, **19**, II132–II136.

Wacker, J., Muller, J., Grischke, E. M. *et al.* (1994) Antihypertensive therapy of pregnancy-induced-hypertension (PIH) with urapidil. (Antihypertensive Therapie bei schwangerschaftsinduzierter Hypertonie (SIH) mit Urapidil.) *Zentralbl. Gynäkol.*, **116**, 271–273.

Walker, J. J. (1991) Hypertensive drugs in pregnancy. Antihypertension therapy in pregnancy, preeclampsia, and eclampsia. *Clin. Perinatol.*, **18**, 845–873.

Walker, J. J., Mathers, A., Bjornsson, S. *et al.* (1992) The effect of acute and chronic antihypertensive therapy on maternal and fetoplacental Doppler velocimetry. *Eur. J. Obstet. Gynecol. Reprod. Biol.*, **43**, 193–199.

Walters, B. N. and Redman, C. W. (1984) Treatment of severe pregnancy-associated hypertension with the calcium antagonist nifedipine. *Br. J. Obstet. Gynaecol.*, **91**, 330–336.

WideSwensson, D., Montal, S. and Ingemarsson, I. (1994) How Swedish obstetricians manage hypertensive disorders in pregnancy. A questionnaire study. *Acta Obstet. Gynecol. Scand.*, **73**, 619–624.

WideSwensson, D., Montan, S., Arulkumaran, S. *et al.* (1993) Effect of methyldopa and isradipine on fetal heart rate pattern assessed by computerized cardiotocography in human pregnancy. *Am. J. Obstet. Gynecol.*, **169**, 1581–1585.

Wisdom, S. J., Wilson, R., McKillop, J. H. and Walker, J. J. (1991) Antioxidant systems in normal pregnancy and in pregnancy-induced hypertension. *Am. J. Obstet. Gynecol.*, **165**, 1701–1704.

# MANAGEMENT OF SEVERE HYPERTENSION IN PREGNANCY AND/OR ECLAMPSIA – THE GLASGOW/LEEDS EXPERIENCE

*James J. Walker*

## 14.1 INTRODUCTION

Preeclampsia and eclampsia is still associated with significant maternal mortality and morbidity in the UK (Turnbull *et al.*, 1989; DHSS, 1991). Although the number of hypertensive pregnant women seen remains around 15% of the total pregnancies, the incidence of many of the major complications of hypertension has markedly reduced over the last 50 years. This is particularly true of eclampsia, which now occurs in around 3/10 000 deliveries. This means that the average obstetrician will only see one case of eclampsia every 4 years. Therefore, in the UK, eclampsia is not the main presentation of pregnancy hypertension, unlike other parts of the world (Chapter 16). The incidence of proteinuric hypertension is around 4% but the number of those with severe hypertension requiring crisis management is lower, at around 1–2%. Around 60% of severely preeclamptic patients will present acutely, often out of hours. Because of this, it is important to have management protocols available in the labor ward of all hospitals aimed at the main sequelae of hypertension in pregnancy (Walker, 1992). Delay in the treatment of these women can contribute to the maternal mortality and morbidity.

## 14.2 MATERNAL SEQUELAE OF SEVERE PREECLAMPSIA–ECLAMPSIA

Maternal morbidity from this condition remains high because of the requirement for admission to hospital, various forms of treatment to lower blood pressure and prevent convulsion, and increased induction of labor and cesarean section. There also remains more serious complications such as cerebrovascular accident and cardiorespiratory failure which remain the main causes of maternal mortality (DHSS, 1991, 1994). It is not just maternal death but significant morbidity that can occur (Table 14.1) which can lead to long-term sequelae, both physical and psychological.

It should not be forgotten that after an event of severe hypertension many patients are very reluctant to embark on future pregnancy because of the fear of suffering such experiences again. There is, therefore, a fear factor involved in this condition, not only at the time of presentation but relating to the possibility of future pregnancy. Therefore, the

*Hypertension in Pregnancy*
Edited by J.J. Walker and N.F. Gant. Published by Chapman & Hall, 1997 ISBN 0 412 30910 6

**Table 14.1** Maternal sequelae of severe hypertension in pregnancy

**Major**
- Cerebral vascular accident
- Occipital lobe blindness
- Convulsions
- Pulmonary edema
- Aspiration syndrome
- Haemolysis, elevated liver enzymes and low platelets (HELLP)
- Hemorrhage
- Renal failure
- Deep venous thrombosis

**Complications of treatment**
- Sedation and aspiration
- Cesarean section

management of this condition should consist of the accurate assessment of the maternal condition (Chapter 9), lowering of the blood pressure in a smooth and predictable way, prevention of further convulsions if eclampsia has occurred, delivery at the appropriate time in the appropriate way, continued vigilance postpartum with close and adequate long-term follow-up.

## 14.3 FETAL SEQUELAE OF SEVERE PREECLAMPSIA–ECLAMPSIA

As far as the baby is concerned perinatal mortality and morbidity is increased because of placental insufficiency (Table 14.2).

**Table 14.2** Fetal sequelae of severe hypertension in pregnancy

- Direct effect of the disease itself
- Intrauterine growth restriction
- Resulting from the necessary intervention
- Premature delivery
- Ventilation
- Cerebral hemorrhage
- Pneumothorax
- Cerebral palsy

The level of maternal blood pressure is not a significant factor. There is also a greatly increased incidence of prematurity, with the concomitant need for ventilatory support, cerebral hemorrhage and long-term developmental problems. When looking at the epidemiology of hypertension in pregnancy it is clear that the majority of patients present between 32 weeks and term. However, the majority of the severe problems present at gestations earlier than 32 weeks with the increased risk to the baby because of the earlier gestation. There is a need, therefore, to be able to differentiate between the patients who are at risk of the severe complications of hypertension in pregnancy and those who can be easily controlled and have a more benign course.

## 14.4 THE STEPWISE MANAGEMENT OF HYPERTENSION IN PREGNANCY

The basis of the management of hypertension in pregnancy is comprehensive antenatal care. In most countries throughout the world where mortality from hypertension is high, it is related to poor antenatal care or unbooked patients. It is important that when designing the future of maternity services in this country that we maintain this level of vigilance. There is therefore a stepwise system of management in pregnancy hypertension (Table 14.3).

## 14.5 ASSESSMENT OF RISK

The main problem in the management of hypertension in pregnancy is the assessment of risk (Table 14.4).

It is obvious that certain groups of patients including primigravidae, people with preexisting hypertension and people with either a past history or family history of hypertension in pregnancy, are at increased risk of developing the condition. However, it is also clear that many of the patients developing this condition have no prodromal signs and therefore

**Table 14.3** The stepwise management of pregnancy hypertension

- Screen antenatal patients for the risk or signs of hypertension in pregnancy
- Monitor those thought to be at risk in a antenatal day unit (Chapter 9)
- Early involvement of senior medical staff
- Early treatment with antihypertensive drugs if required
- Give prophylactic steroids if the pregnancy is under 34 weeks
- Continuing close monitoring of those selected and/or treated to look for signs of progression
- Delivery of the baby on the best day and the best way
- Continuing close monitoring of the mother postdelivery with particular care concerning the fluid balance
- Arrange long-term follow-up to make sure that the blood pressure resolves and to discuss the problems of the pregnancy
- Offer a prepregnancy visit prior to embarking on the next pregnancy to assess the risk and design a pregnancy care plan

we will remain dependent on the normal antenatal care system to pick up many of the patients with early disease. Any patient with an elevation of blood pressure to a diastolic above 90, especially if that has been a sudden change of at least 15 mmHg should be referred for closer assessment. Similarly, the development of proteinuria and increasing edema merits closer scrutiny. Any clinical symptoms such as headache, visual disturbance and abdominal pain in the presence of even mild hypertension should put that patient into the high-risk category requiring immediate referral for more intensive assessment. This close assessment can be carried out in the antenatal day assessment unit (Chapter 9). The majority of the hypertensive women can be managed as outpatients with no intervention apart form monitoring. However, around 35% of hypertensive patients are found to have persistent hypertension and

are admitted to hospital for further management. There is evidence that antihypertensive agents may be beneficial in this group.

## 14.6 THE USE OF ANTIHYPERTENSIVE AGENTS

From 1950–1980 there was no reduction in the maternal mortality from hypertension in pregnancy. During the 1980s the first fall was seen in deaths from this condition (DHSS, 1991). This correlates with an increased use of antihypertensive drugs among obstetricians in the management of hypertension in pregnancy (Hutton *et al.*, 1992). The antihypertensive therapy may be associated with the apparent reduction of death from cerebrovascular accident.

The mainstay of therapy in hypertension in pregnancy in this country and throughout the world has always been the use of anticonvul-

**Tale 14.4** Women at particular risk of developing preeclampsia and its complications

- Primigravidae
- Women with a family history of preeclampsia
- Women with a past history of preeclampsia
- Women with a history of essential hypertension
- Multiple pregnancy

sant therapy to prevent eclampsia. Eclampsia now is a rare occurrence in hypertension in pregnancy, occurring in approximately 1/300 of all pregnant patients with hypertension. If people do convulse, the majority of patients convulse once and do not convulse again. The risks to the mother and baby from eclampsia appears to be more related to the degree of preeclampsia preceding the convulsion than to the eclampsia itself (Nelson, 1955). Therefore, it would seem logical that the first-line therapy in patients with hypertension in pregnancy would be to lower blood pressure rather than use any form of sedation or anti-convulsant. The latest meta-analysis of anti-hypertensive drug usage shows that there is a reduction in the incidence of hypertensive crisis and perinatal death (Collins and Duley, 1994). Such protocols are now well established in the UK, where the use of prophylactic anti-convulsants is no longer recommended. The use of antihypertensive drugs depends on the gestation of presentation.

### 14.6.1 PRESENTATION PRIOR TO 20 WEEKS

If the patient presents below 20 weeks it is our normal policy to observe the blood pressure, as it normally will fall in the second trimester. If the blood pressure falls to subnormal levels, we would normally stop therapy and then continue to monitor the patient to see whether therapy should be started at a later date. Some drugs are contraindicated in pregnancy, such as ACE inhibitors, and if at all possible these always are stopped. If the blood pressure rises with a persistent blood pressure of over 100 mmHg antihypertensive therapy is (re)started. If someone presents for the first time with hypertension before 20 weeks it always should be remembered that it may be due to underlying renal disease.

### 14.6.2 PRESENTATION AFTER 20 WEEKS

If a patient presents after 20 weeks with hypertension in pregnancy the assumption is

that the diagnosis is preeclampsia until the assessment suggests otherwise. The antihypertensive policy is basically the same as prior to 20 weeks. Close monitoring is carried out and if the blood pressure rises with a persistent diastolic over 100 mmHg antihypertensive therapy is commenced. Even with this apparently liberal approach to the use of antihypertensive therapy, fewer than 17% of our hypertensive patients are actually given antihypertensive therapy. That's about 1.7% of our pregnancy population. Therefore, despite this relatively low level of diastolic blood pressure being used for a reason for commencement of antihypertensive therapy, relatively few patients would appear to require it. After antihypertensive therapy has been started close vigilance has to be maintained as antihypertensive therapy lowers blood pressure and should not be expected to do anything else. Close monitoring, particularly of maternal urates and platelet count as well as the cardiotocograph and fetal growth should be used to see whether the condition is progressing and the effect it has on the mother and baby.

In the UK, the drugs commonly used for the treatment of hypertension in pregnancy are methyldopa, labetalol and nifedipine (Hutton *et al.*, 1992). The regime used in the Glasgow Royal Maternity Hospital (GRMH) and St James's University Hospital, Leeds (SJUH) consists of oral labetalol with a starting dose of 200 mg t.i.d. (Table 14.5).

This can be increased steadily to a maximum of 300 mg q.i.d. If control is not achieved, 10 mg oral nifedipine retard is given twice a day and this is increased to a maximum of 20 mg twice a day. It is rare for us to increase antihypertensive doses above this level.

If acute blood pressure reduction is required or oral therapy is not successful, intravenous labetalol 50 mg given by slow bolus would appear to be successful in the majority of patients and this can be followed up by labetalol infusion. It is rare, however, to

**Table 14.5**   The recommended antihypertensive regime

**Acute management**
- Labetalol 200 mg orally repeated hourly until control is achieved
  or
- Nifedipine 10 mg orally
  or
- Labetalol 50 mg by slow IV bolus
  followed by
- Labetalol infusion starting at a rate of 60 mg/h, doubling every 15 minutes until control is achieved or a maximum of 480 mg is reached.

**Starting daily dose for chronic therapy**
- Labetalol 200 mg three times daily
  increasing to
- Labetalol 300 mg four times daily
  with the addition of
- Nifedipine retard 10 mg twice a day
  increasing to
- Nifedipine retard 20 mg twice a day

require intravenous therapy as most patients will achieve blood pressure control starting with oral treatment. Of all the patients who present with a diastolic blood pressure of greater than 100 mmHg, with or without proteinuria, about 60% of them are easily controlled in the short term with an average prolongation of the pregnancy of at 15 days. About 30% of patients have reasonable control achieved but there is steady deterioration of both mother and baby and therefore delivery is normally required within a week following commencement of therapy. Around 10% of patients do not achieve adequate blood pressure control and although lowering of blood pressure can be achieved for a number of hours delivery is soon necessary. Similar results have been found by others (Mabie *et al.*1987; Sibai *et al.*1987).

After blood pressure is controlled, the situation should be reassessed and a management plan instigated by a senior doctor (Table 14.6).

**Table 14.6**   Management plan for the continuing care of women with severe preeclampsia

**Maternal management**
- Keep blood pressure controlled with antihypertensive drugs
- Close monitoring of the blood pressure at least four times a day
- Serum uric acid twice weekly
- Platelet count twice weekly
- Test for the presence of proteinuria quantification

**Fetal management**
- Prophylactic steroids given if the gestation is below 34 weeks
- An initial ultrasound assessment of fetal weight
- Doppler ultrasound assessment of umbilical blood flow twice a week
- Daily cardiotocographs
- Daily ultrasound for liquor volume

It is important to monitor blood pressure regularly using daily averages to assess control. If delivery within the next few days is thought to be a possibility, and the gestation is less than 34 weeks, prophylactic steroids are given to encourage fetal lung maturity. Dexamethasone 12 mg given twice 12 h apart is given. An attempt is then made to prolong the pregnancy for at least 48 h to achieve maximum effect. Delivery should be carried out if there is strong maternal or fetal reasons prior to 48 h being completed. At 48 h, a decision needs to made on whether further prolongation for more than a week is achievable. If it does not appear likely that this will be achieved, delivery when the mother is stable and the baby is well should be carried out. Transfer of the mother prior to delivery may be necessary for the optimum care for mother or her newly born (probably premature) baby.

If the pregnancy is prolonged, proteinuria should be quantified and serial uric acid levels and platelet counts taken on a twice-weekly basis. A cardiotocograph (NST) is completed daily and weekly ultrasounds are carried out partly for fetal growth but also for umbilical Doppler and liquor volume estimations, which can be done daily if the volume is thought to be low. Serial levels are required because it is the change of level of any given parameter that tells you whether the condition is deteriorating or not. Occasionally you can get an improvement in parameters particularly of platelet count and levels of proteinuria. This is due to the effect of lowering blood pressure with labetalol. It is affect of the drug itself and is not a sign that the condition is improving. Although the mainstay of therapy of hypertension in pregnancy should be in lowering blood pressure, is there a place for prophylactic anticonvulsant therapy?

## 14.7 ANTICONVULSANT THERAPY

Some 50 years ago in the GRMH the approximate risk of eclampsia occurring in the preeclamptic patient was 1/30. This is similar to the rate found in the Johns Hopkins Hospital in the USA (Chesley, 1971). Over the last 10 years the risk appears to have fallen to about 1/300; therefore, the risk of eclampsia is small (Walker, 1991). In North America magnesium sulfate is a commonly used preparation for both prophylaxis and treatment of convulsion (Pritchard, 1955). The use of magnesium sulfate appears to be increasing in the UK for the management of established convulsions. Until recently, it had never been subjected to a randomized, placebo-controlled trial to assess whether it has any benefit either as prophylaxis or in the treatment of eclampsia. Different therapies have been compared and it is obvious that irrespective of which anticonvulsant is used, convulsions can occur on any therapy (Dommisse, 1990; Crowther, 1990; Duley *et al.*, 1995). So no therapy will prevent convulsions completely. However, it now appears clear that magnesium sulfate is the drug of choice for the treatment of established convulsions as it has been proved to be superior to both phenytoin and diazepam (Duley *et al.*, 1995). However, it is still not proven as a prophylactic agent in severe preeclampsia. Moodley in Durban, South Africa, carried out a randomized study in severe preeclampsia, giving either magnesium sulfate or antihypertensive therapy alone (Moodley and Moodley, 1994). In over 200 patients only one convulsion occurred and that was in a patient treated with magnesium sulfate (Chapter 16). In a further study magnesium sulfate was compared with phenytoin as prophylactic treatment in severe preeclampsia to prevent convulsions. There were over 2000 preeclamptic women in the study and it showed magnesium to be superior to phenytoin (Lucas, Leveno and Cunningham, 1995). Only ten women convulsed and they were all in the phenytoin group. Although this suggests that magnesium is superior to phenytoin, it also demonstrates that the risk of convulsion is low, at around 1/200. This means that a regime of routine prophylaxis in severe preeclampsia may medicate many women who do not benefit from it.

Whatever is decided, it is important for each unit to have clear guidelines as to what protocols it wishes to follow. In the GRMH and St James's Hospital in Leeds, we do not routinely use prophylactic anticonvulsants and many units are also following this line. Although evidence of prodromal signs, particularly of headache and abdominal pain, are present in many patients who go on to convulse, about 20% of patients will convulse unexpectedly, often with normal blood pressure, and no sign is specific for the development of eclampsia. The widely used clinical assessment of hyperreflexia has never been demonstrated as being an accurate predictor, although it is widely used as such.

If an anticonvulsant therapy is to be used either prophylactically or after convulsions have occurred, there can be no doubt that magnesium sulfate is now the drug of choice (Duley *et al.*, 1995) even though the majority of obstetricians in the UK have no experience of it (Hutton *et al.*, 1992). The regime followed in St James's Hospital in Leeds is that of Zuspan (1978) (Table 14.7). This consists of a loading dose of 5 g given intravenously over 10 min followed by an infusion of 1 g/h for 24/48 h.

Two other commonly used preparations are infusions of diazepam and chlormethiazole. These preparations are sedation agents and not anticonvulsants and therefore to work the patients must be sedated to a semiconscious state. Although this may be effective, it produces many side-effects such as a marked respiratory depression in both the mother and baby resulting in orthostatic pneumonia and the need for ventilation in both mother and neonate, and therefore its use is not encouraged. Magnesium sulfate can be used both to treat the convulsion as well as preventing further seizures. Once the patient has been stabilized with both antihypertensive drugs and anticonvulsants, if required, consideration should be given to the next line of action.

## 14.8 CONTINUATION OF THE PREGNANCY

There is no doubt that the best intensive care unit consists of the uterus, but in certain circumstances the uterine environment is not beneficial for the baby or the maternal condition is such that it would be dangerous for the pregnancy to continue and therefore delivery is expedited. In the presence of convulsions there have been reported cases of successful continuation of pregnancy with a satisfactory

---

**Table 14.7** Anticonvulsant therapy to be used in the eclamptic patient (magnesium sulfate is supplied in solution containing 1 g/2 ml)

**IV regime (Zuspan)**
- Loading dose of 4/5 g intravenously (IV) over 20 min
- Infusion of 1 g/h for 24 h

**For recurring convulsion**
- A further 2–4 g was given IV over 20 min
- Make sure: respiratory rate > 16/min
  urine output > 25 ml/h,
  knee jerks are present

**If magnesium toxicity is suspected**
- Suggested by the absence of reflexes
- 1 g IV of calcium gluconate should be given

outcome for mother and baby. However, these cases are rare and usually from centers that receive many more eclamptics than are normally seen in centers in the UK. Therefore continuation of pregnancy after convulsion has occurred cannot be justified in the UK setting.

In the absence of convulsions prolongation of the pregnancy may be possible and this may improve the outcome for the premature fetus (Table 14.8).

It is gestation of onset that influences the outcome of the baby more than any other parameter. It is important, however, that the mother's condition is stable so that prolongation of pregnancy does not jeopardize her life. Lengthening of the pregnancy may be for a few hours which allows the pediatric unit to be organized to take the baby or the transfer of the patient to a unit which is better suited for looking after both the mother and the baby since intensive care therapy for either or both may be required. If pregnancy can be prolonged for a few days it may be possible to use steroids to mature fetal lungs in a baby of less than 34 weeks gestation. Since the benefits to the baby are at a maximum between 48 h and 6 days, it is important to reconsider whether further prolongation is advantageous 48 h after each steroid administration. If the patient is not well controlled and the probability is that she will require delivery over the next 2 or 3 days and a planned delivery at a time suiting all the professionals involved should then be decided upon.

It is important to emphasize that if pregnancy is going to be continued close monitoring of the mother and baby is required. A particular area of concern is that of liver impairment and that of HELLP syndrome (Table 14.1). Therefore, it is important that regular liver function tests or a minimum of at least the ALT should be carried out on a twice-weekly basis. This, along with platelet counts, should be able to pick up early signs of HELLP syndrome. If there is any concern that HELLP syndrome is developing, a blood film looking for fragmented red cells and evidence of hemolysis along with a full coagulation screen should be carried out. It is important to note that if the platelet count is above 100, the probability of an abnormal coagulation screen is virtually nil. Therefore, it is not necessary to do a full coagulation screen in all patients with hypertension in pregnancy on a regular basis.

## 14.9 THE MAIN MATERNAL RISKS AFTER DELIVERY

Govan in 1961 produced data from patients who died of eclampsia in the Royal Maternity Hospital in the 1940s and 50s (Govan, 1961). In reviewing 116 patients, he showed that 68 were primigravidae and 48 were multips. This emphasizes the problems of eclampsia are also present in the parous hypertensive women and are not limited to primigravidae. A total of 35% of the patients died from cerebral lesions, whereas the highest cause of fatality was cardiorespiratory failure, accounting for 43% of the patients. The patients who died in the hospital of cerebral lesions died generally within 24 h of eclampsia or delivery, whereas those dying from cardiorespiratory causes did so about 24 h after this. Both

---

**Table 14.8**  Benefits for the mother and baby of prolonging the pregnancy

- Stabilization and improvement of maternal condition
- Transfer to a unit more experienced and equipped for management
- The use of antenatal steroids
- Planned delivery in controlled conditions

groups had an average of seven seizures. The conclusion from this data is that control of the convulsions would not necessarily reduce the incidence of cerebral lesion and that the risk of cardiorespiratory failure was present in the 1940s prior to intravenous fluids or intensive care units and is probably due to various underlying mechanisms within the hypertensive woman (Table 14.9).

Only a very small number (< 5%) died of renal impairment and this was at a time where there were no renal units or dialysis and demonstrates the fact that renal failure is a relatively small risk in this group of patients. It is obvious, therefore, that the mainstay of care for these patients should be lowering blood pressure and the monitoring of fluid balance.

## 14.10 DELIVERY

The delivery of these patients should be at the best way on the best day and performed in the best place and by the best team. Therefore, the main problems are where, when and how to deliver the baby.

Timing affects the outcome for both mother and baby. If the mother is unstable, many people think that it is important to deliver her immediately in the maternal interest. However, a rushed delivery in an unstable patient probably adds to her risk rather than reduces it. On the other hand, a delay in delivery for too long in a patient who is sick can be treacherous. It is important in any situation of crisis to stabilize the blood pressure and convul-

---

**Table 14.9** The reasons women with preeclampsia are prone to pulmonary edema

- Low plasma osmolality
- Increased peripheral resistance
- Increased perfusion pressure
- Capillary leakage
- Increased venous return postdelivery

---

sions before any delivery decision is made. Once it is decided to deliver the baby, transfer to a more specialized unit may be prudent both for the baby's sake and also for the mother. Access to an intensive care unit may be equally as important for the mother as it is for the baby. Transfer of the pregnancy should be at an early stage before any evidence of deterioration and communication should be between relevant consultants rather than junior staff. It is important that *in utero* transfers organized by the pediatricians are also approved by the obstetricians, as the care of the sick mother in these situation can require much skill, time and effort.

If delivery has been decided before 32 weeks, it is our policy to carry out elective cesarean section. If it is after 34 weeks a vaginal delivery is aimed at, particularly when the chances of this being successful have been greatly increased by the use of vaginal prostaglandins. Antihypertensive therapy is continued throughout the procedure and throughout labor to help control blood pressure. The choice of anesthetic in cesarean section is important. General anesthetic can add to the risk to the mother, since intubation and extubation can cause a rise in both systolic and diastolic blood pressure as well as heart rate (Ramanathan *et al.*1988). This has led to cases of maternal mortality and cardiac failure in patients with severe disease. Therefore, an epidural block or spinal would seem by far the more sensible, allowing delivery to take place with the patient awake and speeds recovery from the procedure. Care should be taken prior to epidural that fluid load is kept to a minimum and it is often better to use a colloid solution than to use crystalline, which passes quickly across the capillaries into the interstitial space. During labor an epidural also is beneficial but not to control blood pressure, as this is a pathological effect of epidural rather than a physiological one. However, by relaxing the patient and allowing adequate pain relief it can stop unexpected rises of blood pressure often associated with painful labors. It also allows planned delivery and easy transition to cesarean section if this is thought necessary.

### 14.11 AFTER DELIVERY

After the patient has been delivered, close vigilance must be maintained. Many maternal deaths occur at this time. Fluid management is the most crucial aspect of this care (Table 14.10).

It is often found that antihypertensive therapy can be reduced steadily postdelivery although occasionally at 24–48 h there may be a need to increase treatment again. If antihypertensive therapy is stopped too quickly a rebound hypertension can occur. Postdelivery a relative oliguria is not uncommon, occurring in about 30% of patients with severe disease. This does not require therapy as urine output will recover in its own time. Anuria, on the other hand, is extremely concerning and if urine is not passed over a 2 h period active measures of assessment of plasma creatinine and the response to a test dose of frusemide should be carried out to check for the presence of renal failure. If there is any doubt about renal function, a urinary osmolality should be carried out. If the urine is concentrated, then renal function is satisfactory. If it is not then renal failure is present and a renal failure regime should be put in place. There is no evidence, however, that oliguria, especially in the presence of concentrated urine leads to renal failure.

Fluid challenges are potentially dangerous in preeclampsia, as much of the fluid will be lost from the cardiovasculature vessels into the interstitial fluid. If fluid is to be given, colloid is most sensible and a maximum of 500 ml should be given and not repeated unless an adequate response has been achieved. Although invasive monitoring is commonly used in the USA (Chapter 5) this is rarely deemed necessary in the UK outside an ICU setting. Not only is it often not helpful, it can be misleading. In preeclampsia, pulmonary edema, because of increased interstitial fluid, can occur in the presence of a low central venous pressure (CVP). If a CVP line is used, it is important not to transfuse fluid to produce a CVP level of more than 5 mmHg or 7 cmH$_2$O. If the CVP is higher than this, active measures using diuretics should be used to reduce it. One of the best methods of assessing pulmonary edema is arterial blood gasses and continuous measurements can be carried out using a pulse oximeter.

It is far safer and sensible to run a patient 'dry' and restrict intravenous fluids than to run the risk of pulmonary overload. Total fluid replacement should not exceed an hourly rate of 50 ml plus the previous hour's output. If the patient is in positive balance or there is evidence of pulmonary edema, active measures using 40 mg of frusemide followed

---

**Table 14.10**   Postpartum fluid management

**Monitoring**
- Assess both input and output
- Use a pulse-oximeter

**Fluid replacement**
- Fluid used should be Hartmann's solution or similar, not dextrose
- Hourly replacement of 50 ml plus the previous hour's output
- If patient in positive balance of over 2 liters or has low oxygen saturation, 40 mg frusemide followed by 20 g of mannitol
- Treat signs of pulmonary overload, not oliguria

by 20 g of mannitol should be used to help to reduce the fluid overload. Most of the problems of fluid overload begin around 16 h after delivery, with severe problems occurring between 24 and 48 h. This is associated with a failure of the normal postpartum diuresis. The active diuretic management, in the absence of diuresis in the overloaded patient, will reduce the probability of pulmonary edema, increase oxygen saturation, reduce cerebral edema and improve blood pressure control.

Postdelivery, the majority of people who will convulse do so within the first 24 h so it is rarely required to continue anticonvulsant therapy for more than 48 h postdelivery. If the patient is well, especially if prophylactic anticonvulsant is being used in the absence of any convulsions, it is probably safe to stop this therapy within 24 h.

## 14.12 FOLLOW-UP

The diagnosis of the underlying cause of the hypertension in pregnancy may not be apparent until after the pregnancy is over. It is therefore important to follow the patient up until normal blood pressure has returned. If normotension is not achieved by 6 weeks postpartum, the patient should be referred for further investigation of the underlying cause.

If severe preeclampsia has been suffered, especially if significant complications have occurred, the women and her partner should be seen for postpregnancy counseling. This has two purposes. An explanation of the events should be given but also advice regarding any future pregnancy is also required. There appears to be a risk of around 10% of recurrence of severe disease with a further 10–15% of people experiencing a milder form of hypertensive problem. It is rare for any mother to lose a second baby because of pregnancy hypertension. If recurrent problems are found, screening for a connective tissue disorder should be carried out as well as for antiphospholidin antibody syndrome.

## 14.13 CONCLUSION

Most patients with hypertension in pregnancy should emerge unscathed with a healthy baby at the end of pregnancy but all patients who present with an elevated blood pressure should be monitored closely and abnormal clinical signs and symptoms should be noted. The early use of antihypertensive drugs, optimum timing of delivery and strict fluid balance by experienced staff and specialist teams will help to increase the chances of a successful outcome. Early consideration of transfer of the patient to a specialist center or the seeking of specialist advice should be considered by clinicians not experienced in the management of this condition. Major maternal complications are more likely to be associated with a lack of or delay in treatment than the wrong treatment.

## REFERENCES

Chesley, L. C. (1971) Johns Hopkins Hospital figures, quoted in Hypertensive disorders of pregnancy, in *Williams Obstetrics*, 14th edn, (eds L. M. Hellman and J. A. Pritchard), Appleton-Century-Crofts, New York, p. 747–747.

Collins, R. and Duley, L. (1995) Any antihypertensive therapy for pregnancy hypertension, in *Pregnancy and Childbirth Module* (eds M. W. Enkin, M. J. N. C. Keirse, M. J. Renfrew and J. P. Neilson), Cochrane Database of Systematic Reviews, review no. 04426. Published through Cochrane Updates on Disk, Update Software, Oxford.

Crowther, C. (1990) Magnesium sulphate versus diazepam in the management of eclampsia: a randomized controlled trial. *Br. J. Obstet. Gynaecol.*, **97**, 110–117.

DHSS, Welsh Office, Scottish Home and Health Department (1991) *Report on Confidential Enquiries into Maternal Deaths in the United Kingdom 1985–87*, HMSO, London.

DHSS, Welsh Office, Scottish Home and Health Department (1994) *Report on Confidential Enquiries into Maternal Deaths in the United Kingdom 1988–90*, HMSO, London.

Dommisse, J. (1990) Phenytoin sodium and magnesium sulphate in the management of eclampsia. *Br. J. Obstet. Gynaecol.*, **97**, 104–109.

Duley, L., Carroli, G., Belizan, J. *et al.* (1995) Which anticonvulsant for women with eclampsia – evidence from the collaborative eclampsia trial. *Lancet*, **345**, 1455–1463.

Govan, A. D. T. (1961) The pathogenesis of eclamptic lesions. *Pathol. Microbiol.*, **24**, 561–565.

Hutton, J. D., James, D. K., Stirrat, G. M. *et al.* (1992) Management of severe preeclampsia and eclampsia by UK consultants. *Br. J. Obstet. Gynaecol.*, **99**, 554–556.

Lucas, M. J., Leveno, K. J. and Cunningham, F. G. (1995) A comparison of magnesium-sulfate with phenytoin for the prevention of eclampsia. *N. Engl. J. Med.*, **333**, 201–205.

Mabie, W. C., Gonzalez, A. R., Sibai, B. M. and Amon, E. (1987) A comparative trial of labetalol and hydralazine in the acute management of severe hypertension complicating pregnancy. *Obstet. Gynecol.*, **70**, 328–333.

Moodley, J. and Moodley, V. V. (1994) Prophylactic anticonvulsant therapy in hypertensive crises of pregnancy – the need for a large, randomized trial. *Hypertens. Pregn.*, **13**, 245–252.

Nelson, T. R. (1955) A clinical study of pre-eclampsia: part 1. *J. Obstet. Gynaecol. Br. Emp.*, **62**, 48–52.

Pritchard, J. A. (1955) The use of the magnesium ion in the management of eclamptogenic toxaemias. *Surg. Gynecol. Obstet.*, **100**, 131–135.

Ramanathan, J., Sibai, B. M., Mabie, W. C. *et al.* (1988) The use of labetalol for attenuation of the hypertensive response to endotracheal intubation in preeclampsia. *Am. J. Obstet. Gynecol.*, **159**, 650–654.

Sibai, B. M., Gonzalez, A. R., Mabie, W. C. and Moretti, M. (1987) A comparison of labetalol plus hospitalization versus hospitalization alone in the management of preeclampsia remote from term. *Obstet. Gynecol.*, **70**, 323–327.

Turnbull, A., Tindall, V. R., Beard, R. W. *et al.* (1989) *Report on Confidential Enquiries Into Maternal Deaths in England and Wales 1982–1984*, DHSS, London, vol. 34, p. 1–166.

Walker, J. J. (1991) Hypertensive drugs in pregnancy. Antihypertension therapy in pregnancy, preeclampsia, and eclampsia. *Clin. Perinatol.*, **18**, 845–873.

Walker, J. J. (1992) What can current management offer?, in *Maternal Mortality – the Way Forward*, (ed. N. Patel), Royal College of Obstetricians and Gynaecologists, London, p. 21–34.

Zuspan, F. P. (1978) Problems encountered in the treatment of pregnancy-induced hypertension. A point of view. *Am. J. Obstet. Gynecol.*, **131**, 591–597.

*John R. Barton and Baha M. Sibai*

## 15.1 INTRODUCTION

Although the incidence varies according to the population studied and the criteria used for diagnosis, hypertension complicates about 7–10% of all pregnancies. Apart from being the most common medical complications of pregnancy, hypertensive disorders are the leading cause of maternal morbidity and mortality worldwide (Rubin, 1987; Melrose, 1984). Further, hypertensive disorders are a major factor in perinatal morbidity and mortality. The incidence of these complications will depend on time of onset, presence of maternal target organ damage and presence of associated medical problems. Clearly, these complications are more common with increasing severity of hypertension but they may be positively affected by the quality of management. Severe hypertension may result from different pathological processes with various underlying causes and may present any time during pregnancy or in the puerperium. This chapter reviews the diagnosis and current management recommendations for pregnancies complicated by severe hypertension as carried out at the University of Tennessee, Memphis.

## 15.2 SEVERE HYPERTENSION: PREPREGNANCY AND FIRST TRIMESTER

Management of the patient with chronic hypertension should begin prior to pregnancy. The patient is encouraged to have her blood pressure checked several times before pregnancy to establish the cause and the severity of her hypertension in the non-pregnant state. The patient is advised to seek prenatal care once pregnancy is confirmed to ensure accurate determination of gestational age and assess the severity of her hypertension in the first trimester. For patients who are seen for the first time during pregnancy, the first step in management should include evaluation of the hypertension. Attention is paid to the duration of hypertension, use of antihypertensive medications, history of cardiac or renal disease, diabetes or thyroid disease, and the outcome of previous pregnancies (superimposed preeclampsia, abruptio placentae, perinatal outcome, congestive heart failure or renal failure) (Table 15.1).

The physical examination should include a careful evaluation of the optic fundi, auscultation of the flanks for a renal artery bruit, and auscultation of chest as well as assessment of dorsalis pedis pulses for detection of coarctation of the aorta. Baseline laboratory studies should be obtained for the organ systems that are likely to be affected by chronic hypertension or that are likely to deteriorate during pregnancy. Studies should include urinalysis, urine culture, serum electrolytes, uric acid, glucose and a 24-hour urine evaluation for creatinine clearance and protein. If hyper-

*Hypertension in Pregnancy*
Edited by J.J. Walker and N.F. Gant. Published by Chapman & Hall, 1997 ISBN 0 412 30910 6

**Table 15.1**  Initial evaluation of women with severe hypertension

- Evaluation prior to pregnancy
  - Establish severity
  - Document the etiology
  - Establish duration
- Counseling regarding medications used
- Presence of associated medical complications
  - Diabetes, renal disease
  - Cardiac disease, thyroid disease
  - Asthma, stroke, aneurysms
  - Antiphospholipid antibodies
- Outcome in previous pregnancies
  - Preeclampsia in second trimester
  - Abruptio placentae
  - Perinatal loss
  - Congestive heart failure
  - Renal failure

glycemia or wide blood pressure swings are evident, a 24-hour urine for vanillylmandelic acid and metanephrines is indicated to rule out pheochromocytoma. For patients with severe hypertension or significant proteinuria in the first trimester, a chest X-ray, electrocardiogram, antinuclear antibody and serum complement are indicated. If the patient is likely to have left ventricular hypertrophy from severe or long-standing hypertension, or if she has signs or symptoms of heart failure, an echocardiogram should be performed (Table 15.2). In addition, patients with a history of poor pregnancy outcome (repetitive mid-pregnancy losses) and those with recent thromboembolic disease should be evaluated for the presence of lupus anticoagulant and anticardiolipin antibodies.

Pregnancies in patients with chronic hypertension and renal insufficiency are associated with increased perinatal loss and increased incidence of superimposed preeclampsia, preterm delivery and fetal growth retardation. These risks are increased in proportion to the severity of the renal insufficiency. In addition, women with severe renal insufficiency, particularly those with primary glomerular disease, are at increased risk

for rapid progression to end-stage renal disease during pregnancy or in the postpartum period. Thus, women with renal disease desiring pregnancy should be counseled to conceive before renal insufficiency becomes severe. In women with hypertension and severe renal insufficiency in the first trimester, the decision to continue the pregnancy should not be made without extensive counseling. These women should be counseled

**Table 15.2**  Severe hypertension with cardiac disease prior to pregnancy and/or first trimester

- Maternal evaluation
  - Chest X-ray
  - Electrocardiogram
  - Echocardiography
- Coarctation of the aorta
  - Auscultation of chest
  - Check dorsalis pedis pulses
  - Risk of dissection and rupture
- Left ventricular disease
  - Abnormal systolic function (FS < 25%)
  - Hypertrophy (diastolic dysfunction)
  - Dilated cardiomyopathy
  - Antepartum heart failure
  - Postpartum pulmonary edema

regarding the potential maternal and fetal risks, particularly the potential need for dialysis during the course of pregnancy. Women who elect to continue with their pregnancies must be observed and managed at a tertiary care center with adequate maternal–neonatal intensive care facilities.

Early onset of prenatal care and frequent prenatal evaluation are paramount for successful outcome for patients with severe hypertension. These women require close monitoring throughout pregnancy and may require multiple hospital admissions for control of maternal blood pressure and/or for the management of associated medical complications. At the initial prenatal visit, patients should be seen by a dietitian and instructed on nutritional requirements, weight gain and sodium intake (2 g/d). In addition, they should be advised to avoid smoking and caffeine and encouraged to have adequate bed rest during the day.

Antihypertensive drugs such as thiazide diuretics, minoxidil and angiotensin converting enzyme (ACE) inhibitors should be discontinued in patients receiving them because of the potential adverse maternal and fetal side-effects. These patients are then restarted on methyldopa or nifedipine as needed. The initial dose of methyldopa is usually 250 mg every 8 h and for nifedipine it is 10 mg every 6 h. This dose is subsequently increased every 48 h as needed to maintain the diastolic blood pressure consistently below 100 mmHg for women with essential hypertension, and below 90 mmHg for women with target organ damage such as diabetes mellitus, renal disease and cardiac dysfunction. If maternal blood pressure is inadequately controlled with maximum doses of methyldopa (4 g/d) and nifedipine (120 mg/d), then a third drug such as labetalol may be added. The initial dose of labetalol is usually 200 mg every 8 h, which can be increased to a maximum dose of 2400 mg per day. In some of these patients, blood pressure control may demand the use of multiple oral drugs as well as occasional intravenous therapy.

During the course of pregnancy, the patient is to be seen every 2 weeks during the first and second trimester and then weekly thereafter. The timing of prenatal visits is then adjusted based on maternal and fetal conditions. Fetal evaluation should include serial ultrasonography for fetal growth, and antepartum fetal testing with the use of the non-stress test (NST) and/or the biophysical profile (BPP). Fetal testing is to be started at 26 weeks gestation and then repeated weekly or more often depending on fetal condition (superimposed preeclampsia, suspected fetal growth retardation). The biophysical profile needs to be performed only when the NST is non-reactive. When indicated, amniocentesis is performed to assess fetal pulmonary maturity.

The pregnancy may then be continued to term or until onset of superimposed preeclampsia (uric acid > 6 mg/dl and proteinuria > 1g/24 h), or until development of fetal growth retardation or fetal distress. The development of superimposed preeclampsia is an indication for immediate hospitalization. Subsequent management will depend on severity of the preeclampsia and fetal gestational age. The development of severe superimposed preeclampsia is an indication for delivery in all patients with a gestational age above 34 weeks. If superimposed preeclampsia develops before this time, then the pregnancies may be followed conservatively, with daily evaluation of maternal and fetal wellbeing. As stated previously, pregnant patients with chronic hypertension are at increased risk for superimposed preeclampsia, abruptio placentae, fetal growth retardation and preterm delivery. In addition, these patients may require frequent hospitalization for various obstetric and medical complications. Thus, it is advisable that such patients be delivered at a tertiary care center.

## 15.3 SEVERE PREECLAMPSIA: SECOND TRIMESTER

Severe preeclampsia developing in the second trimester is an obstetric dilemma. The timing of delivery in women who develop severe preeclampsia in the second trimester is a very difficult decision for the women and the obstetrician. Aggressive management with immediate delivery will result in extremely high neonatal mortality and morbidity whereas attempts to prolong pregnancy may result in fetal demise and may expose the mother to severe morbidity and even mortality. Sibai (1985) reviewed pregnancy outcome in 60 such patients that had conservative management over a 7-year period. The mean gestational age at time of management was 24.8 weeks (range 17–27) and the average length of pregnancy prolongation was 11.4 days (range 3–40). The perinatal outcome for these pregnancies was poor, with 31 of the 60 resulting in fetal demise and 21 ending in neonatal death, for a total perinatal mortality of 87%. In addition, maternal morbidity was significantly high. This study was retrospective, the majority of patients were managed at level 1 hospitals and a few of these pregnancies had antepartum fetal evaluation.

Pattinson, Odendaal and Dutoit (1988) described the results of conservative management in 34 patients who had severe preeclampsia before 28 weeks. The patients were managed by bed rest, antihypertensive drugs and intensive fetal and maternal monitoring. A total of 11 patients presented before 24 weeks, all of them resulting in perinatal deaths. The remaining 34 were between 24 and 27 weeks gestation, with 13 (38%) resulting in a surviving infant. Maternal complications included three (9%) patients with pulmonary edema and one (3%) with pleural effusion.

Recently, Sibai *et al.* (1990) described the results of individualized management in 109 women with severe preeclampsia at 19–27 weeks gestation. All women received exten-sive counseling regarding the risks and benefits of expectant management. In addition, pregnancy termination was recommended for 25 women with gestation age less than 24 weeks. Ten of these 25 women accepted termination, and the other 15 elected to continue with the pregnancies and thus were managed expectantly for an average of 19.4 days. These 15 pregnancies resulted in 13 fetal deaths and three neonatal deaths, for an overall perinatal survival of 6.7%. In addition, three women developed the syndrome of hemolysis, elevated liver enzymes and low platelets (HELLP syndrome), two developed abruptio placentae and one had eclampsia. The authors concluded that expectant management is not justified in these women. Expectant management was recommended for the other 84 women, with a gestational age beyond 24 weeks. Of the 84, 30 had immediate delivery, either because of patient's desire or because of attending staff desire. These women received continuous maternal and fetal monitoring, magnesium sulfate to prevent convulsion, antihypertensive drugs to maintain diastolic blood pressure below 110 mmHg and steroids for fetal lung immaturity. All were delivered within 48 h of initiation of management. The other 54 women were managed expectantly with antihypertensive drugs (intravenous hydralazine, oral labetalol, oral nifedipine) and daily evaluation of maternal and fetal conditions (daily biophysical profile). Pregnancy outcome in the two management groups is listed in Table 15.3.

The authors found that the expectantly managed group had significantly higher perinatal survival and lower acute and long-term neonatal morbidities. In addition, maternal complications were infrequent in both groups. In summary, the three described trials note that perinatal survival is extremely poor when severe preeclampsia develops before 24 weeks gestation (2%), whereas it is 50% when the disease develops between 25 and 27 weeks gestation (Table 15.4). Expectant management for women with severe preeclampsia

**Table 15.3** Perinatal survival (*n*; % in brackets) in conservative management of severe preeclampsia in the second trimester

| Gestation (weeks) | < 24 | 25–27 | > 27 |
|---|---|---|---|
| Sibai *et al.*, 1985 | 1/25 (4) | 7/35 (20) | 8/60 (13.7) |
| Pattinson, Odendaal and Dutoit, 1988 | 0/11 (0) | 13/34 (38) | 13/45 (29) |
| Sibai *et al.*, 1990a | 1/15 (6.7) | 42/55 (76) | 43/70 (61.4) |
| All studies | 2/51 (2) | 62/124 (50) | 64/175 (36.6) |

in the second trimester should be selective and should be practiced only in a tertiary care center with adequate intensive care facilities.

## 15.4 SEVERE HYPERTENSION: THIRD TRIMESTER

Severe elevations of blood pressure during the third trimester are usually caused by preeclampsia, or due to exacerbation of known chronic hypertension or of a silent renal disease. As a result, management of these women will depend on the etiology, gestational age and the presence or absence of associated medical or fetal complications.

Management of patients with severe preeclampsia prior to 35 weeks gestation is highly controversial. Some authors consider delivery as the definitive therapy for all patients regardless of gestational age; others recommend an expectant-management approach. However, the results of two recent randomized trials of expectant management were associated with a favorable perinatal outcome. Odendaal and co-workers (1990) described the results of individualized management in 58 patients with severe preeclampsia at 28–34 weeks gestation. The patients were initially treated with magnesium sulfate, hydralazine and steroids. All patients received antenatal testing with the non-stress test and ultrasound evaluation of the fetus. Of the 58 patients, 20 were delivered for maternal and/or fetal reasons within 48 h of hospitalization. The other 38 patients were subsequently randomized to either delivery (*n* = 20) or conservative management (*n* = 18). The active management group received steroids for fetal lung maturity and were delivered within 48 h after randomization. The conservatively managed group were managed by bed rest and blood pressure was controlled with prazosin 3–20 mg per day. During therapy, the blood pressure was

**Table 15.4** Pregnancy outcome in immediate delivery versus expectant management of severe preeclampsia at 25–27 weeks gestation; data presented as mean s.d. (Source: modified from Sibai *et al.*, 1990a)

| | Immediate delivery (*n* = 30) | Expectant management (*n* = 54) |
|---|---|---|
| Pregnancy prolongation (d) | 2.0 ± 0.2 | 13.2 ± 8.1* |
| Gestational age at delivery (weeks) | 26.3 ± 0.8 | 28.0 ± 1.2* |
| Birth weight (g) | 709 ± 159 | 880 ± 212* |
| Neonatal intensive care stay (d) | 115 ± 94 | 70 ± 32 |
| Perinatal deaths – *n* (%) | 20 (64.5) | 13 (23.6) |
| Abruptio placentae – *n* (%) | 2 (6.7) | 3 (5.6) |
| Eclampsia – *n* (%) | 1 (3.3) | 3 (5.6) |

* $p < 0.02$

maintained between 140/90 and 150/100 mmHg. Fetal evaluation included ultrasound for fetal growth and non-stress tests were performed at least three times daily. The patients were delivered either at 34 weeks gestation or for maternal or fetal distress.

Table 15.5 compares the pregnancy outcome between the active and the conservative management groups.

The total average length of pregnancy prolongation in the conservatively managed group was 9 days and the average length of pregnancy prolongation following randomization was 7.1 days (range 2–18). Only one patient in this group achieved 34 weeks gestation prior to delivery, however, neonatal complications and number of days spent in the neonatal intensive care unit were lower in this group as compared to the actively managed group. As a result, the authors concluded that conservative management may improve perinatal outcome in a select group of patients with severe preeclampsia at this gestation. It is important to note that such management requires intensive maternal and fetal evaluation.

In the second recent study (Fenakel *et al.*, 1991), a randomized clinical trial was conducted in which patients with severe preeclampsia between 26 and 36 weeks gestation were assigned to be treated with either nifedipine ($n = 24$) or hydralazine ($n = 25$). Patients assigned to the nifedipine group received 10–30 mg sublingually initially, then 40–120 mg per day orally. Those assigned to the hydralazine group received 6.25–12.5 mg

intravenously initially, then 80–120 mg per day orally until delivery. Maternal evaluation included frequent measurements of blood pressure, heart rate, patellar reflexes, urine output and laboratory tests. Fetal evaluation included daily fetal heart rate monitoring, biophysical profile three times a week and weekly ultrasonographic assessment of fetal growth. The authors found better control of blood pressure and a lower incidence of fetal distress in the group managed with nifedipine. In addition, the group receiving nifedipine had a better perinatal outcome than those receiving hydralazine. They concluded that nifedipine is a safe and effective drug in the management of patients with severe preeclampsia remote from term.

At the University of Tennessee, Memphis, all patients with severe preeclampsia are admitted to the labor and delivery area for close observation of maternal and fetal condition. All patients receive intravenous magnesium sulfate to prevent convulsions and bolus doses of hydralazine (5–10 mg) intravenously or nifedipine (10–20 mg) orally as needed to maintain diastolic pressure below 110 mmHg. All patients with persistent severe hypertension or other signs of maternal or fetal deterioration are usually delivered within 24 h irrespective of gestational age or fetal lung maturity. In addition, women with gestational age beyond 35 weeks and those with evidence of fetal lung maturity at 33–35 weeks are usually delivered within 24 h. Patients at 33–35 weeks with immature fluid receive

**Table 15.5** Pregnancy outcome in randomized management of severe preeclampsia at 28–34 weeks (Source: adapted from Odendaal *et al.*, 1990)

|  | *Active group (n = 18)* | *Conservative group (n = 20)* |
|---|---|---|
| Gestational age at delivery (weeks) | 30.1 ± 2.1 | 31.8 ± 1.9 |
| Pregnancy prolongation (days) | 1.3 ± 1.1 | 7.1 ± 5.1 |
| Birth weight (g) | 1272 ± 357 | 1420 ± 350 |
| Perinatal deaths – *n* (%) | 5 (25) | 3 (16.7) |
| Abruptio placentae – *n* (%) | 3 (15) | 4 (22.2) |

steroids to accelerate fetal lung maturity and are then delivered.

For pregnancies at 28–32 weeks gestation with severe preeclampsia, the management is dependent upon their clinical response during the observation period. Some of these women will demonstrate marked diuresis and improvement in blood pressure during observation. If the blood pressure remains below 100 mmHg diastolic (without antihypertensive therapy) after the observation period, magnesium sulfate is discontinued and the patients are followed closely in the hospital until fetal maturity is achieved. During hospitalization, they undergo frequent evaluation of maternal and fetal wellbeing. Steroids are administered for enhancement of fetal lung maturity. It is the authors' experience that the majority of these patients will require delivery within 2 weeks after hospitalization. However, some patients may continue with their pregnancy for more than 2 weeks. Recent work has suggested that with judicious use of antihypertensive drugs and careful monitoring many pregnancies can be prolonged safely for an average of 15 days (Sibai *et al.*, 1994)

Severe hypertension in pregnancy may be associated with functional derangement of multiple organ systems such as pulmonary, renal, hematological, hepatic and central nervous systems. The remainder of the chapter will focus on these manifestations and their management.

## 15.5 PULMONARY EDEMA

Capillary–interstitial fluid exchange in the lungs is governed by the Starling forces that regulate fluid movement across the pulmonary capillaries. As a result, alveolar pulmonary edema may develop secondary to various mechanisms that may be operating alone or, more often, in combination. Table 15.6 summarizes some of the mechanisms leading to pulmonary edema in severe preeclampsia.

Cardiogenic pulmonary edema due to systolic dysfunction (impaired myocardial contractility) may occur in patients with severe hypertension due to increased afterload or in patients with underlying heart disease, e.g. peripartum cardiomyopathy, idiopathic dilated cardiomyopathy or coronary artery disease. Impaired left ventricular systolic function

---

**Table 15.6** Mechanisms associated with pulmonary edema in preeclampsia

- Decreased plasma colloid oncotic pressure
  - Use of large amount of crystalloids
  - Blood loss during and after delivery
  - Loss of albumin in urine and interstitium
- Increased capillary wedge pressure
  - Iatrogenic fluid overload
  - Postpartum mobilization of extravascular fluid
  - Impaired renal function or renal failure
- Capillary endothelial damage
  - Increased permeability
  - Increased interstitial oncotic pressure
  - Sepsis
- Left ventricular dysfunction
  - Systolic
  - Diastolic
  - Both systolic and diastolic

results in increased left atrial pressure, with a concomitant increase in pulmonary capillary wedge pressure and a decrease in the oncotic–hydrostatic pressure gradient.

Diastolic dysfunction or impaired ventricular relaxation has been described in obese, chronically hypertensive women with superimposed preeclampsia (Mabie *et al.*, 1988) These women with stiff ventricles require high filling pressure and are thus predisposed to develop pulmonary edema with the expanded blood volume of pregnancy. Diastolic dysfunction occurs in patients with left ventricular hypertrophy and often coexists with normal systolic function. Combined systolic and diastolic dysfunction occurs later in the course of disease and is seen primarily in elderly multiparae with long-standing, severe hypertension.

Non-cardiogenic pulmonary edema develops either as a result of alterations in the alveolar–capillary membrane or reductions in the colloid osmotic pressure (COP)–pulmonary capillary wedge pressure (PCWP) gradient. Pulmonary edema due to alveolar–capillary membrane injury has been reported in preeclamptic patients who had normal wedge pressures and normal COP–wedge gradients. The second mechanism of non-cardiogenic pulmonary edema, narrowing of the COP–wedge gradient, has been well described in the obstetric literature (Benedetti, Kates and Williams, 1985) The normal gradient during pregnancy in the third trimester is approximately 14 mmHg. Reduction of this gradient to 4 mmHg or less is associated with an increased risk of pulmonary edema. In patients with severe preeclampsia, changes in the plasma COP (usually decreased) and in PCWP (usually increased with the use of crystalloids and postpartum) will result in a narrowing of this gradient, thus increasing the risk of pulmonary edema.

The work of several authors has clarified the mechanisms for narrowing of the COP–wedge gradient in preeclampsia. Pulmonary edema occurs in the postpartum period in 70–80% of the cases (Sibai *et al.*, 1987). Serum albumin decreases as a result of renal losses, impaired liver synthesis and blood loss with crystalloid replacement. Wedge pressure increases as a result of delayed mobilization of extra vascular fluid; in other words, beginning 24–72 h postpartum edema fluid is mobilized and is then returned to the intravascular space faster than the diseased kidneys can excrete it (Hankins *et al.*, 1984). Iatrogenic fluid overload may also contribute to raising the wedge pressure; however, elevations in filling pressure are often not significant enough to account for pulmonary edema without simultaneous lowering of intravascular oncotic pressure (Benedetti, Kates and Williams, 1985; Sibai *et al.*, 1987; Hankins *et al.*, 1984)

In 1980, Strauss *et al.* (1980) were the first to report Swan–Ganz data in preeclamptic patients with pulmonary edema. They described three cases of cardiogenic pulmonary edema with wedge pressures of 22–33 mmHg, systemic vascular resistances of 1710–2130 dyn.s/cm$^5$ and cardiac outputs of 4.6–4.8 l/min. They believed that pulmonary edema was secondary to isolated left ventricular systolic dysfunction, the result of increased afterload, and advocated nitroprusside therapy.

Sibai *et al.* (1987) retrospectively reviewed 37 cases of pulmonary edema in severe preeclampsia–eclampsia during a 9-year period. The incidence of pulmonary edema in preeclampsia–eclampsia was 2.9%. A total of 11 patients (30%) had antepartum pulmonary edema, with ten of these having chronic hypertension. The other 26 patients (70%) had postpartum pulmonary edema, with an average onset at 71 hours postpartum. There were four maternal deaths and morbidity was significant. Table 15.7 summarizes the associated maternal complications and maternal and perinatal outcome from this study. Sibai *et al.* pointed out that pulmonary edema usually does not occur as an isolated complication of preeclampsia, but is seen more com-

**Table 15.7** Associated maternal complications, maternal and perinatal outcome in 37 cases of pulmonary edema in severe preeclampsia-eclampsia (Source: adapted from Sibai *et al.*, 1987)

|  | n (%) |  |
| --- | --- | --- |
| Metritis – sepsis | 17 (46) |  |
| Abruptio placentae | 12 (32) |  |
| Disseminated intravascular coagulopathy | 18 (49) |  |
| Acute renal failure | 10 (27) |  |
| Cardiopulmonary arrest | 5 (14) |  |
| Hypertensive crisis | 6 (16) |  |
| Maternal death | 4 (11) |  |
| Perinatal death | 18/39 (49) |  |
| Mean gestational age |  | 32.4 ± 0.9 weeks |
| Mean birth weight |  | 1775 ± 183 g |

monly in association with multiple organ dysfunction.

Important considerations on the management of acute pulmonary edema are outlined in Table 15.8.

Acute pulmonary edema in preeclampsia usually responds to oxygen, morphine and furosemide (frusemide). If severe hypertension is present, a vasodilator such as hydralazine, nifedipine, nitroglycerin (Cotton *et al.*, 1986) or short-term nitroprusside may be needed. Digoxin is usually not required except in patients with impaired left ventricular systolic function or mitral stenosis with atrial fibrillation or supraventricular tachycardia. Aminophylline is occasionally useful in refractory pulmonary edema for its positive inotropic, mild diuretic and bronchodilating effects. Rotating tourniquets and phlebotomy are cumbersome and rarely used today. Intubation and mechanical ventilation, including the use of positive end-expiratory pressure, may be needed for the treatment of severe pulmonary edema.

## 15.6 ACUTE RENAL FAILURE

Acute renal failure is a dramatic syndrome characterized by a sudden decrease in renal function accompanied by rapidly progressing azotemia. Oliguria, although frequent, is not mandatory for the diagnosis. Acute renal fail-

**Table 15.8** Management of pulmonary edema

- Check arterial blood gas, follow $O_2$ saturation with pulse oximetry
- Supplemental oxygen
- Positive pressure ventilation (CPAP mask avoids intubation but if respiratory distress is severe, intubate and ventilate)
- Reduce sodium in intravenous fluids
- Reduce intravenous fluid rates
- Discontinue any agents associated with pulmonary edema development (i.e. beta-sympathomimetics)
- Swan–Ganz catheter to differentiate cardiogenic versus non-cardiogenic pulmonary edema
- Intravenous diuretics
- Afterload reduction, if needed
- Intravenous nitroglycerin

ure is an extremely rare complication of preeclampsia–eclampsia and its development is usually a result of either acute tubular necrosis or, rarely, bilateral cortical necrosis. The pathogenesis of acute renal failure continues to be the subject of extensive investigation and several pathological mechanisms have been implicated as possible etiological factors (Sibai, Villar and Mabie, 1990). The occurrence of acute renal failure is usually associated with preeclampsia–eclampsia complicated by abruptio placentae and disseminated intravascular coagulopathy (DIC). As a result, these pregnancies are associated with increased maternal–perinatal mortality and morbidity (Sibai, Villar and Mabie, 1990). In addition, it has been reported that patients who progressed to acute renal failure as a result of preeclampsia–eclampsia had a higher incidence of residual renal function impairment (Biggs *et al.*, 1967; Riff *et al.*, 1967)

Sibai, Villar and Mabie (1990) described the short-term pregnancy outcome, subsequent pregnancy outcome and remote prognosis in 31 cases of acute renal failure complicating pregnancy. A total of 18 patients had 'pure' preeclampsia and 12 patients (13 pregnancies) had chronic hypertension, parenchymal renal disease or both before pregnancy. There were three immediate maternal deaths (two in the pure preeclampsia group and one in the other group). Nine patients (50%) in the 'pure' group required dialysis during hospitalization and all 18 patients had acute tubular necrosis. Five patients (42%) in the other group required immediate dialysis and three patients had bilateral cortical necrosis. The majority of pregnancies in both groups were complicated by abruptio placentae and hemorrhage. Associated maternal complications and maternal and perinatal outcome from this study are summarized in Table 15.9.

All 16 surviving patients in the pure preeclampsia group had normal renal function on long-term follow-up (average $4.0 \pm 3.1$ years). Conversely, nine of the 11 surviving patients in the second group required long-term dialysis on follow-up and four of them ultimately died of end-stage renal disease.

Therapeutic principles in the management of acute renal failure include supportive and dialytic treatment until renal function recovers. Once the maternal condition is stabilized, if the fetus is mature, delivery should be effected. Successful peritoneal dialysis and hemodialysis (Hov, 1987) have been reported for the treatment of acute renal failure in pregnancy. Peritoneal dialysis is associated with a lower risk of hypotension and rapid fluid shifts.

**Table 15.9** Associated maternal complications, maternal and perinatal outcome in 31 cases of acute renal failure occurring with hypertensive disorders of pregnancy (Source: adapted from Sibai, Villar and Mabie, 1990)

|  | *Pure preeclampsia (%)* *(n = 18)* | *Chronic hypertension* *Renal disease (%)* *(n = 13)* |
|---|---|---|
| Abruptio placentae | 50 | 54 |
| Pulmonary edema | 61 | 54 |
| Cerebral edema/injury | 17 | 8 |
| Postpartum hemorrhage | 93 | 85 |
| Malignant hypertension | 22 | 54 |
| Cardiac arrest | 11 | 8 |
| Maternal death | 11 | 8 |
| Perinatal death | 29 | 57 |
| Mean gestational age | 33.1 weeks | 28.0 weeks |

Although numerous authors have reported threshold laboratory values of serum BUN as an indication for dialysis, our current management at the University of Tennessee, Memphis, does not. We prefer to manage the patient with close observation of fluid status, aided by central hemodynamics and serial evaluation of serum electrolytes. Dialysis is performed for life-threatening hyperkalemia, hypermagnesemia, fulminant volume overload, or markedly increased serum creatinine. Acute renal failure, as a consequence of preeclampsia–eclampsia, resolves completely following delivery in well-managed cases in our experience. The risks of hemodialysis or peritoneal dialysis may therefore be unjustified in the absence of severe volume overload or electrolyte abnormalities.

## 15.7 ECLAMPSIA

Eclampsia is defined as the development of convulsions and/or coma unrelated to other cerebral conditions during pregnancy and the postpartum period in patients with signs and symptoms of preeclampsia. It is primarily a disease of young primigravidae, with an increased incidence seen in the single indigent woman. In recent years, the reported incidence of eclampsia has ranged from 1/110–1/3448 pregnancies (Richards *et al.*, 1986; Moller and Lindmark, 1986). Its occurrence is significantly increased in twin pregnancies with a reported incidence of 1.5–3.6% (Long and Oats, 1987; Lopez-Llera, De la Luna Olsen and Niz Ramos, 1989). Although not all cases of eclampsia are preventable, the incidence and severity in a specific population may be reduced by early and adequate prenatal care as well as astute medical judgment.

The diagnosis of eclampsia requires the development of convulsions, in the presence of hypertension and proteinuria and/or generalized edema, after the 20th week of gestation or within 48 hours postpartum. About 75% of eclampsia cases develop before delivery, while 25% occur after delivery. Eclampsia

has rarely been diagnosed prior to 20 weeks of gestation (Sibai, Abdella and Taylor, 1982) or beyond 48 hours postpartum (Sibai *et al.*, 1980). Several risk factors for eclampsia have been established. These include nulliparity, multiple gestation, molar pregnancy, preexisting hypertension or renal disease, previous severe preeclampsia–eclampsia and nonimmune hydrops fetalis. Patients with any of these risk factors should have close observation for weight gain, edema and elevation in blood pressure, and frequent prenatal visits.

The clinical course prior to the development of eclampsia is most commonly characterized by a prolonged and gradual process beginning with the development of preeclampsia. Although hypertension is the hallmark for the diagnosis of eclampsia, it does not necessarily have to exist in the severe range (more than 160 mmHg systolic and/or more than 110 mmHg diastolic). Indeed, relative hypertension (120–140/80–90 mmHg) has been reported in about 20% of eclamptic patients (Sibai *et al.* 1983). Furthermore, although the diagnosis of eclampsia is usually associated with significant proteinuria (more than 2+ on dip stick), 20% of eclamptic patients do not have proteinuria (Sibai *et al.*, 1983). Symptoms prior to an eclamptic convulsion vary, but headache (83%) and visual disturbances (44%) are the most commonly noted (Sibai *et al.*, 1981).

The most common cause of convulsions developing in association with hypertension and proteinuria during pregnancy is eclampsia. Rarely, other etiologies producing convulsions in pregnancy may mimic eclampsia. The differential diagnosis for eclampsia is summarized in Table 15.10. These diagnoses are especially important in 'atypical' eclampsia, where convulsions occur prior to the 20th week of gestation or more than 48 h after delivery.

Eclamptic convulsions constitute a life-threatening emergency. The basic principles in the management of eclampsia involve the following measures:

Table 15.10   Differential diagnosis of eclampsia

**Cerebrovascular accidents**
- Intracerebral hemorrhage
- Cerebral venous thrombosis
- Cerebral arterial occlusion
- Cerebral arterial embolism
- Arteriovenous malformation
- Ruptured berry aneurysm

**Space-occupying central nervous system lesions**
- Brain tumor
- Brain abscess

**Hypertensive disease**
- Hypertensive encephalopathy
- Pheochromocytoma

**Epilepsy**

**Metabolic disease**
- Hypoglycemia
- Hypocalcemia
- Water intoxication

**Infectious disease**
- Meningitis
- Encephalitis

**Thrombotic thrombocytopenic purpura**

1. support of cardiorespiratory function;
2. control of convulsions and prevention of recurrent convulsions;
3. correction of maternal hypoxemia and acidemia;
4. control of severe hypertension;
5. control of increased intracranial pressure;
6. initiation of the process for delivery.

### 15.7.1 CARDIORESPIRATORY STATUS

During an eclamptic seizure, the first action is to assess and establish airway patency and ensure maternal oxygenation. The head is lowered and turned to one side to maintain an open airway and prevent aspiration. If possible, a padded tongue blade should be carefully inserted to prevent tongue injury. The tongue blade should not be forced to the back of the throat as this can result in stimulation of the gag reflex, vomiting and possible aspiration. Suction should be used as needed and the patient should be protected from injury by making sure the bed side-rails are elevated and padded. Oxygen should be administered to improve maternal oxygen concentration and increase oxygen delivery to the fetus, compromised as a result of the convulsion. Most eclamptic convulsions resolve in 60–90 s. The patient will be lethargic initially but should begin respirations that are most commonly rapid and deep.

### 15.7.2 PHARMACOLOGICAL ANTICONVULSANT THERAPY

Eclampsia is frightening. The natural tendency for those caring for an eclamptic patient is to provide therapy to immediately abolish the seizure activity. This philosophy is not only unwise, it is potentially dangerous to the patient. Although medications such as diazepam will stop or shorten a convulsion, they can produce apnea or cardiac arrest or both (Oradell, 1990). Parenteral magnesium sulfate ($MgSO_4.7 H_2O$, USP) does not cause any significant maternal or neonatal central nervous system depression when used properly and is the drug of choice to treat and prevent convulsions in the USA (Sibai, 1990). Magnesium causes relaxation of smooth muscle by competing with calcium for entry into cells at the time of cellular depolarization. The exact mechanism of action of the magnesium ion in the control of eclamptic convulsions is unknown. However, it is speculated that it works as an anticonvulsant by causing central nervous system depression and suppressing neuronal activity. Its efficacy in the prevention and control of eclamptic convulsions has been well documented over the past 80 years. During its administration, the mother is awake and alert with intact laryngeal reflexes, which helps to protect against aspiration.

Currently, the most commonly used regimens of magnesium sulfate administration (Table 15.11) are the standard intramuscular regimen of Pritchard, Cunningham and Pritchard (1984) and the intravenous regimen of Zuspan (1978).

**Table 15.11** Specific magnesium sulfate regimens to treat eclamptic convulsions

---

**Pritchard, Cunningham and Pritchard, 1984**
Loading dose: 4 g IV over 3–5 min and 10 g IM
Maintenance dose: 5 g IM every 4 h

**Zuspan, 1978**
Loading dose: 4 g IV over 5–10 min
Maintenance dose: 1–2 g/h IV

**Sibai, 1986**
Loading dose: 6 g IV over 20 min
Maintenance dose: 2–3 g/h IV

---

Both of these regimens are reported to be clinically safe and effective. In addition, a modified intravenous regimen has been introduced by Sibai (1986). In that report, the author describes the various clinical regimens in use, mechanism of action of the drug, serum magnesium levels achieved with the various regimens, effects on labor, maternal–fetal–neonatal side-effects and toxicity (Sibai, 1986).

In many centers outside the USA, eclampsia is treated similarly to status epilepticus, using such drugs as diazepam, chloromethiazole and phenytoin. In the UK and Australia, the usual approach is to administer intravenous diazepam (10 mg) to terminate a convulsion. Following a convulsion, the most common practice is to give a loading dose of phenytoin 10 mg/kg intravenously over 15–20 min. Slater *et al.* (1987) evaluated a regimen of phenytoin based on maternal weight in 26 patients (seven had severe preeclampsia, 17 had mild disease and two had eclampsia). They reported no seizures after the initiation of phenytoin (750–1250 mg intravenously at a rate of up to 25 mg/min), and they noted no major maternal or neonatal side-effects. Moosa and El-Zayat (1987) used phenytoin 100 mg three times a day in 50 preeclamptic women and compared the pregnancy outcome to that in another 50 patients who received similar management except for not receiving phenytoin. They suggested that phenytoin had a favorable effect on maternal blood pressure and fluid balance in addition to its anticonvulsant effects. On the other hand, Tufnell *et al.* (1989) reported that three (17%) of 18 preeclamptic–eclamptic women developed a further convulsion after the administration of the recommended dose. A similar experience was also reported by Slater *et al.* (1989) in their subsequent report, in which two (25%) of eight eclamptic patients developed another seizure following the initiation of the phenytoin infusion.

Friedman and associates (1993) reported a prospective, randomized clinical trial comparing a standardized regimen of intravenous phenytoin ($n = 45$) to intravenous magnesium sulfate ($n = 60$) as seizure prophylaxis in preeclampsia–eclampsia. No seizures occurred in preeclamptic patients who received either drug, but subsequent convulsions developed in the two eclamptic patients assigned to the phenytoin group. The authors noted lower maternal side-effects, shorter duration of active phase of labor and lower amount of estimated blood loss at vaginal delivery in the phenytoin group. There are two randomized studies comparing the use of magnesium sulfate to phenytoin or diazepam in eclampsia. Dommisse (1990) reported on 22 patients with eclampsia who were randomly allocated to receive intravenous phenytoin or intravenous magnesium sulfate. None of 11 patients managed with magnesium sulfate had further convulsions, while four of 11 patients treated with phenytoin had further convulsions. All four patients that failed phenytoin therapy subsequently were effectively treated with magnesium sulfate and the author suggested that magnesium sulfate is a more effective agent in eclampsia. Crowther (1990), in a randomized controlled trial, compared the use of magnesium sulfate with diazepam as an anticonvulsant in 51 eclamptic patients. She noted that the use of magnesium sulfate was associated with less serious morbidity but the difference was not statistically significant. A further large randomized controlled trial of many thousands of patients with eclampsia has demonstrated that magnesium sulfate is superior to both diazepam and phenytoin (Duley *et al.*, 1995). This confirms the review of the literature by Sibai (1990a). There can now no doubt that magnesium sulfate is the ideal anticonvulsant in preeclampsia–eclampsia and should be widely accepted throughout the world (Chapter 14).

At the University of Tennessee at Memphis, a standardized treatment protocol has been established for all women with preeclampsia–eclampsia. Patients receive an intravenous loading dose of 6 g of magnesium sulfate

($MgSO_4.7 H_2O$) prepared as 6 g diluted in 150 ml $D_5W$ administered by infusion pump over 20–30 min. Magnesium sulfate is available as a 50% solution, containing 1 g ($MgSO_4.7 H_2O$) per 2 ml. The medication is usually supplied in 10 ml (5 g) vials or ampoules. If the patient develops recurrent convulsions after the initial infusion of magnesium sulfate, then a further dose of 2–4 g can be infused over 5–10 min. A more rapid infusion or administration of magnesium sulfate by an intravenous push should be avoided because of the risk of magnesium toxicity, including respiratory arrest. If convulsions recur, a short-acting barbiturate such as sodium amobarbital should be given in an intravenous dose of up to 250 mg over 3 min. Upon completion of the magnesium loading infusion, a maintenance infusion of 2 g per hour (40 g magnesium sulfate in 1000 ml $D_5$ Ringer's lactate) is infused at 50 ml per hour. It is essential that magnesium sulfate be administered slowly to avoid toxic levels and maternal morbidity.

The infusion rate of magnesium sulfate should be adjusted on the basis of serial serum magnesium levels and physical exam. Maternal serum magnesium levels in a range from 4–8 mg/dl are considered therapeutic. The first sign of magnesium toxicity is loss of patellar reflexes which occurs at serum magnesium levels of 10–12 mg/dl. Hence, any order for administration of the drug should include checking patellar reflexes before continuing the maintenance dose. Other early signs and symptoms of magnesium toxicity include nausea, a feeling of warmth, flushing, slurred speech and somnolence, which occur at serum levels of 9–12 mg/dl. Table 15.12 outlines more severe side-effects associated with increased maternal serum levels of magnesium.

Patients receiving magnesium sulfate therapy require monitoring for evidence of drug toxicity. Magnesium is excreted by the kidneys and renal dysfunction may cause toxic accumulation. Magnesium toxicity can be avoided by:

**Table 15.12** Clinical findings associated with increasing maternal serum levels of magnesium

| Serum magnesium level (mg/dl) | Clinical findings |
|---|---|
| 1.5–2.5 | Normal pregnancy level |
| 4–8 | Therapeutic range for seizure prophylaxis |
| 9–12 | Loss of patellar reflex |
| 15–17 | Muscular paralysis, respiratory arrest |
| 30–35 | Cardiac arrest |

1. confirming adequate renal function with hourly urinary output assessment;
2. serial evaluation for presence of patellar deep tendon reflexes;
3. close observation of respiratory rate;
4. monitoring serial serum magnesium levels.

If magnesium toxicity is suspected, the physician is notified, the magnesium infusion should be discontinued immediately, supplemental oxygen should be administered and a serum magnesium level should be assessed. If magnesium toxicity is recognized, 10 ml of 10% calcium gluconate is administered (1 g total) as a slow intravenous push. Calcium competitively inhibits magnesium at the neuromuscular junction, but its effect is only short-term. Symptoms of magnesium toxicity can recur following calcium gluconate if the magnesium level remains elevated. If respiratory arrest is identified, prompt resuscitation measures, including intubation and assisted ventilation, are indicated (Bohman and Cotton, 1990). The items described in Table 15.13 should be readily available or at the bedside, if hospital policies allow. Oxygen and suction should be present at the bedside and assured to be in working order.

### 15.7.3 MATERNAL METABOLIC STATUS

Maternal hypoxemia and/or acidemia may result from repeated convulsions, respiratory depression from the use of multiple anticonvulsant agents, aspiration or a combination of these factors. Supplemental oxygen may be administered by face mask or face mask with an oxygen reservoir at 8–10 l/min. At 10 l/min, the oxygen concentration delivered approaches 100%, using a face mask with an oxygen reservoir. Maternal oxygenation can be monitored non-invasively by transcutaneous pulse oximetry while acid–base status may be assessed by arterial blood gas analysis. Correction of hypoxemia and acidemia is a necessary step prior to administration of anesthetic drugs or anticonvulsant drugs with

**Table 15.13** Emergency supplies to be available or kept at the bedside of patients receiving magnesium sulfate

- Padded tongue blade
- Medium plastic oral airway
- Ambu bag with mask
- 10 ml ampoules of 10% calcium gluconate
- 10 ml vial of 50% magnesium sulfate
- Several 10 ml syringes with 18–20 gauge needles
- Suction (wall or portable) with suction catheter and tubing
- Oxygen supply (cylinder or piped wall oxygen) and connecting tubing

potential myocardial depressant effects. Normalization of maternal metabolic status reduces the likelihood of toxic side-effects. Pharmacological buffers such as sodium bicarbonate are rarely needed and should be administered only as directed by arterial blood gas analysis.

### 15.7.4 ANTIHYPERTENSIVE THERAPY

Following control of convulsions and adequate maternal oxygenation, the next step in management should involve maintenance of maternal blood pressure within a reasonable safe range (systolic blood pressure below 160 mmHg and/or diastolic pressure below 110 mmHg). The objective of treating severe hypertension is to prevent maternal cerebrovascular accidents and congestive heart failure without compromising cerebral perfusion or jeopardizing uteroplacental blood flow, already reduced in eclampsia.

Although the underlying causative factors are not completely delineated, hypertension in preeclampsia is clearly a consequence of a generalized arterial vasoconstriction. Desirable antihypertensive agent properties for use in hypertensive emergencies in pregnancy include a rapid onset of action following administration and short duration of action in the event of overtitration. Severe elevations in blood pressure associated with preeclampsia–eclampsia constitute a hypertensive emergency. Profound rapid reductions in blood pressure are not desirable because of the need to maintain adequate uteroplacental blood flow. Continuous fetal monitoring should therefore be employed during antihypertensive medication titration to assess fetal well being. Further, the therapy goal is not the return of normal blood pressure but rather reduction of blood pressure to a level associated with a decreased risk of cerebral vascular accidents or loss of cerebral autoregulation.

Autoregulation of the cerebral circulation is a mechanism for the maintenance of constant cerebral blood flow during changes in blood pressure, and may be altered in preeclampsia–eclampsia. Through active changes in cerebrovascular resistance at the arteriolar level, cerebral blood flow normally remains relatively constant when cerebral perfusion pressure ranges between 60 and 120 mmHg (Strandgaard, 1978). In this normal range, vasodilatation of cerebral vessels occurs in response to elevations in blood pressure while vasoconstriction occurs as blood pressure is lowered. Once cerebral perfusion pressure exceeds 130–150 mmHg, however, the autoregulatory mechanism fails. In extreme hypertension, the normal compensatory vasoconstriction may become defective and cerebral blood flow increases. As a result, segments of the vessels become dilated, ischemic and increasingly permeable. Thus, exudation of plasma occurs, giving rise to focal cerebral edema and compression of vessels resulting in a decreased cerebral blood flow. Hypertensive encephalopathy (a possible model for eclampsia) is an acute clinical condition that results from abrupt severe hypertension and subsequent severe increases in intracranial pressure (ICP). Management of increased intracranial pressure will be discussed later in this chapter.

The three parenteral agents labetalol, hydralazine and sodium nitroprusside are currently the most widely used antihypertensive agents for acute reductions of elevated blood pressure related to preeclampsia. Labetalol, a competitive antagonist at both postsynaptic alpha-1- and beta-adrenergic receptors, lowers arterial pressure by reducing systemic vascular resistance. Recent research indicates that it may also have a beta-2-receptor-stimulation-mediated vasodilatory action. Available in oral and intravenous form, parenteral labetalol has a rapid onset of action and produces a smooth reduction in blood pressure with rare overshoot hypotension. It is, however, contraindicated in patients with a greater than first-degree heart block. Mabie *et al.* (1987) compared bolus labetalol to bolus hydralazine in a randomized trial involving 60 peripartum patients. Hydralazine lowered mean arterial pressure more than did labetalol (33.3 ± 13.2 *versus* 25.5 ± 11.2 mmHg, mean ± s.d.), but labetalol had a more rapid onset of action. There was considerable interpatient variability in the dosage of labetalol required to control blood pressure. The duration of antihypertensive action also varied in the labetalol group, with the shortest duration occurring in those patients who required the highest dosage for blood pressure control. No fetal or neonatal problems ascribable to drug treatment were noted in the 13 instances in which labetalol was given before delivery. However, fetal distress due to overshoot hypotension occurred in two of the six cases involving antenatal hydralazine.

Hydralazine is a direct arteriolar vasodilator which causes a secondary baroreceptor-mediated sympathetic discharge resulting in tachycardia and increased cardiac output. Introduced in 1951, it is a safe and dependable agent for the control of hypertension in preeclampsia. Intravenous hydralazine has an onset of action in 10–20 min with a peak effect in 60 min and a duration of action of 4–6 h. Its long duration of action, therefore, makes it poorly suited for use in a continuous infusion. The drug should be administered in intermittent bolus injections with an initial dose of 5 mg. Blood pressure should then be recorded every 5 min. If an inadequate reduction in blood pressure is present 20–30 min following the initial dose, then a repeat dose or one increased to 10 mg in increments every 20–30 min should be given.

Sodium nitroprusside is an extremely effective agent for the emergent treatment of patients in hypertensive crises. Because of its immediate onset of action and very short duration of action (1–10 min), it must be given as a continuous intravenous infusion. Pharmacologically, it relaxes both arteriolar and venous smooth muscles equally by interfering with both influx and the intracellular activation of calcium. It is hepatically metabo-

lized and renally excreted. As preeclamptic patients have a propensity for depleted intravascular volume, they are especially sensitive to its effects. The initial infusion dose should therefore be 0.2 μg/kg/min rather than 0.5 μg/kg/min as is standard in non-pregnant patients. Cyanide and thiocyanate are both metabolic products of sodium nitroprusside metabolism. Thiocyanate toxicity, manifested as tinnitus delirium or blurred vision, should be monitored. Further, although cyanide intoxication is rare, it can be of particular concern in the neonate in patients treated intrapartum.

Two oral agents, nifedipine and captopril, have recently been successfully employed for the emergent reduction of severe hypertension. The calcium channel antagonist nifedipine (a dihydropyridine derivative), has potent peripheral arterial vasodilating properties. Extensive reviews (Houston, 1987) indicate that single-dose nifedipine is associated with a 25% reduction in systolic blood pressure, diastolic blood pressure and mean arterial pressure in 98% of cases. Given sublingually, 10 mg of nifedipine has an onset of action within 3 min with a peak effect within 1 h (Angeli *et al.*, 1991). Captopril, a competitive inhibitor of angiotensin I converting enzyme, has also been shown to produce a rapid reduction of blood pressure. Given sublingually, 25 mg of captopril has an onset of action within 5 min with a hypotensive effect lasting an average of 4 h (Angeli *et al.*, 1991). Because of reports of adverse effects on fetal renal perfusion, this drug should be reserved for use in postpartum patients.

## 15.7.5 INCREASED INTRACRANIAL PRESSURE

Increased intracranial pressure (ICP) is a severe complication of eclampsia and should be considered in patients who remain persistently comatose following their seizure or those with oval pupils or papilledema. If increased ICP is suspected, cranial computed tomography is indicated to assess for intracranial hematoma, tumors or cerebral contusions. If an intracranial hematoma is detected, then neurosurgical consultation is mandatory to determine if immediate surgery or conservative management is indicated.

Once increased ICP is suspected, then direct measurement of ICP with a subarachnoid monitor, epidural monitor, intraparenchymal fiberoptic transducer or through an intraventricular catheter is indicated. The intraventricular catheter offers the advantage of serving as a port for withdrawal of cerebrospinal fluid (CSF). If increased ICP is confirmed, then immediate treatment is warranted. Because of the occurrence of tissue ischemia noted with ICP above 40 mmHg, treatment is recommended at ICP above 20 mmHg. A suggested treatment protocol includes:

1. elevation of the head of the bed (30–45°) to improve venous drainage
2. intubation and hyperventilation to reduce the arterial $P\text{CO}_2$ (target $P_a\text{CO}_2$ of 3.3–4 kPa);
3. correction of hyponatremia or hypo-osmolality, if present;
4. administration of osmotic or loop diuretics;
5. withdrawal of CSF, if an intraventricular catheter is used.

Hyperventilation producing hypocapnia causes cerebral vasoconstriction. This vasoconstriction leads to a reduction of cerebral blood volume and secondarily a lowered ICP. Hypocapnia may also promote reduction in CSF formation. Hyponatremia and hypo-osmolality would result in movement of water into the cerebral extravascular space. Careful monitoring of electrolytes and judicious use of appropriate intravenous fluids will avoid these conditions exacerbating increased ICP.

### 15.7.6 DELIVERY MANAGEMENT

All eclamptic patients should undergo continuous cardiac monitoring and transcutaneous pulse oximetry, and have an indwelling urinary catheter with a urimeter inserted to assist in accurate fluid management. The fluid intake and output should be monitored very closely during labor and delivery as eclamptic patients are at increased risk of pulmonary edema from fluid overload and compromised renal function (Sibai *et al.*, 1987) Ideally, all intravenous lines are placed on pumps to assure accurate delivery of fluids or medications. Parenteral magnesium sulfate should be continued throughout labor and delivery and for at least 24 h postpartum. If the patient has oliguria (less than 100 ml/4 h), the rate of both fluid administration and dose of magnesium sulfate should be reduced. The patient should be placed in the left lateral decubitus position to maximize uterine blood flow and venous return. The patient's blood pressure, urine output, proteinuria and edema are continually assessed, documented and reported appropriately (Gilbert and Harmon, 1986). Specially designed preeclampsia–eclampsia nursing flowsheets for these patients are beneficial. It is advisable that all such patients, especially those less than 36 weeks gestation should be managed at tertiary care centers.

For patients with eclampsia, uterine hyperactivity (increased frequency and tone) and fetal heart rate changes usually appear during and after an eclamptic convulsion. These changes are usually transient, lasting from 3–15 min. Such changes may include fetal bradycardia, transient late decelerations, decreased beat-to-beat variability and compensatory tachycardia (Boehm and Growdon, 1974). Most of these changes will resolve spontaneously following the termination of convulsions and/or the correction of maternal hypoxemia and acidosis. The patient should not be rushed for an emergency cesarean section based on these findings, especially if the maternal condition has not been stabilized. Such an approach might prove detrimental to both mother and neonate. If the above changes persist despite corrective measures, the presence of abruptio placentae or fetal distress should be considered, especially in the preterm or growth-retarded fetus.

Because evacuation of the uterus is the definitive treatment of preeclampsia–eclampsia, patients are evaluated for delivery once stabilized. Vaginal delivery, unless obstetrically contraindicated, is the preferred method of delivery. An oxytocin infusion for induction or augmentation of labor may be administered simultaneously with the magnesium sulfate infusion. Total fluid intake is limited to 100 ml per hour. The protocol for oxytocin infusion for preeclampsia–eclampsia is the same as for routine patients yet, due to fluid restrictions, oxytocin may need to be more concentrated and dosages per minute to be adjusted accordingly. Continuous fetal monitoring should be employed.

Maternal analgesia can be provided by the intermittent use of small doses (25–50 mg) of intravenous meperidine. Local infiltration anesthesia with pudendal block may be used in most cases of vaginal delivery; a balanced general anesthesia can be used for abdominal deliveries, but probably the anesthesia of choice is epidural. There has been controversy regarding the use of epidural analgesia–anesthesia, with some authors against its use because of the potential maternal hypotension and reduced uteroplacental blood flow (Lindheimer and Katz, 1985), but other authors reported no adverse maternal or fetal outcome when epidural analgesia was used in such patients (Abboud *et al.*, 1980). This subject was recently reviewed by Jones and Joyce (1987). It must be emphasized that the use of epidural analgesia in such patients requires the availability of central hemodynamic monitoring and personnel with special expertise in obstetrical anesthesia.

At delivery, neonatal side-effects of maternal administration of magnesium sulfate include hypotension, hypotonia, respiratory depression, lethargy and decreased suck reflex. The pediatrician and newborn nursery should be informed of patients receiving magnesium sulfate. Calcium gluconate may also be administered to the newborn if magnesium toxicity is suspected.

Following delivery, the patient should be monitored in the recovery room or intensive care unit under close observation for a minimum of 24 hours. During this time, magnesium sulfate should be continued and maternal vital signs and intake-output should be monitored hourly. Some of these patients may require intensive and invasive hemodynamic monitoring as they are at increased risk for the development of pulmonary edema from fluid overload, fluid mobilization and compromised renal function (Sibai *et al.*, 1987). Magnesium sulfate administration should continue until improvements in blood pressure, urine output and sensorium are noted.

In a review of 704 cases of eclampsia from Mexico, Lopez-Llera (1982) reported that 17% of cases occurred after delivery. Some of the postpartum cases occurred as much as 2 weeks after delivery. Similarly, 25 (25%) of the 71 cases of eclampsia reported by Moller and Lindmark (1986) occurred in the postpartum period (19 occurred within 12 h). Late-onset postpartum eclampsia is defined as convulsions occurring more than 48 h after delivery in patients with signs and symptoms of preeclampsia. In a review of the literature through 1979, Sibai *et al.* (1980) found more than 50 cases of postpartum eclampsia developing between 3 and 23 days after delivery. Extensive neurological evaluation in such patients to rule out the presence of other cerebral pathology is indicated. If eclampsia is confirmed, then management is as previously noted for antepartum convulsions. More vigorous control of blood pressure is possible, however, since there is no longer concern about compromising the uteroplacental circulation in the postpartum patient. Further, magnesium sulfate therapy should be continued for 24–48 h from seizure onset.

## 15.8 HELLP SYNDROME

Hemolysis, abnormal liver function tests and thrombocytopenia have been recognized as complications of preeclampsia–eclampsia for many years (Chesley, 1978; Goodlin, 1982; McKay, 1972). In 1982, Weinstein described 29 cases of severe preeclampsia–eclampsia complicated by thrombocytopenia, abnormal peripheral smear and abnormal liver function tests. He suggested that this collection of signs and symptoms constituted an entity separate from severe preeclampsia and coined the term HELLP syndrome: H for hemolysis, EL for elevated liver enzymes and LP for low platelets. The presence of this syndrome has become a major cause of litigation against obstetricians involving cases of alleged misdiagnosed preeclampsia. The remainder of this chapter will review the diagnosis and current management recommendations for pregnancies complicated by HELLP syndrome.

### 15.8.1 TERMINOLOGY AND DIAGNOSIS

This syndrome has been recognized as a complication of severe preeclampsia–eclampsia for many years. A review of the literature by Sibai *et al.* (1986) revealed considerable differences concerning the terminology, incidence, cause, diagnosis and management of this syndrome. The reported incidence ranges from 2–12%, reflecting the different diagnostic criteria and methods used in studies describing this syndrome. In addition, there are considerable differences regarding its time of onset and the type and degree of laboratory abnormalities used to make the diagnosis. Evidence of hemolysis was documented in few studies and the definition of thrombocytopenia ranged from $< 75\,000/mm^3$ to $< 150\,000/mm^3$. Moreover, there is no consensus in the literature regarding which liver function test abnormalities should be used to diagnose the HELLP syndrome. Many authors now advocate that lactic dehydrogenase (LDH) and bilirubin values should be included in the diagnosis of hemolysis. In addition, the degree of liver enzyme abnormality should be defined as a certain number of standard deviations from the normal values for each hospital. At our institution, we use a cutoff value of more than 3 s.d. above the mean to indicate abnormality. Our criteria for the diagnosis of the HELLP syndrome include the following laboratory findings, summarized in Table 15.14.

### 15.8.2 CLINICAL PRESENTATION

The incidence of severe preeclampsia–eclampsia complicated by hemolysis, low platelets and elevated liver enzymes has been reported to range from 2–12%. In the series reported by Sibai *et al.* (1986), patients with

---

**Table 15.14**   University of Tennessee, Memphis, criteria for HELLP syndrome

**Hemolysis**
- Abnormal peripheral smear
- Total bilirubin $> 1.2\,mg/dl$
- Lactic dehydrogenase (LDH) $> 600\,U/l$

**Elevated liver functions**
- Serum aspartate aminotransferase (AST) $> 70\,U/l$
- Lactic dehydrogenase (LDH) $> 600\,U/l$

**Low platelets**
- Platelet count $< 100\,000/mm^3$

HELLP syndrome were significantly older (mean age of 25 years) than patients with severe preeclampsia–eclampsia without features of HELLP syndrome (mean age of 19 years). The incidence of the syndrome was significantly higher among the white population and multiparous patients. Coincidentally, medical complications (notably diabetes and lupus nephritis) were no more common among the patients with HELLP syndrome. Other authors have made similar observations (MacKenna, Dover and Brame, 1983; Thiagarajah *et al.*, 1984; Weinstein, 1985)

Patients with HELLP syndrome may present with a variety of signs and symptoms – none of which are diagnostic and all of which may be found in patients with severe preeclampsia–eclampsia without HELLP syndrome. Sibai (1990b) noted that the patient usually presents remote from term complaining of epigastric or right upper quadrant pain (90%) some will have nausea or vomiting (50%) and others will have non-specific viral-syndrome-like symptoms. The majority of patients (90%) will give a history of malaise for the few days prior to presentation. In Weinstein's reports, nausea and/or vomiting and epigastric pain were the most common symptoms. Right upper quadrant or epigastric pain is thought to result from obstruction to blood flow in the hepatic sinusoids, which are blocked by intravascular fibrin deposition.

Patients with HELLP syndrome usually demonstrate significant weight gain with generalized edema. It is important to appreciate that severe hypertension (systolic blood pressure $\geq$ 160 mmHg, diastolic blood pressure $\geq$ 110 mmHg) is not a constant finding in HELLP syndrome. Although 66% of the 112 patients studied by Sibai *et al.* (1986) had a diastolic blood pressure of 110 mmHg or more, 14.5% had a diastolic blood pressure of less than 90 mmHg. In Weinstein's (1952) initial report of 29 patients, less than half (13) had an admission blood pressure equal to or more than 160/110 mmHg. Thus, these patients may present with a variety of signs and symptoms, none of which are diagnostic

of severe preeclampsia. As a result, they are often misdiagnosed as having various medical and surgical disorders, including appendicitis, gastroenteritis, glomerulonephritis, pyelonephritis and viral hepatitis.

Acute fatty liver of pregnancy (AFLP) is a rare but potentially fatal complication of the third trimester of pregnancy. In its early presentation, AFLP may be difficult to differentiate from HELLP syndrome. Patients with AFLP typically present with nausea, vomiting, abdominal pain and jaundice. HELLP syndrome and AFLP are both characterized by elevated liver function tests, but the abnormalities tend to be greater in HELLP syndrome. Further, prothrombin time and partial thromboplastin time are usually prolonged in AFLP while normal in HELLP syndrome. Table 15.15 details laboratory differentiation of AFLP from HELLP syndrome.

Microscopic examination of the liver is the definitive diagnostic test for determining AFLP. Diffuse low-grade panlobular microvesicular fatty change (steatosis) is pathognomonic for AFLP. The management of AFLP includes immediate delivery with correction of hypoglycemia or coagulopathy, if present.

### 15.8.3 HELLP MANAGEMENT

Patients with HELLP syndrome who are remote from term should be referred to a tertiary care center and initial management should be as for any patient with severe preeclampsia. The first priority is to assess and stabilize the maternal condition, particularly coagulation abnormalities (Table 15.16).

The next step is to evaluate fetal wellbeing using the non-stress test or biophysical profile, as well as ultrasonographic biometry for assessment of possible intrauterine growth retardation. Finally, a decision must be made as to whether immediate delivery is indicated. Amniocentesis may be performed in these patients without risk of bleeding complications.

A review of the literature highlights the confusion surrounding the management of

**Table 15.15**    Laboratory differentiation of AFLP and HELLP syndrome

|  | *AFLP* | *HELLP* |
|---|---|---|
| **Serum chemistries** |  |  |
| Glucose | Low | Normal |
| Uric acid | High | High |
| Creatinine | High | High |
| Ammonia | High | Normal |
|  |  |  |
| **Hematological** |  |  |
| Platelet count | Low or normal | Low |
| Fibrinogen | Low | Normal to increased |
| Prothrombin time (PT) | Prolonged | Normal |
| Partial thromboplastin time (PTT) | Prolonged | Normal |

this syndrome (Sibai, 1990b) Some authors consider its presence to be an indication for immediate delivery by cesarean section, while other recommend a more conservative approach to prolong pregnancy in cases of fetal immaturity. Consequently, there are several therapeutic modalities described in the literature to treat or reverse the HELLP syndrome. Most of these therapeutic modalities are similar to those used in the management of severe preeclampsia remote from term.

If the syndrome develops at or beyond 34 weeks gestation, or if there is evidence of fetal lung maturity or fetal or maternal jeopardy before that time, then delivery is the definitive therapy. Without laboratory evidence of DIC and absent fetal lung maturity, the patient can be given two doses of steroids to accelerate fetal lung maturity and then delivered 48 h later. However, maternal and fetal conditions should be assessed continuously during this period.

---

**Table 15.16**    Management outline of antepartum HELLP syndrome at less than 35 weeks gestation (stabilization of maternal condition and delivery is recommended for patients at 35 weeks gestation or more, with documentation of HELLP syndrome)

1. **Assess and stabilize maternal condition:**
   (a) If DIC present, correct coagulopathy
   (b) Antiseizure prophylaxis with magnesium sulfate
   (c) Treatment of severe hypertension
   (d) Transfer to tertiary care center if appropriate
   (e) Computed tomography or ultrasound of the abdomen if subcapsular hematoma of the liver is suspected

2. **Evaluate fetal wellbeing**
   (a) Non-stress testing
   (b) Biophysical profile
   (c) Ultrasonographic biometry

3. **Evaluate fetal lung maturity if less than 35 weeks gestation**
   (a) If mature expedite delivery
   (b) If immature give steroids, then deliver

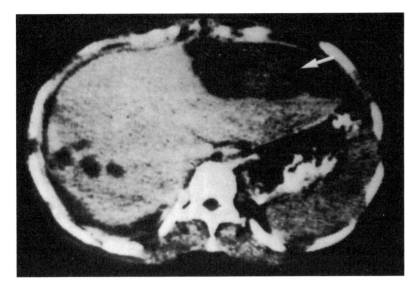

**Figure 15.1** A computed axial tomographic scan of the liver in a patient who had HELLP syndrome at 23 weeks gestation. Subcapsular hematoma of the liver (large white arrow heads) with rupture (small white arrow heads) and intraparenchymal hemorrhage (black arrow heads). (Source: reproduced with permission from Sibai, 1990b.)

The presence of this syndrome is not an indication for immediate delivery by cesarean section. Such an approach might prove detrimental to both mother and fetus. Patients presenting with well-established labor should be allowed to deliver vaginally in the absence of obstetric contraindications. Otherwise, labor may be initiated with oxytocin infusions as for routine induction in all patients with gestational age of more than 32 weeks, irrespective of the extent of cervical dilatation or effacement. A similar approach is used for patients at less than 32 weeks if the cervix is favorable for induction. In patients with an unripe cervix and gestational age less than 32 weeks, elective cesarean section is the method of choice for delivery. A management protocol for the HELLP patient requiring cesarean delivery is presented in Table 15.17.

Maternal analgesia during labor can be provided by intermittent use of small doses (25–50 mg) of intravenous meperidine. Local infiltration anesthesia can be used for all vaginal deliveries. The use of pudendal block or epidural anesthesia is contraindicated in these patients because of the risk of bleeding into these areas. General anesthesia is the method of choice for cesarean sections.

Patients presenting with shoulder pain, in shock or with evidence of massive ascites or pleural effusions should have ultrasound or computed axial tomography of the liver to rule out the presence of subcapsular hematoma of the liver (Figure 15.1).

---

**Table 15.17** Management of HELLP syndrome in a patient requiring cesarean section for delivery

- General anesthesia
- 10 units of platelets prior to surgery if platelet count less than 50 000/mm$^3$
- Leave vesicouterine peritoneum (bladder flap) open
- Subfascial drain
- Secondary closure of skin incision or subcutaneous drain
- Postoperative transfusions as needed
- Intensive monitoring for 48 h postpartum

Rupture of a subcapsular hematoma of the liver is a life-threatening complication of HELLP syndrome. In most instances, rupture involves the right lobe and is preceded by the development of a parenchymal hematoma. The condition usually presents with severe epigastric pain that may persist for several hours prior to circulatory collapse. Patients frequently present with shoulder pain, in shock or with evidence of massive ascites, respiratory difficulty or pleural effusions, and often with a dead fetus.

The presence of ruptured subcapsular liver hematoma resulting in shock is a surgical emergency requiring acute multidisciplinary treatment. Resuscitation should consist of massive transfusions of blood, correction of coagulopathy with fresh frozen plasma and platelets, and immediate laparotomy. Options at laparotomy include packing and draining (preferred), surgical ligation of the hemorrhaging hepatic segments, embolization of the hepatic artery to the involved liver segment and/or loosely suturing omentum or surgical mesh to the liver to improve integrity. Even with appropriate treatment, maternal and fetal mortality is over 50%. Mortality is most commonly associated with exsanguination and coagulopathy. Initial survivors are at increased risk for developing adult respiratory distress syndrome, pulmonary edema and acute renal failure in the postoperative period.

Surgical repair has been recommended for hepatic hemorrhage without liver rupture. However, more recent experience suggests that this complication can be managed conservatively in patients who remain hemodynamically stable. Management should include close monitoring of hemodynamics and coagulation status. Serial assessment of the subcapsular hematoma with ultrasound or computed tomography is necessary, with immediate intervention for rupture or worsening of maternal status. It is important with conservative management to avoid exogenous sources of trauma to the liver such as abdominal palpation, convulsions, or emesis and to use care in transportation of the patient. Indeed, any sudden increase in intra-abdominal pressure could potentially lead to rupture of the subcapsular hematoma.

Any algorithm for the management of a subcapsular hematoma of the liver in pregnancy must emphasize the potential need for large amounts of blood products and the need for aggressive intervention if rupture of the hematoma is suspected. Our algorithm, employed at the University of Tennessee, Memphis, is presented in Table 15.18.

Our experience is in agreement with the recent observations of Smith *et al.* (1991), in that a stable patient with an unruptured subcapsular hematoma may be managed conservatively. Constant monitoring must continue during this management, however, as patients can rapidly become unstable following rupture of the hematoma. Survival is clearly associated with rapid diagnosis and medical and surgical stabilization. Coagulopathy must be aggressively reversed as failure to do so is associated with an increased incidence of renal failure. In addition, these patients should be managed in an intensive care unit facility with close monitoring of various hemodynamic parameters and fluid states to avoid the potential of pulmonary edema and/or respiratory compromise.

Platelet transfusions are indicated either before or after delivery if the platelet count is less than 20 000/mm³. Correction of thrombocytopenia is particularly important before cesarean section. However, repeated platelet transfusions are not necessary since consumption occurs rapidly and the effect is transient. Our policy is to administer 10 units of platelets in all patients with a platelet count less than 50 000 mm³ prior to intubating the patient for cesarean section. Generalized oozing from the operative site is very common and to minimize the risk of hematoma formation the bladder flap should be left open and a subfascial drain should be used for 24–48 h. The wound may be left open from the level of the fascia or a subcutaneous drain may be

**Table 15.18**   Management of patients with documented subcapsular hematoma of the liver

**General considerations**
1. Have the blood bank aware of the potential need for large amounts of fresh frozen plasma, packed red blood cells and platelet concentrate
2. Consult a general or vascular surgeon
3. Avoid direct and indirect manipulation of the liver
4. Close monitoring of hemodynamic status

**If the hematoma is unruptured**
1. Conservative management with serial computed tomography scans or ultrasound if hemodynamically stable

   or
2. Surgical repair and evaluation

**If the hematoma is ruptured**
1. Massive transfusions
2. Immediate laparotomy
   (a) If bleeding is minimal:
       (i)   Observation
       (ii)  Draining area
   (b) If bleeding is severe:
       (i)   Applying laparotomy sponges as packs for pressure
       (ii)  Surgical ligation of hemorrhaging hepatic segment
       (iii) Embolization of the hepatic artery to the involved liver segment
       (iv)  Loosely suture omentum or surgical mesh to the liver to improve integrity

placed and the skin closed. All wounds that are left open can be successfully closed within 72 h. Failure to adhere to these recommendations will result in about 20% incidence of hematoma formation.

Following delivery, the patient should be monitored very closely in an intensive care facility for at least 48 h. Most patients will show evidence of resolution of the disease process within 48 h after delivery. Some, however (especially those with DIC), may demonstrate delayed resolution or even deterioration. Such patients may require intensive monitoring for several days. These patients are at risk for development of pulmonary edema from transfusions of blood and blood products, fluid mobilization and compromised renal function (Sibai *et al.*, 1987).

HELLP syndrome may also develop in the postpartum period. Sibai noted in a review of 304 patients with HELLP syndrome that 95 (31%) had only postpartum manifestation. In the postpartum group, the time of onset of the manifestations ranges from a few hours to 6 days, with the majority developing within 48 h postpartum. Further, 75 patients (79%) had evidence of preeclampsia prior to delivery. However, 20 patients (21%) had no such evidence either antepartum or intrapartum. Patients in this group are at increased risk for the development of pulmonary edema and acute renal failure (Weinstein, 1985). Management is similar to the antepartum patient with HELLP syndrome – including the need for antiseizure prophylaxis. Hypertension control may be more aggressive, however, since there is no longer concern about compromising the uteroplacental circulation in the postpartum patient. The differential diagnosis in these cases should include thrombotic thrombocytopenic purpura, hemolytic uremic syndrome and exacerbation of systemic lupus.

Patients with delayed resolution of HELLP syndrome (including persistent severe thrombocytopenia) represent a management dilemma. Exchange plasmapheresis with fresh frozen plasma has been advocated as a treatment by some authors (Schwartz, 1986; Martin *et al.*, 1990) Since the majority of these patients will have spontaneous resolution of their disease, however, early initiation of plasmapheresis may result in unnecessary treatment. Schwartz (1986) suggested that serial studies indicating a progressive elevation of bilirubin or creatinine associated with hemolysis and thrombocytopenia be considered an indication for plasmapheresis. Martin *et al.* (1990) reported the use of plasma exchange with fresh-frozen plasma in seven women in the postpartum period with HELLP syndrome that persisted for more than 72 h following delivery. All patients had persistent thrombocytopenia, rising lactic dehydrogenase and evidence of multiorgan dysfunction. Sustained increases in mean platelet count and reduction in LDH concentrations were associated with plasma exchange. The authors recommended that a trial of plasma exchange with fresh-frozen plasma be considered in HELLP syndrome that persists past 72 hours from delivery and in which there is evidence of a life-threatening microangiopathy. Potential adverse effects of this technique include plasma-transmitted infections, volume overload, cardiac arrhythmia and hemorrhage. Ultimately, the question remains of how many patients would spontaneously improve without benefit of plasmapheresis.

## 15.9 SEVERE HYPERTENSION: POSTPARTUM MANAGEMENT

Patients with severe hypertension in pregnancy are at risk for hypertensive encephalopathy, pulmonary edema and renal failure in the postpartum period. These risks are particularly increased in patients with underlying cardiac disease and chronic glomerular renal disease, patients requiring multiple drugs for control of their hypertension, patients with superimposed preeclampsia in the second trimester and those with abruptio placentae complicated by disseminated intravascular coagulopathy. As a result, patients with the above listed complications should receive intensive management for a minimum of 48 h after delivery. In addition, these patients should receive intravenous hydralazine or labetalol for control of severe hypertension as needed. Moreover, diuretic therapy should be used in women who are at risk for delayed onset of postpartum circulatory congestion and pulmonary edema (massively obese older women with long-standing hypertension and those with previous antepartum congestive heart failure).

Occasionally a woman may develop severe hypertension for the first time in the postpartum period (Table 15.19). Management of such women will depend on the etiological factor. It is important to emphasize that preeclampsia may develop as late as 4–6 weeks after delivery.

Oral antihypertensive drugs may be needed for control of maternal blood pressure after delivery. Some women may wish to breast feed their infants while receiving these drugs. Unfortunately, there are limited data concerning the excretion of these drugs into human breast milk, as well as their effects on the infants. In addition, there are no published reports describing the long-term effects of any antihypertensive drug on

---

**Table 15.19**  Severe hypertension postpartum

- Preeclampsia
- Exacerbated chronic hypertension
- Exacerbation of systemic lupus erythematosus
- Drug-induced
  - Methergine
  - Cocaine
  - Bromocriptine?

breast feeding infants exposed to these drugs. In general, most of the published data on the subject have described the milk/plasma ratio after a single measurement of the drug concentration. Moreover, the data in the literature indicate that all studied antihypertensive agents are excreted into human breast milk; however, there are differences among these drugs regarding the milk/plasma ratio. The available data also indicate that there are no short-term adverse effects on the breast feeding infant exposed to methyldopa, hydralazine, nifedipine or beta-blockers. On other hand, thiazide diuretics should be avoided during lactation since their use has been reported to decrease or inhibit the production of milk.

## 15.10 SUMMARY

Prompt hospitalization is the optimum management of all patients with severe preeclampsia. The development of this disease after 34 weeks gestation in an indication for maternal stabilization and delivery. Expectant management is possible, however, for patients remote from term. The success rate of expectant management will depend on both fetal gestational age and the state to which the disease has progressed at the time of hospitalization. Maternal and perinatal complications are significantly increased in patients with severe preeclampsia. Patients with evidence of maternal or fetal compromise, including HELLP syndrome, eclampsia, acute renal failure or severe intrauterine growth retardation, should be treated aggressively regardless of gestational age, primarily with delivery.

## REFERENCES

Abboud, T., Artal, R., Sarkis, F., *et al.* (1980) Sympathoadrenal activity, maternal, fetal and neonatal responses after epidural anesthesia in the preeclamptic patient. *Am. J. Obstet. Gynecol.*, **144**, 915.Angeli, P., Chieza, M., Caregarao, L. *et al.*

(1991) Comparison of sublingual captopril and nifedipine in immediate treatment of hypertensive emergencies. *Arch. Intern. Med.*, **151**, 678–682.

Benedetti, T. J., Kates, R. and Williams, V. (1985) Hemodynamic observations in severe preeclampsia complicated by pulmonary edema. *Am. J. Obstet. Gynecol.*, **152**, 330–334.

Boehm, F. H. and Growdon, J. H. Jr (1974) The effect of eclamptic convulsions on the fetal heart rate. *Am. J. Obstet. Gynecol.*, **120**, 851–852.

Bohman, V. R. and Cotton, D. B. (1990) Supralethal magnesemia with patient survival. *Obstet. Gynecol.*, **76**, 984–986.

Briggs, J. D., Kennedy, A. C., Young, L. N. *et al.* (1967) Renal function after acute tubular necrosis. *Br. Med. J.*, **iii**, 513–516.

Chesley, L. C. Disseminated intravascular coagulation, in *Hypertensive Disorders in Pregnancy*, (ed. L. C. Chesley), Appleton-Century-Crofts, New York, p. 88.

Cotton, D. B., Jones, M. M., Longmire, S. *et al.* (1986) Role of intravenous nitroglycerin in the treatment of severe pregnancy-induced hypertension complicated by pulmonary edema. *Am. J. Obstet. Gynecol.*, **154**, 91–93.

Crowther, C. (1990) Magnesium sulphate versus diazepam in the management of eclampsia: a randomized controlled trial. *Br. J. Obstet. Gynaecol.*, **97**, 110.

Dommisse, J. (1990) Phenytoin sodium and magnesium sulphate in the management of eclampsia. *Br. J. Obstet. Gynaecol.*, **97**, 104.

Duley., L., Carroli, G., Belizan, J. *et al.* (1995) Which anticonvulsant for women with eclampsia – evidence from the collaborative eclampsia trial. *Lancet*, **345**, 1455–1463.

Fenakel, K., Fenakel, E., Appleman, Z. *et al.* (1991) Nifedipine in the treatment of severe preeclampsia. *Obstet. Gynecol.*, **77**, 331–337.

Friedman, S. A., Lim, K. H., Baker, C. A. and Repke, J. T. (1993) Phenytoin versus magnesium sulfate in preeclampsia: a pilot study. *Am. J. Perinatol.*, **10**, 233–238.

Gilbert, E. S. and Harmon, J. S. (1986) *High-Risk Pregnancy and Delivery: Nursing Perspectives*, 1st edn, C. V. Mosby, St Louis, MO.

Goodlin, R. C. (1982) Beware the great imitator – severe preeclampsia. *Contemp. Obstet. Gynecol.*, **20**, 215.

Hankins, G. D. V., Wendel, G. D., Cunningham, F. G. and Leveno, K. J. (1984) Longitudinal evaluation of hemodynamic changes in eclampsia. *Am. J. Obstet. Gynecol.*, **150**, 506–512.

Houston, M. C. (1987) Treatment of severe hypertension and hypertensive crisis with nifedipine. *Clin. Med.*, **146**, 701–704.

Hov, S. (1987) Pregnancy in women requiring dialysis for renal failure. *Am. J. Kidney Dis.*, **9**, 368.

Jones, M. M. and Joyce, T. H. (1987) Anesthesia for the parturient with pregnancy-induced hypertension. *Clin. Obstet. Gynecol.*, **30**, 591–600.

Lindheimer, M. D. and Katz, A. L. (1985) Hypertension in pregnancy. *N. Engl. J. Med.*, **313**, 675.

Long, P. A. and Oats, J. N. (1987) Preeclampsia in twin pregnancy – severity and pathogenesis. *Aust. NZ J. Obstet. Gynaecol.*, **27**, 1.

Lopez-Llera, M. M. (1982) Complicated eclampsia. Fifteen years' experience in a referral medical center. *Am. J. Obstet. Gynecol.*, **142**, 28.

Lopez-Llera, M., De la Luna Olsen, E. and Niz Ramos, J. (1989) Eclampsia in twin pregnancy. *J. Reprod. Med.*, **34**, 802.

Mabie, W. C., Gonzalez, A. R., Sibai, B. M. and Amon, E. (1987) A comparative trial of labetalol and hydralazine in the acute management of severe hypertension complicating pregnancy. *Obstet. Gynecol.*, **70**, 328–333.

Mabie, W. C., Ratts, T. E., Ramanathan, K. B. and Sibai, B. M. (1988) Circulatory congestion in obese hypertensive women: a subset of pulmonary edema in pregnancy. *Obstet. Gynecol.*, **72**, 553–558.

McKay, D. G. (1972) Hematologic evidence of disseminated intravascular coagulation in eclampsia. *Obstet. Gynecol. Surv.*, **27**, 399–417.

MacKenna, J., Dover, N. L. and Brame, R. G. (1983) Preeclampsia associated with hemolysis, elevated liver enzymes, and low platelets-an obstetric emergency? *Obstet. Gynecol.*, **62**, 751–754.

Martin, J. N. Jr, Files, J. C., Black, P. G. *et al.* (1990) Plasma exchange for preeclampsia. I. Postpartum use for persistently severe preeclampsia–eclampsia with HELLP syndrome. *Am. J. Obstet. Gynecol.*, **162**, 126–137.

Oradell, N. J. (1990) Medical economics, in *Physician's Desk Reference*, 45th edn, p. 1874–1875.

Melrose, E. B. (1984) Maternal deaths at King Edward VIII Hospital, Durban. *S. Afr. Med. J.*, **65**, 161–165.

Moller, B. and Lindmark, G. (1986) Eclampsia in Sweden, 1976–1980. *Acta Obstet. Gynecol. Scand.*, **65**, 307.

Moosa, S. M. and El-Zayat, S. G. (1987) Phenytoin infusion in severe pre-eclampsia. *Lancet*, **ii**, 1147.

Odendaal, H. J., Pattinson, R. C., Bam, R. *et al.* (1990) Aggressive or expectant management for patients with severe preeclampsia between 28–34 weeks' gestation: a randomized controlled trial. *Obstet. Gynecol.*, **76**, 1070–1074.

Pattinson, R. C., Odendaal, H. J. and Dutoit, R. (1988) Conservative management of severe proteinuric hypertension before 28 weeks' gestation. *S. Afr. Med. J.*, **73**, 516–518.

Pritchard, J. A., Cunningham, F. G. and Pritchard, S. A. (1984) The Parkland Memorial Hospital protocol for treatment of eclampsia: evaluation of 245 cases. *Am. J. Obstet. Gynecol.*, **148**, 951–963.Richards, A. M., Moodley, J., Graham, D. I. and Bullock, M., R. R. (1986) Active management of the unconscious eclamptic patient. *Br. J. Obstet. Gynaecol.*, **93**, 554.

Riff, D. P., Willson, D. M., Dunea, G. *et al.* (1967) Renocortical necrosis: partial recovery after 49 days of oliguria. *Arch. Intern. Med.*, **119**, 618–621.

Rubin, P. (1987) Hypertension in pregnancy. *J. Hypertens.*, **5**(suppl 3), S57–S60.

Schwartz, M. L. (1986) Possible role for exchange plasmapheresis with fresh frozen plasma for maternal indications in selected cases of preeclampsia and eclampsia. *Obstet. Gynecol.*, **68**, 136–139.

Sibai, B. M. (1986) Magnesium sulfate in preeclampsia–eclampsia. *Contemp. Obstet. Gynecol.*, **29**, 155–170.

Sibai, B. M. (1990a) Magnesium sulfate is the ideal anticonvulsant in preeclampsia–eclampsia. *Am. J. Obstet. Gynecol.*, **162**, 1141–1145.

Sibai, B. M. (1990b) The HELLP syndrome (hemolysis, elevated liver enzymes, and low platelets): much ado about nothing? *Am. J. Obstet. Gynecol.*, **162**, 311–316.

Sibai, B. M., Abdella, T. N. and Taylor, H. A. (1982) Eclampsia in the first half of pregnancy. Report of three cases and review of the literature. *J. Reprod. Med.*, **27**, 11.

Sibai, B. M., Villar, M. A. and Mabie, B. C. (1990) Acute renal failure in hypertensive disorders of pregnancy: pregnancy outcome and remote prognosis in thirty-one consecutive cases. *Am. J. Obstet. Gynecol.*, **162**, 777–783.

Sibai, B. M., Schneider, J. M., Morrison, J. C. *et al.* (1980) The late postpartum eclampsia controversy. *Obstet. Gynecol.*, **55**, 74.

Sibai, B. M., McCubbin, J. H., Anderson, G. D. *et al.* (1981) Eclampsia I. Observations from 67 recent cases. *Obstet. Gynecol.*, **58**, 609.Sibai, B. M., Anderson, D. G., Abdella, T. N. *et al.* (1983) Eclampsia III. Neonatal outcome, growth, and development. *Am. J. Obstet. Gynecol.*, **146**, 307–315.

Sibai, B. M., Taslimi, M., Abdella, T. N. *et al.* (1985) Maternal and perinatal outcome of conservative management of severe preeclampsia in midtrimester. *Am. J. Obstet. Gynecol.*, **152**, 32–37.

Sibai, B. M., Taslimi, M. M., El-Nazer, A. *et al.* (1986) Maternal–perinatal outcome associated with the syndrome of hemolysis, elevated liver enzymes, and low platelets in severe preeclampsia–eclampsia. *Am. J. Obstet. Gynecol.*, **155**, 501–509.

Sibai, B. M., Mabie, B. C., Harvey, C. J. and Gonzalez, A. R. (1987) Pulmonary edema in severe preeclampsia–eclampsia: analysis of thirty-seven consecutive cases. *Am. J. Obstet. Gynecol.*, **156**, 1174–1179.

Sibai, B. M., Akl, S., Fairlie, F. and Moretti, M. (1990) A protocol for managing severe preeclampsia in the second trimester. *Am. J. Obstet. Gynecol.*, **163**, 733–738.

Sibai, B. M., Mercer, B. M., Schiff, E. and Friedman, S. A. (1994) Aggressive versus expectant management of severe preeclampsia at 28–32 weeks gestation – a randomized controlled trial. *Am. J. Obstet. Gynecol.*, **171**, 818–822.

Slater, R. M., Wilcox, F. L., Smith, W. D. *et al.* (1987) Phenytoin infusion in severe preeclampsia. *Lancet*, **i**, 1417.

Slater, R. M., Wilcox, F. L., Smith, W. D. and Maresh, M. J. A. (1989) Phenytoin in preeclampsia. *Lancet*, **ii**, 1224.

Smith, L. G. Jr, Moise, K. J. Jr, Dildy, G. A. and Carpenter, R. J. Jr. (1991) Spontaneous rupture of the liver during pregnancy: Current therapy. *Obstet. Gynecol.*, **77**, 171–175.

Strandgaard, S. (1978) Autoregulation of cerebral circulation in hypertension. *Acta Neurol. Scand.*, **57**(supp 66), 1.

Strauss, R. G., Keefer, J. R., Burke, T. and Civetta, J. M. (1980) Hemodynamic monitoring of cardiogenic pulmonary edema complicating toxemia of pregnancy. *Obstet. Gynecol.*, **55**, 170–174.

Thiagarajah, S., Bourgeois, F. J., Harbert, G. M. and Caudle, M. R. (1984) Thrombocytopenia in preeclampsia: associated abnormalities and management principles. *Am. J. Obstet. Gynecol.*, **150**, 1–7.

Tufnell, D., O'Donovan, P., Lilford, R. J. *et al.* (1989) Phenytoin in preeclampsia. *Lancet*, **ii**, 273.

Weinstein, L. (1982) Syndrome of hemolysis, elevated liver enzymes, and low platelet count: a severe consequence of hypertension in pregnancy. *Am. J. Obstet. Gynecol.*, **142**, 159–167.

Weinstein, L. (1985) Preeclampsia/eclampsia with hemolysis, elevated liver enzymes, and thrombocytopenia. *Obstet. Gynecol.*, **66**, 657–660.

Zuspan, F. P. (1978) Problems encountered in the treatment of pregnancy-induced hypertension. *Am. J. Obstet. Gynecol.*, **131**, 591–596.

# MANAGEMENT OF SEVERE HYPERTENSION IN PREGNANCY/ECLAMPSIA IN AFRICA

*Jack Moodley*

## 16.1 INTRODUCTION

Epidemiological studies of hypertension in pregnancy have almost exclusively been performed in the Western world. It is reported that hypertension complicates nearly 10% of all pregnancies in these countries (Decker and Van Geijn, 1992). The frequency of severe hypertension in pregnancy requiring parenteral antihypertensives is reported to be 3% of all patients (Reti *et al.*, 1987), but eclampsia is now a rare event in developed countries. In Africa, data on hypertension in pregnancy is hospital-based. Therefore, this may not be representative of the population as a whole. Many women in developing countries deliver their babies at home or in primary health care clinics. Nonetheless, Moodley (1991) quotes a frequency of preeclampsia of 18% of all deliveries at King Edward VIII Hospital (KEH), Durban, South Africa.

The incidence of severe hypertensive crisis in pregnancy in Africa is also more frequent. During 1991, 126 eclamptic patients were admitted to KEH (unpublished data), while there were approximately 14 200 deliveries during the same period. These high figures are probably due to inadequate prenatal care, late hospitalization, inappropriate use of antenatal facilities and lack of health education.

Obstetric care in much of Africa is based on community clinics staffed by midwives. Such clinics and their referral (district) hospitals have limited facilities and are understaffed. The district hospitals rarely have specialist obstetricians in attendance. Women attend for antenatal care late in their pregnancies and often with severe disease. Transport systems are usually not well developed. Consequently, delay is a feature of referrals and accounts for much of the maternal and perinatal morbidity and mortality. Tertiary hospitals are burdened with both high-risk obstetric patients and high cesarean section rates. Thus, although there exist good models for basic obstetric care in parts of Africa, e.g. the midwifery obstetric units in Cape Town, much more effort is needed to improve the efficiency of such health care systems elsewhere in Africa.

## 16.2 PREVENTION

The goal in the management of preeclampsia is to detect the disease at an early stage and to effect cure or at least ameliorate its progression in an attempt to achieve fetal maturity. Preventative strategies that are currently receiving attention include the use of low-dose aspirin, calcium and magnesium supplementation and prepregnancy counseling of

*Hypertension in Pregnancy*
Edited by J.J. Walker and N.F. Gant. Published by Chapman & Hall, 1997 ISBN 0 412 30910 6

women with chronic hypertension. The most promising of these strategies is the use of low-dose aspirin, but its use in Africa may be limited by the fact that most women 'book' for antenatal care late in their pregnancies. The use of procedures such as the roll-over test and measurement of maternal weight gain, which would be of value in developing countries, remains controversial. The measurement of maternal weight gain has not been shown to be useful for the detection of women who will develop hypertension (Dawes and Grudzinkas, 1991) while a report from Nigeria found a sensitivity of only 10% and a false-negative rate of 33% for the roll-over test (Okonofua *et al.*, 1991).

Early preeclampsia in Africa should be detected by establishing a history of previous hypertension, eliciting edema and measuring blood pressure and proteinuria. Furthermore, use of the symphysis–uterine-fundus height measurement is valuable in detecting the failure of fetal growth. Once detected, it is important for the health worker in Africa to convince women to be referred for hospitalization. Most women with eclampsia are remarkably well during the early stages of the disease. Because facilities for outpatient care are virtually non-existent, frequent visits to an antenatal clinic may bring social and financial hardships to patients. Therefore, they need appropriate counseling and advice as regards hospitalization.

## 16.3 DEFINITION OF SEVERE HYPERTENSION IN PREGNANCY (BLOOD PRESSURE LEVELS AT OR ABOVE 170/110 MMHG)

In the non-pregnant patient, a hypertensive crisis is arbitrarily defined as a severe elevation in blood pressure, generally considered to be a diastolic blood pressure above 120–130 mmHg This definition is based on the fact that patients with chronic hypertension can tolerate much higher elevations in blood pressure than previously normotensive individuals. Encephalopathy, for example, rarely develops in patients

with long-standing hypertension until the diastolic blood pressure exceeds 150 mmHg. Young women, however, may develop an encephalopathy with diastolic blood pressures of 110 mmHg or less (Finnerty, 1972; Calhoun and Oparil, 1990). Thus, in pregnancy, severe hypertension (blood pressures at or above 170/110 mmHg) should be treated, especially when it is well documented that cerebral hemorrhage is the most common cause of death in preeclampsia (Redman, 1991).

A severe elevation in blood pressure is considered an emergency if there is evidence of rapid or progressive central nervous system, myocardial, hematological or renal deterioration. In such circumstances, an immediate reduction in high blood pressure, generally effected by means of intravenous therapy in an intensive-care setting, is warranted. In patients who have no evidence of progressive end-organ injury, only a gradual reduction in blood pressure over 24–48 h is required.

The goal of therapy in hypertensive emergencies is to effect a prompt but gradual decrease in high blood pressure. A reasonable goal is to lower the mean arterial pressure by approximately 25% or to reduce the diastolic blood pressure to between 100 and 110 mmHg over a period of several minutes to several hours, depending on the clinical situation (Garcia and Vidt, 1987). Rapid reductions in high blood pressure and reductions to normotensive or hypotensive levels should be avoided as they may provoke end-organ ischemia (Franklin, 1984). Fetal distress following hypotension due to parenteral dihydralazine administration has been reported and is probably due to a reduction in uteroplacental blood flow resulting from rapid lowering of high blood pressure. The reduction in uteroplacental blood flow mainly affects the growth retarded fetus (Vink, Moodley and Philpott, 1980) Furthermore, excessive lowering of high blood pressure may have untoward effects on cerebral blood flow (Moodley, Naicker and Mankowitz, 1983; Richards *et al.*, 1986)

## 16.4 CRITERIA OF SEVERE PREECLAMPSIA (TABLE 16.1)

Calhoun and Oparil (1990) list severe preeclampsia–eclampsia as an important cause of a hypertensive emergency. However, it is important to note that preeclampsia is a multisystem disorder; which organ system is going to be affected predominantly cannot be predicted. Thus hypertension is only one sign, albeit the commonest one, of preeclampsia. The concept of 'normotensive preeclampsia' is well recognized. Women may present with clinical manifestations that are not typical of preeclampsia; for instance patients may present with abnormal hemostats and have minimal or absent hypertension but abnormal liver function tests and low platelet counts (the HELLP syndrome – H = hemolysis, EL = elevated liver enzymes, LP = low platelets). The Working Group on High Blood Pressure (1990) states that the HELLP syndrome constitutes an emergency that requires prompt termination of pregnancy.

## 16.5 MANAGEMENT OF HYPERTENSIVE EMERGENCIES

The management of severe hypertension is summarized in Figure 16.1.

The clinical course of severe preeclampsia–eclampsia is characterized by progressive deterioration in both maternal and fetal status. These pregnancies are associated with increased rates of maternal and perinatal morbidity and mortality. The ultimate goal of therapy must always be safety of the mother first, and then consideration for optimum perinatal outcome. This is of particular importance in Africa, where facilities for neonatal care are lacking, where many single women in the urban areas have unplanned pregnancies and where neonatal and infant mortality rates for low birthweight babies are extremely high.

### 16.5.1 PATIENTS PRESENTING AT 34 WEEKS GESTATION AND GREATER

There is universal agreement to deliver all patients presenting with severe preeclampsia beyond 34 weeks or, if there is evidence of fetal lung maturity and/or fetal jeopardy, prior to that time. This method of treatment is based on the fact that the only cure for preeclampsia is delivery of the placenta. Temporization in such circumstances is associated with maternal and fetal complications. Therefore, control of the blood pressure to levels between 100 and 110 mmHg should be achieved and labor induced.

### 16.5.2 PATIENTS PRESENTING BEFORE 24 WEEKS GESTATION

There is also agreement among researchers that in this specific group of patients, termination of pregnancy should be advised. Sibai *et*

---

**Table 16.1**  Criteria for severe preeclampsia

- **Blood pressure** readings with the patients at rest, of at least 160 mmHg systolic or 110 mmHg diastolic on two occasions at least 6 h apart
- **Proteinuria** levels of at least 5 g in a 24 h urine collection (or 3+ to 4+ on semiquantative assay)
- **Oliguria** (24 h urine output of less than 400 ml), cerebral or visual disturbances such as altered consciousness, headache, scotomata or blurred vision
- **Pulmonary edema** or cyanosis
- **Epigastric** or right upper quadrant **pain**
- Impaired liver function of unclear etiology
- Thrombocytopenia

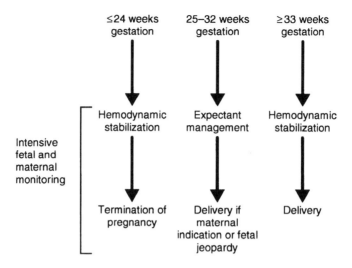

**Figure 16.1**   Proposed management of severe hypertension.

*al.* (1985), in a study of preeclampsia in the midtrimester, found that the perinatal survival rate was 3% for those developing severe disease before 25 weeks gestation compared to 24% for those developing disease at or after 25 weeks. Odendaal, Pattinson and Du Toit (1987), working in Cape Town, South Africa, also found no fetal survivors in 11 pregnancies with severe preeclampsia at less than 24 weeks gestation. Further, Moodley and Koranteng (unpublished data), working with an indigent and underprivileged Black community in Durban, found no fetal survivors in 12 pregnancies with severe preeclampsia. Therefore, in such situations, termination of pregnancy with vaginal prostaglandins is recommended, but hysterotomy should be resorted to in those patients who are 'toxic', in whom hypertension is uncontrollable or in whom the labor is going to be of long duration.

### 16.5.3 PATIENTS PRESENTING BETWEEN 24 WEEKS AND 32 WEEKS GESTATION

The management of severe preeclampsia between 24 and 32 weeks gestation remains a difficult clinical problem. Aggressive management with immediate delivery may result in high neonatal mortality, while expectant management may lead to an unacceptably high maternal complication rate and convert stillbirths into neonatal deaths. Recent studies performed by Sibai *et al.* (1990) and Odendaal *et al.* (1990) suggest that expectant treatment in specialized units providing intensive maternal and fetal monitoring can result in a high percentage of fetal survivors with a low maternal complication rate. Sibai *et al.* (1990) studied 109 patients with severe preeclampsia diagnosed at or before 27 weeks of gestation. They devised a protocol whereby patients at 24 weeks gestation or less were counseled for termination of pregnancy and were divided into two groups: those who accepted termination and those who refused termination. A second group of patients presenting between 24 and 27 weeks were counseled for expectant management or delivery. The outcomes then were studied among the four groups.

Among the 25 patients in the group that were at 24 weeks gestation or less, 15 (60%) refused termination and pregnancies were allowed to proceed. After aggressive maternal and fetal monitoring, the overall perinatal survival rate in this group was only 6.7% (one of 15), with significant maternal morbidity of 27%. These authors reconfirmed that expectant management of patients with severe pregnancy-induced hypertension at 24 weeks gestation or less is of little potential benefit. Among the 84 patients that were at gestations between 24 and 27 weeks who were counseled for conservative management, 30 (36%) had immediate delivery because of refusal of expectant management, either by the patient or the attending physician. A total of 54 patients underwent expectant management, which was associated with an average prolongation of pregnancy of 2 weeks with a significant improvement in both perinatal mortality and morbidity. There was no significant increase in maternal morbidity when compared with the group who had immediate delivery. They found a perinatal survival rate of 76.4% in the expectant group compared with 35.5% in the group that underwent immediate delivery.

Thus treatment with aggressive fetal and maternal monitoring at this tertiary perinatal center improved perinatal outcome in patients with severe preeclampsia with gestational ages between 24 and 27 weeks. Similarly, Odendaal *et al.* (1990), working in Cape Town, South Africa, showed that intensive maternal care and frequent fetal monitoring can improve perinatal outcome. This group studied 58 women with severe preeclampsia between 28 and 34 weeks, randomly assigning women to an aggressive management group (control of high blood pressure and betamethasone for 48 h and then elective delivery) or an expectant treatment group (delivery indicated by maternal or fetal jeopardy). Expectant treatment resulted in prolongation of the gestational age by a mean of 7.1 days, improving neonatal outcome without an increase in maternal morbidity. The same group of researchers in Cape Town, South Africa (Pattinson, Odendaal and Du Toit, 1988) also described the results of expectant management in 34 patients with severe preeclampsia before 28 weeks. The patients were managed by bed rest, frequent fetal monitoring and antihypertensive drugs. All 11 pregnancies presenting before 24 weeks resulted in perinatal deaths. The remaining 34 presented between 24 and 27 weeks, with 13 (38%) resulting in a surviving infant. Maternal complications included three (9%) with pulmonary edema and one (3%) who had a pleural effusion. Thus expectant management with aggressive monitoring of the mother and fetus is possible in patients beyond 24 weeks.

It should be remembered that the prerequisites for expectant management of early onset severe preeclampsia are timely referral to a perinatal center with obstetricians and neonatologists experienced in this field and facilities for intensive fetal and maternal monitoring. In circumstances where maternal and neonatal facilities are lacking, as is the case in the most of Africa, it may be safer in the interests of the mother to advocate delivery after hemodynamic stabilization. Sibai *et al.* (1985) initially reported a poor perinatal outcome and a high maternal complication rate in 60 women with severe preeclampsia treated conservatively. Most of these women were managed at local hospitals with limited facilities for fetal and maternal monitoring and few had antenatal fetal evaluations. Further referrals after the onset of maternal complications to the tertiary perinatal center was a feature in a large number of the cases. These features are typical of the hospitals in Africa and it may be more appropriate to regard fetal viability in Africa as 28 weeks and above. Moodley and Koranteng (1992, unpublished data), working in Durban, South Africa, managed 23 patients with early-onset preeclampsia at 27–29 weeks gestation expectantly and the fetal survival rate was approximately 30%.

Perinatal outcome in the patients between 28 and 32 weeks is relatively good and it is recommended that in such patients an expectant approach to management is followed and steroids are used to accelerate fetal lung maturity. Pregnancy is then continued until the development of either maternal or fetal jeopardy.

## 16.6 TREATMENT OF HYPERTENSIVE EMERGENCIES

### 16.6.1 LOWERING OF HIGH BLOOD PRESSURE

Current treatment strategies of severe hypertension in pregnancy vary. Because of the life-threatening complications – cerebral hemorrhage and congestive cardiac failure – treatment of a diastolic blood pressure persistently greater than 110 mmHg at any stage of pregnancy constitutes a maternal indication for parenteral antihypertensive therapy. When this approach is taken, the usual choice of antihypertensive agent is parenteral dihydralazine. Its popularity stems from ease of administration, being used mainly in intermittent boluses without intra-arterial monitoring, and the vast experience of its use in pregnancy. Its effect is predominantly on arterial vessels with minimal effect on the capacitance vessels. In practice, dihydralazine frequently precipitates fetal distress with reported rates as high as 58% (Vink, Moodley and Philpott, 1980; Spinnato, Sibai and Anderson, 1986). The risk of fetal distress is lowered with correction of hypovolemia and low doses of bolus injections of dihydralazine (Vink and Moodley, 1982)

Dihydralazine is satisfactorily administered in small boluses of 5 mg injections every 10 min (Mabie *et al.*, 1987). The drug is also administered by infusion. This may be hazardous because dihydralazine is a long-acting drug with a relatively long time to maximum effect (20 min) and is difficult to titrate and control (Spinnato, Sibai and Anderson, 1986). While the use of dihydralazine is not without hazard, (headache, flushing mimicking symptoms of preeclampsia, hypotensive episodes) the risks are well defined and can be minimized by proper dosing (5–10 mg every 20

min to a diastolic of approximately 100 mmHg) and adequate hydration (Silver, 1989).

Labetalol is another antihypertensive agent that is used in pregnancy. It is a unique adrenoceptor antagonist as it has both alpha-adrenoceptor-antagonist and non-selective beta-adrenoceptor-antagonist properties. The beta-blocking effect of labetalol is four times less potent than that of propranolol. It appears to produce its hypotensive effects without compromising the maternal cardiovascular system by producing peripheral vasodilation. This may help to maintain renal and uterine blood flow (Lund-Johansen, 1984). Labetalol also has antiarrhythmic properties and this may be of specific value in hypertensive emergencies of pregnancy. Bhorat, Naidoo and Moodley (1991) have shown that such women have a high incidence of ventricular arrhythmias and that these arrhythmias may be the cause of sudden unexplained deaths associated with eclampsia.

Results with the use of intravenous labetalol in severe preeclampsia have been variable. While in some reports the ability to achieve a diastolic blood pressure of less than 100 mmHg with labetalol reaches 90% (Mabie *et al.*, 1987), in others this goal was obtainable in only 40% (Ashe *et al.*, 1987). In all studies of the use of intravenous labetalol in pregnancy, there were no cases of maternal hypotension and therefore no iatrogenic fetal distress, as is commonly seen with direct vasodilators. Walker (1991) recommends either an oral dose of 200 mg of labetalol or alternatively a slow intravenous injection of 50 mg labetalol, which is followed by an infusion pump delivering a solution containing 300 mg of labetalol in 60 ml, or 5 mg/ml. This infusion can be started at 12 ml per hour and increased or decreased depending on the blood pressure response. The author recommends the infusion method. Overall, the results with labetalol are good and despite unpublished reports from the Netherlands (Dekker and Van Geijn, 1992) of fatal cardiogenic shock in the early neonatal period, this drug may become more widely used for hypertensive emergencies.

The calcium channel blockers have been added to the acute antihypertensive regimen. The most commonly used agent is the dihydropiridine calcium channel agonist nifedipine. Although animal studies have reported that its use is associated with decreased uteroplacental bloodflow and fetal hypoxemia, Moretti *et al.* (1990) failed to show any effect on fetal and uteroplacental Doppler waveforms with the use of oral nifedipine. Two randomized studies (Seabe and Moodley, 1989; Fenakel *et al.*, 1990) that compared nifedipine with dihydralazine suggest that nifedipine is associated with fewer episodes of hypotension and causes less of a tachycardia than dihydralazine. Although, Fenakel *et al.* (1990) used concomitant magnesium sulfate, nifedipine did not appear to result in severe maternal hypotension. Concern, however, still exists over the combined use of these drugs as both agents depress cardiac performance and the synergistic effects may have a cumulative depressive effect on cardiac function (Thorpe *et al.*, 1990). A number of cases, have been reported where magnesium sulfate and nifedipine used together resulted in marked hypotension (Waisman *et al.*, 1988). Nifedipine, by virtue of its oral or sublingual route, rapid onset of action and relatively short duration of action (3–5 h), is attractive for use during referral or the postpartum period, especially in developing countries with limited facilities.

Other agents, such as sodium nitroprusside and nitroglycerin, have a rapid onset of action and short duration of action (3–5 min). They have to be given by intravenous titration and, because of this, intra-arterial blood pressure monitoring is required.

Once the high blood pressure is lowered to 100–110 mmHg diastolic pressure, most patients will be delivered. There will be a proportion, however, in whom pregnancy will be prolonged and who will require long-term oral antihypertensives under close and frequent maternal and fetal monitoring. Methyldopa is still the most frequently used drug for this purpose.

## 16.6.2 HYPOVOLEMIA

Much has been written recently about the intravenous infusion of volume expanders (e.g. albumin, Dextran) as supportive therapy for hypertension in pregnancy. These observations are based on hemodynamic studies with Swan–Ganz catheters, which show that plasma volume, cardiac output and pulmonary capillary wedge pressure may be decreased in this condition. Although there is no doubt that blood pressure is lowered transiently and vasodilation is produced by such infusions, the mechanism of action is still poorly understood (Gallery, Mitchell and Redman, 1984). There is also evidence of increased capillary permeability in preeclampsia and excessive administration of volume expanders may lead to pulmonary edema. This form of therapy is therefore not recommended for general use. Central venous catheterization is useful, to correct any hypovolemia with Ringer's lactated solution (60–150 ml/h) prior to parenteral antihypertensive therapy. However it has been shown that central venous pressure may have a poor correlation with LAP, particularly at the lower values often seen in preeclampsia. Pulmonary capillary wedge pressure measurements are of benefit in selected cases, such as patients in pulmonary edema or patients who are oliguric despite fluid challenge.

## 16.6.3 PROPHYLACTIC ANTICONVULSANTS

The choice of drug to prevent convulsions in eclampsia is controversial as are the appropriate indications for routine seizure prophylaxis in preeclampsia. In the USA parenteral magnesium sulfate is widely used both for prophylaxis against and treatment of convulsions. In the UK, magnesium sulfate is not used for prophylaxis nor for treatment of eclamptic seizures. Chau and Redman (1991) reported their results on a policy of not routinely prescribing anticonvulsants in severe preeclampsia. Of 78 patients with severe preeclampsia entered into the study, in whom sublingual nifedipine was supplemented if necessary with dihydralazine to lower high blood pressure, only one patient developed eclampsia. It would be difficult to establish whether prophylactic anticonvulsants are of value because of the large number of patients required for a randomized trial in such a situation. Moodley and Moodley (1994), working in Durban, South Africa, recently randomized 228 patients with severe hypertension in pregnancy to receive either prophylactic anticonvulsant therapy in the form of magnesium sulfate therapy or no anticonvulsant therapy. All patients in the study had immediate lowering of high blood pressure. There was only a single patient who had a convulsion in the study and this occurred in the magnesium sulfate group ($n = 114$) within 10 min of initiating anticonvulsant therapy. In developing countries, with limited facilities, it would be safer to use fewer drugs in the management of severe preeclampsia. Polypharmacy was one of the factors identified as a cause of death in women with eclampsia (Moodley, Naicker and Mankowitz, 1983). Therefore, the author recommends that the aim should be to lower blood pressure to between 100 and 110 mmHg diastolic blood pressure and to induce labor as soon as practical. In situations where patients are 'toxic', prophylactic anticonvulsants should be used.

### 16.6.4 COAGULATION DEFECTS IN PREECLAMPSIA

The most often occurring hemostatic abnormalities in preeclampsia appear to be a rise in factor VIII R:Ag (Redman *et al.*, 1977) and a low antithrombin III concentration (Mobbs, Moodley and Kenoyer, 1985). In some cases of

severe preeclampsia, thrombin action may be markedly increased by comparison to that in normotensive pregnancy. However, the mechanisms designed to limit the spread of hemostatic reactions (antithrombin III, protein C and the fibrinolytic system) are rarely overwhelmed and the occurrence of the clinical syndrome of disseminated intravascular coagulation is an exception in preeclampsia. On the other hand, episodes of platelet activation and consumption are rather common and platelet activation is not thrombin- but rather surface-mediated (Brook *et al.*, 1984). The spiral arteries in the placental bed constitute a likely site of such platelet activation.

Selective platelet destruction in preeclampsia, sometimes accompanied by microangiopathic hemolysis but usually without signs of increased thrombin action, shows a striking similarity with that found in thrombotic thrombocytopenic purpura and in the hemolytic syndrome (Harlan, 1983). The concept of a defective vascular prostacyclin synthesis that appears to explain most of the pathophysiological features has also been applied to these disorders (Remuzzi, Imperti and De Gaetano, 1981).

Hemolysis, defined as the presence of microangiopathic hemolytic anemia, is the hallmark of the HELLP syndrome. The reported incidence of this syndrome ranges from 2–12% (Sibai, 1990) and it is said to be an early 'marker' of severe preeclampsia. It usually occurs in the antepartum period but 30% of the cases first present postdelivery. The natural history of thrombocytopenia (100 000 platelets/mm³) with preeclampsia was reported by Katz *et al.* (1990). Of 375 women with preeclampsia, 61 had thrombocytopenia. By postpartum day 3, 90% of these women had rising platelet counts and by postpartum day 4, 59 of the 61 women had platelet counts greater than 100 000/mm³. These data suggest that this type of thrombocytopenia should resolve by postpartum day 4 and if it is not resolved by this time, other causes of thrombocytopenia should be investigated.

## 16.7 ANESTHESIA/ANALGESIA FOR SEVERELY HYPERTENSIVE PREGNANT WOMEN

There is no doubt that epidural analgesia is of benefit for vaginal and operative delivery in preeclampsia. The benefits are the prevention of increases in catecholamine release, thereby preventing further increases in high blood pressure during uterine contractions, and permitting a gentle controlled delivery during the second stage by abolishing excessive maternal bearing down. Further evidence of the advantages of epidural analgesia was demonstrated by Ramos-Santos *et al.* (1991), who studied the effects of epidural anesthesia on Doppler velocimetry of umbilical and uterine arteries in normotensive and hypertensive patients during active labor. After epidural block, uterine artery systolic/diastolic ratios fell significantly in pre-eclamptic, chronic hypertensive and normotensive women. This study suggests that a well-controlled and effective epidural can provide additional benefits to the pre-eclamptic mother and fetus by improving uteroplacental perfusion. However, there are problems, which require careful technique, and there are situations where it is relatively or absolutely contraindicated.

Prerequisites for epidural anesthesia are the exclusion of a coagulopathy and the assessment and correction of cardiac preload prior to anesthesia. More recently concern has been expressed as regards patients on low-dose aspirin, given to reduce the incidence of perinatal and maternal morbidity associated with preeclampsia (Schiff *et al.*, 1989), who are presenting to labor wards where epidural techniques are practiced. The safety of regional anesthesia in patients on aspirin is uncertain (Douglas, 1991) and, while epidural hematoma is rare, potential neurological sequelae are serious. The bleeding time is recommended as the screening test prior to regional anesthesia (MacDonald, 1991), but this test has come under increasing scrutiny (Rodgers and Levin, 1990). These authors, in a review of 1000 publications using meta-analysis, concluded that bleeding time could not be used to predict the risk of hemorrhage. In a recent study, comparing the thromboelastograph with bleeding time on blood samples taken prior to and after 4 weeks of therapy with 75 mg aspirin daily, Payne *et al.* (1991) found that, although the bleeding times were prolonged, none was greater than 10 min. There were no changes in the thromboelastograph measurements. Therefore, they suggest that low-dose aspirin does not markedly affect bleeding time and that the thromboelastogram, which gives a view of the whole coagulation system, should be used prior to epidural anesthesia.

In Africa, epidural analgesia in preeclampsia is of special significance because of the lack of specialist anesthetists and the risks of general anesthesia, e.g. exacerbation of hypertension during intubation and at extubation, laryngeal edema and hypovolemia.

## 16.8 STEROIDS IN SEVERE PREECLAMPSIA

Steroid therapy is recommended if there is no fetal or maternal jeopardy and the pregnancy is between 26 and 32 weeks gestation. Maximum benefit is achieved when steroids are given in appropriate doses and the last dose is given at least 24 h before delivery.

## 16.9 ECLAMPSIA IN AFRICA

Eclampsia, the onset of convulsions associated with preeclampsia, is not an uncommon condition in Africa. Moodley, Naicker and Mankowitz (1983), working in Durban, South Africa, quote an 'eclampsia rate' of 2.3/1000 deliveries and a mortality rate of 11.9%. They also state that 80% of their patients with eclampsia had no antenatal care and that most had five convulsions or more prior to admission to hospital. In addition, they highlighted risk factors associated with maternal mortality and morbidity. Delay in hospitalization, late referrals to tertiary hospitals and lack of transport were emphasized as risk factors. The typical profile of the patient at risk was the unbooked, parous patient above the age of 30 admitted in an unconscious state. If, in addition, polypharmacy was used and labor was prolonged with hemorrhage and/or operative shock, the chances of maternal death were high.

Appropriate prenatal care and early hospitalization of patients with preeclampsia will prevent most cases of eclampsia. In Sweden, a country with good antenatal services, the incidence is 1/3448 pregnancies (Moller and Lindmark, 1988). Other factors, apart from the lack of provision of antenatal services, account for the high incidence of eclampsia in Africa. Socioeconomic uplift, community empowerment and education on health matters are needed. This will take time to develop, given the poor economic conditions in Africa. In the meantime, guidelines are necessary for the management of such patients (Table 16.2).

### 16.9.1 IMMEDIATE MANAGEMENT

#### (a) Minimal or no impairment of consciousness

Management of eclamptic patients with minimal or no impairment of consciousness requires control of convulsions, lowering of high blood pressure and appropriate investigations. For control of convulsions and prevention of further convulsions, magnesium sulfate is recommended. The dosage regime of Pritchard (1979) should be used in Africa. A loading dose of 14 g is given; 4 g in 200 ml of lactated Ringer's solution is infused over 15 min and 10 g by deep intramuscular is given concurrently, 5 g into each buttock. Then 5 g is given intramuscularly every 4 h. Before each dose, ensure:

1. that the urine output is greater than 30 ml per hour;
2. that the patellar reflexes are present;
3. that respiration is adequate.

If any of these parameters is not within the normal range, the next dose of magnesium sulfate is withheld.

Magnesium sulfate can also be administered by continuous intravenous administration. Sibai (1990) recommends 6 g IV slowly, followed by a maintenance dose of 2–3 g per hour. Continuous administration is advocated because the intramuscular injections are painful and repeated injections lead to abscess formation. This has not been the experience in Durban. Continuous infusions also entail an absolute necessity for close monitoring and use of appropriate equipment because of the

---

**Table 16.2** Principles of management of eclampsia

1. Immediate care – attend to airway, turn patient on her side
2. Termination of convulsion (if appropriate) – Diazepam 10 mg IV
3. Prevention of further convulsions – magnesium sulfate
4. Lower high blood pressure to between 95–105 mmHg diastolic
5 Coagulation screen, renal function tests, Foley urinary catheter
6. Delivery following hemodynamic stabilization with 6–8 h
7. Intensive care for 24–48 h postpartum. Nurse in 'head up' position to decrease cerebral edema

**Note:** Ventilation for 24 h at least:
- the unconscious eclamptic
- the eclamptic with poor blood gases
- the extremely restless eclamptic

risk of respiratory arrest. This is not always possible in Africa, even in tertiary hospitals. Further, Lipsitz (1977) has shown that the newborn is unlikely to be compromised using the intramuscular regimen, whereas signs of hypermagnesemia may be expected if continuous intravenous infusion is used, especially if used for 24 h and more. It is best to use a regimen that one is familiar with and that suits a particular hospital.

Diazepam should only be used for termination of a convulsion (10 mg IV slowly) because of the excessive sedative effects on both mother and baby associated with its long-term use. Further, Crowther (1990) reported on 51 patients with eclampsia who were randomly allocated to receive either magnesium ($n = 24$) or diazepam ($n = 27$). Recurrent convulsions occurred more often in the diazepam group (26%) than the magnesium sulfate group (21%). Magnesium sulfate was also reported to have significant clinical advantages for the mother and fetus.

Rapid and excessive lowering of high blood pressure may be disadvantageous to both mother and fetus, while polypharmacy is to be avoided wherever possible. The main dangers of severe hypertension are maternal cerebrovascular accidents and congestive heart failure. Excessive lowering of high blood pressure may exacerbate maternal cerebral ischemia, by lowering cerebral perfusion, and jeopardize fetal wellbeing by decreasing placental perfusion. The aim of control of severe hypertension is to lower high blood pressure to levels within the range of 140–150 mmHg systolic and 90–100 mmHg diastolic pressure. Hydralazine in small bolus doses (6.25 mg IV) is a safe and effective drug for this purpose. Alternatively, or where the maternal pulse rate is 120/min or more, labetalol should be used. Agents such as sodium nitroprusside, nitroglycerin and diazoxide are seldom required, being mainly used prior to endotracheal intubation at the time of general anesthesia. Note should be taken of drug interactions. Davey, Moodley and Soutter

(1981) have reported on the extreme lowering of blood pressure when diazoxide and hydralazine are used in combination. Further, magnesium sulfate and the calcium channel blockers may have a summative effect.

### (b) Monitoring of the cardiovascular system

The eclamptic patient is hemodynamically unstable and ventricular arrhythmias have been demonstrated in such circumstances (Bhorat, Naidoo and Moodley, 1990). The heart rate should be measured continuously using an ECG monitor. The blood pressure should also be monitored continuously, using an automatic non-invasive technique, as marked changes in blood pressure levels may occur from minute to minute in eclampsia. In patients who are extremely restless or deeply unconscious, direct intra-arterial pressure monitoring is recommended.

Central venous pressure should be monitored in all patients. A drum cartridge catheter (Abbott) is inserted via an antecubital vein and a bedside chest radiograph is performed to check the position of the catheter tip. The temptation to overcome hypovolemia associated with eclampsia persists because of reports that cardiac output, intravascular volume and filling pressures are often suboptimal and that volume expansion may be beneficial. Overenthusiastic use of hyperosmotic fluids may result in circulatory overload unless there is concomitant relief of the vasospasm that is responsible for the decreased capacity of the intravascular compartment. Central venous pressure monitoring is therefore essential to prevent dangerous overfilling or underfilling. Ringer's lactate solution is recommended as intravenous fluid and an infusion rate of 100 ml per hour is prudent, and is the best way to avoid postpartum pulmonary edema.

The indications for the use of Swan–Ganz catheterization to measure pulmonary artery wedge pressures are rare. They are associated with mortality (Robin, 1987) and in Africa both the equipment and the required expertise for these techniques are lacking. In most cases, women with eclampsia can be treated without invasive monitoring. From a clinical point of view, blood pressure, pulse rate and central venous pressure should be measured every 15 min.

### (c) Marked impairment of consciousness

Particular attention should be given to preventing the excessive lowering of high blood pressure. Therefore, following magnesium sulfate therapy, high blood pressure should be lowered gradually to between 100 and 110 mmHg diastolic pressure. Such patients have raised intracranial pressure (Richards *et al.*, 1986) and excessive lowering of the blood pressure may lead to a decrease in the cerebral perfusion, with retention of metabolites and a further increase in intracranial pressure.

If it is difficult to maintain an airway or, if ventilation is required, the patient should be intubated and ventilated if necessary. Such patients should have arterial blood gas analysis performed as a routine. Following hemodynamic stabilization, cesarean section is resorted to as soon as possible. Ventilation should be continued for at least 24 h postdelivery. In such patients the use of steroids and/or diuretics should be considered, to reduce cerebral edema (Marshall, 1978). At King Edward VIII Hospital, Durban, dexamethasone 32 mg IV *statim* and 8 mg 6-hourly is used for 24 h in such circumstances. A group of patients with eclampsia, despite being fully conscious, display extreme restlessness. This makes close monitoring difficult and leads to an overuse of sedative and anticonvulsant drugs. Such patients may have adequate arterial gases; nevertheless, they should be sedated and ventilated for 24 h. Their restlessness is due to cerebral edema and hyperventilation will not only reduce cerebral edema but will allow appropriate monitoring of all vital parameters.

Computed axial tomography is not necessary in the routine management of such patients. Its use should be limited to patients with 'localizing' central nervous system signs and those with atypical eclampsia, e.g. convulsions occurring 3 or more days following delivery, to rule out cerebral pathology.

### (d) Further steps in management

Urine output should be monitored closely by inserting an indwelling catheter, blood should be drawn for urea and electrolytes and a coagulation screen (platelet count, PI, PTT fibrinogen levels) should be performed. Thrombocytopenia may occur in up to 50% of cases with hypertensive crises of pregnancy (Giles and Inglis, 1981) and if the platelet count $< 50 \times 10^9/l$ then platelet concentrate should be transfused immediately prior to any operative procedure. Platelet counts between 50 and $150 \times 10^9/l$ require a platelet function test performed before any operative procedure.

### (e) Management of labor

All deeply unconscious patients should be delivered by cesarean section, unless delivery is imminent. A cesarean section should be performed in all other eclamptic patients only if delivery is unlikely to occur within 6–8 h, fetal distress is present, convulsions persist, hypertension is refractory to therapy or oliguria supervenes. It goes without saying that continuous fetal rate monitoring should be performed.

Continuous epidural blockade is the method of choice of pain relief for those patients able to cooperate, provided that there is no coagulation defect. However, general anesthesia is usually recommended for cesarean section. The anesthetist should be aware of all drugs used and modify the anesthetic technique according. The dangers of a marked hypertensive response to laryngoscopy, airway suctioning, intubation and extubation, and laryngeal edema must be taken into account. Consequently the presence of an obstetric anesthetist is required.

## (f) Postpartum management

Although delivery will eventually cure the women of preeclampsia, the risk may still be present for some days postpartum. Therefore, continuous close monitoring of blood pressure and pulse rate are maintained, and magnesium sulfate therapy is continued for at least 24 h. Antihypertensives are usually required during this period and hydralazine should be given in small intravenous boluses. Decreased urine output is also a feature of this period and, once hypovolemia is corrected, renal doses of dopamine are recommended.

## 16.10 SPECIAL PROBLEMS IN AFRICA

The major problem in Africa is that most patients present at primary or secondary levels of health-care systems. The key issue therefore is maternal transport. Ideally there needs to be communication between the referral clinic/hospital and the tertiary center prior to transfer. Patients should be stabilized at the referral center by administration of magnesium sulfate and antihypertensive therapy. Following hemodynamic stabilization, the patient should be accompanied by a nurse or doctor during transfer in an ambulance.

In Africa, because of lack of drugs, facilities, health personnel, communication and ambulances, and vast distances, this ideal is virtually impossible. It is suggested that magnesium sulfate therapy be administered and the patient be transferred on her side, accompanied by a health worker.

## 16.11 FUTURE PREGNANCIES

Postnatal examination and discussion are a vital part of management. The patient should be encouraged to attend a postnatal clinic and any persistence of proteinuria and hypertension will require further investigation. The patient should be advised against pregnancy until she is normotensive and her renal function has been assessed as being satisfactory.

The patient should also be encouraged to report early in her next pregnancy and be warned that intensive antenatal care will be instituted to detect the earliest evidence of preeclampsia, and that low-dose aspirin may be administered from the end of the first trimester of pregnancy in an attempt to prevent the onset of preeclampsia.

In Africa, an improvement in socioeconomic standards is required to lower the incidence of eclampsia. In addition, mortality and morbidity can be reduced by:

1. formation of regional centers with the necessary expertise to attend to hypertensive crises of pregnancy;
2. selective booking of primigravidae in tertiary centers;
3. early referral of patients with the mildest hypertension to the tertiary centers;
4. provision of adequate numbers of antenatal beds for prolonged hospitalization if necessary;
5. aggressive management of severe hypertension;
6. provision of appropriate antenatal services.

## 16.12 SUMMARY

Severe preeclampsia–eclampsia is a complex problem and requires the expertise of a fetomaternal specialist, an obstetric anesthetist and a neonatologist to be involved in a health-care team making decisions at all stages of management.

Delivery remains the cure, but antihypertensive agents are used to prevent complications. Patients at risk for preeclampsia should be detected at an early stage and referred timeously to a tertiary center. Once the diagnosis of severe hypertension is made, the aim of the therapy is to stabilize the mother to reduce the risks to her, and to allow either prolongation of pregnancy or delivery in a controlled manner. High blood pressure (160/110 mmHg) should be lowered following correction of hypovolemia, coagulopathy should be excluded and delivery carried out, if necessary for maternal or fetal reasons. The method of delivery depends on the individual case. Generally vaginal delivery is preferred if the patient is beyond 32 weeks gestation. Many of the complications of severe hypertension occur following delivery; observations need to be maintained and treatment continued for some weeks. If blood pressure does not settle, then referral for further investigations is necessary.

In Africa, longer periods of hospitalization and earlier recourse to termination of pregnancy are necessary because of limited monitoring facilities and the high maternal complication rate.

## REFERENCES

Ashe, R. G., Moodley, J., Richards, A. M. *et al.* (1987) Comparison of labetalol and dihydralazine in hypertensive emergencies of pregnancy. *S. Afr. Med. J.*, **71**, 354–356.

Bhorat, I., Naidoo, D. P. and Moodley, J. (1991) Continuous electrocardiographic monitoring in hypertensive crises in pregnancy. *Am. J. Obstet. Gynecol.*, **164**, 530–535.

Brook, Z., Wietz, J., Owen, J. *et al.* (1984) Fibrinogen proteolysis and platelet granule release in pre-eclampsia/eclampsia. *Blood*, **63**, 525–527.

Calhoun, D. A. and Oparil, S. (1990) Treatment of hypertensive crises. *N. Engl. J. Med.*, **323**, 1177–1183.

Chua, S. and Redman CWG. (1991) Are prophylactic anticonvulsants required in severe pre-eclampsia? *Lancet*, **337**, 250–251.

Crowther, C. (1990) Magnesium sulphate versus diazepam in the management of eclampsia. *Br. J. Obstet. Gynaecol.*, **97**, 110–114.

Davey, M., Moodley, J. and Soutter, P. W. (1981) Adverse effects of a combination of diazoxide and hydralazine therapy. *S. Afr. Med. J.*, **59**, 496–497.

Dawes, M. G. and Grudzinkas, J. G. (1991) Patterns of maternal weight gain in pregnancy. *Br. J. Obstet. Gynaecol.*, **98**, 195–201.

Dekker, G. A. and Van Geijn, H. P. (1992) Hypertensive diseases in pregnancy. *Curr. Opin. Obstet. Gynecol.*, **4**, 10–27.

Douglas M J. (1991) Coagulation abnormalities and obstetric anaesthesia. *Can. J. Anaesth.*, **38**, R17–R21.

Fenakel, K., Fenakel, E., Apleman , Z. *et al.* (1991) Nifedipine in the treatment of severe preeclampsia. *Obstet. Gynecol.*, **77**, 331–337.

Finnerty, F. A. J. (1972) Hypertensive encephalopathy. *Am. J. Med.*, **52**, 672–678.

Franklin, S. A. (1984) The case of more rapid lowering of blood pressure, in *Controversies in Nephrology and Hypertension*, (ed. R. G. Narins), Churchill Livingstone, New York, p. 241–252.

Gallery, E. D. N., Mitchell, M. D. and Redman, C. W. G. (1984) Fall in blood pressure in response to volume expansion in pregnancy associated hypertension. Why does it occur? *J. Hypertens.*, **2**, 177–182.

Garcia, J. Y. Jr and Vidt, D. G. (1987) Current management of hypertensive emergencies. *Drugs*, **34**, 263–278.

Giles, C. and Inglis, T. C. M. (1981) Thrombocytopenia and macrothrombocytosis in gestational hypertension. *Br. J. Obstet. Gynaecol.*, **88**, 1115–1119.

Harlan, J. M. (1983) Thrombocytopaenia due to non-immune platelet destruction. *Clin. Haematol.*, **12**, 39–41.

Katz, V. L., Thorp, J. M., Rozas, L. and Bowes, W. A. (1990) The natural history of thrombocytopenia associated with pre-eclampsia. *Am. J. Obstet. Gynecol.*, **163**, 1142–1143.

Lipsitz, P. J. (1977) The clinical and biochemical effects of excess magnesium in the newborn. *Paediatrics*, **47**, 501–504.

Lund-Johansen, P. (1984) Pharmacology of combined a-13 blockade. *Drugs*, **28**, 35–40.

Mabie, W. C., Gonzalez, A. R, Sibai, B. M. *et al.* (1987) Comparative trial of labetalol and hydralazine in the acute management of severe hypertension in complicating pregnancy. *Obstet. Gynecol.*, **70**, 328–331.

MacDonald, R. (1991) Aspirin and epidural blocks. *Br. J. Anaesth.*, **66**, 1–3.

Marshall, M. (1978) Intracranial pressure, cerebral blood flow and metabolism, in *Neuroanaesthesia*, (eds S. A. Friedman and C. F. Scurr), Edward Arnold, London, p. 1–21.

Mobbs, C., Moodley, J. and Kenoyer, G. (1985) Antithrombin III in eclampsia. *Clin. Exper. Hypertens.*, **B4**(2&3), 105–106.

Moller, B. and Lindmark, G. (1988) Eclampsia in Sweden, 1976–80. *Acta Obstet. Gynecol. Scand.* **65**, 307-314.

Moodley, J. (1991) Hypertension in pregnancy. *S. Afr. Med. J. C. M. E.*, **9**(1), 72–80.

Moodley, J. and Moodley, V. V. (1994) Prophylactic anticonvulsant therapy in hypertensive crises of pregnancy – the need for a large, randomized trial. *Hypertens. Pregn.*, **13**, 245–252.

Moodley, J., Naicker, R. S. and Mankowitz, E. (1983) Eclampsia – a method of management. *S. Afr. Med. J.*, **63**, 530–535.

Moretti, M. M., Fairlie, F. M., Akl, S. *et al.* (1990) The effect of nifedipine therapy on fetal and placental Doppler waveforms in pre-eclampsia remote from term. *Am. J. Obstet. Gynecol.*, **163**, 1844–1848.

Odendaal, H. J., Pattinson, R. C. and Du Toit, R. (1987) Fetal and neonatal outcome in patients with severe pre-eclampsia before 34 weeks. *S. Afr. Med. J.*, **71**, 555–558.

Odendaal, H. J., Pattinson, R. C., Bam, R. *et al.* (1990) Aggressive or expectant management for patients with severe pre-eclampsia between 28 and 34 weeks gestation. A randomised controlled trial. *Obstet. Gynecol.*, **76**, 1070–1075.

Okonofua, F. E., Odunsi, A. O., Hussain, S. and O'Brien, P. M. S. (1991) Evaluation of the roll-over test as a predictor of gestational hypertension in African women. *Int. J. Gynecol. Obstet.*, **35**, 37–40.

Pattinson, R. C., Odendaal, H. J. and Du Toit, R. (1988) Conservative management of severe pre-eclampsia before 28 weeks gestation. *S. Afr. Med. J.*, **73**, 516–518.

Pritchard, J. A.(1979) The use of magnesium sulphate in pre-eclampsia–eclampsia. *J. Reprod. Med.*, **23**, 107–109.

Ramos-Santos, E., Devoe, L. D., Wakefield, M. L. *et al.* (1991) The effects of epidural anaesthesia, on the Doppler velocimetry of umbilical and uterine arteries in normal and hypertensive patients during active term labour. *Obstet. Gynecol.*, **77**, 20–26.

Redman, C. W. G. (1991) Drugs, hypertension and pregnancy. *Prog. Obstet. Gynaecol.*, **9**, 83–97.

Redman, C. W. G., Denson, K. W. E., Beilin, L. J. *et al.* (1977) Factor VIII consumption in pre-eclampsia. *Lancet*, **ii**, 1249.

Remuzzi, G., Imperti, L. and De Gaetano, G (1981) Prostacyclin deficiency in thrombotic microangiopathy. *Lancet*, **ii**, 1 22.

Reti, L. L., Ross, A., Kloss, M. *et al.* (1987) The management of severe pre-eclampsia with intravenous magnesium Sulphate, hydralazine and central venous catheterisation *Aust. NZ J. Obstet. Gynaecol.*, **27**, 102–105.

Richards, A. M., Moodley, J., Graham, D. I. and Bullock, M. R. (1986) Active management of the unconscious eclamptic patient. *Br. J. Obstet. Gynaecol.*, **93**, 554–562.

Robin, E. D. (1987) Death by pulmonary artery flow directed catheter: time for a moratorium? *Chest*, **92**, 727–731.

Rodgers, R. P. C. and Levin, J. (1990) A critical reappraisal of bleeding time. *Semin Thromb. Haemostasis*, **16**, 1–20.

Seabe, S. J. and Moodley, J. (1989) Nifedipine in acute hypertensive emergencies in pregnancies. *S. Afr. Med. J.*, **76**, 248–250.

Sibai, B. M., Taslima, M., Abdella, T. N. *et al.* (1985) Maternal and perinatal outcome of conservative management of severe pre-eclampsia in the mid-trimester. *Am. J. Obstet. Gynecol.*, **152**, 32–37.

Sibai, B. M., Sherif, A., Fairlie, F. and Moretti, M. (1990) A protocol for managing severe pre-eclampsia in the second trimester. *Am. J. Obstet. Gynecol.*, **163**, 733–738.

Silver, H. (1989) Acute hypertensive crisis in pregnancy. *Med. Clin. North Am.*, **73**, 623–637.

Spinnato, J. A., Sibai, B. M. and Anderson, G. D. (1986) Fetal distress after hydralazine therapy for severe pregnancy-induced hypertension. *S. Afr. Med. J.*, **79**, 559.

Thorpe, J. M., Speielman, F. J., Valea, F. A. *et al.* (1990) Nifedipine enhances the cardiac toxicity of magnesium sulfate in the isolated perfused toxicity of magnesium sulphate in the isolated perfused Sprague–Dolly rat heart. *Am. J. Obstet. Gynecol.*, **163**, 655–656.

Vink, G. and Moodley, J. (1982) The effects of low dose dihydralazine in the treatment of maternal hypertension. *S. Afr. Med. J.*, **62**, 475–7.

Vink, G., Moodley, J. and Philpott, R. H. (1980) Effect of dihydralazine on the fetus in the treatment of hypertension in pregnancy. *Obstet. Gynecol.*, **55**, 519–522.

Waisman, G. D., Mayorga, L. M,. Camera, M. I. *et al.* (1988) Magnesium plus nifedipine potentiation of hypotensive effect in pre-eclampsia? *Am. J. Obstet. Gynecol.*, **159**, 308.

Walker, J. J. (1991) Hypertensive drugs in pregnancy. *Clin. Perinatol.*, **18**, 845–867.

Working Group on High Blood Pressure (1990) National High Blood Pressure Education Program Working Group report on high blood pressure in pregnancy: consensus report. *Am. J. Obstet. Gynecol.*, **163**, 1689–1712.

# HYPERTENSION IN PREGNANCY – MANAGEMENT OF THE NEWBORN INFANT

*J. Stewart Forsyth*

## 17.1 INTRODUCTION

If hypertension develops during pregnancy, the influence that this may have upon the fetus and the newborn infant will depend upon the severity and duration of the hypertension, the presence of preexistent hypertensive disorder or accompanying proteinuria, the gestational age and the degree of intrauterine growth retardation (Derham *et al.*, 1989). Information on the presence of any of these factors should be made available to the pediatric staff in order that the most appropriate arrangements can be made for receipt of the infant. Mild hypertension during the final weeks of pregnancy is unlikely to jeopardize the clinical progress of the infant during the newborn period, but the infant who is the product of a pregnancy complicated by severe prolonged hypertension will require careful management throughout the perinatal and postnatal period. Any measure of outcome of pregnancy hypertension must include the eventual health and wellbeing of the baby.

## 17.2 PLANNING THE DELIVERY

Once the decision to deliver the infant has been made, obstetric and pediatric management is aimed at preventing or reducing infant morbidity, which may be a consequence of the hypertensive disease in the mother or organ immaturity in the infant.

### 17.2.1 ANTENATAL STEROIDS

Delay of the delivery may allow time for the administration of antenatal steroids. Although beta-mimetics can be used to suppress premature labor (King *et al.*, 1988), their administration in women with hypertensive disease should be used with caution as the hypertension may be exacerbated. The importance of the value of antenatal steroids was highlighted in an overview of the results of 12 controlled trials, which demonstrated that the administration of corticosteroid therapy to women at increased risk of early delivery significantly reduced the risk of respiratory distress syndrome, by approximately 50%. The greatest benefit in respect of respiratory distress syndrome was seen when the time interval between the start of treatment and delivery was more than 24 h and less than 7 days. Nevertheless, some babies born before or after this optimal time interval still derived benefit (Crowley, Chalmers and Keirse, 1990).

*Hypertension in Pregnancy*
Edited by J.J. Walker and N.F. Gant. Published by Chapman & Hall, 1997 ISBN 0 412 30910 6

## 17.2.2 MODE OF DELIVERY

The effect of the mode of delivery of the infant on subsequent outcome is probably more a reflection of the skill of the nurse or doctor than of the route of delivery. Delivery by cesarean section may be associated with a higher risk of respiratory distress syndrome than vaginal delivery (Tubman *et al.*, 1990), but confirmation from properly controlled trials is lacking, and therefore a decision to deliver by cesarean section should be based on obstetric criteria. If there are significant signs of fetal distress antenatally, cesarean section is preferable unless an easy vaginal delivery can be achieved. Discussion concerning the mode and timing of delivery should involve the pediatrician from an early stage.

## 17.2.3 PLACE OF DELIVERY

It is important that the infant is delivered in a hospital that has the facilities and the expertise to resuscitate and support the infant. If these standards cannot be met by the local obstetric unit, *in utero* transfer to a hospital with intensive obstetric and neonatal facilities is mandatory.

## 17.3 CARE OF THE NEWBORN

### 17.3.1 RESUSCITATION

Important goals for effective resuscitation include adequate oxygenation of the infant, employing active respiratory support if required, maintenance of blood glucose and acid–base homeostasis and prevention of hypothermia. To achieve these goals different levels of resuscitation may be required (Figure 17.1).

### 17.3.2 ENDOTRACHEAL INTUBATION

In the absence of fundamental data on the advantages and disadvantages of routine endotracheal intubation of low-birthweight infants, acceptable practice would be to refrain from routinely intubating all infants, even the most premature infants, provided they are breathing effectively, and intubate those infants who are cyanosed or making inadequate respiratory effort.

### 17.3.3 HYPOTHERMIA

Hypothermia is a preventable complication which if prolonged may cause serious long-term neurodevelopmental sequelae (Davies and Tizard, 1975). In the Scottish Low Birthweight Study of infants born in 1984, 38% of infants with birthweight less than 1000 g had a temperature of less than 34° on admission to the neonatal unit (McIlwaine *et al.*, 1989). Follow-up of these infants at 2 years of age showed that mortality in this hypothermic group was 87% and only 4% of survivors were alive and not impaired. Although the temperature on admission may have reflected the duration and the intensity of resuscitation required by these infants, such marked and preventable hypothermia undoubtedly contributes to mortality and morbidity (Stewart and Reynolds, 1974). To prevent low body temperatures occurring in growth-retarded infants the thermal environment must be meticulously controlled in the labor ward, draughts being avoided. Drying and covering of the infant immediately after delivery will prevent evaporative and radiant heat loss and if transfer to the neonatal unit is required this should be undertaken in a transport incubator with an ambient temperature appropriate for the infant's body weight – 1 kg: 36°, 2 kg: 34°, 3 kg: 32–33° (Hey, 1971).

### 17.3.4 HYPOGLYCEMIA

Infants who are stressed during pregnancy and delivery, and especially those who are growth-retarded, are at considerable risk of developing hypoglycemia. In the normal fetus, glucose readily crosses the placenta and glycogen is deposited in the liver. The

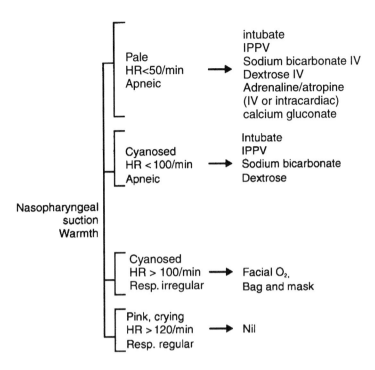

**Figure 17.1** Resuscitation procedures (N.B. If history of maternal pethidine, especially within 4 h of delivery, reverse with IV or IM naloxone).

deposition increases markedly during the latter part of pregnancy and at term the normally grown fetus has a higher liver glycogen concentration than at any other time in his/her life (Cornblath and Schwartz, 1966). In infants in whom there has been preceding hypertension during pregnancy and intrauterine growth retardation has ensued, there will be a markedly reduced hepatic glycogen load. After birth, when the constant infusion of glucose from the placenta stops abruptly, the blood glucose levels in the infant will fall rapidly. In normal circumstances, a surge of glucagon production will lead to glycolysis of the hepatic glycogen stores. In the case of the small-for-dates infant these stores are rapidly depleted and the infant becomes hypoglycemic. In normal infants a lack of glycogen will be compensated for by gluconeogenic mechanisms but in small-for-dates

infants there is evidence that gluconeogenesis may be defective (Williams *et al.*, 1975).

Clinical hypoglycemia may present with jitteriness, poor feeding, cyanosis or convulsions. Although the definition of neonatal hypoglycemia has been hotly debated (Aynsley-Green, 1982), a blood glucose level below 2.5 mmol/l merits active therapy and an acceptable management strategy for these infants is outlined in Figure 17.2.

### 17.3.5 RISK OF RESPIRATORY DISEASE

Traditional teaching indicates that meconium aspiration and pulmonary hemorrhage are the principal lung pathologies that occur in infants who have endured a stressful intrauterine environment and are growth-retarded at birth, but in clinical practice these conditions are now relatively uncommon (Jones and

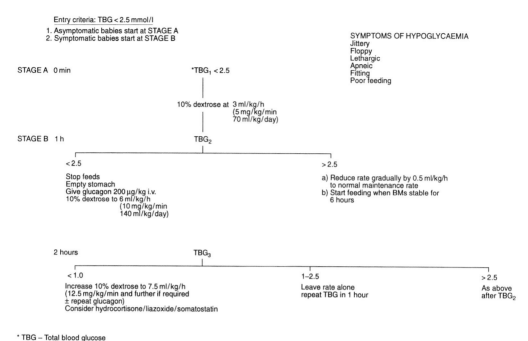

**Figure 17.2**   Guidelines for management of a baby with hypoglycemia

Roberton, 1984), and as many of these infants are born prematurely the respiratory disorder that causes the greatest concern is surfactant-deficient respiratory distress syndrome.

### 17.3.6 RESPIRATORY DISTRESS SYNDROME

The effect of hypertension in pregnancy on the incidence of neonatal respiratory distress syndrome remains controversial. Although evidence from a number of studies strongly supports the widely accepted view that maternal hypertensive disease protects against the development of respiratory distress syndrome (Chiswick and Burnard, 1973; Chiswick, 1976; Yoon, Khol and Harper, 1980), some workers have found an increase in the incidence of respiratory distress syndrome in infants of mothers with hypertension (White,

Shy and Benedette, 1986; Bowen *et al.*, 1988) A recent investigation of the association between maternal hypertension and the incidence of respiratory distress syndrome in a large group of very-low-birthweight babies, birthweight less than 1500 g and gestation less than 34 weeks, showed that after adjustment for birthweight, gestational age, growth retardation and membrane rupture greater than 24 h, the risk of developing respiratory distress syndrome was significantly greater in babies of hypertensive mothers (Tubman *et al.*, 1990). However, significance was lost after adjustments were made for the confounding variables, presence of labor before delivery and the mode of delivery, suggesting that the increased incidence of respiratory distress syndrome in babies of hypertensive mothers is related to the higher elective cesarean section rate and not the presence of hypertensive disease. Confirmation of this hypothesis will require a large randomized controlled study of the effect of different management policies for labor and delivery on the principal outcome measure respiratory distress syndrome.

### 17.3.7 RESPIRATORY SUPPORT

All infants at risk of respiratory distress syndrome should be closely monitored for clinical and blood gas evidence of respiratory failure. Respiratory support may vary from increased ambient oxygen concentration to continuous positive airway pressure and in the more severely affected infants to intermittent positive pressure ventilation. Frequent monitoring of blood gases is essential, especially during the acute stages of respiratory distress syndrome, this being most reliably achieved through umbilical artery catheterization or by indwelling peripheral arterial cannulae. Alternatively, non-invasive methods such as transcutaneous $P_{O_2}$ or $P_{CO_2}$ monitors or pulse oximetry are of value, particularly in determining trends, but preferably they should only be used in conjunction with arterial blood sampling. It is recommended that the pH is maintained at 7.25 or above, and the $P_a O_2$ 6–10 kPa. Provided that the pH is greater than 7.25, an elevated $P_a CO_2$ is not in isolation a great concern. Unless there is a specific reason for inducing hypocarbia then the lower limit of $P_a CO_2$ should be above 5 kPa. Continuous positive airway pressure may reduce the severity of the disease and improve blood gas tensions (Baum and Roberton, 1974). Although there is no clear agreement as to when, how and at what pressure CPAP should be applied, there is some evidence that it is more effective if introduced early (Avery *et al.*, 1987), and pressures of 3–6 cmH$_2$O are commonly used. If the condition of the infant deteriorates despite CPAP, intermittent positive pressure will be required. The aim is to use the lowest peak and mean airway pressure required to maintain acceptable

$P_a O_2$ and $P_{CO_2}$ levels. Pressure-limited, time-cycled, constant flow ventilators are commonly used in RDS and the application of a positive end expiratory pressure (PEEP) of 3–6 cmH$_2$O is thought to conserve surfactant on the alveolar surface (Wyszogrodski *et al.*, 1975). There is no consensus view on neonatal ventilator management, the two traditional methods commonly employed being those referred to as slow rate ventilation (30–40 breaths/min) and fast rate (60–120 breaths/min). Evidence from randomized controlled trials indicates that both methods are equally effective in achieving oxygenation but the incidence of pneumothoraces is lower in infants receiving the higher ventilation rates (Heicher, Kasting and Harrod, 1981). There is no evidence to suggest that ventilator rates above 150 breaths/min or the use of oscillatory ventilation techniques provide additional benefit (HIFI Study Group, 1989). The role of patient trigger ventilators is still being evaluated. Preliminary evidence suggests that this technique is particularly effective in larger more mature infants with RDS (Mitchell, Greenough and Hird, 1989).

Extracorporeal membrane oxygenation (ECMO) is a pulmonary bypass procedure that can be used to treat persistent pulmonary hypertension of the newborn, which may be associated with severe RDS or other lung pathology such as meconium aspiration. Initial experience of this technique is encouraging but it has been limited to infants with birthweight greater than 2000 g (O'Rourke *et al.*, 1989). The need for systemic heparinization makes this method potentially hazardous for more immature infants.

### 17.3.8 SURFACTANT THERAPY

In recent years the use of surfactant in RDS has been shown to reduce the risk of death from the disease. Meta-analysis of 34 randomized controlled trials of surfactant replacement comprising over 6000 babies showed significant reductions in the risk of neonatal death, both when the surfactant was given early (prophylactically) and when used for established RDS (rescue therapy) (Soll, 1991). These analyses show conclusively that surfactant therapy also reduces the risk of pneumothorax. Further research is required to determine whether prophylactic administration has any advantage over rescue therapy, whether the synthetic or natural form of surfactant is the most effective, whether surfactant is equally effective in infants below 26 weeks gestation and whether surfactant is cost-effective in infants over 31 weeks gestation. Further well-defined controlled studies are required to answer these questions.

The presence of RDS increases the risk of complications in other systems including the circulation (hypotension, patent ductus arteriosus) the bowel (necrotizing enterocolitis) and the brain (periventricular hemorrhage and/or leukomalacia).

### 17.3.9 CARDIOVASCULAR STABILIZATION

It is essential to closely monitor blood pressure in infants of hypertensive mothers as they may respond adversely to the effects of maternal medication (Boutry *et al.*, 1982). Systemic hypotension is a common occurrence in infants with severe respiratory distress syndrome (Skinner *et al.*, 1992) and if unrecognized and untreated the associated cerebral hypoperfusion may precipitate cerebral parenchymal injury and intraventricular hemorrhage (Mehrabani, Gowen and Kopelman, 1991). Intravascular blood pressure monitoring should be available but non-invasive BP measurement using the Doppler technique may give a reliable estimate of systolic pressure. The level of blood pressure at which hypotension is diagnosed depends on the maturity of the infant but a systemic blood pressure of less than 40 mmHg will usually require therapy (Emery, Greenough and Gamsu, 1992). Hypotension due to hypovolemia may be treated with colloid, plasma or blood the choice depending upon the clinical

circumstances. Inotrope infusion, although not fully evaluated in the preterm infant, may be effective after hypovolemia has been excluded or treated.

Patent ductus arteriosus is more common in infants with RDS requiring ventilation (Skinner *et al.*, 1992). There is no evidence to suggest that this condition is more likely to occur in infants of hypertensive mothers. Clinically there is a systolic murmur which is heard maximally below the left clavicle and conducted through to the back, and classically the peripheral pulses are full and bounding. If signs of heart failure are present (tachycardia, tachypnea, hepatomegaly, generalized edema and deteriorating blood gases) medical treatment with the prostaglandin antagonist indomethacin is usually successful in closing the duct and surgical ligation is rarely required (Rennie and Cooke, 1991).

### 17.3.10 NUTRITION

The importance of optimal nutrition for low-birthweight infants, especially those that are growth-retarded at birth, is being increasingly realized. The work of Barker and colleagues has shown that infants of low birthweight and low weight at 1 year of age are at increased risk of the chronic adult diseases of ischemic heart disease (Barker *et al.*, 1989a), hypertension (Barker *et al.*, 1989b) and diabetes mellitus (Hales *et al.*, 1991). Lucas and colleagues in Cambridge have shown that enhanced nutrition for a relatively short period of time, median 21 days, resulted in improved neurodevelopmental scores at age 18 months and 5 years (Lucas *et al.*, 1989; 1991) This evidence, indicates that optimum nutrition during the immediate postnatal period is associated with a reduction in both neurodevelopmental impairment in childhood and serious illness in adulthood.

### 17.3.11 CURRENT NUTRITIONAL CONCERNS

The provision of optimal nutrition is especially difficult with the more premature and intrauterine-growth-retarded infants. This is reflected in the data from Australia demonstrating that the time taken to regain birthweight is directly proportional to the degree of prematurity (Gill *et al.*, 1986). The nutritional management of the sick, ventilated infant is particularly complex. Enteral feeds are frequently not tolerated and total parenteral nutrition (TPN) is required. The TPN regimes at present in use were originally based on the composition of breast milk (Cockburn, 1976) and were designed for full-term infants recovering from gastrointestinal surgery. Recognized complications occurring during the administration of these regimens to premature ventilated infants include hyperglycemia, acidosis and lipidemia, each of which will necessitate a reduction in the prescribed volume of the relevant parenteral fluid. This inevitably results in the infant receiving a suboptimal caloric intake. To date, modifications to neonatal parenteral nutrition regimes have tended to be *ad hoc* rather than scientifically based.

## 17.3.12 DETERMINING OPTIMAL NUTRITION

Attempts to determine more specific nutritional requirements of the preterm infant have hitherto concentrated on healthy growing infants, their energy expenditure and nutritional balance being estimated during the administration of enteral and parenteral feeding regimens (Reichman *et al.*, 1983; Pineault *et al.*, 1988). Indirect calorimetry has been the method of choice as it is practicable and accurate for the spontaneously breathing infant. This method provides an estimate of oxygen consumption and carbon dioxide production from which the energy expenditure and respiratory quotient (RQ) can be calculated. If simultaneous measurement of urinary nitrogen is made, fat, carbohydrate and protein utilization can be calculated. From these studies on healthy premature infants it has been suggested that the total energy intake for enterally fed infants should be in the region of 110–160 kcal/kg per day (Wharton, 1987) and 60–80 kcal/kg per day for infants receiving parenteral nutrition (Pineault *et al.*, 1988) .

## 17.3.13 SICK VENTILATOR-DEPENDENT INFANTS

It cannot be assumed that this data is meaningful for the sick ventilator-dependent infant. The overall work of breathing in these infants will be influenced by the contribution of ventilator support, the frequency of spontaneous respirations and the compliance of the lungs. In adults, oxygen consumption is increased in trauma and sepsis (Stoner, 1987), both of which are frequently present in sick infants. In healthy premature infants 15–20% of energy expenditure may be due to spontaneous activity (Wharton, 1987) and this is likely to be reduced in the sick and the more premature infant. The overall effect of all of these factors on total energy expenditure in sick ventilated infants is at present unknown.

The lack of calorimetry data for sick ventilator-dependent infants is related to the difficulties of measuring gas exchange in infants being ventilated with continuous flow ventilators. The dilutional effect of the gas flow precludes the use of standard calorimetry systems. Systems of greater accuracy and precision have recently been developed and preliminary data indicate that the resting energy expenditure of ventilated infants during the first week of life may not differ significantly from non-ventilated preterm infants (Forsyth and Crighton, 1992). Of particular interest, the respiratory quotient is frequently in excess of 1.0, indicating that excess carbohydrate which is being administered to the infant is being converted to fat. A reduction in carbohydrate intake in these infants may therefore decrease carbon dioxide production and thus allow a reduction in ventilator support (Askanazi *et al.*, 1980). Recognizing that available information on the parenteral nutrition requirements of sick ventilated infants is extremely limited, a regimen based on current knowledge is outlined in Table 17.1.

It has been traditional practice to gradually increase the amino acid and fat content over the first few days of life; however, this practice has recently been questioned and studies have indicated that both these nutrients are tolerated from day 1 (Gilbertson *et al.*, 1991). There have been reports that intravenous fat infusions may be associated with an increased risk of chronic lung disease (Cooke, 1991; Hammerman and Aramburo, 1988), but recent evidence indicates that fat emulsions may protect the lung from hypoxic damage (Sosenko, Innis and Frank, 1991).

Enteral feeds should be commenced as soon as clinical circumstances permit. During the period of feeding by TPN it is advantageous to simultaneously give a small volume of milk feed, as this increases the secretion of specific gastrointestinal hormones that promote intestinal growth and maturation. This priming of the gut is thought to enable an earlier tolerance of full enteral feeds (Lucas, 1989).

Whether expressed breast milk or a special low-birthweight formula should be offered to these infants is still uncertain. The previous concern that breast milk may not meet the nutritional demands of fast-growing preterm infants has now to be balanced against recent reports that formula-fed infants are at increased risk of necrotizing enterocolitis and allergic disease (Lucas and Cole, 1990; Lucas *et al.*, 1990). An acceptable approach is to encourage mothers to express milk for their infants and to continue with this form of nutrition provided growth velocity is satisfactory. If nutritional supplementation is required this can be given either as an energy supplement or as complementary energy and protein-enriched formula feed (Table 17.2).

The timing of full enteral feeds in growth-retarded infants, particularly those infants in whom umbilical artery flow abnormalities have been detected, has recently been questioned. Doppler studies have shown a strong association of necrotizing enterocolitis occurring in infants with absent or reversed umbilical artery end-diastolic frequencies prior to delivery (Fairlie *et al.*, 1991), and reduced superior mesenteric artery blood flow velocity following delivery (Malcolm *et al.*, 1991) . The additional metabolic demand of an enteral feed on an already compromised gut is thought to precipitate the development of narcotizing enterocolitis. Special caution has therefore been recommended for these infants and it has been suggested that, if breast milk is not available, the introduction

**Table 17.1**  A neonatal parenteral nutrition regimen

| Nutrient (per kilogram body weight/24 h) | Days | | | | |
|---|---|---|---|---|---|
| | *1* | *2* | *3* | *4* | *5* |
| Amino acid (g) | 0.5 | 1.0 | 1.5 | 2.0 | 2.5 |
| Carbohydrate (g) | 8 | 10 | 10 | 12 | 14 |
| Fat (g) | 1.0 | 1.0 | 2.0 | 3.0 | 3.5 |
| Sodium (mmol) | 3.0 | 3.0 | 3.0 | 3.0 | 3.0 |
| Potassium (mmol) | 2.5 | 2.5 | 2.5 | 2.5 | 2.5 |
| Calcium (mmol) | 1.0 | 1.0 | 1.0 | 1.0 | 1.0 |
| Magnesium (mmol) | 0.25 | 0.25 | 0.25 | 0.25 | 0.25 |
| Phosphate (mmol) | 0.6 | 0.6 | 0.6 | 0.6 | 0.6 |
| Energy (kJ) | 172 | 205 | 244 | 315 | 367 |
| Non-protein energy (kJ) per gram of nitrogen | 2150 | 1281 | 1016 | 984 | 917 |

Additional supplements – trace elements, fat- and water-soluble vitamins of artificial formula should be delayed for 7–10 days. (Lucas and Cole, 1990).

## 17.4 CEREBRAL MORBIDITY

Cerebral morbidity occurring in infants of hypertensive mothers may be related to intrauterine malnutrition or cerebral insults, which are associated with prematurity. Intrauterine malnutrition, if severe, will impair fetal brain growth and place the infant at increased risk of neurodevelopmental impairment. Infants with subnormal head size at 8 months were recently shown to have poor cognitive function and academic achievement at 8 years of age (Hack *et al.*, 1991). Those infants, in whom the brain has been spared from intrauterine malnutrition, are still at risk of cerebral morbidity because depleted glycogen and fat stores place them at greater risk of hypoglycemia and the metabolic consequences of birth asphyxia.

Cerebral hemorrhage (intraventricular/periventricular) and ischemia (periventricular leukomalacia) occur in premature infants who have suffered hemodynamic or acid–base disturbance pre- or postnatally. In preterm infants the subependymal germinal matrix contains a rich vascular network of thin-walled capillaries. This, coupled with the fact that the cerebral blood flow in the preterm infant is pressure-passive, means that these vessels are likely to rupture during acute blood flow surges. Once the hemorrhage occurs it may extend because of increased fibrinolytic activity in this area of the brain. Hemorrhage of greater than 1–2 mm can be detected as increased echogenicity in the germinal matrix on the floor of the lateral ventricles. Echogenic areas in the ventricles and the parenchyma in the periventricular areas indicate more extensive hemorrhage. There is consistent agreement that echoes apparently confined to the region of the germinal matrix alone carry no increased risk of adverse outcome whereas hemorrhage that is associated with ventricular dilatation or has extended into the parenchyma is associated with significant neurodevelopmental sequelae.

Periventricular leukomalacia (PVL) appears to be caused, at least in part, by ischemic injury to the periventricular white matter, this being an arterial watershed zone. It is possible to diagnose these lesions with cranial ultrasound. PVL appears as an echodense triangle with its apex at the lateral border of the lateral ventricles and then later as echo-free cavities, representing cyst formation. The prognosis is worse if the lesions are cystic and bilateral. On a more optimistic note, if the cranial ultrasound scan is normal at 40 weeks postconception, a good prognosis can be given to the parents (Levene, 1990)

## 17.5 INFANTS OF BORDERLINE VIABILITY

Recent advances in perinatal medicine have permitted very small babies to survive who previously would have been considered non-viable. Unfortunately the cost of this success can be heavy and the dilemma that is now facing neonatal clinicians is that as smaller

**Table 17.2** Differences in major nutrient composition (per 100 ml of milk) between human milk, standard formula and low-birthweight formula

|                  | Human milk | Standard formula | Low-birthweight formula |
|------------------|------------|------------------|-------------------------|
| Carbohydrate (g) | 7.2        | 7.2              | 8.6                     |
| Protein (g)      | 1.2        | 1.5              | 2.0                     |
| Fat (g)          | 3.6        | 3.6              | 4.4                     |
| Sodium (mg)      | 16         | 16               | 32                      |
| Calcium (mg)     | 34         | 44               | 100                     |

and smaller babies receive intensive care there is a diminishing return in healthy survivors and an increasing risk of moderate or severe handicap. Reports that some units have made an active decision not to resuscitate babies below a specific birthweight has provoked considerable discussion (Pemberton, 1987). Adoption of such policies places doctors and nurses in the unenviable position of deciding which babies should live and which babies should die. This practice can only be acceptable if there are recognized criteria that can accurately predict survival or risk of serious handicap.

Attempts to identify specific factors that may indicate the likely prognosis have so far proved to be unreliable. A major concern among some is that, once active treatment has been initiated, it will be impossible to discontinue at a later stage. Throughout the care of the baby, decisions should be made on the basis of what is best for the infant and active treatment should be continued when there is a medical consensus that there is a net benefit to the infant (Forsyth, 1988). The baby's medical condition should be the sole focus of any decision-making process. Active treatment should not be discontinued for the primary purpose of improving the psychological, economical or social wellbeing of others, no matter how poignant or overwhelming these needs may be. On the other hand, automatic prolongation of life with high technology is clinically irresponsible. When the medical facts reveal the futility of further curative efforts the decision to discontinue life support and to provide a more conservative approach should be made. To prolong life artificially at this stage is simply prolonging dying. Care should continue to be provided but should now be directed towards making the baby comfortable, avoiding unnecessary and painful interventions and providing support to the parents and family.

## REFERENCES

Askanazi, J., Rosenbaum, S. H., Hyman, A. I. *et al.* (1980) Respiratory changes induced by the large glucose loads of total parenteral nutrition. *J. A. M. A.*, **243**, 1444–1447.

Avery, M. E, Tooley, W. H., Keller, J. B. *et al.* (1987) Is chronic lung disease in low birthweight infants preventable? A survey of 8 centres. *Pediatrics*, **79**, 26–30.

Aynsley-Green, A. (1982) Hypoglycaemia in infants and children. *Clin. Endocrin. Metab.*, **11**, 159–194.

Barker, D. J. P., Winter, P. D., Osmond, C. *et al.* (1989a) Weight in infancy and death from ischaemic heart disease. *Lancet*, **ii**, 577–580.

Barker, D. J. P., Osmond, C., Golding, J. *et al.* (1989b) Growth in utero, blood pressure in childhood and adult life, and mortality from cardiovascular disease. *Br. Med. J.*, **298**, 564–567.

Baum, J. D. and Roberton, N. R. C. (1974) Distending pressure in infants with the respiratory distress syndrome. *Arch. Dis. Child.*, **49**, 771–781.

Boutry, M. J. H., Vert, P., Bianchetti, G. *et al.* (1982) Infants born to hypertensive mothers treated by acebutolol. *Dev. Pharmacol. Ther.*, **4**(suppl), 109–115.

Chiswick, M. L. (1976) Prolonged ruptured membranes, pre-eclamptic toxaemia, and respiratory distress syndrome. *Arch. Dis. Child.*, **51**, 674–679.

Chiswick, M. L and Burnard, E. (1973) Respiratory distress syndrome. *Lancet*, **i**, 1060.

Cockburn, F. (1976) Intravenous feeding of the newborn. *Clin. Endocrinol. Metab.*, **5**, 191–219.

Cooke, R. W. I. (1991) Factors associated with chronic lung disease in preterm infants. *Arch. Dis. Child.*, **66**, 776–779.

Cornblath, M. and Schwartz R. *Disorders of Carbohydrate Metabolism*, 1st edn, W. B. Saunders, Philadelphia, PA.

Crowley, P., Chalmers, I. and Keirse, M. J. N. C. (1990) The effects of corticosteroid administration before preterm delivery: an overview of the evidence from controlled trials. *Br. J. Obstet. Gynaecol.*, **97**, 11–25.

Davies, P. A. and Tizard, J. P. (1975) Very low birthweight and subsequent neurological defect (with special reference to spastic diplegia). *Dev. Med. Child Neurol.*, **17**, 3–17.

Derham, R. J., Hawkins, D. F., De Vries, L. S. *et al.* (1989) Outcome of pregnancies complicated by severe hypertension and delivered before 34 weeks: stepwise logistic regression analysis of prognostic factors. *Br. J. Obstet. Gynaecol.*, **96**, 1173–1181.

Emery, E. F., Greenough, A. and Gamsu, H. R. (1992) Randomised controlled trial of colloid infusions in hypotension preterm infants. *Arch. Dis. Child.*, **67**, 1185–1188.

Fairlie, F. M., Moretti, M., Walker, J. J. and Sibai, B. M. (1991) Determinants of perinatal outcome in pregnancy-induced hypertension with absence of umbilical artery end-diastolic frequencies. *Am. J. Obstet. Gynecol.*, **164**, 1084–1089.

Forsyth, J. S. (1988) Dilemmas in the neonatal management of extremely low birth weight babies. *Scot. Med. J.*, **33**, 356–357.

Forsyth, J. S. and Crighton, A. (1992) An indirect calorimetry system for ventilator dependent very low birthweight infants. *Arch. Dis. Child.*, **67**, 315–319.

Gilbertson, N., Kovar, I. Z., Cox, D. J. *et al.* (1991) Introduction of intravenous lipid administration on the first day of life in the vey low birthweight neonate. *J. Pediatr.*, **119**, 615–623.

Gill, A., Yu, V. Y. H., Bajuk, B. and Astbury, J. (1986) Postnatal growth in infants born before 30 weeks gestation. *Arch. Dis. Child.*, **61**, 549–553.

Hack, M., Breslau, N., Weissman, B. *et al.* (1991) Effect of very low birth weight and subnormal head size on cognitive abilities at school age. *N. Engl. J. Med.*, **325**, 231–237.

Hales, C. N., Barker, D. J. P., Clark, P. M. S. *et al.* (1991) Fetal and infant growth and impaired glucose tolerance at age 64. *Br. Med. J.*, **303**, 1019–1022.

Hammerman, C. and Aramburo, M. J. (1988) Decreased lipid intake reduces morbidity in sick premature neonates. *J. Pediatr.*, **113**, 1083–1088.

Heicher, D. A, Kasting, D. S. and Harrod, J. R. (1981) Prospective clinical comparisons of two methods for mechanical ventilation of neonates: rapid rate and short inspiratory time versus slow rate and long inspiratory time. *J. Pediatr.*, **98**, 957–961.

Hey, E. The care of babies in incubators, in *Recent Advances in Paediatrics 4*, (ed. D. M. T. Gairdner), J. & A. Churchill, London, p. 171–216.

HIFI Study Group. (1989) High frequency oscillatory ventilation compared with convential mechanical ventilation in the treatment of respiratory failure in premature neonates. *N. Engl. J. Med.*, **320**, 88–93.

Jones, R. A. K. and Roberton, N. R. C. (1984) Problems of the small for dates baby. *Clin. Obstet. Gynecol.*, **11**, 499–521.

King, J. F, Grant, A., Keirse, M. J. N. C. and Chalmers, I. (1988) Beta-mimetics in preterm labour: an overview of the randomized controlled trials. *Br. J. Obstet. Gynaecol.*, **95**, 211–122.

Levene, M. (1990) Cerebral ultrasound and neurological impairment: telling the future. *Arch. Dis. Child.*, **65**, 469–471.

Lucas, A. (1989) Ontogeny of gut hormones and hormone-related sustances. *Acta Paediatr. Scand. Suppl.*, **351**, 80–87.

Lucas, A. Does early nutrition programme long-term outcome? Guest lecture, 63rd Annual Meeting, British Paediatric Association, University of Warwick, April, 1991.

Lucas, A., Morley, R., Cole, T. J. *et al.* (1989) Early diet in preterm babies and developmental status in infancy. *Arch. Dis. Child.*, **64**, 1570–1578.

Lucas, A., Brooke, O. G., Morley R. *et al.* (1990) Early diet of preterm infants and the development of allergic or atopic disease: randomised prospective study. *Br. Med. J.*, 837–840.

McIlwaine, G., Mutch, L., Pritchard, C. and Fletcher, D. V. (1989) *The Scottish Low Birthweight Study: The Pregnancies, Neonatal Progress and Outcome at Two Years*, Scottish Home and Health Department, Edinburgh.

Malcolm, G., Ellwood, D., Devonald, K. *et al.* (1991) Absent or reversed end diastolic flow velocity in the umbilical artery and necrotising enterocolitis. *Arch. Dis. Child.*, **66**, 805–807.

Mehrabani, D., Gowen, C. W. Jr and Kopelman, A. E. (1991) Association of pneumothorax and hypotension with intraventricular haemorrhage. *Arch. Dis. Child.*, **66**, 48–51.

Mitchell, A., Greenough, A. and Hird, M. (1989) Limitations of patient. triggered ventilation in neonates. *Arch. Dis. Child.*, **64**, 924–929.

O'Rourke, P. P., Crone, R. K., Vacanti, J. P. *et al.* (1989) Extracorporeal membrane oxygenation and conventional medical therapy in neonates with persistent pulmonary hypertension of the newborn: a prospective randomized study. *Pediatrics*, **84**, 957–963.

Pemberton, P. J. (1987) The tiniest babies – can we afford them? *Med. J. Aust.*, **146**, 63.

Pineault, M., Chessez, P., Bisaillon, S. and Brisson, G. (1988) Total parenteral nutrition in the newborn: impact of the quality of infused energy on nitrogen metabolism. *Am. J. Clin. Nutr.*, **47**, 298–304.

Reichman, B., Chessex, P., Verellen, G. *et al.* (1983) Dietary composition of macronutrient storage in preterm infants. *Pediatrics*, **72**, 322–328.

Rennie, J. M. and Cooke, R. W. I. (1991) Prolonged low dose indomethacin for persistent ductus arteriosus of prematurity. *Arch. Dis. Child.*, **66**, 55–58.

Soll, R. F. (1991) Overviews of surfactant trials, in *Oxford Data Base of Perinatal Trials. version 1. 2, disk issue 5,* (ed. I. Chalmers), Records 5206, 5207, 5252, 5253.

Sosenko, I. R. S., Innis, S. M. and Frank, L. (1991) Intralipid increases lung polyunsaturated fatty acids and protects newborn rats from oxygen toxicity. *Pediatr. Res.*, **30**, 413–417.

Stewart, A. L. and Reynolds, E. O. R. (1974) Improved prognosis for infants of very low birthweight. *Pediatrics*, **54**, 724–735.

Stoner, H. B. (1987) Why is energy expenditure increased by trauma and sepsis? *Care Critically Ill*, **3**, 108–109.

Tubman, T. R. J., Rollins, M. D., Patterson, C. and Halliday, H. L. (1990) Increased incidence of respiratory distress syndrome in babies of hypertensive mothers. *Arch. Dis. Child.*, **66**, 52–54.

Wharton, B. A. (1987) *Nutrition and Feeding of Preterm Infants,* Blackwell Scientific Publications, Oxford.

White, E., Shy, K. K. and Benedette, T. K. (1986) Chronic fetal stress and the risk of infant respiratory distress syndrome. *Obstet. Gynecol.*, **67**, 57–62.

Williams, P. R, Fiser, R. H., Sperling, M. A. and Oh, W. (1975) Effects of oral alanine feeding on blood glucose, plasma glucagon, and insulin concentrations in small for gestational age infants. *N. Engl. J. Med.*, **292**, 612–614.

Wyszogrodski, I., Kyei-Aboagye, K., Taeusch, H. W. and Avery, M. E. (1975) Surfactant inactivation by hyperventilation: conservation by end-expiratory pressure. *J. Appl. Phys.*, **38**, 461–466.

Yoon, J. J., Khol, S. and Harper, R. G. (1980) A relationship between hypertensive disease of pregnancy and the incidence of respiratory distress syndrome. *Pediatrics*, **65**, 735–739.

# Index